W9-BXP-315

# 1000
# Cures for
# 200
# Ailments

Copyright © 2007 Marshall Editions
A Marshall Edition
Conceived, edited, and designed by Marshall Editions
The Old Brewery
6 Blundell Street
London N7 9BH

FIRST EDITION
ISBN-10: 0-06-112029-4
ISBN-13: 978-0-06-112029-9

07 08 09 10          10 9 8 7 6 5 4 3 2 1

Cover originated in Hong Kong by Modern Age
Printed and bound in China by Midas Printing International Limited

Publisher: Richard Green
Commissioning Editor: Claudia Martin
Art Direction: Ivo Marloh
Editor: Johanna Geary
Design: Lapiz Digital and Sarah Robson
Proofreader: Chris McNab
Indexer: Vanessa Bird
Production: Nikki Ingram

The information in this book is not a substitute for professional medical or health care. The advice in this book is based on the training, experience, and information available to the authors. Each personal situation is unique. The authors and publisher urge the readers to consult a qualified health professional when there is any question regarding the presence or treatment of any health condition. Unless otherwise specified the treatments recommended are for use by adults. Pregnant women should always consult a qualified health professional before using any treatments recommended in this publication. The publisher does not advocate the use of any particular treatment.

Because there is always some risk involved, the editors and publisher are not responsible for any adverse effects or consequences resulting from the use of any of the preparations or procedures described in the book. Please do not use this book if you are unwilling to assume the risk. For personalized advice, please consult a physician or other qualified health professional. Even your own opinion as to your condition and treatment should be confirmed with the second and third opinions of medical professionals.

Research studies and institutions cited in this book should in no way be construed as an endorsement of anything in this book. The authors and publisher expressly disclaim responsibility of any adverse affects arising from the use or application of the information contained herein.

# 1000 Cures for 200 Ailments

Integrated Alternative and Conventional Treatments for the Most Common Illnesses

## Consultant Editor **Dr. Victor Sierpina**

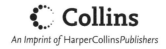

**Collins**

An Imprint of HarperCollins*Publishers*

# AUTHORS

**Consultant Editor: Dr. Victor S. Sierpina**, MD, ABFP, ABHM, is the WD and Laura Nell Nicholson Family Professor in Integrative Medicine, Professor of Family Medicine, and Principal Investigator of CAM Education and Mind-Body Projects at the University of Texas Medical Branch, Galveston, Texas. His teaching and medical practice integrate allopathic, holistic, alternative, and complementary approaches to wellness and health care. His publications include *Integrative Health Care: Complementary and Alternative Therapies for the Whole Person*.

**General Editor: Sarah Wilson** has over 15 years of experience as a journalist on consumer magazines and books. Her specialist areas are complementary health, nutrition, and parenting. Sarah was the editor of *Here's Health* magazine and is now a freelance journalist and health writer. Her books include *Natural Health for Kids*.

**Conventional Medicine: Dr. Christine Gustafson**, MD, has a private integrative medical practice in Alpharetta, Georgia. Her practice combines traditional and complementary medical therapies and investigates the effects of nutrition on disease and health. She is board-certified in holistic medicine, and graduated from the Program in Integrative Medicine at the University of Arizona. She is a member of the American Holistic Medical Association and the American Association of Integrative Medicine.

**Traditional Chinese Medicine: Dr. Zhuoling Ren**, TCMD, is a doctor of TCM with over 20 years' experience and is also a fellow of AAIM. Dr. Ren is the president and founder of the American Foundation of Integrated Medicine. She is also the president and founder of the China Institute of Traditional Chinese Medicine with clinics in Minneapolis and St. Paul, Minnesota. Before establishing the China Institute she was doctor-in-charge and head of the acupuncture department at Xiyuan Hospital in Beijing.

**Naturopathy: Dr. Geovanni Espinosa**, ND, LAc, RH(AHG), earned his Doctor of Naturopathic Medicine degree and Masters degree in Acupuncture from the University of Bridgeport in Connecticut. He is currently a clinical research coordinator, co-investigator, and a complementary medicine practitioner at Columbia University Medical Center in New York. Dr. Espinosa is a member of the American Association of Naturopathic Physicians and the American Herbalist Guild.

**Homeopathy: Beth MacEoin**, MNCHM, RSHom, trained at the Northern College of Homeopathic Medicine before setting up her own practice and becoming a registered member of the Society of Homeopaths. She has numerous books to her credit, and acts as an advisor to magazines, newspapers, and television programs on general health topics. Beth also teaches a course on complementary therapies to medical students in Newcastle, England.

**Herbalism: Dr. David Kiefer**, MD, is a board-certified family physician and a graduate of the Program in Integrative Medicine at the University of Arizona in Tucson, Arizona. His research and teaching activities are in the areas of herbal medicine, integrative medicine, and ethnobotany. The herbalism section was co-written by Angila Jaeggli, ND, and Josh Holexa. Dr. Jaeggli is a naturopathic physician and recently completed her residency at Bastyr University near Seattle, Washington. Josh Holexa is a medical student at the University of Arizona, College of Medicine.

# CONTENTS

# FOREWORD

Home remedies are truly the first line of primary care—and this book provides over 1000 of them. It has been a pleasure acting as consultant editor on this project as it has allowed me to broaden and deepen my knowledge of alternative medicine. My own interest in complementary therapies was incited by my parents' use of home remedies. Our home pharmacopoeia was replete with apple cider vinegar, fish oil, vitamins and minerals, ginger, and a broad variety of other herbal and nutritional prescriptions. All of these were administered with confidence and traditional ritual. Working on *1000 Cures*, I feel as though I have come full circle in my connection with medicine—from home remedies to medical school, to practice, to academia, and now back to home remedies with this book.

*1000 Cures* is an ambitious work that offers the reader a broad perspective on over 200 very common medical conditions. Experts in the fields of conventional western medicine, traditional Chinese medicine, naturopathy, homeopathy, and herbal medicine have each contributed sections on how to treat a plenitude of acute conditions, from hangovers to strep throat, colic, earaches, fevers, and many more. The book also suggests holistic, natural treatments for some chronic illnesses such as high blood pressure, diabetes, high cholesterol, and asthma.

*1000 Cures* has the potential to decrease the cost of your family's health care by making office or emergency room visits to treat minor conditions unnecessary and by minimizing the need for expensive prescription medications when simpler treatment measures will suffice. However, it is important to recognize the limits of self-diagnosis and self-prescribing. *1000 Cures* always advises the reader when consultation with an expert is necessary, when medication is likely to be more helpful than homeopathic, herbal, or nutritional approaches, and when a problem clearly requires emergency evaluation and treatment. *1000 Cures* is not a substitute for standard medical care and cannot replace an evaluation by a trained professional. Readers must heed the warnings included in each section to protect their own and their families' health. With this caveat in mind, *1000 Cures* will be a rich treasury of health information for readers.

The strength of *1000 Cures* lies in its flexibility and in the variety of the natural treatment choices it offers its readers. Each ailment is clearly defined and the symptoms that most commonly occur are described so that readers can more accurately diagnose conditions. For those who prefer to treat ailments using a conventional medical approach, conventional remedies are described thoroughly and succinctly. However, advice on conventional treatment is always given alongside recommendations from practitioners of complementary therapies, allowing you to explore how other traditions approach the same condition. By considering opinions on health conditions from five different traditions of healing, the reader can develop a more holistic view of how the body can be healed.

As a guide to home remedies, *1000 Cures* is unparalleled in its depth and sophistication. Each treatment suggestion is complete with advice on appropriate doses, whether of herbs, supplements, or medication, and clear instructions on how to prepare teas, infusions, poultices, compresses, and herbal decoctions. Each remedy is carefully explained, and all have been verified for safety and accuracy by the authors. Although the book primarily focuses on physical and biological treatments such as herbs and diet modification, it also gives sound preventive advice on healthy lifestyle changes and mind-body therapies.

*1000 Cures* provides the tools and techniques to effectively treat ailments at home, but don't wait to get sick: take a look at some common problems that you or your family have had in the past and see how they might be approached more naturally. Many of the recommendations, particularly in the naturopathy sections, provide good general advice on how to lead a healthy life and protect yourself against illness. As an ancient Chinese sage once said, "The superior doctor treats the disease before it occurs." With *1000 Cures* you are in for a vast, exciting learning and healing experience.

Dr. Victor S. Sierpina
University of Texas Medical Branch

# INTRODUCTION

*1000 Cures* is an invaluable integrated medical resource that provides real choices in an easy-to-use, at-a-glance format. Over 200 ailments are grouped according to type (for example, conditions that affect the skin and hair, or those that require first aid) and listed alphabetically within each group. For each condition, a diagnosis, the most common symptoms, and the goal of treatment are clearly set out. Remedies are then provided from five different fields of healing—conventional medicine, traditional Chinese medicine, naturopathy, homeopathy, and herbalism—allowing you to compare approaches to the same condition, and choose the remedy that is right for you.

## CONVENTIONAL MEDICINE

The practice of medicine involves using science as an evidence base in the application of medical knowledge and clinical judgment to determine a treatment plan for an ailment. Medical doctors undergo extensive training at university and within the hospital system to enable them to diagnose illnesses accurately.

A patient–doctor relationship involves first gathering data, by taking a case history, performing a physical examination, and carrying out any necessary tests, including X-ray, blood, or urine tests. This data is then analyzed and assessed to develop a treatment plan. A doctor follows the patient's progress and alters the plan as necessary. The type of treatment offered often includes pharmaceutical drugs, which require a prescription.

## TRADITIONAL CHINESE MEDICINE

According to TCM theory, illness occurs when a person's inner balance is disturbed. This balance inlcudes the body's Qi (the internal energy), blood, and body fluid. Good health also involves being in harmony with nature; for example the four seasons and the elements of heat, cold, dampness, dryness, and wind. As such, a red and inflamed rash is "hot" and is treated by using cooling remedies, while a phlegmy cough is "damp" and requires herbs that dispell dampness.

TCM treatment usually involves combining herbal remedies with acupuncture and/or acupressure. Acupuncture is the practice of inserting and manipulating needles into meridian points on the body by a well-trained practitioner. Acupressure involves using fingers, hands, arms, elbows, or feet to place pressure on acupoints. The treatment principle is to promote the circulation of Qi, blood, and body fluids, to relieve the pathogenic factors (cold, heat, dampness, etc.), and to rebuild the balance between internal and external organs.

## NATUROPATHY

Naturopathy was founded on the principle of "nature cure," which asserts that the body is essentially self-healing if provided with the right diet, environment, and habits, such as meditation. Naturopathic medicine concentrates on healing the whole person by identifying and resolving the underlying cause of a condition, rather than only treating symptoms. Practitioners will determine the most natural, non-toxic, and least invasive therapies necessary for achieving a cure.

The doses and cures outlined in the naturopathic sections of this book are primarily intended for adults. However, if an ailment predominantly affects children (for example, chickenpox) the recommended doses are appropriate for children. If an ailment affects adults and children equally, the doses suggested are for adults unless otherwise indicated. The remedies outlined for each ailment (both herbs and supplements) can generally be taken at the same time, and any contraindications are specified in each section.

## HOMEOPATHY

At the heart of homeopathy lies the principle of "the law of similars." Much like the process of immunization, homeopathy involves administering a highly dilute amount of a substance to stimulate the body to heal. To determine the most appropriate homeopathic treatment, make a note of your symptoms and assess the speed with which they have come on, whether there have been any obvious triggers, the location and severity of pain, the time of day that pain is most intense, and any emotional reactions to feeling ill. Then match your symptoms to those described in the homeopathic sections of this book. If a close match does not exist, the remedy will not improve your symptoms.

Homeopathic remedies are available in "first aid" potencies of 6c, 30c, 6x, or 30x. Mild symptoms that have recently developed should respond well to an appropriately selected remedy in a 6c. Established problems that have developed slowly and insidiously over a few days rather than a few hours will respond better to a stronger 30c potency. Work along the same lines with 6x and 30x potencies if these are the only ones available to you. Unlike conventional medicine, which advocates completing a course of treatment, homeopathy involves taking the appropriate remedy for strictly short-term use.

## HERBALISM

Herbalism is a traditional medical practice based on the use of plants and plant extracts. Much of modern-day pharmacology owes a debt to herbal medicine as many of the drugs available to Western physicians are derived from plants that have a long history of use as herbal remedies. Opinions on acceptable doses of herbs to ingest, and the appropriate quantity of plant material to use to make an infusion or decoction, vary. Dosage depends on a patient's specific symptom and its severity, personal taste, and/or the form of the plant available (for example, fresh versus dried plant material). The quantities of plant material or liquid recommended in the recipes in this book are approximate. Consult a medical herbalist regarding the specific amount to be used to treat a particular remedy.

There are also different philosophies regarding the use of herbs, or any medication for that matter, during pregnancy or lactation, and in children. But years of experience with herbs has illustrated that some plants can be helpful and safe to take in these situations to ease a variety of complaints. For instance, slippery elm root bark powder is often used to treat heartburn in pregnant women and is considered quite safe because the herb is minimally absorbed by the body. Nonetheless, if you are pregnant or breastfeeding, or considering using herbal medicine to treat your children, consult a medical herbalist for specific direction.

# SKIN
# AND
# HAIR

# ABSCESS

## DIAGNOSIS

Abscesses are pus-filled lumps that form when a follicle, pore, or gland becomes infected, or an injury to the skin is neglected. Although they usually occur on the skin, they can occur anywhere on the body and occasionally affect internal organs. They are often found in the mouth and are a common cause of dental pain (see p. 227). They include smaller superficial abscesses such as styes, boils, and pimples, which are more common in moist areas of the body such as the armpit and groin, and more serious internal abscesses of the liver or brain, which require surgical treatment.

Abscesses usually either burst, are drained by a doctor under local or general anesthetic, or clear up of their own accord without draining. Depending on the size and severity of the abscess, you may or may not need to seek medical help. Antibiotics may be needed to make sure the infection does not spread. There is a danger that an abscess may release pus and bacteria into the bloodstream causing blood poisoning (septicemia). This is what happens when an abscess in the appendix bursts, causing the condition of peritonitis (inflammation of the abdominal lining). Some people are more prone to skin abscesses, and this may be an indication of lowered resistance to infection.

## SYMPTOMS

- Red painful swelling that fills with pus
- Skin feels hot to the touch
- Sense of discomfort
- Build-up of pressure in the affected area
- Fever and sweating
- Feeling generally unwell
- Swollen, tender glands

## TREATMENT GOAL

To work on the infection that has caused the abscess and bring rapid relief from the symptoms.

## CONVENTIONAL MEDICINE

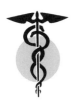

**Antiseptic wash:** External abscesses usually give obvious warning through pain and inflammation prior to formation. They are generally formed from a boil or furuncle (the inflammation of a hair follicle and the skin around it) and then a carbuncle (a group of furuncles coming together). When they present like this, prior to complete abscess, they can be treated and abscess formation can be prevented. At the first sign of skin inflammation or irritated hair follicles, clean the area with an antiseptic wash. Try an over-the-counter product such as Betadine® solution, which is like iodide, or an antiseptic scrub solution.

**Antibiotic ointment:** After you have cleaned the infected area, apply Neosporin®, a topical, over-the-counter antibiotic ointment, or tea tree oil three times a day.

**Epsom salt compress:** Soak a gauze pad or clean washcloth in 1 cup of hot water and 2 tbsp of salt. Apply the gauze to the infected area as a compress three times a day for 15 minutes to help relieve the infection.

**When should I see my doctor?** If your symptoms do not improve within seven days, see your doctor. If redness around the area progresses, or if the pus under the skin accumulates, the abscess probably needs to be lanced and drained. This is a procedure that, depending on the location of the abscess, can usually be performed in the doctor's office.

**Antibiotics:** If there are any systematic signs of infection—if you have a fever and are generally feeling under the weather—you may need a course of antibiotics. Cephalosporin is the kind of antibiotic most commonly used to prevent or treat early infection. If you are put on antibiotics, be sure to use a good strong probiotic to replace the beneficial flora in the gut that antibiotics can kill. Florastore™, a product that contains the probiotic *Saccharomyces boullardii*, is available through health care practitioners. Probiotics known as mixed *Bifidus* and *Lactobacillus species* can be found in many health food store products.

## TRADITIONAL CHINESE MEDICINE

**Herbs:** The herbs listed below are available from Chinese pharmacies or online.
• Watermelon frost: This dry powder made from watermelon will help to reduce the infection and eliminate pain. Gather some watermelon frost on the tip of a cotton wool bud and dab it on the surface of the abscess. Repeat every couple of hours to bring relief.

• Chuan Xin Lian: This traditional Chinese medicine has heat and fire toxicity cleaning actions. Take 9 g of the powder three times a day for three to five days. The herb has an extremely bitter taste, and you may prefer to take it in capsule form.

• Niu Huang Shang Qin Wan: Take this patent Chinese herbal pill according to instructions for one week. If your condition does not improve, see a doctor.

**Acupuncture:** This will reduce the infection and eliminate pain. You may see immediate relief after one or two treatments, but for acute pain you may need daily treatments. For chronic pain, you may need acupuncture once or twice a week for a few months.

**Acupressure:** Use the tip of your thumb to apply strong pressure to the Hegu points, which are located on your hands in the depression between the thumb and the index finger, for one to two minutes. Repeat on the other hand. It will relieve the pain temporarily.

**Diet:** Generally, light, fresh food is recommended. Include plenty of turnips, celery, spinach, aubergine, and mung beans in your diet. Foods to be avoided include ginger, chilies, mustard greens, and mutton. These pungent and irritating foods increase your body heat, which may make the abscess worse.

## NATUROPATHY

**Diet:** Eat plenty of multicolored vegetables to obtain the nutrients and phytochemicals needed to strengthen the immune system. Avoid all foods that decrease your immunity, such as junk food, anything containing hydrogenated oils and trans-fatty acids, simple carbohydrates, and sugars. Eliminate foods to which you may be allergic or intolerant, such as dairy products, wheat, and corn, which can cause inflammation and decrease your immunity.

**Herbs and spices:** Add herbs and spices to your cooking that enhance the immune system and have antiseptic properties, such as garlic and ginger. Burdock root is a great skin detoxifier; take 500 mg of the capsule or 4 ml of tincture three times a day. Take 500 mg in capsule form or 4 ml of tincture of goldenseal three times a day for its antibacterial, anti-inflammatory, and immune-enhancing properties.

**Detox:** A three-day juice fast will help eliminate impurities, reduce inflammation, and provide you with the nutrients you need to boost your immune system. Drink juices primarily from green vegetables or carrots. Celery and cucumbers are great for juicing because their high water content yields plenty of juice.

**Topical:** Tea tree oil is an effective antibacterial agent. Apply it as a cream, or 10–15 drops of the oil diluted in a ½ oz of water, two to three times a day. Oregano oil can also be used topically for its antibacterial effects. Use the oil directly on the abscess once or twice a day.

**Supplements:** Take 1,000 mg of vitamin C with bioflavonoids three times a day. These nutrients work synergistically to support the immune system and reduce skin inflammation. Zinc also supports skin function and the immune system. Zinc can deplete the body's stores of copper, so 3 mg of copper should be taken with this supplement.

**Hydrotherapy:** Apply hot and cold water (three minutes hot, followed by 30 seconds cold) to the affected area to drain pus. Do not use extreme temperatures, and do not use this treatment in areas where there is any numbness due to nerve damage.

## HOMEOPATHY

For a remedy to work effectively, match the remedy with your symptoms as closely as possible. Also choose a remedy based on the stage of the abcess, as some remedies are best suited to the early stage of inflammation, while others help resolve a more established condition. If no relief occurs after a period of 24–48 hours, seek conventional care.

**Belladonna:** Belladonna is useful in the early stages of inflammation where heat, redness, and throbbing pains are characteristic, but where there is little or no swelling. The affected area will be tender to the touch and sensitive to contact with cold air.

**Hepar sulph:** This is the most common remedy for abscesses, especially when the patient is irritable and chilly. When there are "drawing," sticking, or splintering pains in the affected area, Hepar sulph helps to speed up pus formation to resolve the abscess.

**Silica:** Silica can be helpful where an abscess has been developing slowly and insidiously, often in deep tissue. Use this remedy if the lymph glands in the area near the abscess are swollen and tender, and if there is a tendency for the abscess to be disinclined to resolve itself. This remedy can be especially useful where an abscess has been incised, but isn't healing very well, or if the abscess has resulted from a foreign body embedded in the skin.

**Mercurius:** This is used if there is swelling, tenderness, and inflammation of the glands near the abscess, plus a noticeable increase in the amount of saliva produced, and a nasty metallic taste in the mouth. If pains associated with the abscess are pulsating, and if contact with heat or cold makes the pain more intense, use Mercurius.

## HERBALISM

**Tea tree oil:** Apply this antibacterial and antifungal oil to the abscess. Tea tree oils can be "cut" with any number of inert oils. Oil that is 15% tea tree oil would likely provide the best results. If the skin becomes irritated, dilute the oil with vegetable oil to reduce its strength.

**Calendula:** Calendula is valued for its anti-inflammatory and wound-healing properties. Steep calendula flowers in hot water, let them cool, and then soak a clean cloth or piece of gauze in the liquid and apply it to the affected area as a compress. Calendula cream, available from health food stores, pharmacies, or naturopathic doctors, can also be used.

**Comfrey:** Also known as knitbone, comfrey contains allantoin, which helps to dissolve pus. To make a decoction, add 50 g of fresh, peeled root to 4 cups of water and boil for five to seven minutes. Add 50–100 g of fresh leaves and let them steep for 5–10 minutes. When the decoction has cooled to a warm temperature, strain it and soak a clean cloth or piece of gauze in the liquid. Hold the cloth against the abscess for 10–15 minutes.

**Arnica:** Steep a few ounces of dried arnica flowers, available from herb stores, in 1–2 cups of hot water. Soak a clean cloth in the liquid and apply it as a compress to the affected area.

**Garlic:** Crush some garlic to make a poultice and apply it to the abscess for its anibacterial properties. Alternatively, make a garlic syrup by soaking garlic cloves in a 50:50 vinegar to water solution. Dip a clean cloth in the mixture and apply it directly to the abscess.

**Marshmallow:** Chop up a whole marshmallow plant and let 25–30 g stand in 4 cups of cold water for a few hours. Apply this thick mixture to the abscess as a poultice or soak a clean cloth or piece of gauze in the mixture and apply it as a compress several times a day.

**Walnut:** Add 5 tsp of plant material to 200 ml of water. If using primarily root material, chop it into small pieces and boil for 10 minutes; if using leaves, chop and boil them for a few minutes. Allow the plant to steep for a few minutes and strain the liquid. Soak a clean cloth or piece of gauze in the liquid and apply it to the abscess several times a day.

**Peppermint essential oil:** Apply a few drops to the abscess for its antibacterial and antiseptic qualities.

**Goldenseal:** Take goldenseal in capsule form (500 mg) or as a tincture (4 ml) three times a day. This herb has antibacterial, anti-inflammatory, and immune-enhancing properties.

**Burdock root:** This plant is a great skin detoxifier. Infuse the roots to make a tea or a tincture and take 4 ml, or take 500 mg in capsule form, three times a day. Also, a salve of burdock can be applied to the skin. Macerate the burdock root and mix it with either a small amount of water to make a thick paste or with anti-inflammatory oils such as castor. Apply the mixture two to three times a day until there is less swelling or redness.

**Echinacea:** Echinacea stimulates the immune system. A pre-made tincture of Echinacea can be added to a compress or poultice of the plants mentioned above. It can also be purchased as a cream and applied to the abscess to speed up the healing process.

# ACNE

## DIAGNOSIS

Acne is a common skin disorder affecting young people during puberty, with boys tending to be more prone to it than girls due to hormonal activity. It is caused by the inflammation of the oil-producing sebaceous glands, which become overactive, flooding the pores with grease. Acne is also linked with an increased number of bacteria (Propionibacterium acnes) on the skin that become trapped inside hair follicules and oil ducts. Bacterial enzymes break down sebum into a range of free fatty acids, resulting in inflammation. Pus cells become attracted to the area and release potent chemicals to fight the infection, making the inflammation worse.The severity of acne increases and, typically, reaches its peak in the late teens. For most people, acne tends to subside by the time they reach their mid-20s; however, some may continue to have problems well into their 40s.

Triggers include stress and emotional tension, squeezing or picking at the pimples, and a reaction to some medicines and chemicals. There seems to be no clear evidence to support the theory that cutting out fatty foods and chocolate prevents acne breakouts, but a healthy balanced diet including plenty of fresh fruit and vegetables should certainly help to improve matters. If pimples are squeezed and the skin is damaged, there is a danger of infection, which can cause permanent scarring.

## SYMPTOMS

- Small, tender, red spots
- Blackheads and whiteheads
- Pus-filled pimples
- Spots on the face, back of the neck, upper back and chest, and occasionally in the armpits and on the buttocks
- Inflammation lasting a few days or weeks, depending on the severity
- Psychological stress

## TREATMENT GOAL

To bring relief from the socially debilitating symptoms of this condition, help with the stress of dealing with it, and act quickly to minimize the risk of any long-term scarring.

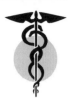

## CONVENTIONAL MEDICINE

**To treat non-inflammatory acne (blackheads):** A topical retinoid is usually prescribed to prevent and resolve the condition. Tretinoin, adapalene, and tazorotene are common retinoids. Azelaic acid, with its antimicrobial properties, is a more natural option. Salicyclic acid used topically is also effective. Antibiotics are not necessary for this type of acne.

**To treat pustular, mildly inflamed acne (whiteheads):** Antibiotics (oral or topical) may be used to inhibit the growth of bacteria, thus decreasing the concentration of free fatty acids and the resulting lesions. Topical antibiotics such as erythromycin or clindamycin are usually the first choice. They may be combined with benzoyl peroxide. Topical metronidazole or flagyl is useful for other types of bacteria. Dapsone topical gel 5% was approved by the FDA in August 2005 for the treatment of mild-to-moderate acne. Oral antibiotics are used if topical agents are not working. Doxycycline, minocycline, and tetracycline, which have anti-inflammatory properties, are the most effective.

**To treat severely inflamed acne:** A topical antibiotic such as benzoyl peroxide is prescribed with an oral antibiotic. These contain tetracyclines (or erythromycin for pregnant women, young children, or others unable to tolerate tetracyclines). Occasionally an injection of corticosteroids is effective for treating individual painful and unsightly lesions.

**If acne does not respond to the above treatments:** Oral isotretinoin is highly effective in treating all types of acne and leads to a prolonged remission. It may not be used by women of reproductive years without contraception as it harms developing babies.

**Oral contraceptives:** These can be prescribed for women when not contraindicated and when acceptable to the patient (especially when using isotretinoin). It is effective in treating moderate inflammatory acne caused by excessive androgen (male hormone) secretion.

**Natural alternatives:** As a rich source of chromium, brewer's yeast may be a natural alternative for treating acne. Zinc has also been shown to treat acne.

**To treat excessive scarring:** Cryotherapy, dermabrasion, laser resurfacing, chemical peels, punch grafting, and collagen injections can reduce the appearance of scars.

---

**TIP:** AVOID MEDICATIONS THAT TRIGGER LESIONS
Medications with iodine (found in cough medicines) and some prescription drugs such as lithium, corticosteroids, anabolic steroids, and oral contraceptives with a high androgen content can exacerbate acne lesions.

## TRADITIONAL CHINESE MEDICINE

**Herbs:** Chrysanthemum, available from Chinese pharmacies, dispells body heat and relieves body toxicity. Add 6–8 g of dried flowers to 2–3 cups of boiled water. Let them steep for a few minutes, strain the liquid, and refill once or twice more. Drink the tea throughout the day. It usually takes six to eight weeks for acne to clear.

**Acupuncture:** The main acupoints for treating acne are located on the large intestine and stomach meridians. Local facial points are also used. Usually an accupuncture practitioner will give you treatment once a week for three to six months. Acupuncture and Chinese herbal medicine can be combined to treat acne. You can expect some improvement after as few as two sessions: The acne will start fading and fewer new breakouts will occur.

**Acupressure:** To improve local circulation, self-massage the Yang Bai point, located on the forehead, directly above the pupil, 1 inch above the eyebrow. The Yang Bai point is especially useful for treating acne on the forehead. If there is more acne on the cheeks, press the Quan Liao point, located about 3 inches from the nostril, in the depression directly below the cheekbone.

**Diet:** Drink sufficient water daily. Eat plenty of fresh fruit and vegetables, and avoid food that has heating or warming properties, such as hot chili peppers, beef, and lamb. Also steer clear of deep-fried, fatty, and greasy food since they create more heat.

## NATUROPATHY

**Diet:** Eat plenty of dark green and orange vegetables for their high beta carotene content. They are best eaten steamed or lightly cooked so that they retain nutrients and fiber. Eat meat products once a day only, or make sure they are organic and free range, and are hormone- and antibiotic-free. Eat plenty of high-yielding proteins—especially those that are high in omega-3 fatty acids, such as cold-water fish. Raw almonds, walnuts, and pumpkin seeds are a good source of skin-healthy vitamin E and essential fatty acids. If you are taking antibiotics, eat plenty of unsweetened cultured foods such as kefir, yogurt, and raw cabbage. Antibiotics destroy the healthy bacteria in your digestive tract that are important for good health. Ground flaxseeds provide an adequate amount of fiber for regulation and essential fatty acids. Mix 2 tbsp with food or take it with a glass of water. Avoid junk foods, which have high amounts of toxins that contribute to acne formation. Simple carbohydrates and sugars encourage oil production and feed bacteria and yeast. Also, the sugar-regulating hormone insulin increases skin inflammation. Avoid food allergens such as wheat, milk, and corn and any foods to which you may be intolerant.

**Supplements:** Take 50 mg of zinc picolinate three times a day for one to three months to enhance the immune system, nourish the skin, and reduce build-up of dihydrotestosterone (DHT). Take 10,000 IU of vitamin A twice a day to reduce sebum production. A high dosage (up to 50,000 IU a day) is needed to be effective against acne, which is best taken under the supervision of a doctor because of its potential toxicity. Pregnant women should not take more than 10,000 IU of vitamin A a day—a dosage that may be too low to treat acne. Vitamin E (taken at 400 IU daily) increases the benefits of vitamin A and selenium. Selenium (taken at 200 mcg daily) works with vitamin E to reduce inflammation.

**Topical treatment:** Tea tree oil is a natural antiseptic. Apply 5 drops of a 5–15% solution in diluted water to a cotton ball and dab on the affected area.

## HOMEOPATHY

The following remedies can speed up recovery and healing from a fairly mild, recently occurring episode of acne. However, bear in mind that recurring acne breakouts suggest a more deep-seated problem, which can benefit from treatment by a homeopathic practitioner.

**Belladonna:** Taken at the first sign of inflammation, belladonna can stop large, red spots from occuring, or bring them to a head. Use this remedy if there is a rapid onset of symptoms with heat, redness, and throbbing tender spots.

**Pulsatilla:** This remedy is ideal for spots that have emerged in response to a rich and fatty diet. Spots may be noticeably worse at times of major hormonal shifts, such as during puberty, around the time of a period, after pregnancy, and approaching the menopause.

**Natrum mur:** This can help resolve spots that emerge as a result of excess oil and sebum production. Spots are usually preceded by blocked pores and blackheads. Although greasy in patches, the skin is generally dry and cracked, especially around the lips and mouth.

**Nux vomica:** Use this detoxing remedy to treat itchy, burning spots that result from getting too little sleep, and consuming too much junk food, alcohol, caffeine, and cigarettes.

**Hepar sulph:** This is useful for slow-healing skin, where scars of large, yellow, pus-filled sensitive spots remain for a long time. This remedy can also encourage "blind" spots to come to a head and resolve themselves.

**TIP:** TREAT SKIN GENTLY
Avoid using harsh cleansing and exfoliating products that can aggravate the problem by encouraging the skin to produce more oil to redress the balance.

## HERBALISM

**Fumitory:** Take 30 drops of a tincture of this plant, available from health food stores, pharmacies, and naturopathic doctors, three times a day. It contains anti-inflammatory compounds like quercetin and rutin, and compounds that may act as an antiviral or immunity stimulant.

**Burdock root:** This can be boiled and the tea drunk to act as a blood purifier to improve acne. One method is to boil 2 g of the root and take this tea three or four times daily. However, some people may develop dermatitis from the use of burdock.

**Black walnut leaves:** These are used medicinally for their astringent, tonifying, antiseptic, laxative, and wound-healing properties. Make a decoction by boiling cut or powdered leaves to take internally or use in a compress. Add 5 tsp of plant material to 200 ml of water. If primarily adding root material, chop it into small pieces and boil for 10 minutes; if using primarily leaves, chop and boil them for a few minutes. Let the plant steep for a few minutes before straining and drinking the liquid. Drink a small glassful two to three times daily. If diarrhea develops, reduce the amount being consumed.

**Arnica flowers:** A 20–25% ointment or tincture of the flower should be applied twice a day, but should never be used on open skin; there are compounds that can be toxic to the liver if they enter the body. Or use a homeopathic ointment that has been diluted to avoid the adverse effects. There is a slight chance of an allergic reaction to arnica.

**Peppermint essential oil:** Use peppermint essential oil for its antibacterial, anti-inflammatory, analgesic, and antiseptic properties. Apply a couple of drops to a piece of cotton wool and quickly run water over it to dilute it slightly. Dab on the site of acne.

**Calendula:** Also called marigold, calendula is valued for its anti-inflammatory, astringent, antifungal, and wound-healing properties. Use a cold cream containing calendula.

**Eliminating toxins:** Persistent acne may require herbal treatments to assist the body in eliminating toxins by using blood-purifying and gastrointestinal tract stimulants. Try drinking a cup of tea containing nettles, dandelion root and herb, rosehip, frangula bark, senna leaf, and anise fruit twice daily to assist the body in blood purification. Mix equal ratios of the dry plants and fill a tea ball with the mixture. Let the plants steep in hot water for five minutes before drinking.

## DIAGNOSIS

Allergies are often a sign of infection, but can also be a reaction of the immune system when it comes into contact with a substance in the environment that it views as an invader. These substances are called allergens, and it is common to see an inflammatory response in the skin—in fact, the skin is often the first part of the body to react. Some allergies can affect anyone, not just those prone to them—for example, contact dermatitis, where the skin reacts to a particular substance. Generally, skin allergies fall into three categories: eczema (p. 73), urticaria (p. 159), and contact dermatitis (p. 56). Triggers and irritants can include house dust; animal fur; pollen; synthetic fabrics such as elastic and latex; certain foods such as wheat, dairy, eggs, seafood, berries, and chocolate; chemicals in soap or fabric conditioners; nickel; fragrances and household cleaners; and emotional states such as upheaval, stress, and anxiety.

**DANGER**: Any escalating symptoms of an allergic skin reaction that are combined with any hint of swelling of the face, lips, or throat require immediate emergency treatment. This need becomes even more pressing where there is any sign of breathing difficulties or distress.

## SYMPTOMS

- Itchy skin and a red or pink rash
- Patches of rough, flaky red skin after contact with an allergen. This suggests contact dermatitis (p. 56)
- Patches of dry, scaly red skin on the face and in the skin folds. This suggests atopic eczema (p. 73)
- Itchy red patches with white heads resembling nettle stings. This suggests urticaria (p. 159)
- Headaches, dizziness, and a general feeling of being under the weather

## TREATMENT GOAL

To identify triggers and develop methods of coping with skin allergies, as well as easing any immediate symptoms.

## CONVENTIONAL MEDICINE

Skin allergies, or contact dermatitis, are very common. There are two types of contact dermatitis: an allergy and an irritant, which people often call an allergy. Allergic contact dermatitis is a reaction to a substance to which one has previously been exposed and is therefore sensitized. The most common skin allergens are nickel, poison ivy, and latex. Irritant contact dermatitis requires no previous exposure. Common causes include soaps and solvents that contain alkaloids. Treatment aims to decrease dryness and inflammation and to prevent recurrence. Identification of the allergen or irritant and avoiding re-exposure are vital.

**Emollients:** Use emollients and non-detergent soap substitutes to relieve dryness. Cool, moist compresses with isotonic saline are another popular treatment.

**Oral antihistamines:** This class of drugs, also called histamine one blockers, such as Benadryl® and Atarax®, can relieve itchiness. Calamine used topically is also useful.

**Hydrocortisone cream:** For moderate cases, this topical corticosteroid, should be tried first. It is available over the counter. It should not be used over large areas of the body.

**Potent topical corticosteroids:** Stronger potency topical corticosteroids, such as clobetasol or betamethasone dipropionate, are used for more severe rashes. These are obtained with a prescription and are very effective in treating small areas of moderate allergic contact dermatitis; systemic corticosteroids such as prednisone may be used in more severe cases.

**Topical tacrolimus or pimecrolimus:** These may be an option for patients who cannot use, or whose dermatitis is unresponsive to, corticosteroids. They should only be used when other therapies have failed due to potential increased risk of immunosuppression— a condition where the immune system does not work well because there are not enough white blood cells to fight infection—and cancer. Always try the lowest concentration first.

## TRADITIONAL CHINESE MEDICINE

**Herbs:**
• Yin Qiao Jie Tu Pian: To help relieve itching and rashes, try Yin Qiao Jie Tu Pian, the pill form of a combination of herbs, available from Chinese pharmacies or online. Take as indicated with warm water.
• Peppermint and lychee: Drink peppermint and lychee tea to clear toxins that cause itchy skin from the body. Add 10 g of dried peppermint and

10 g of dried lychee fruit, available from Chinese pharmacies or online, to boiling water. Take three times a day for 7–10 days. The tea can be taken for longer periods depending on the condition.

• Fang Fen Tong Shen Wan: To treat an acute condition, take Fang Fen Tong Shen Wan. It is mostly available in pill form but can also be taken as a powder. Take 6 g of the powder three times a day for one to two weeks. If the condition is chronic, consult a doctor for the correct dosage and treatment.

**Acupuncture:** You can have acupuncture treatment for both acute and chronic stages of skin allergies. For acute conditions, the treatment will focus on skin rashes. Traditional Chinese medicine sees all itchiness as the result of pathogenic wind. To let go of the "wind" poison, the practitioner will use needling techniques that release toxins to stop itchiness and prevent the condition from becoming chronic. At a chronic stage, the treatment will be to regulate your immunity, or rebuild your internal balance, by tonifying some of your deficient organs or reorganizing energy. In a chronic treatment plan, patients can undergo treatments for a few months or even years depending on the severity of the condition.

**Acupressure:** Use your thumb to press the Feng Chi point 2 inches from the center point of the base of the skull at the back of the head. Start with gentle pressure and gradually increase. Press and release 20 times. The Feng Chi point is important for dispelling wind and stimulating the immune system. When skin is terribly itchy don't scratch. Instead relieve itchiness by pressing your palm on the skin right next to where the rashes are or directly press on rashes with vertical pressure, avoiding rubbing.

**Diet:** Eat food that has a gentle property and will strengthen the immune system, such as organic green vegetables, aubergine, radish, mung beans, bitter melon, purslane, and pear. Green tea is also good since it has a gentle cleansing effect. Avoid seafood and anything that is fatty or spicy.

**TIP:** STAY CALM
At the acute stage of a skin allergy, keep yourself mentally calm and relaxed. This will help your body be in the right state for healing.

## NATUROPATHY

**Diet:** Eat plenty of non-mucus-forming foods, such as fresh vegetables and fruits, healthy cold pressed oils, seeds, and nuts (except peanuts, which are a legume and should be avoided as well as any other nut to which you might be allergic). Eat lean proteins such as antibiotic- and hormone-free chicken and grass-fed meats, tofu, and seafood. Try juicing green vegetables for a daily drink to raise immunity and flush out toxins from the body. Avoid mucus-forming foods, such as processed sugars, dairy products, and items made with flour. Also avoid foods that decrease immunity, such as hydrogenated oils and trans-fatty acids. Steer clear of any foods to which you are intolerant or allergic, such as wheat, dairy, or corn.

**Supplements:** Take 50 mg of zinc picolinate twice a day to enhance the immune system and nourish the skin. Take 4 g of fish oil to reduce skin inflammation. Take 1,000 mg of vitamin C three times a day to help boost the immune system (if stools soften, cut back to 1,000 mg twice a day).

**Herbs:** Burdock root is an excellent skin detoxifier. Take 500 mg of the capsule or 3 ml of tincture three times a day.

**Exercise:** Exercise regularly to help circulate toxins out of the body.

**TIP:** USE AN AIR FILTER
Use a high-energy particulate air (HEPA) filter to reduce your exposure to allergen triggers such as mold and dust. Place the filter where you spend the most time, such as your bedroom.

## HOMEOPATHY

Mild symptoms of redness, itchiness, blotchiness, and irritation may respond well to any of the following homoeopathic remedies. However, severe or recurrent problems will require professional treatment in order to help the body deal with the underlying imbalance that is at the root of the problem.

**Apis:** Use this remedy if rashes are blotchy, pinkish, and raised in nature. It is called for when rashes tend to erupt very quickly with lots of irritation and stinging pains that cause great distress and irritability. The discomfort is temporarily soothed by contact with cool air and cool bathing, while exposure to heat in any form intensifies restlessness and distress.

**Urtica:** If skin rashes come on as a result of marked temperature changes, use Urtica. Characteristic symptoms include itchy, stinging swellings of the fingers and/or blotchiness of the face. When trying to imagine the sensations that are eased by this remedy, think of a rash that feels like it has been set off by contact with stinging nettles.

**Rhus tox:** If an allergic rash is blistery, intensely itchy at night (to the point of preventing sleep), with burning itchiness triggering compulsive scratching, use Rhus tox. Rashes may develop in response to getting damp and chilled, and react very badly to getting hot in bed at night. Rashes are worse after getting wet or when you are feeling stressed.

**Arsenicum album:** This is a strong candidate to consider where distressingly itchy and burning rashes are temporarily soothed by contact with warmth. This could take the form of warm compresses or warm bathing. Compulsive scratching only makes the itchiness more intense. When this remedy is strongly indicated there is also likely to be a great deal of mental, emotional, and physical restlessness and anxiety.

**Natrum mur:** If an allergic rash looks large, red, and blotchy, having a strong tendency to appear on the areas of skin covering the joints, use Natrum mur. These eruptions are likely to feel much more irritated and uncomfortable if you get overheated by exercising, especially in hot, sunny conditions.

## HERBALISM

**Herbs:** Aloe vera, slippery elm bark, marshmallow root, fenugreek, chickweed, and comfrey leaves or roots can be used as poultices, creams, and lotions to soothe inflamed red, itchy skin. In addition, chamomile and calendula can calm a skin allergy when applied topically. Both chamomile and calendula can be incorporated into creams and lotions.

**Oats or oatmeal:** These can effectively soothe the redness of a skin allergy and calm the itchiness. Mix about 1 cup of oats with enough cool water to create a mash, which should be left to macerate for 5–10 minutes. Dab the liquid from the mash onto affected skin with a clean washcloth several times a day. A film will form on the skin, which is calming, but the treatment can also stick to clothing, so be careful what you wear. The mash itself can also be placed directly on the skin for 10–15 minutes, rather like a poultice. A cup of oats can also be added to bathwater to provide a soothing layer to the whole body.

**Figwort:** Figwort can work in two ways to help with skin allergies and itchiness. Taken as a tincture internally, it is a blood purifier, helping to cleanse the body and remove toxins and other allergens that could be contributing to the outbreak. A figwort extract can also be added to ointments and salves that, when applied directly to the skin, can calm allergies, possibly because of flavanoid compounds; flavanoids are often effective as an antioxidant and anti-inflammatory. Figwort tinctures and extracts can both be found in health food stores.

# ATHLETE'S FOOT

## DIAGNOSIS

Athlete's foot is a very common fungal infection and can affect anyone, although small children do not appear to be at risk. We all have one or more of the fungi that can cause athlete's foot to be present on our bodies. They feed on dead skin cells and are usually harmless. The fungi love warm, moist places; and athlete's foot is primarily a problem for people who suffer from sweaty feet, wear trainers for long periods of time, or do not dry their feet properly. It is also more common in those who do not wash their feet as frequently as they should. It is usually picked up through communal changing rooms and other damp environments. The condition is contagious. It can spread quickly by direct skin-to-skin contact and indirectly through towels. The fungus thrives in the damp conditions between the toes, where it multiplies, eating the dead skin that is shed by the body every day.

## SYMPTOMS

- Irritation and itchiness between the toes and around the base of the foot
- A red, itchy rash in the spaces between the toes (often between the fourth and fifth toes)
- Small pustules (sometimes, but not always)
- Peeling skin and blisters
- Unpleasant odor
- Often a small degree of scaling
- Painful cracks between the toes
- Toenails can become infected too, sometimes separating from the nail bed
- The infection can spread to the rest of the foot and other parts of the body

## TREATMENT GOAL

To clear up the condition using conventional and complementary therapies without recourse to a dermatologist.

## CONVENTIONAL MEDICINE

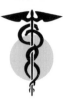

**Prevention:** Athlete's foot is a superficial fungal infection known as tinea pedis. There are about five fungal organisms that produce athlete's foot, all of which thrive in moist, warm places. For this reason keeping the feet dry and cool is important in prevention and treatment. Over-the-counter powders such as Tinactin® are effective in prevention and in early treatment, as is tea tree oil. Avoiding communal changing areas and showers is advisable. Changing socks daily or whenever they are damp and keeping up a diet rich in antioxidants also helps.

**Fungicidal agents:** Treatment consists of applying an over-the-counter fungicidal agent such as terbinafine, naftifine, or butenafine for four weeks. These agents are associated with higher cure rates and quicker response times than some of the older topical treatments. Sometimes a once-weekly internal antifungal medicine called Diflucan (fluconazole) is used, especially in severe cases.

## TRADITIONAL CHINESE MEDICINE

**Herbs:** The herbs below are all available from Chinese herbalists.
• Herbal footbath: Add 30 g of Ku Shen (sophora root), 30 g of Huang Bai (phellodendron), 18 g of Ma Zhi Xian (dried purslane), 20 g of Cang Zhu (atractylodes rhizome), 30 g of Bai Xian Pi (dictamnus root bark) to 6 cups of fresh water in a ceramic herb cooking pot. Boil the herbs for five minutes. Turn down the heat and simmer for 30 minutes, then strain the herbs. You will get approximately 4 cups of liquid. Pour 2 cups into a pan, add hot water, and soak your feet in the herbal footbath for 20 minutes once a day before going to bed.
• Herbal powder formula: Ask a Chinese herbalist to mix the following powders well: 10 g of Huang Lian (coptis root), 10 g of Huang Bai (phellodendron), and 6 g of Da Huang (rhubarb root/rhizome). Store the herbs in a sealed container. Wash your feet with warm water and dry them thoroughly. Apply an adequate amount of powder—about 1 tsp—to the affected area with a cotton wool bud. Leave the herbal powder on for up to 12 hours. Apply twice a day for three days. Stop for one day, then use again for three days. Repeat this procedure for one month. If your skin feels irritated, stop using the powder and consult your doctor.

**Acupuncture:** To treat athlete's foot, you will receive acupuncture on your arms and legs, in addition to treating local foot points, because the healing involves draining damp toxins from the body. Needles will remain in your body for 20–30 minutes. Treatment once or twice a week for a few months is common.

**Moxibustion:** Some practitioners may also practice moxibustion for athlete's foot. This technique involves burning a dried herb over a particular acupuncture point to produce a very penetrating heat to influence the flow of Qi and blood. Moxibustion can also be combined with acupuncture.

**Diet:** Those with athlete's foot should avoid hot, fatty and greasy foods, which can aggravate this condition. Sweet foods should also be avoided.

## NATUROPATHY

**Diet:** Eat plenty of fresh vegetables, lean protein, and whole grains. These foods will support your immune system. Add unsweetened cultured foods to your diet such as kefir, yogurt, miso, and raw sauerkraut, which contain friendly bacteria that fight off systemic fungus. Avoid sugar and processed carbohydrates, which fuel yeast and help athlete's foot to reproduce. Avoid or reduce fruits and avoid fruit juice altogether. Most fruits and all fruits juices are too high in sugar and fuel yeast. Drink 10 glasses of water a day to assist in flushing out yeast toxins. Drink two glasses a day of a green drink made from spirulina, wheat grass, and barley grass powder. These substances will help raise your immunity levels and feed healthy bacteria.

**Topical:** Tea tree oil has antifungal properties and can be applied directly to the infected area. If the toenail is infected, cut the nail back as much as possible and apply pure tea tree oil to the infected area.

**Herbs:** Use oregano oil for its strong antifungal effects. Take 5 drops of liquid under the tongue or mixed with a glass of water. Undiluted drops may be too strong for some people and you may belch the oregano. You can also take oregano oil in capsule form at 500 mg a day. Garlic fights fungus and boosts the immune system; take 500 mg twice a day. Grapefruit seed extract has antifungal properties. Take 200 mg twice a day. Caprylic acid is a fatty acid shown to have antifungal properties; take 1,000 mg three times a day. Undecylenic acid is a derivative of castor bean oil and has been shown to have strong antifungal properties. Take 200 mg three times a day. Pau d'Arco tea, available in bulk or as tea bags at health food stores, has strong antifungal properties. Take 2 cups of the tea a day.

**Supplements:** Take 1,000 mg of vitamin C twice a day for its immune-enhancing functions. Take a high-potency multivitamin. It will provide many nutrients that will support immune function.

## HOMEOPATHY

Any of the following remedies can be effective in easing the symptoms of a mild, recently developed flareup of athlete's foot. However, if symptoms are severe or have a tendency to recur, the best results will be obtained by consulting a homeopathic practitioner who will aim to treat and strengthen the whole system. Always bear in mind when considering the following remedy choices that you need to select the remedy that matches your symptoms most closely for relief.

**Causticum:** If there is severe itchiness between the toes, with a tendency for recently healed-over cracks to re-open easily, use Causticum. It is helpful in relieving soreness and rawness that develop in folds of skin. It can also help remedy sleeplessness due to a sensation of "restless legs" at night that makes it almost impossible to keep the feet and legs still.

**Rhus tox:** If the rash looks blistery and crusty, and feels very itchy at night, use Rhus tox. It is especially helpful for moist athlete's foot that is made more noticeably distressing, irritating, and distracting if it gets cold, damp, or wet.

**Sepia:** For athlete's foot that has a tendency to flare up periodically (for instance, during seasonal changes), use Sepia. Symptoms will include intense blistery eruptions that settle in the folds of skin between the toes. Along with this condition, there may be a noticeable tendency to develop dry, cracked skin, and you may feel run down and drained.

**Mezereum:** If irritation and itchiness quickly change location on being scratched, or are much more distressing after a warm bath, use Mezereum. Other symptoms include marked sensitivity to cold air, with itching, burning, and smarting sensations of the affected area.

**Calc carb:** Use Calc carb if your feet have a tendency to be cold, clammy, and sweaty; if the skin is generally cold and damp to the touch, while also tending to chap and crack very readily; if the least physical effort sets off a bout of sweating, with irritation of the feet being made worse by bathing, socks, and contact with cold air; or if it improves in dry, warm weather, and becomes temporarily more comfortable for being carefully rubbed.

## HERBALISM

Athlete's foot can be treated fairly easily with herbal medicine in addition to proper foot hygiene. Almost all herbal remedies used for athlete's foot are applied topically, directly to the infected area. This method increases effectiveness and limits unwanted side-effects. However, if symptoms do not resolve, it is advisable to seek medical attention as a more aggressive mode of therapy may be indicated.

**Garlic:** Garlic is antiseptic, antifungal, and a diuretic, plus it acts as an expectorant and stimulant. It contains the compound ajoene, known to have powerful antifungal properties, and has been shown to work just as well as over-the-counter antifungal medications. Garlic has virtually no side-effects when used topically, although minor irritation is sometimes reported. When taken internally at high, therapeutic doses, garlic may interfere with certain antithrombotic drugs. Crushed raw garlic can be applied directly to the affected area two to three times a day for one to two weeks, although the odor can act as a deterrent. A more effective and tolerable method of delivery is a garlic gel, which can be purchased from local health food stores. Look for a gel containing 1% ajoene if possible. Apply twice daily for 7–10 days.

**Tea tree oil:** There are many competing recommendations regarding the dosage and effectiveness of tea tree oil for use in treating athlete's foot. It can be used topically as an antifungal and antibacterial agent and has been shown to work well to relieve symptoms. Apply a 5–15% tea tree oil solution or a 5–15% tea tree oil cream topically to the infected area. A much stronger dose of either the solution or cream is needed to produce a cure. Recommendations range from applying a 25–100% strength oil or cream two to three times daily. Dermatitis is the only significant side-effect associated with the prolonged and repeated topical use of tea tree oil.

**Calendula:** Also referred to as marigold, calendula is easily accessible and can be applied topically as an ointment or tincture. Dosing recommendations are highly varied, and consultation with a local herbal therapist may be warranted. Calendula has very few contraindications or adverse reactions when used topically. There is a small potential for an allergic reaction, most likely in people who have an allergy to other plants in the daisy family.

**Cloves:** When applied topically, cloves have known antifungal properties. Use this herb as an essential oil or salve, available over the counter, several times a day. There are several potential adverse reactions to the topical application of cloves, including dermatitis and mucous membrane irritation. Do not take this herb internally to treat fungal infections.

# BOILS

## DIAGNOSIS

A boil is a skin infection that results in an inflamed lump under the surface of the skin. It starts as a painful red lump that then swells and fills with pus, which hardens to form a yellow head. It is very tender and can be very distressing, particularly if it is noticeable. Boils usually appear on the face, neck, buttocks, back, armpits, or groin but can also appear on other areas of the body. They are caused by bacteria entering the skin, and can also result from conditions such as eczema and scabies. Some people are prone to recurrent infection, and boils can spread if you are in close contact with someone who is infected. Boils can often be left alone until they discharge of their own accord. If it is large and particularly painful, a boil can be lanced. Antibiotics may be prescribed, particularly if there is recurrent infection. As soon as the pus is released and the core of the boil is gone, the skin should start to heal.

## SYMPTOMS

- A hard, sore lump under the surface of the skin
- Soreness around the affected area
- Swollen glands
- Fever
- Enlarged lymph glands
- Infected hair follicle
- Infected sebaceous gland
- Impaired resistance to infection
- Feeling rundown/general poor health
- Constipation
- Diabetes

## TREATMENT GOAL

Boils usually run their natural course and are best left alone. But there are ways you can help relieve the symptoms and prevent the infection from spreading.

## CONVENTIONAL MEDICINE

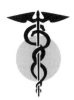

**Prevention:** Boils can be caused by a virus, bacteria, fungus, chemical irritation, or a physical impact to the skin. However, they are usually bacterial, caused by staphylococcus and streptococcus, both of which live naturally on the skin. They are more common in diabetics and those with weakened immune systems, and in those who are obese, have poor hygiene, perspire a great deal, or wear overly tight clothing. Losing weight, improving hygiene, and wearing looser clothing is a straightforward way to prevent or reduce the occurrence of boils. You should also eliminate any possible mechanical or chemical skin irritants.

**Topical ointments:** Use mupirocin or benzoyl peroxide in conjunction with an oral antibiotic. Usually, cephalexin (Keflex®) is a first choice for common boils. A herpectic boil (caused by the Herpes simplex virus) is treated with acyclovir. If the source of the infection comes from a fungus rather than bacteria, the boil is treated with a topical antifungal such as econazole. Zeasorb™, which comes as a powder as well as an ointment, is topical and available over the counter. It can be useful in decreasing moisture in prone areas.

## TRADITIONAL CHINESE MEDICINE

**Internal herbal formulas:**
• Wu Wei Xiao Tu Yin: To treat boils that look red and may have a current infection, take Wu Wei Xiao Tu Yin for one month. It contains herbs that dispel heat toxicity.
• Tuo Li Xiao Tu Shan: Take this formula for one to three months to treat recurring chronic boils at different stages.

**External herbal formulas:**
• Jin Huang Gao and Si Huang Gao: Apply either of these herbs in cream form once or twice a day on boils that are broken or infected. They have similar benefits.
• Herbal wash: Combine 30 g of Zi Hua Di Ding (Yedeon's violet), 18 g of Pu Gong Ying (dandelion), 30 g of Huang Bai (phellodendron), 30 g of Bai Jiang Cao (patrinia), and 30 g of Jin Yin Hua (honeysuckle flower) in a ceramic pot. Add 6 cups of water and let the mixture boil for five minutes, and then simmer for a further 10 minutes. Strain the decoction, add 6 cups of water to the herbs, and reboil a second time. Repeat the same procedure as above and use the decoction to wash boils once or twice a day.

**Acupuncture:** You may be treated once or twice a week and you will see a gradual improvement. Boils will start drying up with less new breakouts, and the cause of the boils will be evaluated and addressed. Don't give up too quickly—acupuncture treatment not only deals with symptoms, it also regulates your body energy. As it heals the skin, it also heals the internal problem that has contributed to the skin condition.

**Diet:** Light, fresh, cooling foods are beneficial for boils. Eat oyster, crab, clams, mussels, kelp, daikon, water chestnuts, celery, spinach, bamboo shoots, pears, and watermelon. Avoid garlic, onion, chilies, and mustard greens, as well as fatty, greasy food.

## NATUROPATHY

**Diet:** Eat plenty of multicolored vegetables to provide your body with all the nutrients and photochemicals needed to strengthen the immune system. Avoid all foods that depress the immune system, such as junk food, food containing hydrogenated oils and trans-fatty acids, simple carbohydrates, and sugars. Also eliminate foods to which you may be allergic or intolerant, such as dairy, wheat, and corn.

**Herbs and spices:** Add herbs and spices to your cooking that enhance the immune system and have antiseptic properties, such as garlic and ginger. Take 4 ml of burdock root as a tincture or 500 mg in capsule form a day to detoxify the skin. Take 4 ml of goldenseal as a tincture or 500 mg in capsule form a day to benefit from its antibacterial, anti-inflammatory, and immunity enhancing properties.

**Detox:** A three-day juice fast will help eliminate impurities, reduce inflammation, and provide you with the nutrients you need to boost your immune system. The juices should be primarily green vegetables and carrots. Celery and cucumbers are great for juicing because their high water content yields plenty of juice.

**Topical treatments:** Tea tree oil is an effective antibacterial agent. Apply the oil as a cream or 10–15 drops diluted in ½ oz of water two to three times a day. Oregano oil can also be used topically for its strong antibacterial effects. Use the oil directly once or twice a day.

**Supplements:** Take 3,000 mg of vitamin C with bioflavanoids a day—1,500 mg in the morning and 1,500 mg in the evening. These two nutrients work synergistically to support the immune system and reduce skin inflammation. Take 30 mg of zinc twice a day to support skin function and the immune system. Zinc can deplete the body's stores of copper, so 3 mg of copper should be taken with this supplement.

**Hydrotherapy:** Alternate applying hot and cold water (three minutes hot, followed by 30 seconds cold) to drain pus. Be careful not to burn yourself by using extreme temperatures. Do not use this treatment in areas where you have numbness due to nerve damage.

Boils can arise as a sign of being temporarily rundown or can appear as a symptom of a more on-going, underlying problem. Remedies listed below can help speed up recovery from a mild to moderate boil, but recurrent and/or severe episodes will need treatment from a practitioner to understand and eliminate the underlying problem. If no relief occurs after a period of 24–48 hours, seek conventional care.

**Drink plenty of water:** Where your health is concerned, it should always be a priority to guard against dehydration and flush out the system by drinking five large glasses of water a day (ideally filtered tap water or still mineral water). This becomes even more of a priority where there is any disturbance on the skin, and the need rises again if drugs such as antibiotics are being taken. Not only does this support the action of the kidneys, but it also helps guard against constipation and headaches, as well as supporting healthy skin.

**Diet:** Products that contain a substantial amount of white sugar are thought to aggravate boils, so steer clear of foods and drinks that contain a high proportion of refined sugar. These include obvious sources such as cakes, sweets, cookies, and pastries as well as "hidden" sugars in fizzy, carbonated drinks, processed foods (ketchup, canned beans, and even some pizzas can have a surprising amount of added sugar), and fruit bars.

**Belladonna:** Taken early, this remedy can stop the boil developing further, or will move it to the next stage where pus is formed. Belladonna is effective when taken at the first sign of boil formation where throbbing, heat, and redness of the affected area are noticeable.

**Hepar sulph:** This is the most common remedy for this problem, especially when the patient is irritable and chilly. It is useful if the boil has reached the next stage, where there are lots of drawing pains and where suppuration needs to be supported before the boil will resolve itself. The affected area will be hypersensitive to cold air, which aggravates the splintering, sharp pains, and pus when it forms will be yellow in color and thick in texture. This remedy is useful where there is a history of skin being easily infected and slow to heal.

**Silica:** For festering boils that produce a thin, clear discharge, use Silica. It is also useful for treating boil formation in skin that is stubborn to heal, and tends to scar. Scars are also likely to remain sensitive and painful for a lengthy period of time.

**Mercurius:** If boils emerge around the time of menstruation, use Mercurius. Pains in the affected area are characteristically stinging and burning, and very sensitive to the slightest variation of temperature from warmth to cold. Pus formation looks thin with a greenish tinge, or may be blood-tinged.

## HERBALISM

**Arnica:** Apply a 20–25% ointment or tincture of the flower to the skin twice a day, but never on open skin. There is chance of an allergic reaction to arnica, most likely to occur in those allergic to plants in the daisy family.

**Dogwood:** The bark of the root can be used topically to relieve boils and other infections. Boil 5 tsp of plant material in 200 ml of water. Let the plant steep for a few minutes and strain the liquid. Soak a cloth or piece of gauze in the liquid and apply it to the boil.

**Goldenseal:** Take goldenseal in capsule form (500 mg) or as a tincture (4 ml) three times a day for its antibacterial, anti-inflammatory, and immunity enhancing properties. It should be purchased from manufacturers who use cultivated goldenseal as its populations are threatened or endangered in some areas.

**Calendula:** The plant contains flavanoids, carotenes, carotenoid pigments, and volatile oil, which are anti-inflammatory, astringent, and antifungal. Steep the flowers in hot water, let the liquid cool slightly, and then soak a clean cloth or piece of gauze in the liquid and apply it to the affected area. Alternatively, apply warm masses of plant material or a cold cream containing calendula to the affected area.

**Black walnut tree leaves:** These leaves have astringent, tonifying, antiseptic, laxative, and wound-healing properties. To make a strong decoction from the plant, add 5 tsps of plant material to 200 ml of water. If using root material, chop it into small pieces and boil for 10 minutes; if using leaves, chop and boil them for a few minutes. Soak a clean cloth or gauze in the decoction and apply it to the affected area. You can also drink a small glassful of the decoction two to three times a day. If diarrhea develops, reduce the amount consumed.

**Peppermint essential oil:** Gently massage a few drops of the essential oil or linament into the boil for its antibacterial, anti-inflammatory, analgesic, and antiseptic effects.

**Flaxseed:** Make a poultice of ground decocted hot flaxseed to draw out the infection and decrease inflammation. Add boiling water to 1–2 tbsp of ground flaxseed to make a thick paste. Let it cool and apply a warm mass, wrapped in a linen cloth, to the affected area.

# COLD SORES

## DIAGNOSIS

Cold sores are small blisters that usually come up around the mouth and nostrils. They usually appear towards the end of a cold, which explains their name. They are often passed on by kissing, and tend to be more common among teenagers. The first sign is a tingling sensation, followed by a blister, which can be very sore and itchy. After a couple of days the blister will crust over, eventually healing. While irritating and unpleasant to look at, cold sores are not a serious problem. However, once caught, the cold sore virus will lie dormant in the system and can be a recurring problem, causing repeated discomfort. Cold sores are caused by the Herpes simplex virus, to which most of us have a natural immunity that enables us to keep it under control. In susceptible people, a trigger such as a cold or sore throat will cause it to flare up. Extreme weather conditions such as cold weather and sunlight can also cause a reaction. It is thought that there is a tendency for certain families to be susceptible to cold sores.

## SYMPTOMS

- An itchy, tingling sensation
- Small blisters around or on the lips, inside the mouth, around the nostrils, and sometimes elsewhere on the face
- Blisters filled with yellow liquid that feel hot and itchy, and eventually burst
- Tenderness and pain in the affected area
- Feeling rundown

## TREATMENT GOAL

There is no way of removing the virus from your system and once the blisters have formed there is no treatment available to stop them. However, there are steps you can take to help relieve symptoms and stop the cold sore from becoming infected, thus reducing the need for antibiotics.

## CONVENTIONAL MEDICINE

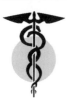

**Prevention:** A cold sore can take up to 26 days to erupt, with four to six days being the average. It takes between one to six weeks for a cold sore to heal. After the first infection, the virus can migrate up a sensory nerve and lie dormant until it is reactivated. A large part of treatment lies in learning the triggers for your cold sores and implementing strategies to prevent outbreaks.

**Nutritional supplements:** Studies have shown that high amounts of vitamin C (500 mg taken daily for seven days), and zinc (at a dose of 25 mg daily) are effective. Zinc can also be obtained over the counter in a lip balm or ointment. This should be applied at the first sign of occurrence or when in UV light and windy conditions to cut down the risk of an outbreak. Supplements or a diet rich in lysine (found in vegetables, beans, fish, turkey, and chicken) and low in arginine (found in chocolate, peanuts, almonds, cashews, and sunflower seeds) also suppress outbreaks.

**Pharmaceuticals:** Acyclovir, famcyclovir, and valacyclovir treat severe cold sore outbreaks by stopping the virus from spreading. Because of this, the medicine must be prescribed at the first sign of outbreak. For recurrences the same medications are used in less frequent doses. For people who have more than six outbreaks a year or very severe symptoms, a prophylactic approach is required. The same medications are used but at about half the dose. However, if outbreaks are occurring this frequently, it is wise to look for an underlying problem with nutrition, stress, or immune function and act accordingly.

## TRADITIONAL CHINESE MEDICINE

**Herbs:**
• Watermelon frost powder: To create a cool feeling to help stop the pain and heal the sores, apply watermelon frost. Do not worry about swallowing the powder when applying to your mouth as it is harmless.
• Niu Huang Jie Du Pian: If the cold sores are infected, take three Niu Huang Jie Du Pian pills three times a day, or as instructed.
• Herbal tea: Combine 3 g of peppermint, 5 g of Da Qin Ye (woad leaf), 5 g of Zi Cao (groomwell root), and 2 g of raw licorice in a teapot. Add 2–3 cups of boiling water, let the mixture steep for five minutes, and strain. Drink a cup of this three to four times a day. The herbal tea can be refilled two to three times. When there is a cold sore outbreak, take the tea daily. This tea is to be used only at the acute stage.

**Acupuncture:** Each treatment should last around half an hour. Treatment twice a week is better than once a week during the acute stage; however, patients with a chronic cold sore condition should have preventive treatment. Having acupuncture once a month when there are no outbreaks of the sores will effectively prevent the sores from recurring.

**Acupressure:** Press the Jia Che points, located at the attachment of the masseter muscles to the jawbone. When the teeth are clenched, you can feel these muscles tense, like a pump. When the mouth is open, there are diagonal depressions on each side of the head above the jawbone. Place your index fingers on each of the depressions. Apply gentle to medium pressure, on and off, 10 times. Press the Hegu points, located between your index fingers and thumbs, with your thumb 10 times on and off. Press these points once or twice a day to treat both acute and chronic conditions.

**Diet:** Avoid acidic, sweet, and greasy foods since they often trigger an outbreak. Also avoid beef, oranges, baked potatoes, shrimps, and cheese. Eat organic vegetables and fruit wherever possible. Radish, celery, cabbage, watermelon, and tofu are healing for cold sores.

**TIP: DAIKON JUICE**
Drinking the juice from daikons, a large, juicy Chinese radish, will help heal cold sores. Wash the radish and cut it into small chunks and juice them in a juicer.

## NATUROPATHY

 **Diet:** Eat plenty of legumes, fish, chicken, eggs, meat (preferably grass fed and organic), and potatoes, and take brewer's yeast (1 tbsp twice a day) for their high levels of the amino acid L-lysine, which inhibits herpes replication. Foods that help with tissue repair, such as cold-water fish, are also suggested. Avoid foods that are high in the amino acid L-arginine, such as chocolate, seeds, almonds, peanuts, gelatin, carob, and raisins, as they may stimulate the replication of the herpes virus.

**Supplements:** Take 2,000 mg of L-lysine three times a day between meals to inhibit the spread of cold sores. To prevent cold sores from forming, take 500 mg two times a day. Vitamin C with bioflavonoids will boost the immune system and decrease the duration of the infection. Take 1,000 mg and 500 mg respectively. Take 30 mg of zinc picolinate a day to inhibit viral replication.

**Herbs:** The herb Lomatium root is helpful for its immune-enhancing and antiviral properties. Take 500 mg three times a day.

Choose the most suitable of the following remedies when complementary medical help is needed to speed up the recovery of a cold sore naturally, gently, and efficiently. The treatments below are effective for cold sores that have appeared as a result of over-exposure to sunshine or are associated with a cold. Cold sores that emerge persistently and severely over an established period of time should be treated by an experienced practitioner, who will tailor treatment to boost and strengthen the body's defenses.

**Calendula:** If cold sores affect the lips or the sides of the mouth, add a dab of calendula cream in order to soothe any soreness, tingling, or itchiness. The cream is an excellent skin salve and also has natural antiseptic properties.

**Natrum mur:** This is the most common remedy used to treat cold sores. It helps relieve eruptions that tingle and numbness of the affected area. This is an especially strong remedy to consider where cold sores have developed after exposure to sunshine, or as a consequence of having a heavy head cold. Areas especially vulnerable to develop cold sores include the mouth and lips. There may be an associated tendency for the lips to be dry, sensitive, and to crack very easily.

**Sepia:** For cold sores that affect the lips and corners of the mouth, Sepia is an especially appropriate remedy. The lower lip may become swollen as well as cracked and dry. Signature symptoms include an overwhelming feeling of being drained mentally, emotionally, and physically.

**Rhus tox:** Consider this remedy if you have associated dry lips that have a tendency to crack and split at the corners. Common sites for cold sores to develop include the mouth and lips, with problems initially developing in the form of a blister. Symptoms characteristically affect only the left side of the face, or move from the left-hand side to the right. Localized crawling sensations in the affected area are aggravated by contact with cold air and jarring movements, and are soothed by warm conditions. Rhus tox is usually used to treat cold sores that develop after exposure to cold, or from being exhausted.

**Phosphorus:** If you have cutting, stitch-like sensations in cold sores that seem to bleed at the slightest provocation, and the discomfort is aggravated by touch and temporarily soothed by bathing in cool water, use Phosphorus. This can be helpful in speeding up recovery from cold sores affecting the area above the upper lip.

**Arsenicum album:** This is a common remedy to treat cold sores that burn. Sufferers tend to feel chilly and anxious.

## HERBALISM

**Echinacea:** Also known as purple coneflower, *Echinacea purpurea* has immuno-modulating effects, changing the behavior or actual counts of any of a number of cells that comprise the immune system. Take 1 dropperful of an echinacea tincture three times daily at the first sign of tingling to help prevent an outbreak.

**Black walnut:** Although some products mention using a powder of black walnut leaves, many experts focus on the hulls of the seeds, which are high in tannins, to help cure cold sores. The tannins are astringent and dry the mucosal tissue, decreasing secretions and causing the body to form a protective layer over the damaged tissue.

**Aloe vera:** The leaves of this plant yield a gel that is used to treat many skin problems, including cold sores. The regular application of aloe vera may decrease the formation of specific chemicals in the blood, thereby increasing circulation to the affected area and helping it to heal.

**Lemon balm:** Water extracts of lemon balm have antiviral properties and are useful in the treatment of cold sores, as are lotions containing lemon balm. A lemon balm lotion or cream should be applied to the lips two to three times a day during an outbreak.

**St. John's wort:** One of the main active constituents in St. John's wort is hypericin, which may have antiviral properties that work against the herpes simplex virus. An ointment or oil of St. John's wort can be used on the sores.

**Garlic:** The antimicrobial effects of garlic may help in the prevention and treatment of cold sores. Take garlic capsules or tinctures, although eating more garlic may be just as effective in preventing outbreaks.

**Licorice:** The antiviral properties of licorice may be helpful internally as well as externally for cold sores. Take a licorice lozenge several times a day.

# CORNS AND CALLUSES

## DIAGNOSIS

Both corns and calluses are a build-up of hard skin that forms in response to pressure or rubbing in a particular area. The skin thickens as a form of protection. Corns are usually found on the feet, particularly on the little toe, on the ball of the foot, and sometimes even the heel. Wearing badly fitting shoes or high heels is a contributory factor. Calluses are found on the feet but may also appear on the hands or knees. They usually develop over a bony prominence. Calluses can affect tennis players, joggers, musicians, and anyone doing manual work. Corns can be pared, or filed down. The skin is dead, so you do not feel anything if the top layers are shaved off. Care is needed, however, and anyone with circulatory problems in their feet, or diabetes, should get expert advice before attempting to remove corns themselves. Both conditions occur most often in people who have a high foot arch, as this increases downward pressure on the toes.

## SYMPTOMS

### CORNS
- Dead skin cells build up causing pain and discomfort
- A small raised bump appears with a hard center
- The affected area looks yellow
- Aching sensation
- Usually appear on the feet

### CALLUSES
- A rough patch of skin develops, usually over a bone
- Skin becomes hard, thick, and raised
- Usually appear on the feet, hands, or knees

## TREATMENT GOAL

While uncomfortable and painful, corns and calluses are harmless. Treatment aims to identify and remove the source of pressure or friction and relieve any immediate discomfort.

## CONVENTIONAL MEDICINE

 **Use a pumice stone:** Usually, a callus or corn can be taken care of at home. Try using a file or a pumice stone to soften and rub away excess skin. Continue to do so until the callus or corn disappears.

**Salicylic acid:** After filing away the callus or corn, apply a plaster of 40% salicylic acid, which is available over the counter, to an area slightly larger than the callus or corn and put a corn ring on top to relieve the pressure. You can also apply a skin softening cream to help skin stay soft.

**For persistent calluses and corns:** Seek advice from a doctor if the callus or corn does not go away within four weeks of removing the cause, or if it tends to crack open as this could cause infection. Medical treatment usually involves surgical paring of the thickened skin by a doctor or surgeon.

## TRADITIONAL CHINESE MEDICINE

 **Herbs:** The external use of herbs is common for corns and calluses. Purchase a powder form of the Chinese herb Ji Yian San. Soak the affected area in warm water until the corn or callus becomes soft. Cover the normal skin around the corns and put Ji Yian San on the top of the affected area. Cover the affected area with a dressing. Repeat this procedure once a day for seven days or until the corn is gone. **Caution:** Make sure Ji Yian San does not come into contact with unaffected skin. It should not be used around eyes or nose, and should never be taken orally.

**Acupuncture:** A skilled acupuncture practitioner will insert a needle directly into the deep center of the corn for 15 minutes. Concentrated acupuncture sessions are necessary, and the treatment should be repeated four to six times, twice a week. If the sessions are spread out, they will not be as effective because the corns can regain their strength in the interval between treatments. If there is no improvement after four to six sessions, it is not necessary to continue long-term treatment. Also, if you are feeling tired or under the weather, you should avoid this treatment.

**Moxibustion:** The practitioner will place and ignite a small Moxa cone (about the size of a grain of rice) on the top of the corn or callus. When the cone burns to near the bottom it will be removed and extinguished. The whole procedure uses three to six cones. Localized skin will feel warm and look reddish. **Caution:** Moxibustion should always be performed by a trained practitioner. When extinguishing burning Moxa, extra caution should be taken to prevent fire.

---

**TIP:** HOT WATER SOAK

Soak your feet in hot water daily for 20 minutes before going to bed. This will help foot circulation and is also relaxing for the whole body.

---

## NATUROPATHY

 **Footwear:** The best way to treat corns and calluses naturopathically is by wearing shoes that fit properly, so as not to cause friction, are activity-appropriate, and are kept in good repair. Socks and stockings should not cramp the toes. Feet should be measured, while standing, whenever buying new shoes. It is best to shop for shoes late in the day, when feet are likely to be swollen. It is also important to buy shoes with toe-wiggling room and to try new shoes on both feet.

**Moleskin pads:** Placing moleskin pads over corns can relieve pressure, and large wads of cotton, lamb's wool, or moleskin can cushion calluses.

**Topical remedy:** Mix 1 tsp of lemon juice with 1 tsp of dried chamomile tea. Crush a clove of garlic and add it to the mixture. Rub this remedy directly on the corn once or more times a day.

**Epsom salt soak:** Soak your feet in a solution of Epsom salts and warm water for at least 10 minutes a day before rubbing the area with a pumice stone. This will remove part or all of your calluses. It is important to see a doctor if the skin of a corn or callus is cut or bleeds because it may become infected. If a corn discharges pus or clear fluid, it is infected.

**Physical medicine:** Standing and walking correctly can sometimes eliminate excess foot pressure. Several types of bodywork can help correct body imbalances. Bodywork is a term used for any of a number of systems, including Aston-Patterning, Alexander technique, Feldenkrais method, and rolfing, that manipulate the body through massage, movement education, or meditational techniques.

**Herbs:** Aloe vera cream is an effective skin softener. Two or three daily applications of calendula salve can also soften skin and prevent inflammation. Apply a paste made by combining 1 tsp of aloe vera gel with half that amount of turmeric and apply the paste to the affected area. Bandage overnight, soak in warm water for 10 minutes every morning, and then massage gently with mustard oil (available from health food stores). Repeat this treatment for seven days. Since turmeric can stain skin and clothing, put on an old pair of socks after you've applied this remedy. Any skin discoloration should wash off in about two weeks.

## HOMEOPATHY

 Since both corns and calluses have a mechanical cause (the build up of layers of hard skin that can cause pain and discomfort when pressure is applied), the first approach to treatment needs to be a visit to a chiropodist or podiatrist. The measures listed below can provide some temporary relief until the offending extra layers of skin have been removed. Although treatment of this kind should be relatively pain-free, some practical measures are also suggested that can relieve any residual discomfort and speed up the healing process.

**Antimonium crudem:** Before treatment try Antimonium crudum. This remedy can provide relief from pain that is caused by thickened skin under the soles of the feet, or sensitive corns that develop under the toenails or on the tips of toes. Nails (especially under the toenail on the big toe) can be particularly susceptible to developing corns that look rather like warts.

**Silica:** Try Silica if feet have a tendency to be sweaty and smelly, with burning sensations developing in the feet and soles in bed at night. Silica is also effective if there is a tendency to develop hard, painful calluses, bunions, or corns (especially under the toenails or between the toes) that give rise to shooting pains.

**Calendula:** After treatment try applying calendula cream daily to areas of hard or dry skin. This multipurpose cream is a moisturizer, antiseptic cream, and healing agent all in one. This makes it an excellent healing cream to apply after any minor trauma has occurred to the skin.

**Hypericum:** Take Hypericum if there is any residual pain and discomfort in the feet and/or toes after a podiatry treatment. It is effective for soothing discomfort in areas that are especially rich in nerves , such as the toes, fingers, and base of the spine. Pains that respond especially well to this remedy are very tender and sore, characteristically shooting away from the affected, sensitive area, especially when touched.

## HERBALISM

**Greater celadine:** This well-known herb can be used safely and painlessly to slowly dissolve a corn. To make a decoction of celadine leaves, boil 25–50 g of the leaves in 3–4 cups of water for 5–10 minutes. Strain the water and let it cool. Soak a clean cotton or linen cloth in the decoction and placed it on the corn. Cover the affected area with paper and tape this onto the skin. Leave the compress on overnight and wash it off in the morning.

**Fig, papaya, and pineapple:** These fruits all contain enzymes that break down skin growths. Patented formulas with extracts of these plants can be purchased and should be used according to instructions on the label. Sometimes a number of treatments are required to obtain the best result.

**Willow:** The bark of this tree is popular for its pain-relieving qualities, and the same constituent responsible for the pain relief also dissolves skin growths. Boil 25–30 g of dried willow bark in strips or chunks in 4 cups of water for 10 minutes, making sure that the water does not evaporate and leave the pan dry. Once it has cooled, apply it to the corn, holding the willow in place with a cloth or gauze for 10 minutes several times a day. Avoid contact with the skin around the corn as the salicylates in the bark can irritate unaffected areas.

**Wintergreen:** The volatile oil of wintergreen also contains salicylates that can be used to dissolve corns. Apply essential oil of wintergreen to the corn, preferably at night, and wash it off in the morning so that the surrounding skin isn't irritated. Synthetic oils of wintergreen have been made and are sold as oil of wintergreen, but these oils do not have the same healing properties as the natural oil.

**Sassafras:** Essential oil of sassafras can be applied to the corn, but it can be irritating and may need to be diluted with vegetable oil or used in a lotion.

# CRADLE CAP

## DIAGNOSIS

This is a common condition that can affect the scalp of babies and young children. Although it looks unpleasant, it is actually a harmless skin irritation. It is caused by the over-production of sebum, the oily substance produced by the skin's sebaceous glands. This causes a build-up of a greasy-like crust on the scalp. Occasionally, cradle cap can spread beyond the scalp, which then becomes known as seborrheic dermatitis. It can also be a precursor to eczema. Although your first reaction may be to cover the affected area as it looks so unpleasant, this is the worst thing you can do. If the child gets overheated and starts to sweat, it can aggravate cradle cap. Steer clear of hats and keep the child's head uncovered and exposed to fresh air whenever possible. Never try to pick off the crusts or rub the scalp vigorously, as this could cause soreness, bleeding, or even an infection of the scalp. Any loose flaky areas can be removed with a soft brush. Cradle cap is best left alone, if it is not severe, to allow the condition to settle down. Cradle cap is not caused by poor hygiene, so avoid overwashing your child's hair as this can aggravate the condition.

## SYMPTOMS

- Dry, scaly, or crusty patches on the scalp. These are yellow, orange, or dark brown, and can eventually become quite hard and thick
- In babies, it usually covers the fontanelles—soft areas of the head
- A build-up of dead skin that looks like dandruff, but is visible to the eye
- Affected areas may be red and sore
- Flaky skin spreads to the forehead, behind the ears, and occasionally even around the eyebrows
- The scales may smell and have a build-up of pus underneath

## TREATMENT GOAL

While unsightly to look at, cradle cap is a harmless condition. Treatment aims to relieve any discomfort caused by the condition and protect against infection.

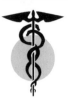

## CONVENTIONAL MEDICINE

The medical term for cradle cap is seborrheic dermatitis. The exact cause of cradle cap is unknown, but it is a common condition. An overgrowth of a yeast organism that usually grows on the skin, pityrosporum ovale, is often present in cradle cap. It also parallels an increase in sebaceous gland activity and tends to run in families. It is more prevalent in cold, dry weather. Although it usually occurs by itself, cradle cap can accompany other medical conditions, such as zinc deficiency, vitamin B deficiency, or any illness that lowers the number or function of the cells that fight infection.

**Non-medicated shampoo:** Cradle cap usually resolves itself within one to eight months. The first choice for treatment is a mild, non-medicated shampoo for scale removal. Tar-based or anti-seborrheic shampoos should not be used on infants as they are too harsh. Using GENTLE friction on the skin to remove the oily scales is essential. Cradle cap often occurs over the soft spot of babies' heads because parents are often reluctant to touch this area.

**Medicated shampoo or cream:** If the condition does not clear up, the second choice for treatment is 1% ketoconazole shampoo or cream. This shampoo kills and stops the fungus from growing. The cream contains sulfites, which can cause allergic type reactions, some of which are serious. Contact with the eyes should also be avoided. With this treatment the cradle cap should clear up in several days. This treatment can be used for children, but other milder treatments are preferred.

## TRADITIONAL CHINESE MEDICINE

**Herbs:** Combine 30 g of almond kernels with 30 g of peach kernels, both available from Chinese herbalists. Boil the herbs in 4 cups of water for 30 minutes, then strain the liquid to remove the cooked herbs. Let the liquid cool until it is a little warmer then body temperature. Soak a clean, dry washcloth in the liquid and place it on the cradle cap, letting it moisten the area for 5–10 minutes. Gently remove the washcloth and dry the area with a clean cotton wool ball. Apply a thin layer of olive oil to the problem area. Repeat this procedure once a day for three days, letting the scales flake off naturally.

**Acupressure:** Press the Feng Chi point, located 2 inches from the center point of the base of the skull at the back of the head. It is level with the hairline, and in the depression lateral to the big muscle on the nape of the neck. Apply gentle pressure with your thumbs, slightly turning them in a small circle to massage the points, for one minute twice a day.

## NATUROPATHY

**Diet:** A nursing mother should eliminate any food allergens and saturated fats from her diet. Eat plenty of cold-water fish such as salmon, mackerel, and herring. A non-nursing child should also eliminate allergenic foods such as cow's milk.

**Topical:** Massage the head with calendula lotion and vitamin E oil alternatively. Allow the oil to remain on the scalp for 15 minutes then shampoo and gently comb away the loosened scales. This treatment works well for adults as well.

## HOMEOPATHY

The homeopathic remedies suggested below can be helpful in clearing up mild cases of cradle cap. Thankfully, there is no age barrier when it comes to the safe use of homeopathic remedies, since they can be administered as appropriately and safely to newborns as to the elderly. Side by side with selecting and administering the remedy that most closely matches the symptoms, it is helpful to avoid over-washing your baby's hair. Too frequent washing can aggravate, rather than improve, the problem as it can stimulate the production of oil or sebum.

**Natrum mur:** For cradle cap that affects the margins of the hairline, use Natrum mur. Skin texture may generally show a tendency to be sensitive and dry, with cracks breaking out around the corners of the mouth or in the center of the bottom lip.

**Graphites:** For moist cradle cap that inclines towards weepiness, Graphites are useful. The scales of cradle cap are characteristically thick, with the head becoming easily sweaty. There may also be a tendency to cracked, dry eruptions in skin folds.

**Lycopodium:** Use this remedy if the cradle cap is typically more irritating and itchy when covered. Eruptions on the head will look typically brownish and scaly, like heavy dandruff. Irritation and itching is eased temporarily be exposing the affected area to fresh air.

**Calc carb:** If the cradle cap occurs in babies who are chubby, pale, and chilly, and who sweat very readily on the head and feet, use Calc carb. Symptoms that indicate that this is an appropriate remedy include a tendency for the developmental milestones to happen later than expected, and for teething to be slow, difficult, and distressing.

**Rhus tox:** If the cradle cap is intensely itchy at night, leading to restlessness and fractiousness, Rhus tox can help. Itchiness and burning of the scalp is more intense when getting too hot, but cold, damp conditions also cause great distress. The child compulsively rubs and scratches at the scalp, leading to a tendency for crusts to become moist and weepy.

## HERBALISM

 The herbal medicine approach to this disorder of the scalp is based on the fact that there are abnormalities in the sebaceous glands involving inflammation of the skin, perhaps also with a fungal infection. There are several herbs that can be useful. Your herbalism practitioner should make sure that there is not a particular fungal infection from Tinea capitis present, which can appear like cradle cap in some infants and children and for which there are other more appropriate treatments.

**Burdock root:** Make a poultice by macerating the burdock root and applying it directly to the skin. This can calm inflammation and promote healing.

**Plantain leaf:** A salve of plantain leaf, available at local health food stores, is healing and soothing when used topically. Depending on the individual case, other plants can be mixed with plantain when making a salve. For example, antifungal herbs can be added if the herbalist suspects that fungus may be an issue.

**Calendula and chamomile:** These topical anti-inflammatory plants can calm the inflammation that is symptomatic of this disorder. Calendula and chamomile flowers are often made into creams that can be easily applied to an inflamed scalp. These plants are gentle enough in their action that they are safe for use on infants.

**Olive oil:** A small amount of olive oil massaged into the affected scalp can be enough to provide some anti-inflammatory and soothing qualities for cradle cap.

### TIP: PLANTAIN AND LAVENDER WASH
Try a gentle wash made from the infusion of plantain leaf combined with the leaves and flowers of violet and lavender flowers. Add equal parts of each plant, about 25–30 g each, to 5 cups of boiling water. Let the leaves steep for five minutes. Strain the water and, when cool, squeeze out the extra liquid from the plant material. Using a soft washcloth, gently wash your baby's head.

# DANDRUFF

## DIAGNOSIS

Dandruff is the most common condition affecting the scalp and anyone is susceptible. Skin is constantly renewing itself and dead cells from the scalp fall off as new cells form beneath them. Everyone loses skin cells in this way, but dandruff occurs when the scaling of this dead skin is excessive and a greater number of cells are shed, often in clumps that are noticeable when they land on clothing. It can be unsightly, and the itchiness it causes on the scalp can be irritating. The scales are more obvious after hair has been brushed and they become loose. Many people think that flaking occurs because the scalp is too dry, and stop using shampoo because they believe it makes the condition worse. This is not true. The flaking occurs due to the increased turnover of skin cells. It is thought that the condition could be hereditary, and that stress and anxiety can play a contributory role. Sometimes dandruff is a symptom of eczema (see p. 73) or psoriasis (see p. 134), so those with severe dandruff should always consult their doctor.

## SYMPTOMS

- Itchy scalp
- A build-up of tiny white flakes of skin on the scalp, and occasionally other hair-covered areas
- Excessively greasy skin and hair
- Angry red patches on the scalp
- Occasionally, skin may crack and ooze liquid
- Occasionally, hard yellow crusts can form
- Red areas of skin on the face, particularly the forehead and eyebrows
- Patches of scaly skin above the ears

## TREATMENT GOAL

While irritating and unpleasant, only severe dandruff—where the condition spreads and skin cracks and becomes sore—requires medical treatment. Bouts of regular dandruff can be successfully treated with a combination of complementary and conventional techniques.

## CONVENTIONAL MEDICINE

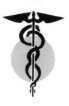

The medical term for dandruff is seborrheic dermatitis. It is a disease that causes flaking of the skin on the scalp in adults and teenagers, most commonly occuring in 30–60 year olds. It can also affect the skin on other parts of the body, making it look greasy and scaly. The cause isn't known. It may be related to hormones, or a fungus present on the skin that grows excessively.

**Shampoos:** The treatment of dandruff depends on the age of the person affected. In adolescents and adults, it is usually treated with an over-the-counter shampoo that has salicylic acid such as X-Seb™ or Scalpicin™. The prescription medicine selenium sulfide is used in low concentrations in Selsun™ and Exsel™, which are over-the-counter products used for dandruff; also pyrithione zinc is used in Head and Shoulders™. All these products should be used as a shampoo twice a week for prevention, or daily to treat an active case of dandruff. Other options are tar shampoos (DHS Tar™, Neutrogena T/Gel™, and Polytar™), which can be used three times a week for prevention, or daily for treatment.

**Steroid cream:** In the rare case that these shampoos are ineffective, a 2% steroid cream is prescribed to be used twice daily for 7–10 days. It is to be used in conjunction with the above shampoo treatment.

**Diet:** Eliminating dairy, eggs, and sometimes gluten can help prevent dandruff. Taking a daily zinc supplement of 40 mg, for adults, as well as ensuring that adequate amounts of vitamin E, A, and C are in your diet, are also helpful for prevention.

## TRADITIONAL CHINESE MEDICINE

**External treatment:** Wash your hair with fresh mulberry leaves. Gather 600 g of fresh white mulberry leaves from a tree (in most cases there are no fresh mulberry leaves available in Chinese herbalists). Rinse the leaves in cold, clean water and mash them up. Press the leaves and gather the juice—or try using a juicer. Add the juice to warm water and wash the hair once a week, for three weeks. Your scalp should become less itchy, and the amount of dandruff should be reduced significantly.

**Acupuncture:** According to traditional Chinese medicine, dandruff could be a secondary symptom of an internal disorder or imbalance. There are many meridians directly connecting the internal systems with the head/scalp. To address dandruff, a traditional Chinese medicine doctor will first evaluate your general health, identifying the cause of the condition. Dandruff could be caused by varying degrees of internal Yin deficiency and excessive heat—an imbalanced condition that is caused by a lack of body fluid or cooling energy. When accompanied with an evaluation of your general health, treating the dandruff is more comprehensive because the treatment is internalized. You may have acupuncture treatment once a week, usually for several months.

**Acupressure:** Press the Feng Chi point, which is located 2 inches from the center point of the base of the skull at the back of the head. It is level with the hairline, in the depression lateral to the big muscle on the nape of the neck. In a sitting position, place your index fingers on the Feng Chi point and apply gentle pressure for about one minute before releasing. Repeat this procedure three times. Next, press the Shuai Gu point. You can locate the Shuai Gu point by drawing a line vertically from the top of your ear straight up about 1½ inches. Apply and release pressure three times for about one minute at a time. Doing this once or twice a day will help local blood circulation to treat and prevent dandruff.

**Diet:** Eat fresh fruit and vegetables. Pears, celery, spinach, daikon radishes, carrots, fish, oysters, mussels, and brown rice are particularly good foods for preventing dandruff.

**TIP:** BE GENTLE
Use mild shampoo, do not wash you hair in water that is too warm, and do not wash your hair too frequently.

## NATUROPATHY

**Home remedy:** Dilute one part of apple cider vinegar and one part of hydrogen peroxide in 10 parts of water. Use this solution like a shampoo and then rinse your hair. After rinsing apply about 20 drops of tea tree oil to the scalp, massage for three to five minutes, and leave overnight. This remedy will eliminate the flakiness and kills the excess yeastlike fungus that contributes to dandruff.

**Diet:** Fried foods should be avoided. Reduce your intake of fats, dairy products, sugar, chocolate, seafood, and peanuts. Increase your intake of green leafy vegetables and raw foods. Eat a whole food diet including foods high in biotin, such as nuts, fruits, brewer's yeast, and brown rice. Do not eat raw eggs or refined foods, or drink too much alcohol, as they deplete the body of biotin.

**Supplements:** Biotin taken in a B-complex has shown to be more effective in treating dandruff than taking biotin alone. Take 100 mg of B-complex with meals and 1,000–3,000 mcg of biotin. Take omega fatty acids, especially omega-6, such as primrose oil and borage oil, as directed on the label to help relieve inflammation. Take 30 mg of zinc to support skin function and the immune system. Zinc can deplete the body's store of copper, so 3 mg of copper should be taken with this supplement.

**Topical:** Dandruff is most often caused by an inflammatory response to an overgrowth of scalp fungus, which causes itchiness and scaling. When this is the case, good results may be obtained by adding a few drops of grapefruit seed extract to your regular shampoo as this kills fungus. Leave the shampoo on for three to five minutes. Fungal infections are also a common cause of dandruff. Use a tea tree oil shampoo or add a few drops of tea tree oil to shampoo for its antifungal properties. Try using a selenium-based shampoo, as it acts as an antifungal agent. Flaxseed oil or vitamin E oil can soothe and nourish the scalp— apply either nightly and wash it off in the morning. Use an old sheet or towel to protect your pillow.

## HOMEOPATHY

This problem can vary in its cause and intensity. Some people may experience on-going problems with severe scaling of the scalp as part and parcel of a chronic skin problem such as psoriasis or eczema. In these situations, dandruff is the tip of the iceberg, and treatment at a deeper level, by a homeopathic practitioner, is needed to clear up the problem for good. If the dandruff scales are infrequent and fairly light in nature, they may be caused by cosmetic triggers, such as failing to rinse the hair thoroughly after shampooing. Traces of shampoo left behind after washing can irritate the scalp, making it increasingly dry, and make hair dull and lifeless. In the absence of an underlying chronic skin condition, selecting and taking one of the following remedies may help clear up mild to moderate dandruff, especially when combined with naturopathic measures to improve scalp and hair quality.

**Arsenicum album:** If the scalp is generally dry and feels irritable and itchy at night, use Arsenicum album. Skin may show a noticeable tendency to dryness, with poor circulation, and often feels chilly. As a result, symptoms can be more pronounced during the winter months. Stress and anxiety can also aggravate problems.

**Natrum mur:** When dandruff is combined with a tendency to dry, sensitive skin, and where dryness and scaling of the scalp are especially noticeable around the margins of the hair, Natrum mur can be helpful. Choose this remedy if the hair shows noticeable features of lankness and poor quality, with a frequent tendency to fall out, especially after emotional stress or trauma.

**Lycopdium:** This can be useful in treating itchy dandruff where the scales cover the whole scalp. The skin may show general tendencies towards dryness and burning itchiness, with symptoms generally appearing, or being made more intense and troublesome, in relation to stress and anxiety. This can be due to an underlying fear of failure under pressure.

**Sulphur:** This is the most common remedy for skin problems, especially when they are accompanied by localized itchiness that is worse at night or after bathing.

## HERBALISM

The herbal approach to this disorder of the scalp is based on the fact that there are abnormalities in the sebaceous glands (sweat glands) involving a mild inflammation of the skin with or without a fungal infection.

**Tea tree oil:** Some practitioners recommend using tea tree oil as a 5% shampoo daily for several weeks. This can work fairly well, but may not completely resolve symptoms, and some people may develop a skin reaction to the tea tree oil. Extra care should be taken not to expose your eyes to the product.

**Aloe vera:** One study found improvements in dandruff following the use of a 30% aloe lotion twice daily for four to six weeks.

**Burdock root:** Topical skin-healing herbs such as burdock root can calm the inflammation and promote healing. A poultice of the root should be applied directly on the scalp for as long as it can be tolerated at least once a day for several weeks. Some herbalists also recommend that burdock be taken internally as 20–40 drops of an alcohol or glycerin tincture, available at local health food stores, several times daily. This may be necessary for particularly severe cases, or for those not responding to topical preparations.

**Eucalyptus and wintergreen essential oil:** An ointment made from the essential oils of eucalyptus and wintergreen is available from health food stores. It acts as a general healer and antiseptic for the skin, making it useful for dandruff.

**Calendula and chamomile:** These topical anti-inflammatory plants can help with redness and inflammation caused by dandruff. A cream made from the flowers from these two plants, and available over the counter, can be easily applied to the inflamed area.

# DERMATITIS

## DIAGNOSIS

Dermatitis is an umbrella term for a variety of inflammatory skin conditions, the most common being contact dermatitis (see skin allergy p. 22) and eczema (see p. 73). Dermatitis is widespread, affects people of all ages, and is often a temporary problem that resolves on its own. The condition manifests itself as an inflammation of the skin due to an over-reaction from contact with an external substance. The result is red and itchy skin, and a strong impulse to scratch that can lead to infection. Specifically, contact dermatitis is an irritant reaction, caused by the direct effect of prolonged exposure to a substance on the skin, one that would cause a reaction in most individuals if applied in sufficient concentration. It usually flares up on the hands, as they are most often exposed to the problem substance. Common irritants include soaps, detergents, and other household chemicals, metals (especially nickel), drugs, and food.

## SYMPTOMS

- Red, itchy, inflamed skin
- A burning sensation
- Blistering and peeling skin
- Occasionally, skin cracks
- Reaction can spread to affect other areas of the body
- A strong urge to scratch
- Skin crusts over

## TREATMENT GOAL

The best way to treat dermatitis is to remove the cause by identifying and avoiding the allergen. While there isn't a cure for dermatitis, treatment aims to control and relieve symptoms.

## CONVENTIONAL MEDICINE

**Prevention:** Dermatitis lends itself to treatment using mind/body therapies, such as meditation, for stress reduction. Elimination diets are very helpful for the condition, with dairy and gluten being predominant offenders.

**Emollients:** Topical emollients and soap substitutes (such as Cetaphil®) should be used to treat dry skin on a daily basis. These emulsifying products keep oil in the skin to relieve itchiness and inflammation caused by dryness.

**Topical steroids:** Many people worry about the effect of topical steroid creams, used to treat dermatitis, on children and are concerned about skin thinning. This complication is prevented by slightly lowering the amount of topical steroid cream used every day over the period of one week. Hydrocortisone (at 0.5% and 1%) and triamcinolone acetonide (0.025%) are mild creams that are suitable for children. A moderate strength cream is triamcinolone acetonide (0.5% and 0.1%). Potent creams are betamethasone dipropionate (0.05%) and fluocinonide (0.05%). These higher potency creams should not be used for more than two weeks continuously, but they can be used intermittently as prescribed. A fingertip unit, the distance from an adult finger tip to the first crease in the palm, is a general dose. This amount usually covers a space twice the size of the adult flat hand.

**Oral steroids:** These are occasionally used for severe flare-ups. They work well but must be used only rarely because of major adverse effects on the endocrine and immune system.

**Newer medications:** Steroids such as tacrolimus ointment and ascomycin ointment are being used with some success. Cyclosporine is very effective but very potent, with renal toxicity (kidney damage) as a side effect and rapid relapse with discontinuation.

**Anihistamines:** Sedating antihistamines can be used at night to decrease itchiness.

## TRADITIONAL CHINESE MEDICINE

If the skin infection is severe, you should see a specialist for treatment.

**Herbs:**
• Internal herbal decoction: Mix 10 g of Ye Ju Hua (wild chrysanthemum flower), 30 g of Huang Jing (Siberian Solomon seal rhizome), 15 g of Huang Bai (phellodendron), and 20 g of Fang Fen (ledebouriella root) in a ceramic pot. Boil the mixture in 3 cups of water for 15 minutes to make about 2 cups of decoction. Take ½ cup three times a day for 10 days to complete one course of treatment. Three courses of treatment may be needed for chronic conditions.

• External herbal formula: Combine 30 g each of She Chuang Zi (cnidium seed), Di Fu Zi (broom cypress), Ma Zhi Xian (dried purslane), Tu Fu Ling (glabrous greenbrier rhizome), and Xin Ren (almond kernels) in a ceramic pot with 6–7 cups of cold water. Bring the mixture to the boil, let it simmer for 30 minutes, and strain the liquid. Add 6 more cups of water to the pot and repeat the process. Wash the affected area with the liquid or add it to warm bath water. Soak the skin in the herbal solution for 20–30 minutes twice a week.

**Acupuncture:** An experienced acupuncture practitioner will stimulate the lung meridian since it is directly related to skin health. It is best to combine treatments with herbs and/or dietary therapy. For chronic dermatitis, have acupuncture treatment once a week, or two to three times a week for acute dermatitis.

**Acupressure:** Press the Feng Chi point, located 2 inches from the center point of the base of the skull at the back of the head with your thumbs, using gentle pressure, for one minute. Close your eyes and press the temple points with your thumbs for one minute. Press the Hegu point (in between the index finger and thumb) for two minutes with your thumb once or twice a day. For chronic dermatitis patients, those pressure points can be used with gentle pressure as long as the condition exists.

**Diet:** Eat fresh food instead of convenience food and drink plenty of fluids. Avoid shrimp, beef, lamb, and chili pepper since they may interfere with your herbal treatment and increase heat in your body.

## NATUROPATHY

 **Diet:** Omit wheat, rye, oats, and barley from your diet. After six weeks add one food at a time and note any changes with the dermatitis. Avoid dairy products, sugar, white flour, trans-fats, omega-6, saturated fats, fried foods, and processed foods as they tend to cause skin inflammation.

**Supplements:** Take vitamin E at 400 IU a day to relieve itchiness and dryness. Vitamin A is essential for smooth skin and helps dryness. Take vitamin A at 100,000 IU for one month, bring it down to 50,000 IU for two weeks, and then take 25,000 IU for maintenance. It is advised that vitamin A be taken under the supervision of a doctor because of its toxic potential. Pregnant women should not take more than 10,000 IU of vitamin A a day. Take 30 mg of zinc three times a day to raise immunity and aid skin healing. Evening primrose oil contains gamma linoleic oil (GLA), which is an essential anti-inflammatory for the skin.

**Burdock root:** Take 4 ml of tincture or a 500 g capsule three times a day to detoxify the skin.

**Hydrotherapy:** Boil 100 g of chopped oat straw, which benefits skin, in 3 quarts of water for 20 minutes. Add this to warm bath water and soak in the bathtub for 30 minutes.

## HOMEOPATHY

 Because of its complex nature, dermatitis should be treated by an experienced homeopathic practitioner. A practitioner will aim to treat the underlying weakness in the constitution that is leaving the patient vulnerable to symptoms of itchiness, soreness, and possible bleeding of the irritated areas of skin as a result of compulsive scratching. With this in mind, the remedies listed below provide an idea of the range of the most common potential homeopathic solutions that a practitioner may consider before prescribing for a patient.

**Identify triggers:** Avoid contact as far as possible with items that are known to trigger a reaction. Consider the toiletries you use. Scented soaps, bath products, body creams, and lotions may be triggers. Always avoid highly-perfumed products that include powerful detergents, which can aggravate skin and cause irritation and dry patches to develop.

**Moisturize:** Keep skin well moisturized, using products that are designed for sensitive, dry skin. These tend to be unperfumed products that aim to put moisture temporarily back into the skin, making it feel superficially more comfortable.

**Petroleum:** If there is a history of rough, dry skin that festers easily and heals very slowly, Petroleum is helpful. Affected areas itch and burn, and skin eruptions tend to settle in folds of skin. Itchiness is so severe that the skin may be broken and bleed as a result of compulsive scratching. This leads to hard, thick crusts developing over sore areas.

**Sulphur:** This is the most common remedy for skin problems, especially when they are accompanied with localized itchiness that is worse at night or after bathing. It is used to treat intensely itchy, inflamed skin that is aggravated by heat in any form. Symptoms include skin that is dry, rough, scaly, and readily infected. Burning sensations after scratching are especially troublesome when getting too warm in bed.

**Graphites:** This is a strong candidate when there is a tendency to develop a thick, honey-colored crust when weeping patches dry out. After scratching, the itchy areas weep a thick, sticky yellow fluid, while the skin feels raw and sore. Affected areas are most likely to include folds of skin (for instance behind the ears or around the nose), with a strong tendency for the skin to crack around mouth, nose, ears, or nipples.

**Arsenicum album:** This is indicated if the skin is dry with associated sore, burning sensations in the eruptions that are unusually soothed by contact with warmth (for instance, in the form of warm compresses or warm bathing). The overall texture of the skin may be dry and rough, while patches of eczema develop blistery eruptions that feel intensely itchy. This sets up an itch-scratch-itch cycle that leads to burning in the affected areas.

## HERBALISM

Treatment will depend on the type of dermatitis, the cause of the inflammation, and the specific symptoms involved. However, some general suggestions for using herbal medicines are mentioned below.

**Calendula:** Use a cream or lotion that includes extracts of calendula, which helps calm the redness and irritation associated with this condition. Alternatively, pour 1 cup of boiling water over 2 tsp of calendula flowers. Let the water sit for 10 minutes, strain it, and soak an absorbent cloth in the mixture. Apply the cloth to the inflamed skin.

**Demulcents:** This category of plant contains mucilaginous compounds that form a protective, soothing layer over the skin, which can improve dermatitis. These plants, which include aloe vera, slippery elm bark, marshmallow root, fenugreek, chickweed, and comfrey leaves or roots, are commonly used as poultices, or in creams and lotions.

**Agrimony:** A poultice of agrimony can be useful for treating dermatitis. Boil the leaves or chopped roots of argrimony in water for a few minutes. Allow the liquid to cool and apply the plant mass to the affected area twice or three times daily. Be careful with sun exposure, as the sun may react with agrimony, used internally or externally, to worsen dermatitis.

**Woodruff:** This is used topically to treat dermatitis. It can also be used internally, but there are some concerns about liver toxicity with chronic internal use; these effects should be avoided if just used externally.

**Witch hazel:** Functioning as an astringent, witch hazel is used on the skin as either an aqueous distillate, an ointment, or a gel, and can be applied up to three times daily. It should not be ingested, and it occasionally can worsen the dermatitis. Keep a close watch on your symptoms to see if the dermatitis is improving.

**Oak:** Another approach to dermatitis is to think of it in terms of a wet or dry condition. Some herbal experts feel that the reason treatment fails is that this principle is applied inaccurately. The herb oak is effective for the beginning stages of contact dermatitis, when it is in the wet form. The bark of the oak tree is astringent in nature because of its high tannin content. To make a decoction, boil 25–50 g of small pieces of oak bark, available from herb stores, in about a quart of water for 15–20 minutes. Apply the liquid as a compress three times daily. Each treatment should be made from fresh water.

**Gumweed:** Tinctures of the flowers and small leaves of gumweed are available from herb stores. They can be applied topically to inflamed skin to calm the reaction and provide relief.

# DIAPER RASH

## DIAGNOSIS

It is not unusual for babies to develop rashes, and diaper rash is one of the most common. Diaper rash is a form of irritant dermatitis that is caused by exposure to urine and heat, and further aggravated by the friction and chafing that results from wearing a diaper. It is usually a harmless rash that affects most babies at one time or another, and is generally something they grow out of. The most common symptom is a red and sore diaper area. Triggers include wearing wet or soiled diapers for long periods of time, skin getting overheated, and overuse of baby wipes or other cleansing agents, such as soap or baby lotion, that may further irritate the sore skin. Some babies develop diaper rash when they begin eating solid food. It can be triggered by a reaction to the new foods, particularly citrus fruit, peas, and raisins, which are not digested easily. Frequent bowel movements and diarrhea can also set the baby on a cycle of diaper rash that can be hard to break, as can teething and taking antibiotics. In some cases, diaper rash can become severe and be very painful and distressing for the baby. Occasionally, the rash can become infected with bacteria or fungus. Diaper rash should always be treated, and can usually be done so simply from the home.

## SYMPTOMS

- Red spots or patches of inflamed skin in the diaper area
- Skin has a tight, shiny appearance
- Scaly skin
- A bright red rash around the anus
- Red, irritated patches in the skin creases of the leg and groin area
- A strong fishy odor
- Pus-filled blisters and spots can develop if the rash becomes infected with bacteria

## TREATMENT GOAL

To identify and eliminate the cause of the rash and bring rapid relief from the symptoms.

## CONVENTIONAL MEDICINE

The four common causes of diaper rash are candida (yeast), irritant dermatitis, bacterial infection, or seborrheic dermatitis. Treatment depends on the cause.

**Prevention:** Change diapers as soon as possible after they are soiled and avoid using plastic pants. Cleanse the skin carefully to remove any urine or feces and dry the skin thoroughly when changing diapers. Check for a bad reaction to a particular brand of diaper. Often a food allergy can aggravate the condition. Eliminating casein (milk protein) from the diet can help. Opt for a soy- or rice-based alternative.

**Topical creams:** To treat irritant or contact dermatitis, zinc oxide can be applied to protect the skin, as can Desitin or A and D ointment. Sometimes a low-potency hydrocortisone cream can be used if the above combination does not work.

**Antibiotics:** If a bacterial infection is diagnosed by the doctor, topical antibiotics such as mupirocin is applied as an ointment. Cases resistant to topical antibiotics are treated with oral erythromycin or penicillin.

**Nystatin cream:** Diaper rashes caused by candida (yeast) are treated with topical nystatin cream. This can be used in conjunction with hydrocortisone cream.

## TRADITIONAL CHINESE MEDICINE

**Herbs:** To reduce itchiness and treat the rash, you can use both internal and external Chinese herbal formulas. The herbs needed for these remedies are all available from Chinese herbalists. They are suitable for babies.

• Internal herbal formula: Add 8 g of Jin Yin Hua (honeysuckle flower), 3 g of Shen Gan Cao (raw licorice root), and 3 g of Bo He (field mint) to 3 cups of boiled water in a teapot. Allow the herbs to steep for 5–10 minutes, then strain the liquid. Feed your baby the tea, diluted in a bottle, three to four times a day for three to five days in a row. If the rash gets worse, stop treatment immediately and see your doctor.

• External formula: Combine 15 g of She Chuang Zi (cnidium seeds), 15 g of Di Fu Zi (broom cypress), 12 g of Jing Jie (schizonepeta stem and bud), 15 g of Fang Fen (ledebouriella root), and 15 g of Xin Ren (almond kernel) in a ceramic or glass cooking pot. Add 4–5 cups of water and bring to the boil. Turn down the heat and let the herbs simmer for 15–20 minutes. Strain the decoction and mix it in warm bath water. Gently lower your baby into the water and keep him or her in the bath for as long as is comfortable/practical. Do not rinse the herbal solution off. Thoroughly dry your baby with a soft cotton towel. Repeat this treatment on a daily basis. If you notice any signs of discomfort, rinse your baby's body with clear water and stop the treatment.

**Acupuncture:** This is an effective treatment for most diaper rashes. You can receive treatment at any stage of the rash. It can be used immediately in acute stages, or for chronic or repetitive rash breakouts. You can also have acupuncture as a complementary treatment.

**Acupressure:** Press the Nei Guan point, which is located in the center of the wrist on the palm side about 2 inches below the crease. The San Yin Jiao point is located about 3 inches above the anklebone on the center of the inside leg. Press this point for about one minute.

**Diet:** Breastfeeding mothers should eat food that is neutral and cooling, such as purslane, mung beans, lotus, lettuce, mango, cucumber, eggplant, spinach, strawberries, and pears. Avoid warm spicy food such as ginger, pepper, chilies, cloves, leeks, and mussels.

## NATUROPATHY

**Diet:** Make sure your baby is getting plenty of fluids, especially water. This dilutes the irritating acids present in the urine and stool. Observe your child carefully when introducing new foods. A breastfeeding mother should reduce or eliminate any food allergens from her diet—especially, dairy, wheat, citrus fruits and juices, sugar, and caffeine.

**Supplements:** Probiotics are essential for infants and for a child's general health. Take 1 tsp of the powder a day mixed with juice or water. A bottle-fed infant can be given ½ a spoon in his or her formula. A breastfeeding mother should take ½ a spoon twice a day. Vitamin E should be applied topically as a cream or oil.

**Herbs:** Calendula has soothing and healing properties. Apply a lotion, gel, or cream to the rash when you change the diaper. Evening primose oil or lotion serves as a gentle anti-inflammatory treatment. Apply it each time you change your baby's diaper.

**General recommendations:** Avoid using diapers as much as possible to allow the baby's bottom to be exposed to the air. Change your baby's diaper as soon as he or she urinates or has a bowel movement. Use diaper wipes that are unscented, or that have witch hazel or calendula. Other diaper wipes contain chemicals that can be irritating to your baby's skin. When washing your baby, avoid using harsh soaps and scrubbing vigorously. Instead, use a mild soap with gentle friction, cleaning well between the skin folds, and pat dry.

## HOMEOPATHY

Any of the homeopathic remedies below can help clear up a recent, fairly mild flare-up of diaper rash. Inflammation, irritation, soreness, and general discomfort should decrease within a day or so. The soothing effect will be further enhanced and supported by following the preventive steps suggested below. However, as with so many other skin conditions, if the diaper rash has approached a more chronic phase where severe, established symptoms have emerged, it should be treated by an experienced homeopathic practitioner.

**Belladonna:** Consider this remedy to treat the first signs of diaper rash, especially if symptoms have developed abruptly and dramatically. Symptoms include spots that look bright red and angry and feel noticeably hot to the touch. Normally calm, placid babies become fractious and irritable.

**Cantharis:** If diaper rash causes particular distress at night, and results in spots that are noticeably sore and burning after urinating, use Cantharis. As a result of poor sleep, the baby becomes drowsy and out of sorts during the day.

> **TIP: TAKE PREVENTIVE STEPS**
> Gently but thoroughly dry the affected area after bathing your baby, and make sure that as much air as possible comes into contact with the affected skin. With this in mind, leave diapers off as often as possible. Change diapers frequently to avoid your baby coming into contact with feces and/or urine for long periods, which can increase the sensitivity of already sore skin.

## HERBALISM

**Salves:** Herbal medicines, in a salve form, can treat diaper rash by serving as a protective barrier between the skin and the diaper, as well as helping to alleviate redness, irritation, and inflammation. Salves that include plantain leaf, violet flowers, and mullein flowers have a combination of antimicrobial, anti-inflammatory, and skin-soothing effects that help to relieve the symptoms of diaper rash. Other preparations with calendula flowers, either in homeopathic form or as extracts added to a lotion or ointment, have many skin-healing properties that can benefit diaper rash. Other treatments for diaper rash are similar to those for dermatitis (see p. 56), such as the use of demulcent herbs to protect and soothe inflamed skin.

# DRY HAIR

## DIAGNOSIS

Dry hair can mean many different things. Hair can be fine and limp but dry, or coarse and curly but dry. It can even be oily at the roots and dry at the ends. Dry, brittle hair is often a sign that your diet is deficient in essential fatty acids. These polyunsaturated fats are vital for locking moisture into skin and hair cells to keep them supple. Good sources of essential fats include oily fish, such as salmon or mackerel, avocados, and nuts. Dry hair can also be caused by a lack of iron or zinc in the diet. Foods rich in iron include wholegrains, fortified cereals, pulses, greens, and dried fruit. Foods rich in zinc include eggs, wholegrains, soya, and chicken. Hair also tends to dry out as you age because the body's natural level of oil production from the sebaceous glands is reduced. In some instances, very dry hair can be an indication of a more serious condition, such as thyroid disease.

## SYMPTOMS

- Dry, brittle hair
- Hair breaks easily
- Frizzy halo effect round the head

## TREATMENT GOAL

To improve the condition of the hair and return its luster.

## CONVENTIONAL MEDICINE

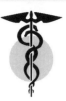

**Moisturize your hair:** Dry hair is not a medical illness as such and is usually a symptom of another condition. It can also be a result of hot dry conditions, exposure to environmental toxins, or chemical processing. In these cases, hair conditioners and moisture packs are appropriate. Also try to avoid exposing the hair to the conditions that cause dryness.

**Diet:** Increase your intake of beneficial oils, such as eicosapentanoic acid (EPA) and docosohexanoic acid (DHA, found in fish oil, which can be taken at 4 g a day), and gamma linolenic acid (GLA, found in evening primrose oil, which can be taken at 3 g). A deficiency of vitamins A, D, and E can affect the condition of hair, so make sure you are getting your recommended daily allowance (RDA). Biotin, found mostly in beans, is also an important vitamin for hair health. Selenium and zinc, found in mushrooms and root vegetables, contribute to good hair condition and should be present in adequate amounts in the diet.

**When should I see a doctor?** The most common diseases associated with dry hair are hypothyroidism, atopic dermatitis, ectoparasitic diseases such as head lice, fungal diseases such as ringworm, chronic protein depletion, chronic malnutrition, and fatty acid deficiency. Today, in the western world, malnutrition is most commonly seen in those with anorexia and occasionally in the elderly. Heavy metal toxicity (particularly lead, zinc, mercury, and cadmium) can also cause dry hair. Certain medications such as oral contraceptives, anti-seizure medication, and steroids can change the texture of your hair. If any of these conditions are suspected, make an appointment to see your doctor.

## TRADITIONAL CHINESE MEDICINE

**Herbs:**
• Internal herbal treatment: According to traditional Chinese medicine, dry hair is usually caused by blood or body fluid deficiency, excessive body heat, or stagnant circulation. Consult a doctor of Chinese medicine for an individual assessment. He Shou Wu (fleece flower root), Dan Shen (salvia root), Shu Di Huang (Chinese foxglove), Mai Men Dong (ophiopogon tuber), and Tian Men Dong (asparagus tuber) can be used in bulk or in powder form to treat dry hair internally by nourishing the blood and body fluid. Peach kernel, Bai Zhi (Chinese angelica root), and Zhi Zi (Cape Jasmine fruit) can be used if dry hair is a result of heat. However, these herbs can cause loose stools. If you have digestive problems or a sensitive stomach, see a TCM practitioner to find out which formula is most suitable.
• External herbal treatment: Add 150 g each of Sang Bai Pi (mulberry root bark) and Ce Bai Ye (biota leaves) to 6 cups of waters in a ceramic pot. Soak the herbs for 30 minutes before bringing them to the boil. After boiling the herbs for 10 minutes, remove the

mixture from the heat and let it cool to a warm temperature. Soak your hair in this decoction and rinse once a week. Your hair should become smoother and shinier after a couple of treatments.

**Acupuncture:** Dry hair can be a symptom of an internal imbalance. It can be a sign of insufficient nourishment from body fluid, blood deficiency, or stagnant circulation. Acupuncture treatment will address these issues. The treatment can take a few weeks to a few months, depending on the individual condition.

**Acupressure:** After showering and before going to bed, press the scalp using the five fingers of both hands like a comb. Comb your scalp with your fingers gently to promote circulation two or three times a day for two to five minutes.

**Diet:** Eat foods that are cooling and nourishing, such as berries, pears, water chestnuts, sponge gourd (available in Asian food markets), and black sesame. Avoid pungent and spicy food and deep-fried food as they are more likely to create heat and dryness.

## NATUROPATHY

**Diet:** The oil in cold-water fish like salmon, herring, and mackerel is rich in omega-3 fatty acids. Eating fish twice a week can help replenish the moisture lost in dry hair. Taking 2 tbsp of flaxseed oil a day can also help replenish hair oils. Drink 10, 8 oz glasses of water a day to replenish some of the body's internal dryness. Consuming good quality protein, such as cold-water fish, organic grassfed meats, and organic chicken, nourishes hair follicles by restoring protein, from which hair is primarily made. Whole grains mixed with legumes are also good sources of protein.

**Supplements:** Fish oils contain fatty acids and have the therapeutic functions mentioned above. Take a maximun of 3 g of EPA/DHA a day. A high-quality multivitamin/mineral is also recommended to sustain overall healthy hair. Follow the instructions on the bottle.

**General recommendations:** Do not overuse chemical products for your hair, for example perms, dyes, etc. Refrain from using a blow-dryer more than once a week. Wash your hair every other day and do not use shampoos with harsh chemicals.

---

**TIP:** WASH YOUR HAIR LESS FREQUENTLY
The natural oils that protect your hair can be lost through overwashing. Depending on the weather and environmental conditions, wash your hair once every three to five days.

## HOMEOPATHY

Dry hair can be a reaction to chemicals found in harsh shampoos or hair dyes. This type of problem can be treated by the short-term use of an appropriate homeopathic remedy, and by making healthy lifestyle changes to rectify any damage. However, the condition of your hair can act as a basic barometer for your health, and dry hair can point to a larger problem. If this is the case, dry hair is best dealt with by a homeopathic practitioner, who will prescribe treatments in an effort to balance the whole system. If dry hair arises at, or beyond, mid-life in combination with unexplained weight gain, tiredness, and dry, cracked skin, have your thyroid gland function tested.

**Calc carb:** If hair appears dry and of poor quality, and if there is a general sense of sweatiness on the head and scalp, Calc carb can be helpful. Those who benefit from this remedy find they have a very slow metabolism with all body processes tending to work very slowly, resulting in easy weight gain, indigestion, constipation, and poor mental focus.

**Thuja:** If hair lacks luster, feels brittle and dry, and is in poor condition, use Thuja. This remedy is helpful for hair that starts to grow very slowly and looks thin in texture, or if dry hair is combined with greasy, unhealthy looking skin that is prone to warty growths.

## HERBALISM

**Burdock root:** For general hair health, the daily consumption of burdock tea may serve as a cleansing tonic that improves the body's ability to grow healthy hair. Make a decoction from 2 g of burdock root and 10 cups of hot water. Ingest the tea three or four times daily. Watch for signs of a skin rash, which may develop as a reaction in some rare instances.

**Horsetail:** This herb (*Equisetum arvense* or *Equisetum telmateia*) is mainly used to fight baldness and brittle fingernails, but it may also help to improve the quality of hair. Take a tincture, available from health food stores, made from the above-ground parts of horsetail. To make a tea, boil 1–2 g of the plant in a few cups of water. Ingest about 6 g of the plant daily. **Caution:** A species related to horsetail, *Equisetum palustre*, has a toxic compound. Make sure that the product you use does not contain this horsetail relative.

**Hair tonic:** There are many different recipes available for hair tonics that combine herbal medicines with other ingredients to create a mixture that promotes strong, healthy hair. One recipe includes nettles as a main ingredient. Simmer a few young leaves of this plant in 10 cups of water. Wash your hair and scalp with this liquid, once it has cooled, to improve hair quality.

# DRY SKIN

## DIAGNOSIS

Dry skin can occur at any age, but it becomes more common as you get older because the number of oil-boosting sebaceous glands becomes reduced, as does the skin's ability to hold moisture. The amount of fat that the outer layer of skin, known as the epidermis, contains determines the skin's ability to retain moisture and how well it protects the body. Genes can also play a role; if relatives suffer from dry skin, you are more likely to develop the condition. Dry skin can point to insufficiencies in your diet, particularly if you don't drink enough water, have a low intake of the essential fatty acids found in oils and fish, or have a vitamin A or B group deficiency. To counter this deficiency, try eating more red- and yellow-colored fruit and vegetables, plus wholegrains and green leafy vegetables, all of which are good sources of vitamins A building blocks (such as cartonoids) and B group vitamins. Other triggers to dry skin include exposure to sunlight, cold weather, and central heating, and the over-use of harsh soaps and cleansing products that strip the skin of its natural oils. When buying skincare products, avoid those that contain alcohol, which is very drying. In extreme cases of dry skin, fish-like scaling of the skin can occur. Very occasionally the condition can get so severe that you should consult your doctor for a prescription-strength cream.

## SYMPTOMS

- Skin is often red, scaly, and itchy
- The problem is usually worse in autumn and winter
- Dry skin is most common on your face, hands, arms, and legs

## TREATMENT GOAL

To improve the condition of dry skin.

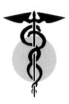

## CONVENTIONAL MEDICINE

**Identify and avoid the cause:** To treat dry, flaky skin first identify the cause. The most common trigger is exposure to a hot, dry environment combined with inadequate fluid intake. Soaps and heat can cause the skin to lose moisture and antiperspirants, perfumes, and hot baths can further irritate the condition. Certain fabrics can also irritate the skin. Many people are sensitive to wool and it should be avoided in most cases.

**Use emollient lotions:** A straightforward case of dry skin generally presents with dryness, itchiness, and some flaking. Scratching the skin generally produces redness and can result in infection in severe cases. Dry skin usually feels better when emollient lotions are applied. For mild symptoms of dry skin without complications, use moisturizers and lotions on a regular basis. Non-fragranced lotions are preferable.

**Use a moisturizing soap:** Use a non-detergent, non-perfumed moisturizing soap, such as Cetaphil®. Pat rather than rub skin dry after bathing. Don't take too many hot baths, and add bath oil to water when you bathe. Protect your hands with gloves when doing the dishes.

**Use a humidifier:** Consider using a humidifier in the home to raise the humidity level in the environment during the winter.

**When should I see a doctor?** Dry skin can be a symptom of certain diseases and can be a side effect of medication. A thyroid abnormality, fatty acid deficiency, malnutrition, anorexia, and kidney disease are accompanied by dry skin. Certain skin illnesses, allergies, and dermatitis cause dry, flaking skin. If you think any of these conditions are the cause of the dry skin, or if you have serious symptoms in addition to dry skin, see your doctor.

## TRADITIONAL CHINESE MEDICINE

**Herbs:**
• Insufficient yin energy can result in dry skin. Mai Men Dong (ophiopogon tuber) and Gou Ji Zi (wolfberry) can tonify body yin energy, creating nutrients to nourish the skin. To make a decoction, combine 30 g of each berry, both available from Chinese pharmacies or online, in a teapot. Let them steep in boiling water for 20 minutes. Strain and drink ½–1 cup three times a day. Continue this treatment three days a week for your long-term nourishment.
• Herbal bath: Boil 50 g of peach kernel, 50 g of almond kernel, 30 g of Dang Gui (Chinese angelica root), 20 g of Jin Yin Hua (honeysuckle) and 20 g of ross tip in 6 cups of water for

30 minutes and then strain the liquid. Add a further 5 cups of water to the herbs and boil them a second time. Strain this liquid and combine it with that of the first batch. Pour all of the liquid into a bathtub and add warm water. Soak the whole body or the affected area in the herbal bath for 20–30 minutes once a week.

**Acupuncture:** Treatment will involve inserting needles into your body meridians for about 20–40 minutes once a week. Treatment will focus on the cause of the condition more than the symptoms, so the course of treatment could last for months.

**Acupressure/massage:** Give the whole body a relaxing massage to boost circulation. Go for a massage once or twice a month or massage the areas you can reach by yourself once or twice a day.

**Diet:** A healthy lifestyle and balanced diet are essential for healthy skin. Drink plenty of water every day to keep skin hydrated. Eat food that is cooling and moistening, such as pears, bananas, lychee, kiwi fruit, cherries, blueberries, sweet rice, sesame, gingko nuts, sweet almonds, fish, and chicken. Avoid deep-fried and baked food. Also avoid hot spices, as they could damage body fluid.

## NATUROPATHY

**Diet:** The oils in cold-water fish such as salmon, herring, and mackerel are rich in omega-3 fatty acids. Eating these types of fish at least twice a week can help replenish lost moisture in skin. Two tbsp of flaxseed oil a day can also help replenish skin oils. Drinking 10, 8 oz glasses of water a day will replenish some of the internal dryness of the body. Eliminate any foods you are allergic to. These foods may include wheat, dairy, corn, eggs, and soy.

**Supplements:** As mentioned above, fish oils contain fatty acids that have therapeutic functions. Take a maximum of 3 g of EPA/DHA a day. Vitamin A, taken at 10,000 IU a day, also nourishes the skin. Although 10,000 IU is a tolerable amount for most people, high amounts of vitamin A can cause toxicity of the liver and you should consult a doctor when taking this supplement. Pregnant women should not take more than 10,000 IU of vitamin A a day. A good multivitamin/mineral is recommended to sustain overall healthy skin. Follow the instructions on the bottle. Vitamin E is also helpful in treating dry skin. Mix 4 oz of jojoba oil or non-scented almond oil with 20 drops of rose oil and 20 drops of lavender (for their pleasant smell) with 10 drops of vitamin E. This mixture will moisturize the skin.

**General recommendations:** Refrain from using soap every day when showering, as it tends to eliminate the natural oils secreted from the glands of your skin. Use a loofa sponge, shower brush, or small towel to scrape the dead cells from your skin every day.

## HOMEOPATHY

Although dry skin can occur at any time of year, it can flare up even more during the autumn and winter months. This results from constantly exposing skin to dry, centrally heated atmospheres and dry, cold winds. There are some simple measures that can be taken to keep your skin supple and well balanced throughout the colder months of the year.

**Calendula:** Calendula cream makes an excellent skin salve that soothes and moisturizes at the same time. Apply the cream to small dry, flaky patches on the face or body.

**Calc carb:** This is a good remedy for dry skin that is also pale, chilly, and sweats easily.

**Natrum mur:** If there is a noticeable tendency for dry, flaky patches of skin to develop around the mouth and the corners of the lips, use Natrum mur. This remedy is likely to be helpful where there's a history of cold sores (often in response to over-exposure to sunlight), spots, and generally hypersensitive skin.

**Graphites:** For small patches of tight, flaky skin that develop into cracks during the cold months, Graphites is a helpful remedy. Sites that can be especially vulnerable include the exposed areas behind the ears, lips, and even the fingertips.

### TIP: USE A CREAM CLEANSER
Avoid washing your face with soap and water throughout the winter. Although this may clean your face, it will strip it of essential oils that help keep skin healthy and supple. Use a gentler cream cleanser, followed by an alcohol-free toning lotion. Or try using a wash-off cleanser that is designed to maintain the oil balance of the skin.

## HERBALISM

**Oats or oatmeal:** A cup of oats can be added to bath water to provide a coating and soothing effect. Small patches of particularly dry skin may respond well to an oat poultice or "mash" (see p. 78).

**Demulcents:** The most useful plants for dry skin are lubricating, soothing plants, such as the demulcents. Common demulcents include aloe vera, slippery elm bark, marshmallow root, fenugreek, chickweed, and comfrey leaves or roots. Decoctions of these plants can be used as skin washes. Each plant will behave differently in hot water. Begin with 25–30 g of plant material in 2–4 cups of water and experiment with different measurements to find the most effective consistency.

# ECZEMA

## DIAGNOSIS

Eczema is an inflammation of the skin that causes itching and discomfort. It is increasingly common and affects around one in 12 people. It usually first appears in early childhood and in many cases the symptoms tend to ease as the child gets older. However, eczema can reappear at a later stage, and can also affect an adult who hasn't previously suffered. It can be triggered by stress, house dust, animal fur, pollen, food allergies, and environmental conditions. It is closely associated with asthma and hay fever. It is an unpredictable disease and there is often no apparent reason for its onset. It can be very upsetting, particularly for children. There are many different types of eczema, with the main ones being contact eczema, caused when an allergen comes into contact with the skin, and atopic eczema, which is passed on genetically. Also see the section on dry skin, p. 69.

## SYMPTOMS

- Patches of rough, flaky, red skin, mainly on face, armpits, elbows, hands, and knees
- Inflamed, itchy skin
- Tiny red pimples
- Patches of dry, scaly skin
- Scratch marks where skin is irritated
- Blisters or cracks, and sometimes bleeding
- Weeping sores, with a thin, watery, or crusty yellow discharge
- Disturbed sleep patterns

## TREATMENT GOAL

To treat the condition both internally and externally. By identifying specific allergens that cause outbreaks and alleviating the discomfort of irritated skin, the itch-scratch-itch cycle can be prevented and potential infection can be avoided.

## CONVENTIONAL MEDICINE

**Identify the triggers:** Avoid any known triggers. Common triggers of eczema include foods (particularly dairy products and gluten), and environmental allergens such as dust mites and pet dander. Food allergy testing can be important in the process of identifying potential food triggers. (See Dermatitis, p. 56, for further treatment options.)

**Diet:** Essential fatty acids (EPA/DHA or fish oil) decrease inflammatory mediators in the body. Eat oily fish two to three times a week, or take 4 g of omega-3 fish oil supplements daily to significantly improve symptoms and reduce outbreaks.

**Mind and body practices:** Meditation, keeping a diary of daily emotions, and deep-breathing exercises, have been proven to reduce stress and the number of flare-ups.

**Topical steroids:** If inflammation continues, topical steroids such as hydrocortisone and triamcinolone acetonide, which are moderate strength ointments, are prescribed. Betamethasone dipropionate and fluocinoninde are more potent steroid creams that can be used if moderate potency steroids are ineffective. The least potent should be chosen, as even topical steroids have side effects.

**Prescription drugs:** Oral prednisone or intramuscular triamcinolone can be used. These have side effects, including immune alteration, emotional changes, weight gain, and glucose intolerance. In the most recalcitrant cases, cyclosporine, a potent chemotherapeutic agent (a drug that can alter the DNA of a cell), can be prescribed. This is for extreme cases only and should be prescribed by a specialist only after alternatives have been explored.

**Antibiotics:** Medical care must be sought in cases of secondary infections occurring from a rash. In this case, doctors do not usually obtain a skin swab for a culture because 90% of patients have skin that is colonized with staph aureus whether it is infected or not. Staph is the most common infecting organism; Streptococcus pyogenes is another common organism that causes infections in an eczema rash. An antibiotic that treats both should be used, such as erythromycin, cephalexin, or dicloxacillin.

### TIP: USE AN EMOLLIENT
For general flare-ups, emollients should be applied liberally and frequently to keep skin from drying and cracking. Emollients can also be used in between steroid cream treatments during the day. A soap substitute such as Cetaphil® is helpful, as are bath oils for retaining the skin's natural moisture. Avoid bathing in extreme temperatures.

## TRADITIONAL CHINESE MEDICINE

To treat eczema, an internal and external herbal treatment is commonly used. The condition often diagnosed is dampness and heat in the body that is disturbing skin health. The treatment principle is to dispel dampness and cleanse blood heat. Before the long-term use of either internal or external treatments, it is recommended that you consult your doctor.

**Herbs:**
• Jin Yin Hua tea: Combine 10 g each of the herbs Jin Yin Hua (honeysuckle flower) and Jin Lian Hua (gold lotus flower) in a teapot. Add 3–4 cups of hot water and let the herbs steep for three minutes. Strain the tea and drink 1 cup three times a day.
• Long Dan Xie Gan Wan pills: Available from a Chinese herbalist, these pills treat chronic eczema. Herbal medicine can be used for several weeks to several months.
• Herbal paste: Mix together the following herb powders: 10 g of Huang Bai (phellodendron), 8 g of Da Huang (rhubarb root and rhizome), 10 g of Huang Lian (coptis rhizome), 10 g of Huang Qin (baical skullcap root), and 15 g of Di Yu (burnet-bloodwort root). Add olive oil to make a paste. Apply this herbal paste on the affected skin once a day for seven days as one course of treatment.

**Acupuncture:** An experienced acupuncturist will insert about a dozen needles into certain meridian points, such as the spleen and stomach meridians. Treatment takes about 25–40 minutes. You will usually receive treatment once or twice a week for several weeks up to several months.

**Diet:** Aim for balanced nutrition. Eat fresh vegetables and reduce your caffeine intake, as it dehydrates the skin. Fruits such as pears, cranberries, blueberries, and bananas are recommended. Mung beans, red or adzuki beans, bamboo shoots, and purslane are also beneficial. Avoid foods that are rich and fatty, as they have a dry and warm property.

## NATUROPATHY

**Diet:** Food allergies appear to be a major cause of eczema, particularly an allergy to milk in infants. In others, an allergy to gluten is a prime culprit. Foods that contain gluten include wheat, oats, rye, and barley. Eliminate these foods, and any others to which you may be allergic, from your diet for six weeks. Reintroduce one type of food each week and take note of any changes in your skin. It is also important to increase the intake of cold-water fish such as herring, salmon, and mackerel. For children, add 1 tsp of fish oil to food twice a day. The types of fats found in fish oil decrease inflammation and moisten the skin. Drink 10 glasses of water every day to keep skin hydrated. Eat plenty of different colored vegetables. They contain high amounts of beta-carotene, which is particularly beneficial to skin.

**Herbs:** Burdock root has a nourishing, cleansing effect on the skin. Adults should take 500 mg in capsule form or 3 ml of tincture a day. Children should take 150 mg or 0.5 ml a day.

**Topical:** Calendula has antiseptic properties and heals broken, damaged skin. Apply calendula cream, available from health food stores, around the affected area twice a day. Neem oil can also be helpful in healing inflamed, red, and itchy skin. Apply it to the affected area twice a day.

**Supplements:** Children should take 1 tsp of fish oil, added to food, twice a day. Adults can take a 3 g total of EPA/DHA combination. Vitamin C with bioflavonoids promotes skin healing and raises immunity; take 1,000 mg three times a day. Adults can take 3,000 mg of evening primrose oil, and children should take 1,000 mg. Gamma-linoleic acid (GLA) is an essential anti-inflammatory for the skin. Vitamin E is useful for the prevention of oxidation of essential oils and for its skin-healing properties; adults should take 400 IU and children should take 100 IU a day.

**TIP:** TAKE PREVENTIVE MEASURES
Keep damaged skin moist using an oil-based cream. Avoiding mental stress is also helpful in reducing the occurrence of eczema.

## HOMEOPATHY

 Due to its complex nature, eczema should be treated by an experienced homeopathic practitioner. He or she will aim to treat the underlying weakness in the constitution that leaves the patient vulnerable to developing the distressing symptoms of itchiness, soreness, and possible bleeding from irritated areas of skin as a result of compulsive scratching. With this in mind, the remedies listed below are suggested with a view to supplying an idea of the range of the most common potential homeopathic solutions that a practitioner may consider before prescribing for a patient.

**Avoid known triggers:** Avoid contact as far as possible with substances or conditions that are known to trigger a sore, itchy, sensitive reaction. Be careful of what toiletries you use. This especially applies to scented soaps, bath products, and body creams and lotions. Always avoid highly perfumed formulas that include powerful detergents. These can aggravate and irritate sensitive skin, and make it more likely for dry, itchy patches to develop.

**Moisturize:** Keep skin well moisturized, using products that are designed for use on sensitive, dry skin. These tend to be unperfumed products that aim to put moisture temporarily back into the skin, making it feel superficially more comfortable.

**Petroleum:** To treat rough, dry skin that festers easily and heals very slowly, use Petroleum. Symptoms include affected areas that itch and burn, with skin eruptions showing a strong tendency to occur in folds of skin, and itchiness that is so maddening that the skin may be broken and bleed as a result of compulsive scratching. This leads to hard, thick crusts developing over the sore areas.

**Sulphur:** To treat intensely itchy, inflamed skin that reacts badly to bathing or showering, and is aggravated by heat in any form, Sulphur is a classic remedy. Use Sulphur on skin that is dry, rough, scaly, and readily infected, and when burning sensations after scratching are especially troublesome if you are too warm in bed.

**Graphites:** If, after scratching, the itchy areas weep a thick, sticky yellow fluid and the skin feels raw and sore, and if a thick, honey-colored crust develops when the weeping patches dry out, use Graphites. Affected areas are most likely to include folds of skin (for instance behind the ears or around the nose), with a strong tendency for the skin to crack around the mouth, nose, ears, or nipples.

**Arsenicum album:** If the skin is dry with associated sore, burning sensations in eruptions that are unusually soothed by contact with warmth (for instance, with warm compresses or warm bathing), use Arsenicum album. The overall texture of the skin may be dry and rough, while patches of eczema develop blistery eruptions that feel intensely itchy. This causes an itch-scratch-itch cycle that leads to burning in the affected areas.

## HERBALISM

**Evening primrose oil:** This oil is an effective anti-inflammatory when ingested, helping to improve skin condition. It is thought to exert many of its effects because it contains the skin boosting omega-6 fatty acid gamma-linolenic acid (GLA). Adults should take 2–5 g a day, which provides approximately 250–500 mg of GLA. This should be taken on a long-term basis for maximum benefits in eczema. Evening primrose oil is a common treatment for atopic dermatitis in adults as well as children. Children should take approximately 3 g of oil a day in divided doses. Topical creams made of 12.5% evening primrose oil have also been shown to improve symptoms of eczema.

**Calendula:** To soothe the skin and help calm redness and irritation, use calendula. Extracts of calendula can be incorporated into creams and lotions, or a poultice can be made from its flowers. Pour a cup of boiling water over 2 tsp of calendula flowers, let them steep for two minutes, and strain the liquid. Soak a clean, absorbent cloth in the liquid and apply it to inflamed skin.

**Demulcents:** Soothing poultices, creams, and lotions can be made from aloe vera, slippery elm bark, marshmallow root, fenugreek, chickweed, and comfrey leaves or roots. The moist properties of the plants will coat the skin, holding in the natural oils and relieving the symptoms of eczema. Each plant will behave differently in hot water, but to make a decoction begin by boiling 25–30 g of plant material in 2–4 cups of water. Experiment with different measurements to find the most effective consistency.

**Burdock oil:** Apply this oil to the skin to relieve itchiness. Tea made from burdock root can also help as it serves as a blood purifier and skin health agent. Boil 2 g of the root and drink the tea three or four times a day. Interestingly, some people may actually develop dermatitis from the use of burdock, so be sure to pay attention to whether your symptoms are improving or getting worse.

**Oats or oatmeal:** Use oats to soothe the inflammation associated with eczema and other forms of dermatitis, and to calm itchiness, redness, and scaling. Mix about 1 cup of oats with enough cool water to create a mash, which should be left to macerate for 5–10 minutes. Dab the liquid from the mash onto affected skin with a clean washcloth several times a day. A film will form on the skin, which is calming, but the treatment can also stick to clothing, so be careful what you wear. The mash itself can also be placed directly on the skin for 10–15 minutes, rather like a poultice. Alternatively, a cup of oats can be added to bathwater to achieve a similar skin-soothing effect.

**To treat wet eczema:** Another approach to eczema is to think of it in terms of whether it is wet or dry. Some herbal experts feel that the reason treatment fails is due to the inaccurate application of this principle. There is a close link between the digestive tract and eczema, so if someone is constipated an internal treatment may be required. One treatment that applies this principle is the use of plants like oak, which is effective for wet eczema. The bark of the oak tree is astringent in nature because of its high tannin content. Make a decoction from the bark by boiling it for 15–20 minutes. Use the liquid to make a compress and apply it three times a day. For best results, the decoction should be made daily and used the same day. A decoction of mallow bark can be used in the same way to treat wet eczema. You can also drink tea made from chamomile flowers for its anti-inflammatory properties. According to some experts, chamomile is inferior to oak bark, but can be used if the eczema is chronic and a change in treatment is required.

# FOLLICULITIS

## DIAGNOSIS

Folliculitis is an inflammatory reaction of the skin around the roots of hair (the follicles), resulting in a rash of red marks and pimples. It is usually triggered by infection, or friction against the affected area. The inflammation is your immune system's response to the invasion of bacteria. Any rash caused by friction or chemicals won't respond unless the underlying skin irritant is identified and avoided. Boils can often develop when bacteria combine with dead skin cells that accumulate in the hair follicle, resulting in a build-up of pus. Boils associated with folliculitis are most often found on the face and scalp, buttocks, thighs, and groin. When men shave they can develop a rash that becomes infected as the razor spreads bacteria. To help this type of folliculitis heal and give the skin a chance to recover, it is best to steer clear of shaving altogether for a few days.

## SYMPTOMS

- A rash of small red dots anywhere hair grows
- Inflamed hair follicles
- Multiple small red bumps, which swell into pimples and boils
- Build-up of painful pressure
- Lymph glands may swell up
- The boils form a head and eventually burst or subside on their own

## TREATMENT GOAL

To ease the symptoms of folliculitis and to avoid the cause of the inflammation.

## CONVENTIONAL MEDICINE

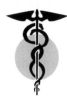

**Identify and eliminate the cause:** Folliculitis commonly exists on its own, but it can also be a component of another skin disease that has spread to the hair. Superficial folliculitis affects the top of the hair follicle and manifests as a tender or painless pustule that eventually heals without scarring. Often the hair cannot even be seen within the pustule. Deeper folliculitis presents as a larger, more painful red bump that eventually forms pus and may scar when it heals. In both cases, the folliculitis can cause skin irritation and itchiness. The most common cause is a bacteria that lives on the skin called staphylococcus. It enters the hair follicle following an injury or wound. Other causes are fungal infections, chemical irritants, pseudomonal folliculitis (caused by a type of bacterium called pseudomonas, which is commonly found in hot tubs), poor razor hygiene, and oral steroids. To prevent folliculitis from occurring, practice good razor and general hygiene and avoid the potential causes listed above.

**Topical powder:** Antiperspirant drying powders are available over the counter. Apply them to moist areas, such as under the breasts and the groin, to keep these areas dry.

**Topical antibiotics:** Treatment of the condition will depend on the cause. Your doctor may perform tests, or may diagnose from observation and history, to determine the cause. Sometimes a skin scraping is taken for diagnosis and occasionally a culture is sent. For common, mild folliculitis a topical antibiotic ointment, such as mupirocin, is used. Benzoyl peroxide may also be helpful.

**Oral antibiotics:** For moderate to severe folliculitis, an oral antibiotic, usually cephalexin (Keflex®), or, if the folliculitis has been caught from a hot tub, ciprofloxin, is used as well as a topical antibiotic. If the folliculitis is associated with a cold sore, an antiviral agen such as acyclovir is used.

**Other topical treatments:** For a fungal folliculitis, a topical antifungal such as econazole is used. Sometimes a mild topical steroid is used for severe itchiness in addition to the above.

## TRADITIONAL CHINESE MEDICINE

**Herbs:**
• Chang Xin Lian Pian: Take 3–5 pills of this patent Chinese herbal medicine three to four times a day. It cleans heat from the body and helps detoxing. You can also take 3–5 Yin Qiao Jie Tu Pian patent herbal pills three times a day. Take the pills for about two to four weeks to complete one course of treatment. You may take these pills together. If the condition is

at an acute stage, take Shan Huang Pian as indicated. You can find the above patent herbal pills at a Chinese herbalist.

• Herbal tea: Combine 5 g of Jin Yin Hua (honeysuckle), 8 g of Ye Ju Hua (chrysanthemum), and 2 g of Shen Gan Cao (raw licorice) in a teapot. Add boiling water and let the herbs steep for three to five minutes. Allow the tea to cool and drink 1 cup three to four times a day. This formula can be taken regularly, but if you have a digestive problem, the tea may be too cold for you. Consult with a Chinese medicine doctor for the formula suitable for your particular condition.

• Herbal bath: Combine 30 g of Jin Yin Hua (honeysuckle), 30 g of Huang Bai (phellodendron), 15 g of Jing Jie (schizonepeta), 30 g of Ku Shen (sophora root), 30 g of She Chuang Zi (cnidium seed), and 30 g of Di Fu Zi (broom cypress) in a ceramic pot. Add 6 cups of water, bring the mixture to the boil, and let it simmer for 30 minutes. Strain the liquid, add it to your bath water, and soak your body in the herbal bath. This formula will cleanse skin toxins, and most of the herbs it includes have been reported as having an antibacterial affect.

**Acupuncture:** An acupuncture practitioner will recommend treatment once a week, or twice a week for an acute condition. Each session should last about 30–40 minutes. Acupuncture can stimulate your body's immune system, and therefore help the body to dispel pathogens.

**Diet:** Eat food that has cooling properties, such as pears, mung beans, grapes, radishes, green beans, watermelon, and duck. Avoid foods that are pungent, greasy, and hot.

## NATUROPATHY

**Diet:** Eat plenty of multicolored vegetables to obtain all the nutrients and photochemicals needed to strengthen the immune system. Avoid all foods that weaken the immune system, such as junk food, foods containing hydrogenated oils and trans-fatty acids, simple carbohydrates, and sugars. Also eliminate foods to which you may be allergic or intolerant, such as dairy, wheat, and corn.

**Herbs and spices:** Consume herbs and spices that enhance the immune system and have antiseptic properties, such as garlic and ginger. Burdock root is a great skin detoxifier; take 4 ml of a tincture or 500 mg in capsule form three times a day. Goldenseal has antibacterial, anti-inflammatory, and immune-enhancing properties; take 4 ml of a tincture or 500 mg in capsule form three times a day.

**Detoxification:** A three-day juice-only fast will help eliminate impurities, reduce inflammation, and provide you with the nutrients you need to raise your immune system. The juices should be primarily green vegetables, combined with one or two carrot sticks. Celery and cucumbers are great for juicing because their high water content yields plenty of juice.

**Topical:** Tea tree oil is an effective antibacterial agent. Apply 10–15 drops of oil diluted in a ½ oz of water, or apply it in cream form, two or three times a day. Oregano oil can also be used topically for its own strong antibacterial effects. Use the oil directly once or twice a day.

**Supplements:** Vitamin C with bioflavanoids works synergistically to support the immune system and reduce skin inflammation. Take 3,000–5,000 mg a day. If stools soften, reduce the dosage by 500 mg at a time until the consistency of the stool returns to normal. Take 30 mg of zinc twice a day to support skin function and the immune system. Zinc depletes the body's store of copper, so 3 mg of copper should be taken with this supplement.

**Hydrotherapy:** Alternate between applying hot and cold water (three minutes hot and 30 seconds cold) to the affected area to drain pus. Be cautious not to burn yourself by using extreme temperatures. Do not use this treatment in areas where you have numbness due to nerve damage.

## HOMEOPATHY

 Any of the following remedies can be helpful in easing symptoms of folliculitis, especially if given at the earliest signs of the condition. It is helpful to know that homeopathic help can be given in a complementary context, in addition to any conventional medication that has been prescribed.

**Belladonna:** Use this remedy for the earliest signs of inflammation, for symptoms of localized or general heat, redness, and throbbing sensations. Belladonna is especially well indicated when symptoms develop with speed and intensity, and when the affected areas feel very tender. It is also appropriate if you feel irritable and peevish in response to the physical discomfort.

**Hepar sulph:** This remedy is helpful for later stages of inflammation, and follows Belladonna very well. It is a strong candidate for skin conditions that are generally slow and sluggish to heal, and for skin that becomes very easily inflamed and infected. If the affected areas of skin are uncomfortably sensitive to drafts of cold air, use Hepar sulph. This remedy can also encourage the resolution of suppuration and pus formation. It is helpful for conditions that tend to be sore, and feel as though a splinter were sticking into the affected areas.

Folliculitis can be treated with plants that combat inflammation and infection.

**Poultices and compresses:** Marshmallow root or leaf, and violet poultices can help to draw out infections and soothe the redness and inflammation associated with irritated skin. Poultices and compresses of calendula, which is valued for its anti-inflammatory, astringent, antifungal, and wound-healing properties, can be made and applied to the affected areas. A poultice of ground and decocted hot flaxseed will help to draw out the infection and decrease inflammation. Place the ground hot flaxseed on a linen cloth and apply it to the affected area.

**Flowering dogwood:** Also known as American boxwood, false box, rose willow, and silky cornel, flowering dogwood can be used topically to alleviate skin infections. A preparation from the bark of the root can be used on the skin, or a tincture of the root bark can be ingested to stimulate the appetite and relieve constipation.

**Tea tree oil:** Apply this antibacterial and antifungal oil directly to the affected area. A 15% tree tree oil solution provides the best results, but if the skin becomes irritated reduce the strength of the oil by diluting with a vegetable oil.

**Goldenseal:** Ingest goldenseal in capsule form (500 mg) or as a tincture (4 ml) three times a day. This herb has antibacterial, anti-inflammatory, and immune-enhancing properties. Be sure to purchase goldenseal from manufacturers who use cultivated goldenseal. If this is not specified, it is possible that the goldenseal has been harvested from the wild where its populations are threatened or endangered.

**Black walnut tree leaves:** These leaves are used medicinally for their, tonifying, antiseptic, hemostatic, antiparasitic, laxative, and wound-healing properties. Make a strong decoction by boiling 25–30 g of cut or powdered leaves in 2–3 cups of water. Apply the plant material as a compress to the affected area. The fluid can also be taken internally; drink a small glassful two to three times a day. If diarrhea develops, reduce the amount being consumed.

**Essential peppermint oil:** This oil has antibacterial, anti-inflammatory, analgesic, and antiseptic actions. The oil or liniment can be applied to the affected area.

# FUNGAL INFECTIONS

## DIAGNOSIS

Fungal skin infections are caused by a variety of fungi that spread and reproduce on the skin, body, and/or nails. The most common of these are yeast and mold infections, which flourish in warm, damp, sweaty places and attack the outer layer of the skin. Athlete's foot (see p. 27), ringworm (see p. 140), and fungal infection of the groin area are other common examples of this type of fungal infection. They can be extremely persistent, but they are also easily treatable. It is possible to catch the conditions from an infected person or animal, or from contaminated showers or changing rooms. Most fungal infections respond well to a cream or ointment containing an antifungal agent. If the scalp or nails are heavily infected an oral drug may be required. Other fungi live inside the body, in the lungs and heart, for example, or deep in tissues, where they set up infections. They are hard to diagnose and are often resistant to treatment.

## SYMPTOMS

- Intense itchiness
- Redness, swelling, scaling, and cracking of the skin
- Multiple patches of infection

## TREATMENT GOAL

To prevent fungal infections from spreading and recurring.

## CONVENTIONAL MEDICINE

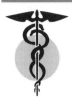

**Prevention:** Fungal infections are quite difficult to treat and are often recurring. The adjacent skin of the nail on the toe is also usually infected. The disease is causes a discoloration of the nail in the form of a yellow or white patch. This usually starts at the tip of the nail, spreads to the sides, and then to the base. The color becomes darker and the nail becomes thick, crumbly, and splits from the nail bed, which can be very painful. The usual cause is a group of fungi called dermatophytes. As you get older, the risk of nail infection increases. Fungus likes to grow in humid, warm places, so keeping the feet dry and cool is important in preventing and treating infections. The fungus can invade the nail plate during exercise, when toes may repeatedly rub against shoes, so special care must be taken after exercise to clean and dry the feet. A drying powder containing a mild antifungal, such as Tinactin, is also useful. Tight footwear should be avoided as it causes crowding of the toes and promotes fungal growth. Fungal organisms can spread quickly in communal pools and showers, and it is important to use separate towels if you are infected.

**Topical treatment:** It often takes months to see any benefit from treatment and resolution of the condition can take up to a year. Medication is almost always prescribed, as spontaneous remission of fungal infections is rare. If the fungus is caught when it appears at the very end of the toenail, topical clotrimazole cream (available over the counter) should be used for 30 days and can be effective. Tea tree oil applied topically can also work wonders in early stages of infection.

**Oral treatment:** If fungal skin infection is persistent or involves the soles of the feet or the nails, a doctor may prescribe a systemic antifungal, typically for a period of two to three months. Oral antifungal drugs include griseofulvin, terbinafine, and itraconazole. Oral antifungals should not be used by pregnant women.

**Caution:** Diabetics, AIDS patients, and those with circulatory problems should seek care immediately and continue treatment until the infection is completely resolved. Check with your doctor if you are prescribed an antifungal medication while taking other medication or herbs (especially St. John's Wort), as complications can be significant.

## TRADITIONAL CHINESE MEDICINE

**Herbs:**
• Herbal decoction: Combine 15 g of Cang Er Zi (cocklebur), 15 g of Di Fu Zi (broom cypress), 15 g of She Chuang Zi (cnidium seed), 30 g of Huang Jing (Siberian Solomon seal), 15 g of Huang Bai (phellodendron), 15 g of Long Dan Cao (Chinese gentian root), and 30 g of Ku Shen

(sophora root). These herbs are all available from Chinese herbalists. Boil the herbs in 5 cups of water for 30 minutes. Strain the liquid and use the decoction to wash the affected area. Soak the infected nail or toenail in the liquid for 15–20 minutes once or twice a day. One course of treatment lasts for 10 days.

• Herbal poultice: Collect 50–100 g each of fresh purslane, which grows throughout the summer, and dandelion leaves. Mash them well while they are still fresh and apply the plant material to the affected area once a day. It will take a couple of months for the herbs to take effect.

**Acupuncture:** Cleaning dampness and heat are the treatment principles for this condition. For fungal infections, combining herbal medicine with acupuncture treatment is much more effective than acupuncture alone. To see long-term effects, long-term, rather than short-term, treatment is required.

**Diet:** Wherever possible, include multigrains rather than wheat in your diet. Choose fresh food over preserved food. Eat green vegetables as well as peppermint, soybean sprouts, bamboo shoots, and cranberries. Coix seeds and wax gourds, available from Chinese herbalists or Asian grocery stores, are also helpful. Avoid foods that are fatty, greasy, and sweet.

---

**TIP:** RICE VINEGAR SOAK

For infected nails, soak your nails two to three times a day in rice vinegar. After soaking, use a towel to scrape away the damaged nail material. Repeat this procedure until the new nail starts to grow.

---

## NATUROPATHY

**Diet:** Eating fresh vegetables, lean protein, and whole grains will support your immune system. Eat plenty of unsweetened cultured foods, such as kefir, yogurt, miso, and raw sauerkraut, which contain friendly bacteria that fight off systemic fungus. Drink 10 glasses of water a day to assist in flushing out yeast toxins. Drink 2 glasses a day of a green drink made from a green powder that consists of spirulina, wheat grass, and barley grass powder. These substances will raise your immunity levels and feed healthy bacteria. Avoid sugar and processed carbohydrates as they fuel yeast, helping it to reproduce. Avoid or reduce fruits and avoid fruit juice altogether. Most fruits and all fruits juices are too high in sugar and fuel yeast. Avoid all alcoholic beverages, as the yeast in these drinks feeds the yeast in your system.

**Detoxification:** Complete a seven-day vegetable juice detoxification fast, supervised by a qualified health practitioner. Drink two juices a day and soup, such as miso and vegetable soup, with plenty of garlic and ginger. After the seven-day detoxification, follow the diet outlined above.

**Supplements:** Garlic fights fungus and boosts the immune system; take 500 mg twice a day. Take 200 mg of grapefruit seed extract twice a day for its antifungal properties. Caprylic acid, a fatty acid shown to have antifungal properties, can be taken three times a day at 1,000 mg. Undecylenic acid, a derivative from castor bean oil, has also been shown to have strong antifungal effects; take 200 mg three times a day. Drink 2 cups of Pau d'arco tea a day for its strong antifungal properties. Vitamin C can be taken at 1,000 mg twice a day for its immune-enhancing functions. You should also take a high-potency multivitamin as it will provide many nutrients that support immune function. Take probiotics with about four billion micro-organisms twice daily, 30 minutes before each meal. These micro-organisms provide you with acidophilus and bifidus, friendly bacteria that prevent yeast overgrowth and fight candida.

---

**TIP:** KEEP YOUR FEET CLEAN

For a foot infection, expose your feet to the open air as often as possible. Keep feet clean and dry and use cotton socks so that your feet can breathe. Change your socks daily.

---

## HOMEOPATHY

 A fungal infection in the foot tends to be a sign of a deeper-seated imbalance in the system. For instance, fungal infections that lead to the distortion of the toenails can be linked to psoriasis, which can trigger thickened, discolored, or brittle toenails. It may be appropriate to try homeopathy as a first resort, but ideally with the blessing and supervision of your medical practitioner or podiatrist, who will be able to judge your progress. However, any sign of a severe, persistent, or spreading fungal infection affecting the feet and/or toes will require treatment from a trained homeopathic practitioner. (Also see Athlete's Foot, p. 27, for further remedies.)

**Keep feet clean and dry:** If there is a mild, underlying tendency to develop fungal infections of the feet, always keep feet as dry as possible. Take sensible precautions, such as drying gently but thoroughly between the toes after washing. Avoid wearing tightly fitting shoes and non-cotton socks that encourage the feet to sweat. This will help keep control the moisture levels that create an ideal breeding ground for infection at bay.

**Calendula:** Dilute one part of calendula tincture in 10 parts of boiling water. Allow the liquid to cool and use it as a soothing wash. Follow this with a light application of calendula cream. The natural antiseptic qualities of calendula can help clear up mild signs of infection.

**Antimonium crudum:** For fungal infections that cause soreness and irritation, with the toenails showing a distinct tendency to become thickened, Antimonium crudum can be helpful. This remedy is suitable if the big toe is especially affected.

**Silica:** This remedy may help ease a low-grade fungal infection of the feet and toes that leads to the toenails becoming weak, brittle, or misshapen, with the appearance of white flecks.

**Graphites:** If fungal infections lead to the development of itchy cracks between the toes, and the irritation is particularly severe at night, Graphites can be helpful. Use this remedy if the toenails show signs of becoming brittle or thickened, and become darkened in color, or if the feet perspire easily, and the skin between the toes exfoliates readily.

## HERBALISM

 Almost all herbal therapies for fungal infections of the skin and nails (as opposed to vaginal yeast infections, see p. 822) are applied topically, directly to the infected area. This method increases the effectiveness of the therapy and limits unwanted side effects. If symptoms don't resolve, worsen, or new symptoms develop within the recommended course of therapy for any of the herbal products listed, seek medical attention, as a more aggressive mode of therapy may be needed.

**Garlic:** An excellent first choice for treating fungal infections, garlic has antiseptic and antifungal qualities, and generally boosts the immune system. Apply crushed raw garlic directly to the affected area two to three times a day for one to two weeks. The odor of this remedy can be unpleasant. Another effective, and more tolerable, method of obtaining garlic is through a garlic gel, available from local health food stores. Ajoene, an organosulfur compound found in garlic, is known to have powerful antifungal properties and has been shown to work just as well as over-the-counter antifungal medications. Look for a gel that contains 1% ajoene and apply it twice a day for one week to 10 days. Garlic can also be taken orally as capsules; take 500 mg twice a day. Garlic has virtually no side effects when used topically, although minor irritation is sometimes reported. When taken internally at high, therapeutic doses, garlic may interfere with certain antithrombotic drugs.

**Tea tree oil:** Used topically as an antifungal and antibacterial agent, tea tree oil has been shown to work well to relieve symptoms, but a complete cure is less likely. Apply a 5–15% tea tree oil solution or cream topically to the infected area. A much stronger dose of either a solution or cream is needed to produce a cure. Recommendations range from applying 25–100% strength, two to three times a day. Dermatitis can be a side effect of prolonged and repeated topical use of tea tree oil.

**Calendula:** Available widely from herb stores, calendula has been shown to be effective in treating fungal infections. It can be applied topically as an ointment or a tincture. Dosage recommendations vary, and a consultation with a medical herbalist may be required. Calendula has very few contraindications when used topically, but there may occasionally be an allergic reaction.

**Oregano oil:** Best taken orally and diluted in water, oregano oil has strong antifungal properties. Drink 3–5 drops of oil diluted in a glass of water two to three times a day. Do not take this remedy if you have an allergic reaction to plants in the mint family. In large doses, oregano oil may cause nausea and can potentially decrease the body's ability to absorb iron.

**Cloves:** When applied topically, cloves have antifungal properties. Available at health food stores, clove oil or salves should be used on the affected area several times daily. Potential adverse reactions to topical application include dermatitis and nasal or vaginal irritation. Do not take cloves internally.

**Alfalfa:** Known for its antifungal properties, alfalfa is best taken as an oil, available from health food stores, in solution or as a tea. To make alfalfa tea, boil 1–2 tbsp of alfalfa in a cup of water. Strain the liquid and drink when it has cooled. In large doses, alfalfa may interact with antithrombotic and hormone drugs, and it has been known to cause sensitivity to light.

# GREASY HAIR

## DIAGNOSIS

Hair requires some natural oil to give it shine, but becomes greasy if too much is produced. Greasy hair is caused by a build-up of the natural secretion known as sebum from glands in the scalp (the sebaceous glands). The sebum passes into the hair follicle and spreads upwards and over the hair shaft. It is not absorbed into the shaft, but instead accumulates on the surface, causing the hair to look dull. It can also affect the skin on the face and give a general impression of ill health. The feel of the hair depends on the volume of grease present. At certain times, such as during puberty, there is a marked change in sebum production due to the presence of higher levels of male hormones (known as androgens). At such times the hair may become greasier and will need to be washed more often. Inadequate removal of the grease aggravates the problem and makes it worse. The best way to deal with hair that gets greasy easily is to wash it more frequently. Aim for once a day. Regular washing will go a long way towards removing excess grease.

## SYMPTOMS

- Hair is oily and looks lank and weighed down
- The scalp produces much the same amount of grease whatever the hair style. However, since very short hair offers a smaller area over which grease can spread, greasiness can be especially troublesome in short hair
- A build-up of grease and other material—environmental dirt and bacteria—on the hair
- When you perspire, the grease combines with sweat and results in lank strands of hair that look unpleasant and may be unmanageable

## TREATMENT

As it is not possible to stop the glands in the scalp from producing grease, treatment aims to keep hair clean and in good condition.

## CONVENTIONAL MEDICINE

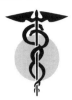

**Identify and eliminate possible causes:** The condition of greasy hair in itself is not a disease and as such there is not a medical treatment. Greasy hair is caused by overactive glands in the scalp producing sebum. This activity naturally increases during puberty, and is sometimes present in infancy due to maternal hormones that are passed on from mother to baby. Usually, elevated masculine hormone activity is associated with greasy hair. For a woman, it can be connected to elevated testosterone or polycystic ovary syndrome. It can also be linked to certain birth control pills that contain androgens. Any condition that causes an elevation in the adrenal hormone DHEA can also result in greasy hair. Seborrheic dermatitis is a skin condition that, when it affects the hair, causes a greasy appearance. Each of these conditions should be evaluated, diagnosed, and treated accordingly if suspected.

**Shampoo:** Greasy hair as an isolated condition can be treated with an over-the-counter shampoo. Frequent washing does not encourage the production of grease. Wash the hair regularly with a shampoo designed for greasy hair and specially formulated to remove natural grease without damaging the hair shaft.

**Diet:** Decreasing your intake of sugar, fat, and dairy produce may reduce sebaceous activity of the hair glands, resulting in less greasy hair.

## TRADITIONAL CHINESE MEDICINE

**Herbs:**
• Zhu Li (dried bamboo sap): Bamboo grows throughout the Yangtze River valley and southern China. Zhu Li is obtained by cutting both sides of a bamboo stalk, heating the bamboo, and then collecting the liquid that drips from it. This sap is often stored in sealed bottles for medicinal use. You may not find this herb in every Chinese pharmacy, but if you search online, you may find suppliers. To treat greasy hair, add 15–25 g of Zhu Li to 3.5 liters of warm water. Soak and wash hair in the water, and let it dry naturally. You can use Zhu Li sap to wash hair three times a week.

**Acupuncture:** See an acupuncturist if the condition is severe. Local points and some points on the large intestine meridian, gallbladder meridian, and triple burner meridian are used to help circulation and detoxification. The skin needle technique, also known as the blossom needle technique, is also effective. This needling method involves lightly tapping certain areas of the skin with a bundle of short needles. Practitioners will use the technique at points or regions that will promote circulation. For this condition, the Feng Chi points, located on either side of the base of the skull, about 2 inches from the center point, are good for the skin needle technique.

**Diet:** Avoid greasy and sweet food. Foods that are particularly good for helping this condition are watermelon, Daikon radish, purslane, fresh dandelion, and water chestnuts.

> **TIP:** USE ALKALINE SOAP
> Try washing hair in warm water with a light alkaline soap rather than shampoo. Consult with your pharmacist about the best brand to use.

## NATUROPATHY

**Diet:** Avoid greasy food. Oily hair sometimes results from having too much fat in your diet, especially saturated fats and hydrogenated oils. These heavy fats work their way into the skin oils, contributing to greasy hair.

**Shampoo:** Wash your hair every day, or even several times a day, with a non-toxic shampoo that does not contain fragrance or chemicals. This will take some of the excess oils off your hair.

**Hormone evaluation:** Greasy hair is hormonally derived. You should have your estrogen, testosterone, and thyroid hormones evaluated.

## HOMEOPATHY

Like healthy skin, healthy hair should show signs of an optimum balance by looking neither too dry nor too greasy. Having hair that looks healthy and of good quality is partly down to genetics and good luck, but the way in which hair is treated can also contribute to its overall condition. This includes taking care when choosing hair products and treatments, and also ensuring that you eat a healthy, balanced diet. There is a positive role to be played by homeopathic treatment, especially if there seems to be a fundamental tendency for hair to be determinedly greasy and lank, no matter how many positive lifestyle changes are put in place. If lackluster, greasy hair is combined with a similar skin condition, it is worth considering getting constitutional treatment from an experienced homeopathic practitioner who will aim to prescribe in order to balance your whole system. For milder, short-term problems try using one of the homeopathic remedies listed below.

**Diet:** It is thought that cutting down on your intake of refined carbohydrates may help improve greasy hair. Offending items include anything that has a high refined white sugar content, such as sweets, chocolates (especially milk chocolates), and fizzy drinks.

**Phos ac:** If hair has become thin and greasy as a result of emotional stress, especially in teenagers who are growing and developing very rapidly, Phos ac can be helpful. There is also likely to be a general sense of nervous exhaustion.

**Sulphur:** This remedy is best used if there is a tendency to be averse to washing in general and if there is a noticeable feeling of heat and sweatiness in the head and scalp. The hair texture may alternate between dry and greasy due to poor or erratic grooming habits.

**TIP:** USE A GENTLE SHAMPOO
Avoid using a shampoo that contains aggressive detergents. Also avoid under- or over-washing as this can backfire by over-stimulating oil production.

## HERBALISM

 **Stinging nettle:** The parts of the plant that grow above ground can be applied topically to the scalp to improve several hair conditions, including the relief of dandruff, improving hair loss, and to help with oily, greasy hair. For oily hair, a decoction of the leaves and stems could serve as a scalp rinse or wash. A concentrated extract, available from health stores, could also be incorporated into a shampoo to wash and improve hair quality. These beneficial effects may be due to compounds in the leaves, such as beta-sitosterol and anti-inflammatory compounds known as flavonoids, such as quercetin and rutin.

# HAIR LOSS

## DIAGNOSIS

Very often there is no specific explanation for hair loss, a very distressing condition that can affect anyone at any time. The scalp is constantly shedding hairs, but the amount of hair shed can vary over time due to a number of factors, stress being one of the most common. The chief causes of hair loss tend to be age and disease, but balding can also be hereditary. It is not unusual to see an increase in hair loss during, for example, exam time or times of similar emotional upheaval. Dieting and poor nutrition can play a role as protein and vitamin deficiencies can lead to hair loss. Pregnancy also affects hair growth. Many women experience extensive hair loss after childbirth, but hair does eventually return to normal thickness. Chemotherapy treatment for cancer can also cause severe hair loss. The best way to keep your hair healthy is to avoid or minimize the use of chemicals such as hair dye, and avoid the harsh heat generated by hair dryers and other styling tools.

Alopecia is the condition where a person suddenly loses his or her hair. This can be a small patch of hair or it can affect the entire scalp (alopecia totalis) and body hair (alopecia universalis). The reasons behind this condition are unknown, but there are indications that it can be triggered by a stressful event. Sometimes the hair falls out completely overnight; at other times it falls out in handfuls over a period of time. Often the hair grows back after a few weeks or months, but in cases of alopecia totalis and alopecia universalis regrowth is highly unlikely.

## SYMPTOMS

- Sudden loss of hair resulting in patches of baldness

## TREATMENT GOAL

Losing hair is very distressing and can be a source of anxiety for men and women alike. Treatment aims to restore hair growth where possible. Permanent hair loss can be concealed through the use of cosmetic products if it causes you distress.

**Identify the type and cause of hair loss:** Treatment of this condition depends on identifying the type and cause of the hair loss. The most common type is male pattern hair loss, which is hormonal, dependent on androgens, and can occur in both men and women. Age and genetic make up are the primary factors in the appearance of this type of hair loss. When it occurs in women along with an increase in hair growth on the face, a more complex medical cause involving the overproduction of male hormones is present. Other types of baldness are alopecia areata, where hair is lost in circular patches, telogen effluvium, which involves general hair loss after experiencing physcial or emotional stress (usually around three months after the event), lupus, and traction alopecia, which results from the direct pulling and damage of the hair (usually from hot rollers and other styling techniques). An unusual cause of hair loss is trichotillomania, which is self-inflicted and more common in children. Some fungal infections, such as ringworm (see p. 140), can also cause patches of hair loss.

**Finasteride:** This drug can be used in men but not in women of reproductive age. It blocks a testosterone hormone that affects the hair follicle. Because of this, it has side effects such as breast tenderness, decreased libido, and testicular pain. Nevertheless, it has an 80% hair regrowth rate after three months. It should be taken indefinitely. Pregnant women should not handle finasteride as it is a hormone modifier and can affect the hormones of the developing fetus.

**Minoxidil:** This drug is not available over the counter. While less effective than finasteride, it is safer and has fewer side effects.

**Surgical techniques:** Hair transplants can permanently restore hair, but it is an expensive procedure and requires many sessions. Scalp reduction is a cosmetic procedure that reduces bald scalp skin. The procedure is repeated every four weeks until hair margins come together or the scalp tissue becomes too thin to continue treatment.

**To treat alopecia areata and traction alopecia:** Steroid injections as well as the topical cream tacrolimus are used to treat this condition. Tacrolimus should be used as a last resort as it has the potential to increase the risk of cancer. To treat traction hair loss, modify your styling techniques.

**To treat trichotillomania:** This condition may be resolved with discussion and understanding. Parental distraction is a technique that sometimes helps. Punitive measures should not be used to treat a child with this problem. It is sometimes associated with obsessive compulsive disease, a condition that benefits from psychotherapy.

## TRADITIONAL CHINESE MEDICINE

**Herbs:**

• He Shou Wu (fleece flower): The name He Shou Wu, which literally means "Why is your hair so dark?" (healthy), comes from an old tale: A 100-year-old man lived in a mountain village. He worked on his farm until he was in his 90s. The village people noticed that not only was he physically strong, but his hair was incredibly shiny, dark, and full. "Why is your hair so healthy? What is your secret?" the people asked. The old man pointed at a fleece flower plant growing on the mountain. "That is why," he replied. Since then He Shou Wu has become known for keeping hair healthy. It has been used for thousands of years as a medicine to nourish the kidney and blood, and therefore nourish hair and treat many of problems that damage it. Clinical research has found that He Shou Wu is an effective herb for promoting circulation to hair. It is available in bulk, powder, or as pills from Chinese herbalists. Take the herb daily as a supplement for three to six months or longer. Those who suffer with diarrhea or other digestive problems should consult their doctor before taking He Shou Wu.

**Acupuncture:** Hair loss and baldness have been successfully treated by acupuncture, since treatment increases scalp blood circulation and tonifies blood. Practitioners will stimulate the local points and related meridian points according to Chinese medicine differentiation diagnosis, the diagnostic method used by a doctor of traditional Chinese medicine to distinguish individual, specific causes of a condition.

**Acupressure:** Use your five fingers as a comb and rake them across your scalp two to three times a day to promote blood circulation. Or, using your fingers, press on the scalp with medium to strong pressure 10 times for 5–10 minutes before you go to bed.

**Diet:** Eat foods that nourish the blood. These include black sesame seeds, red adzuki beans, black beans, radishes, spinach, carrots, and fish. In addition, choose foods that are cooling, such as watermelon, green vegetables, tofu, and Chinese jujube dates. Avoid hot spicy food, such as chilli pepper, garlic, beef, and lamb.

## NATUROPATHY

**Diet:** Hair loss can be caused by undernourishment. Be sure to eat a well-balanced diet that includes fresh fruits and vegetables, whole grains, legumes, and quality protein such as fish, lean chicken, and beans. Eat plenty of green, leafy vegetables as they will provide a base of nutrients required for healthy hair. Eat foods high in biotin (a nutrient that is essential for healthy hair growth), such as nuts, brewer's yeast, brown rice, and oats. Iron is also important for hair growth. Green leafy vegetables, blackstrap molasses, figs, and berries are all foods that are high in iron, which is important for healthy hair.

**Supplements:** As mentioned above, biotin is essential for healthy hair growth; take 3,000 mcg a day. Vitamin C helps with the absorption of iron. Take 2,000 mg of vitamin C a day. Take 50 mg of B-complex twice a day to help relieve stress and contribute to healthy hair. Taking 500 mg of silica a day will help with hair development. A high-quality, high-potency multivitamin will provide a base for hair growth development. Follow the instructions on the bottle.

**Herbs:** Research shows that palmetto is effective against hair loss in men, probably because it balances dihydrotestosterone (DHT), a metabolite of testosterone that contributes to hair loss. Take 320 mg of an 85% liposterolic extract a day.

**Essential oils:** Mix 5 drops of rosemary, thyme, cedarwood, and lavender in your shampoo and massage your head with the mixture for 10 minutes every night. This will help by increasing circulation to your head.

## HOMEOPATHY

 Although it is quite normal and natural to have some degree of hair loss as new hair grows, signs of noticeable or dramatic hair loss can cause a great deal of stress and emotional trauma. Men are more prone to hair loss than women (think of the term male pattern baldness), but this does not mean that women are immune. Common reasons for significant hair loss include stress and emotional trauma, nutritional deficiencies, skin conditions that especially affect the scalp such as psoriasis, taking drugs such as chemotherapy, an imbalance in thyroid gland functioning, pregnancy, and menopause. For any of these cases, it will be beneficial to seek help from a homeopathic practitioner who will target treatment to support the body in coping with the situation. If, however, the problem is a milder one, using the most appropriate homeopathic remedy from those listed below may be helpful.

**Calc carb:** This remedy is appropriate if mild hair loss occurs approaching menopause, together with a noticeable sense that the system is sluggish, easily exhausted, and prone to hot flashes that leave the body feeling chilled and clammy following the slightest physical effort. The head and scalp are likely to be especially prone to feeling sweaty.

**Natrum mur:** This is especially well indicated where mild hair loss sets in after emotional stress or grief, especially if feelings have been suppressed rather than expressed and worked through. Skin will show general tendencies to dry, sensitive patches, while the scalp will be prone to areas of dandruff and scaling, especially around the hairline.

**Sepia:** Consider using Sepia if hair loss follows a phase of major transition in hormone levels, such as following the birth of a baby or during menopause. This remedy is well indicated if there is an overwhelming tendency to feel stressed and exhausted on emotional, mental, and physical levels.

## HERBALISM

Some herbalists feel that hair loss which occurs because of illness or emotional stress is most amenable to treatment by herbal medicines.

**Topical lotions and creams:** The following herbs are used either singly or in combination to address hair loss: nettle leaf, birch leaves, burdock root, gentian tincture, lavender oil, and essential oil from the rhizomes of calamus. The use of alcohol on the scalp may increase hair loss, so it is preferable to boil these plants in water, or olive or almond oil, and then apply the mixture to the scalp. You can also use a lotion that contains one or several of the above plants and apply it regularly to the affected area.

**Bayberry bark:** Boil approximately 50 g of bayberry bark powder in 2 cups of distilled water for 15 minutes. Strain the mixture and allow it to cool. Add enough glycerine to make up 2 full cups. The resulting liquid can be rubbed into the scalp at night with a few drops of lavender oil and washed off in the morning.

> **TIP:** ADD ROSEMARY OIL TO LOTIONS
> Rosemary oil can be added in small amounts to hair lotions to prevent premature male baldness, possibly by helping to stimulate hair growth activity.

# IMPETIGO

## DIAGNOSIS

Impetigo is a common skin disease caused by a bacterial infection. Bacteria infect broken skin by entering through cuts, grazes, and cold sores. It usually first occurs around the nose and mouth, appearing as an area of reddened skin that then develops into a crop of blisters. It sometimes spreads to the rest of the body. Mostly affecting children, impetigo is easily spread through contact, and there tend to be outbreaks in nurseries and schools. If your child has eczema, he or she is particularly at risk of impetigo as it can be a complication that develops from constantly scratching the skin. The condition is not dangerous, but it is highly contagious. It is important to avoid touching the affected area to avoid spreading the infection, and children with the condition should be isolated until it clears up. Keeping the skin clean is also important in treating and preventing impetigo, and in stopping the condition from spreading.

## SYMPTOMS

- First appears as a small scratch or an itchy patch of reddened skin
- A small red, itchy spot develops into a blister containing a clear liquid
- The blister spreads into a small crop of blisters, which become crusty and weep, in the same place or on other parts of the body
- Usually occurs first on the face, especially around the corners of the mouth, the nose, and the back of the ears
- A scabby, itchy yellow crust that forms over the affected area
- In severe cases, feelings of being unwell
- Raised temperature
- Swollen lymph glands

## TREATMENT GOAL

To eliminate the rash, thereby eradicating the infecting organism, and preventing the spread of infection.

## CONVENTIONAL MEDICINE

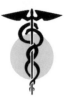

Impetigo is an infection of the skin. There are two types, bullous (with blisters) and non-bullous. They are both caused by the bacterium Staphylococcus aureus. Many physicians choose to treat impetigo with ointment, but in more severe cases oral antibiotics are necessary. However, there are also other simple treatments to control this condition.

**Antibiotics:** Topical antibiotics in the form of a cream or oral antibiotics are prescribed for this condition. The type of antibiotic used depends on how extensive the rash is and what environment the patient is in. Oral antibiotics will prevent the rash from spreading more effectively than topical antibiotics. The most common topical antibiotic used is mupirocin ointment. Success rates are more than 90% with this particular antibiotic if it is used twice a day for a period of two weeks. If the rash is extensive, erythromycin is the antibiotic most frequently used, usually for a period of about seven days. Sometimes the bacteria can become resistant to erythromycin and a cephalosporin is used. Penicillin and amoxicillin are not generally used because impetigo is often resistant to these antibiotics. Symptoms should completely resolve in around 7–10 days.

**Antibacterial soap:** Washing with antibacterial soaps and soaking the affected area with wet compresses to remove the crusts should be practiced in addition to using antibiotics. Good hygiene is also an important part of preventing a recurrence of the condition.

## TRADITIONAL CHINESE MEDICINE

**Herbs:**
• Xia Gu Cao: Literally translated to "summer-withered herb," Xia Gu Cao's pharmaceutical name is *Spica prunellae vulgaris*. This herb grows in most climates and is widely available in powder, bulk, or syrup form from Chinese herbalists. Take 1 tbsp of the syrup three times a day, or drink 1 cup of tea made from 12 g of the dried herb three times a day. Research has shown that Xia Gu Cao has broad antibiotic effects and is anti-staphylococci, which is the pathogen that causes impetigo.
• Shan Huang Shan: This patent powder form may not be carried widely by Chinese herbalists, but is available online. Take 1–3 g of the powder and apply it to the surface of impetigo. Cover the area with a sterilized cloth pad and tape it down to keep the pad in place. Change the pad twice a day. This should help the impetigo to heal and you should see a gradual improvement. If the condition does not seem to be improving after three days, or it is getting worse, make an appointment to see a dermatologist to discuss treatment.

**Acupuncture:** To treat impetigo, an acupuncturist will approach the condition by cleaning the pathogenic heat and stimulating the body's immune system. The points used will be on the arms and legs. You may have acupuncture treatment twice a week, with each session taking about ½ an hour. Combining acupuncture and herbal medicine to treat impetigo is a much better approach than using either method of treatment on its own.

**Diet:** Include plenty of mung beans, red adzuki beans, bean spouts, wax gourd, pears, watermelon, purslane, and duck meat in your diet. These foods are recommended for treating impetigo because they have cooling properties and dispel heat and damp. Avoid rich, fatty foods and deep-fried and roast cooking methods. Also avoid food that has heat and warming properties, such as shrimp, onion, and chili pepper.

## NATUROPATHY

**Diet:** Eat a gluten-free diet for six weeks, omitting wheat, rye, oats, and barley. After six weeks introduce one food at a time and note any changes with the impetigo. Avoid dairy products, sugar, white flour, hydrogenated and saturated fats, fried foods, and processed foods, as they are common food allergens.

**Supplements:** Vitamin E taken at 400 IU a day relieves itchiness and dryness. Take vitamin A at 100,000 IU for one month, then bring the dosage down to 50,000 IU for two weeks, then to 25,000 IU for long-term maintenance. Pregnant women should not take more than 10,000 IU of vitamin A a day. Vitamin A is essential for smooth skin and aids in relieving dryness. It is advised that vitamin A be taken with the supervision of knowledgable doctor as it is potentially toxic in large doses. Take 30 mg of zinc three times a day to raise immunity and aid the skin in healing. Eveing primrose oil contains gamma linoleic oil (GLA), which is an essential anti-inflammatory for the skin.

**Herbs:** Burdock root is a great skin detoxifier. Adults should take 4 ml of tincture or 500 mg in capsule form three times a day; children should take 0.5 ml or 150 mg twice a day. Calendula gel or cream is a mild antiseptic and helps to soothe the skin.

## HOMEOPATHY

This acute bacterial infection of the skin commonly occurs in children, but adults are also susceptible. Any of the following homeopathic remedies can be used to speed up recovery from infection. They can be used as a first resort or in combination with conventional treatment in a complementary, supportive role.

**Calendula:** In addition to taking a homeopathic remedy orally, it can be helpful to apply a diluted tincture of calendula to the infected areas. Dilute one part of tincture in 10 parts of boiled, cooled water and swab the affected areas as often as feels soothing during the day. Calendula can play an important antiseptic role while also speeding up the healing of tissue.

**Arsenicum album:** This remedy should be considered for children who are pale, chilly, and anxious, and prostrated as a result of being "run down." Blisters especially affect the area around the mouth and lips and burn violently. Discomfort from burning may be soothed temporarily by warm compresses.

**Antimonium crudum:** This remedy is especially well indicated where yellow, crusted eruptions affect the cheeks and the chin. The latter may be covered by small, sore, honey-colored granules for cold bathing or for becoming over-heated. Children feel unusually cross, peevish, and weepy when it is time to be washed.

## HERBALISM

**Poultices:** A variety of poultices and compresses have been traditionally used help to draw out infections and soothe the redness and inflammation associated with impetigo. Chop up a whole marshmallow plant and let 25–30 g stand in 4 cups of cold water for a few hours. Either apply this thick mixture to the skin directly (as a poultice) or soak a clean cloth or piece of gauze in this mixture and apply it to the area (as a compress) several times a day. To make a violet compress, add 25–30 g of the flowers to 5 cups of hot water. Let them steep for five minutes, strain the liquid and let it cool until it is hot to the touch, but not hot enough to burn the skin. Soak a clean cloth or piece of gauze in the liquid and apply it to the infected area.

**Flowering dogwood:** Also known as American boxwood, false box, rose willow, and silky cornel, flowering dogwood can be used topically to alleviate infections on the skin. Boil 5 tsp of plant material in 200 ml (about 1 cup) of water. Let the plant steep for a few minutes before straining the liquid. Soak a clean cloth or piece of gauze in the liquid and apply it to the affected area.

**Butternut:** This plant can heal the skin from infections such as impetigo. Boil 2 tbsp of butternut root in 2 cups of water for 10 minutes. Strain the liquid and drink the tea. The tea can also be applied to the infected area as a poultice, or a tincture of the root, available from herb stores, can be taken internally three times a day to facilitate skin healing by, it is theorized, cleansing the blood by improving liver function.

# INGROWN TOENAIL

## DIAGNOSIS

Ingrown nails affect the skin surrounding the nail, causing localized swelling and some pain and discomfort. When one occurs, it usually affects the nail on the big toe. The corner of the nail digs into the skin and breaks the surface, sometimes leading to infection and inflamed tissue. Pus or fluid can ooze from the affected area and there can sometimes also be an unpleasant smell. Although the nail looks like it is growing into the skin, its growth is perfectly normal. This condition arises mainly from neglect of the feet, poor hygiene, and incorrect trimming of the toenails, which should always be trimmed straight across. It is also best to avoid cutting the toenails too short. Unsuitable footwear that is either too tight or too narrow can cause a build-up of pressure around the toes, as can repetitive exercise, which can lead to ingrown toenails. If the condition has progressed too far, a minor operation may be necessary, where the nail is removed and antibiotics are prescribed.

## SYMPTOMS

- Pain and discomfort around a nail
- Localized swelling

## TREATMENT GOAL

To ease the pain of an ingrown nail and bring relief.

## CONVENTIONAL MEDICINE

**Prevention:** To help prevent regrowth, follow up the procedure with proper hygiene and trimming to ensure the nail grows straight. If there are signs of regrowth, a thin piece of cotton wool or a piece or gauze may be used as a wedge under the nail to prevent recurrence.

**Epsom salt soaks:** If it is caught early, an ingrown toenail can be encouraged out of the skin with daily 10-minute epsom salt foot soaks followed by trimming back the nail.

**Have your doctor remove the ingrown nail:** If the nail is too deeply embedded in the skin, you will not be able to rectify the problem simply by clipping. Infection (often with a fungus) of an ingrown nail sometimes necessitates the partial or complete removal of the affected toenail. Usually, this involves a simple 15-minute procedure that can be performed in the doctor's office. The procedure does not require fasting and no special arrangements are needed following the procedure. If you are on blood-thinning medications, such as warfarin or asprin, or a herbal supplement that affects bleeding, such as ginger, garlic, ginkgo, feverfew, ginseng, fish oil, or nattokinase, it should be stopped three days before the procedure. Also, if you are on a steroid or another medication that affects the immune system, consult with your physician about the risks and benefits of having the procedure while on the medication to avoid infection. The procedure itself usually involves numbing the toe with the local anesthetic lidocaine, without epinephrine (adrenaline). Receiving the anesthetic is the most discomfort you will experience during the procedure (much like a dental operation), as it thoroughly numbs the skin so that you cannot feel pain. After the local anaesthetic injection, a special type of scissor is used to lift and cut the nail. The site is then bandaged and a topical antibiotic ointment may be applied daily for five days, or the site can simply be kept clean and dry.

**Phenol:** Sometimes, for recurrent ingrown toenail or for infections, after the nail is clipped a chemical, phenol, is applied to kill the nail bed so that the nail never regrows.

**See a specialist:** Your doctor may refer you to a specialist for treatment of an ingrown toenail if you have peripheral vascular disease, compromised wound healing such as occurs in diabetes, or a condition that requires blood-thinning medication.

**Anti-inflammatories:** Complications of the procedure are very rare, but these may include mild pain within the first 24 hours. This can be treated with an over-the-counter or herbal anti-inflammatory medication. Bleeding may sometimes occur after the procedure, but it should stop within a few hours. If it does not, call the doctor. No sensation changes should occur after the nail has healed.

## TRADITIONAL CHINESE MEDICINE

**Herbal foot soak:** Combine 30 g of Ji Xue Teng (spatholobus or millettia root and vine), 30 g of Xuan Shen (ningpo figwort root), and 20 g of Yan Hu Suo (corydalis rhizome) in a ceramic pot. Boil the herbs in 5 cups of water for five minutes and then simmer for 20 minutes. Strain the liquid and allow it to cool to a warm temperature. Soak your feet in the liquid for 20–30 minutes a day. If the area is infected, add 20 g of Huang Bai (phellodendron) and 20 g of Huang Qin (baical skullcap root) to 1 cup of water. Make a decoction and soak the foot. Treatment can ease the pain caused by an ingrown toenail, and promote local circulation.

**Acupuncture:** Treatment can relieve pain and prevent nails from becoming ingrown by regulating the imbalanced energy and guiding energy flow in the right direction. Moxibustion (see p.29 ) may also be applied for this condition.

**Diet:** Try to choose foods that are rich in vitamin B and which tonify blood and strengthen bones, such as red adzuki beans, kidney beans, soybeans, spinach, dark-green vegetables, fish, seafood, lamb meat, chicken, beef, and pork. It is recommended that you eat soup made from meat bones for natural calcium intake. Use any meat bones. Add water, salt, and a few drops of vinegar and boil on a low heat. You will get a delicious bone broth. Either drink the broth directly or use it for cooking.

**TIP:** VINEGAR FOOT SOAK
Add 2 tbsp of vinegar to 800 ml of warm water. Soak the foot that has an ingrown toenail once a day for 15 minutes. If the skin becomes irritated, use only 1 tbsp of vinegar or discontinue treatment.

## NATUROPATHY

**Prevention:** To prevent ingrown toenails from occurring, practice good nail care, with proper trimming and minimized pressure from shoes.

**Trim the toenail:** Trim the nail in a shallow U-shape across the top, leaving it squared off at the corners. Slip a few fibers of cotton under the edge of the nail to stop it from digging into the flesh. Trim the ends of the cotton short so that they are not in the way, and so they can remain in place for several days, or even weeks. This method of treatment separates the nail from the lateral nail groove, allowing injured tissue to heal, while encouraging the nail to grow normally.

## HOMEOPATHY

Here the main scope of homeopathic support is to act as a complementary treatment to speed up recovery after the offending edge of the nail has been dealt with. Choose from any of the following remedies, depending on how the treated area is feeling.

**Arnica:** This is one of the primary first aid remedies to consider whenever the body has sustained a trauma. It can be given before and after surgery, or to treat any minor accident that results in tenderness and bruising. Use this remedy if there is a great localized tenderness with pain that feels sore and achy in nature.

**Hypericum:** This remedy follows Arnica well and can be used to great effect where there is trauma and injury to areas that are especially well-served with nerve endings, such as the fingers and toes. This remedy is called for if you have sharp, shooting pains that are very sensitive to jarring movements of any kind.

## HERBALISM

Herbal medicines can help to ease the pain, swelling, and possible infection associated with an ingrown toenail. Internal doses of other herbs could be helpful if an obvious infection is present.

**Tea tree oil:** Place 2–3 drops of tea tree oil on a cotton swab and gently press the inflamed skin away from the toenail several times a day. This will not only mechanically help to correct the ingrown skin, but the tea tree oil will infuse the area and its antiseptic properties will address any infection. It is important to buy pure tea tree oil from a reputable manufacturer to avoid using a sub-standard and ineffective product that may have been diluted.

**Burdock root:** A salve of burdock can be applied to the skin over inflamed and infected ingrown nails to help resolve the problem. Macerate the burdock root and mix it with either a small amount of water to make a thick paste, or an anti-inflammatory oil such as castor. Apply the salve to the affected area two or three times a day until there is a reduction in swelling or redness. It may help to cover the paste with an occlusive dressing, such as a thick cloth or even a plastic bag, while you sleep so that the burdock draws out the infection all night.

# JAUNDICE

## DIAGNOSIS

Jaundice is not a disease in itself but the result of a disorder elsewhere in the body, usually the liver, that leads to a yellow appearance of the skin and whites of the eyes. It is a serious condition and should always be investigated by a doctor. The condition arises when the blood contains an excess of the pigment bilirubin, a natural product that arises from the normal breakdown of red blood cells in the body and is excreted in the bile, through the actions of the liver. The relationship between the manufacture and breakdown of red blood cells is normally precisely balanced, but there are several conditions in which the rate of breakdown increases. If the amount of bilirubin released exceeds the liver's capacity to break it down, then jaundice will develop. It is the raised level of bilirubin that gives the skin its distinctive yellow color.

Although jaundice is most often the result of a disorder affecting the liver, it can also be caused by a variety of other conditions affecting, for example, the blood or spleen. It should be thoroughly investigated so that the underlying cause can be identified and treated. It can be an indication of hepatitis, gallstones, cirrhosis of the liver, and cancer. Blood tests may be used to make a diagnosis. The condition is quite common in newborn babies, particularly those that are premature, because their immature livers are not able to cope with the higher than usual rate of breakdown of red blood cells in the first few weeks of life. Light therapy treatment where the baby is exposed to powerful UV light is normally enough to treat the condition.

## SYMPTOMS

- Yellowing of the whites of the eyes
- Yellowing of the skin
- Urine darker than normal

## TREATMENT GOAL

Jaundice is always a sign of a more significant problem in the body and it should never be ignored. Treatment aims to isolate and resolve the cause.

## CONVENTIONAL MEDICINE

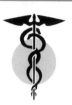

**In newborn babies:** Jaundice is very common in newborns. Sixty percent of newborns develop jaundice during the first week of life. Referred to as physiologic jaundice, it generally progresses from the face to the feet and resolves by itself within 7–10 days. Placing the baby in sunlight (near a window for example) so that skin is exposed, while monitoring temperatures carefully, can help to resolve the jaundice. Helping the baby clear the jaundice through the stool and urine by frequent feedings of breast milk or formula, with feedings of sterile water in between, is a worthwhile therapy. Babies who are breastfed tend to develop a type of jaundice known as feeding jaundice during the first week of life. It is not threatening and usually resolves on its own. The techniques described above can be used to help resolve breastfeeding jaundice. Some rare but dangerous causes of newborn jaundice are severe hemolytic disease of the newborn, some infections, and bilirubin conjugation abnormalities, which are diseases the baby is born with. These are all cases that require medical treatment. The baby should be taken to the doctor as soon as any signs of jaundice are apparent so that the type of jaundice can be determined and the level of the jaundice can be measured. If the level gets too high, whatever the cause, a condition exists in which the brain can be damaged from too high a level of bilirubin. This is called kernicterus. The doctor may just observe the baby, while encouraging frequent feeding and exposure to light. The baby may also be treated with phototherapy, where the baby is placed under artificial lights for at least 12 hours a day. This almost always works and the benefits are usually seen within two days. If this does not work, or if the level of bilirubin is too high even for this procedure, than an exchange transfusion is the treatment of choice. With this treatment, the dangerous blood in the baby's body is replaced with blood that does not have a high level of bilirubin.

**In children or adults:** Adult or early childhood jaundice is usually related to a problem of the liver. These problems are varied and complicated and you should consult your doctor. Treatment depends on the exact nature of the liver problem, but may include phototherapy or addressing liver dysfunction.

## TRADITIONAL CHINESE MEDICINE

Before treating jaundice, a professional consultation is recommended. Herbal treatment should be carried out under the supervision and observation of a medical doctor, and is best combined with acupuncture. Stronger herbal decoctions than those described below can be prescribed by an experienced traditional Chinese medicine doctor.

**Herbs:**
• Yin Chen tea: Yin Chen Hao (artemisia shoots and leaves) and capillaries have proven to be effective herbs for treating jaundice. Since the plant tastes bitter, you can take it with Jin Qian Cao (lysimachia), which has a sweeter taste. To make a tea put 5–6 g of each (one day's dose) in 2–4 cups of boiled water. Drink the tea three or four times a day.
• Long Dan Xie Gan Wan: You can take this patent Chinese medicine pill with the Yin Chen tea. Use Yin Chen tea and/or Long Dan Xie Gan Wan for three to five days.

**Acupuncture:** In traditional Chinese medicine, jaundice is considered a heat and dampness condition. An experienced acupuncturist will treat jaundice with the principle of reinforcing the spleen and reducing liver and gallbladder technique.

**Acupressure:** The Hegu points are located on your hands in the depression between the thumb and the index finger. The Feng Long point is on the front of the shin, half way between the knee and foot and about 1½ inches towards the outside of the large leg bone (tibia). Press the Hegu and Feng Long points with your thumb for five minutes two or three times a day. This will help the body to detox the damp and heat that causes jaundice.

**Diet:** Water and cooked spinach, celery, bamboo shoots, coix seeds, carp, red adzuki beans, and wax gourds induce urination, which is helpful in treating a jaundice condition. Avoid greasy, fatty, spicy, and raw food.

## NATUROPATHY

**Diet:** Eat plenty of unrefined foods. Avoid hydrogenated oils, which tend to form fat around the liver, making it less effective. The over-consumption of alcohol should be avoided as alcohol is a major cause of liver problems.

**Herbs:** Take 4 g of dandelion root or 8 ml three times a day. This herb increases the production and enhances the flow of bile. Milk thistle should be standardized based on its sylimarin content. Take 150 mg three times a day. Milk thistle is the most common and potent protective liver herb known. Artichoke leaves can be taken as a liver tonic. This herb should be standardized to 15% cynarin. Take 500 mg a day.

## HOMEOPATHY

If jaundice develops in adults, it is a sign of an underlying condition, such as hepatitis, or liver or gallbladder disease. Assessment and treatment needs to come from an experienced homeopathic practitioner who may need to work together with your family doctor and/or a hospital consultant. The following are possible remedies that practitioners may consider.

**Chelidonium:** This remedy is thought to have a particular role to play in treating diseases of the liver and gallbladder. As a result, it is used for symptoms of yellowness and biliousness. If pains from the liver move in a backward direction to the area between the shoulder blades, or are especially located around the area of the right shoulder blade, chelidonium may be used. Lying on the stomach helps, while moving around or coughing makes the pain and distress worse.

**Lycopodium:** This remedy also has a reputation for aiding liver function, and can have a positive role to play in cases of hepatitis. Use this remedy if pain and soreness are more intense on the right side, with a great deal of gastric distress including distention, lack of appetite, and burning pains that may settle behind the breast bone or between the shoulder blades.

## HERBALISM

All cases of jaundice need a thorough conventional medicine evaluation to determine the cause. There are many serious maladies associated with jaundice that could be life threatening or cause future disability and suffering if the definitive treatment is ignored or delayed by beginning therapy with botanical medicines. That said, the remedies below can be useful as additional therapies to the conventional medicine approach.

**Treating the gall bladder and bile duct:** There are two categories of herbs that are used in cases of jaundice stemming from problems with the gall bladder or bile duct system: choleretics and cholagogues. Choleretics are plants that cause the liver cells to make more bile and cholegogues are plants that cause the release of bile that has already been formed. Both of these categories of herbs increase the flow of bile that may help to clean out the bile duct system or gallbladder. Examples of choleretics are dandelion root and Culver's root. Examples of cholagogues are dandelion root, tumeric, licorice, Globe artichoke, and tetterwort or celandine. These plants work best if taken 20–30 minutes before meals, and if the person is not constipated. An increase bile flow must be followed by regular bowel movements so that the bile is eliminated from the body and not simply recycled to contribute yet again to bile stagnation and jaundice.

**Treating toxic damage:** Sometimes jaundice occurs because of toxic damage to the liver cells. This can occur from acute or chronic exposure to such toxins as alcohol, chemicals (paints or industrial solvents), or poisonous mushrooms. The primary solution to jaundice of this type, of course, is to stop exposure to these substances. Herbs that can be used to support a person's system and protect the liver until healing is able to occur include tumeric, licorice, schisandra, Globe artichoke, and milk thistle.

# LICE, HEAD

## DIAGNOSIS

Head lice or nits are a very common condition in children, particularly those of nursery and primary school age. They transfer rapidly and easily from head to head by crawling (they can't jump or fly), so children that tend to sit and play in close proximity with other children are more susceptible. A louse is smaller than a match head but still visible. It bites the scalp and feeds on the blood it sucks out. It doesn't matter whether hair is clean or dirty, long, curly, or straight. Lice like warmth so live close to the scalp, clinging to the hair shaft.

Head lice produce a glue-like substance with which they fix their eggs to hair. It is hard to spot the eggs but easier to spot the empty shells once the eggs have hatched, which takes roughly 7–10 days. The empty shells are referred to as "nits." Since head lice transfer easily from head to head, it is usually recommended that the whole family is treated if one member becomes affected, as well as everyone the affected child has been in contact with—don't forget grandparents and childminders.

## SYMPTOMS

- Constant scratching of the head
- A red and irritated scalp
- Specks of white on your child's hair that look similar to dandruff. These are the tiny empty shells attached to the hair shaft near the scalp
- Red rash on the nape of the neck and behind the ears
- Occasionally, swollen glands if the skin becomes infected

## TREATMENT GOAL

Once the presence of lice has been confirmed by inspecting the scalp, treatment aims to rid the affected child of the lice and eggs, and prevent them from spreading to other members of the family.

## CONVENTIONAL MEDICINE

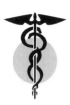

**Wet comb the hair:** Special combs are available to help remove lice and their eggs from the hair. This procedure requires a good light touch and non-tangled hair, so use plenty of conditioner—those containing Neem seed oil are especially good as Neem is a natural, plant-based insecticide and repellent. Use a methodical combing practice, dividing the hair into sections and working through each section systematically to remove lice and eggs.

**Pesticides:** Used topically, the most natural of these are pyrethrins (permethrin), which are derived from chrysanthemums. Malathion is an organophosphate. Although organophosphates are toxic to the environment, no neuro toxicity has been reported in humans as a result of topical lice treatment. Lindane is a strong ohanochloride pesticide. Its use has become less desirable because of several reports of toxicity in the elderly, but it is still a treatment choice for small areas of the skin for less than 10 minutes at a time, which is how it is used to treat head lice. Ivermectin is a newer option that is effective and has virtually no side effects. It is currently being investigated for use on head lice.

## TRADITIONAL CHINESE MEDICINE

**Herbs:** It is not common to treat head lice with herbs, but this external herbal formula is helpful. Combine 50 g Ku Shen (sophora root), 15 g of Bai Pu (stemona root), and 15 g Jing Jie (schizonepeta stem and bud), both available in bulk from Chinese herbalists, in a ceramic pot. Add 5–6 cups of water, boil, and then simmer for 30 minutes. Strain the liquid and soak the hair in the herbal liquid for 10 minutes. The liquid should also be rubbed into the scalp. The scalp will feel less itchy and it will have a cool, refreshing effect. These herbs may also kill the lice and their eggs. Repeat this herbal wash three times, once a day.

**Acupuncture and acupressure:** It is not appropriate to treat head lice with acupuncture, nor acupressue.

## NATUROPATHY

**Anise, ylang ylang, and coconut oils:** Mix 10 drops of ylang ylang, 10 drops of anise, 20 drops of coconut oils, and 1–2 oz of a base oil (such as almond or apricot oil). Combine these oils in a plastic spray bottle and spray the mixture onto the hair twice a day, leaving it in for two hours each time before washing the hair thoroughly. You can cover the hair with a towel or shower cap while the mixture is on. Make sure you comb the hair well after you wash it to make sure the lice and nits are removed.

**Garlic:** Garlic has antiparasitic properties and will help your child's body fight a head lice infestation. Mix 10 drops of garlic oil with 2 oz of olive oil. Rub this mixture into the hair and scalp for five minutes and leave on overnight.

**Goldenseal:** Goldenseal has antimicrobial properties. Mix 20 drops of goldenseal in two cups of water and use to wash the scalp.

**Tea tree oil:** This strong herbal disinfectant will help get rid of head lice. Add 25 drops to 2 oz of olive oil. Rub this mixture into the affected scalp twice a day. Leave it in the hair for two hours each time before washing the hair thoroughly. Make sure you comb the hair after you wash it to make sure that all the lice and nits are removed.

**Prevention:** Vigilant combing with a fine-toothed comb will help treat and prevent infections. Bedding and clothing needs to be washed and preferably dried in a tumble dryer for at least 20 minutes. Brushes, combs, and hair accessories should be soaked in hot water for 20 minutes. Items that cannot be exposed to hot water or to the heat of a dryer may be kept isolated for two weeks to prevent any chance of re-infection from nits that may be present. Vacuum carpets and upholstery.

## HOMEOPATHY

Homeopathic self-prescribing is not the most appropriate measure for isolated instances of head lice, since the first priority should be the localized treatment of the head and scalp. If, once the acute episode has been dealt, you find that your child seems to be especially prone to head lice, consult a homeopathic practitioner.

## HERBALISM

**Anise:** As with scabies, anise essential oil can be used topically. Apply it directly to the scalp two to three times a day, keeping in mind that the most common side effects are irritation and dermatitis. It may help to incorporate essential oil of anise into a gentle shampoo that is easier for the scalp to tolerate but will still kill the head lice.

**Chrysanthemum:** Chrysanthemum produces natural insecticides called pyrethrins. Pyrethrin extracts, in concentrations in the range of 0.15–0.30%, have been used in the treatment of head lice. Many over-the-counter shampoos designed to treat head lice contain pyrethrins as the active component. However, do not ingest or inhale these compounds, and avoid them altogether if your child has asthma or is allergic to plants such as marigolds, daisies, and ragweed. Consult a medical herbalist before this treatment.

# NAIL PROBLEMS

## DIAGNOSIS

The condition of your nails can be a good indication of your general health, with strong, pink, healthy-looking nails being a sign that all is well on the inside. Nail problems are usually caused by inflammation of the skin around the nail, fungus, or by an infection. They can also be symptomatic of other illnesses such as anemia, psoriasis, and fungal infection, and more serious conditions such as heart disease and diabetes. Nutritional deficiencies can cause the condition of your nails to deteriorate, and nails can also be affected by stress. Unsightly nail problems rarely have far-reaching concerns, but nevertheless if you feel that your nails do not look healthy it can indicate a larger problem that requires prompt attention.

## SYMPTOMS

- Itchy inflamed skin around the nail
- Pitted nails
- Blisters around the nail
- Painful nails
- Nails that are thickened and discolored—often yellowed
- Occasionally pus is present

## TREATMENT GOAL

To find the cause of the nail problem and rectify it, at the same time being aware that poor nail condition can be an indication of larger health issues.

Nail abnormalities are a symptom of several diseases and treatment usually involves treating the underlying illness. Nail condition can change for a variety of reasons. Fungal infections of the nail manifesting as thick, yellow, flaking nails are common and generally require oral antifungals once the infection is fully established. If you catch an infection in the early stages, however, tea tree oil can be an effective antifungal.

**If nails are lined:** Many diseases cause changes in the nail. Beau's lines are linear depressions in the nails that appear at the lunula (the moon-shaped area at the base of the nail). They tend to materialize a few weeks after a stressful event interrupts nail formation. Eventually they disappear and no treatment is necessary. They are seen in response to diseases such as syphilis, diabetes, infections of the heart, and diseases that are marked by high fever. They also often occur in response to chemotherapy drugs. Zinc deficiency can cause these lines and can be treated with daily supplementation.

**If nails appear yellow:** Discoloration of the nails (or yellow nail syndrome) occurs in response to some respiratory diseases. Treatment of the disease is needed to reverse the condition, but sometimes spontaneous healing occurs. Mixed tocopherols are the active ingredient in vitamin E. Taking vitamin E as natural mixed tocopherols, rather than just alpha tocopherols, in amounts of about 1,000 IU a day may help. Tea tree oil can be used to prevent progression to fungal infections.

**If nails are spoon shaped:** Spoon shaped nails with a central depression and that curve up at the ends can be normal in children and may persist throughout life, but can also be associated with iron deficiency anemia—the treatment of which is ferrous sulfate. Ferrous gluconate may give fewer gastrointestinal side effects. Copper is needed to help the body utilize iron. Iron should not be given randomly to people with spoon nails since this condition can also occur in people with hemochromatosis, which is an accumulation of iron and in which case iron is contraindicated.

**If nails change color:** Changes in the color of the nail are commonly associated with different toxicities, nutritional insufficiencies, and other organ dysfunction. For example anemia can be associated with diffuse white lines in the nail bed, for which treatment is as described above. Arsenic toxicity gives Mees lines or transverse white lines. This is treated by removing the source of arsenic from the body. Blue nails can be seen with antibiotic treatment, specifically minocycline and in medications used to treat AIDS. Longitudinal black bands are seen in diseases of the adrenal glands. Treatment involves diagnosis and treatment of the specific disease. Longitudinal brown bands are seen normally in about 90% of African Americans and other Afro-Caribbean peoples.

## TRADITIONAL CHINESE MEDICINE

**Herbs:**

• To treat pale nails and thin nails: Combine 10 g of Shan Zhu Yu (Asiatic cornelian cherry fruit), 12 g of Dang Gui (Chinese angelica root), 15 g of Shu Di Huang (Chinese foxglove), 15 g of Dan Shen (salvia root), 12 g of Gou Ji Zi (wolfberry), 12 g of Ji Shen (jilin root), and 15 g of Ji Xie Teng (milletia root). These herbs, available from Chinese pharmacies, are proven to nourish blood and improve circulation, which will benefit nails. To make a decoction, place the herbs in a ceramic or glass pot, add 4 cups of water, and bring the mixture to a boil. Let the liquid simmer for 30 minutes before straining it. Drink 1 cup twice a day. Take this formula for one to three months; nails should become visibly stronger during this time.

• To treat thick and ridged nails: Combine 15 g of Xuan Shen (ningpo figwort root), 12 g of Chi Shao (red peony root), 12 g of Bai Shao (white peony root), 12 g of Shan Zhu Yu (Asiatic cornelian cherry fruit), and 12 g of Dang Gui (Chinese angelica root) in a ceramic or glass pot. Add 4 cups of water, bring the liquid to a boil, and let it simmer for 30 minutes. Strain the liquid and drink 1 cup twice a day. Take this formula for one to three months.

• To treat dry nails that break easily: Combine 18 g of Shu Di Huang (Chinese foxglove), 15 g of Shan Shen (mountain root), 12 g of Du Zhong (eucommia bark), 20 g of Mu Li (oyster shell), 15 g of Mai Men Dong (ophiopogon tuber), and 15 g of Tian Men Dong (asparagus tuber) in a ceramic or glass pot. Add 4 cups of water, bring the liquid to a boil, and let it simmer for 30 minutes. Strain and drink 1 cup of the liquid twice a day for one to three months. These herbs will tonify and strengthen the kidney energy, which is important for healthy nails.

**Acupuncture:** To treat nail problems, a well-trained acupuncturist will collect information on the patient's general health. The practitioner will then treat the underlying problem with some local points that promote circulation to nails.

**Acupressure:** Press Ba Xie and Ba Fen points. The four Ba Xie points are located on the backs of the hands, between the bases of each of the fingers. The four Ba Fen points are found on the instep of the foot between the bases of each of the toes. Use your fingers to press each point with gentle pressure for 30 seconds to one minute, twice a day. This will help to promote circulation to the nails, aiding in the healing process. **Caution:** If you have a fungus infection on your nails, do not use acupressure because it may spread the infection.

**Diet:** Include foods in your diet that may help the blood and kidneys, and nourish the nails, such as duck, liver, loquat, persimmon, pineapple, chives, celery, grapes, lotus, yam, and tangerines.

## NATUROPATHY

**Diet:** Nail problems are often a sign of malnourishment. Look for good sources of protein, high-quality complex carbohydrates, and healthy fats and oils. Make sure you eat a well-balanced diet that includes plenty of fresh fruits and vegetables, whole grains, legumes, and quality protein (fish, lean chicken, and beans) everyday. Eat plenty of green leafy vegetables for their high nutrient content, which will provide a base of nutrients required for healthy nails.

**Supplements:** There is some scientific evidence that the B vitamin biotin may help treat nail problems, especially brittle nails. Preliminary evidence from one study suggests that biotin may increase the thickness of brittle nails, reduce their tendency to split, and improve their structure. Take 1,500 mcg twice a day for 8–12 weeks. Calcium will help treat dry and brittle nails. Take 600 mg of calcium along with 250 mg of magnesium, and 200 IU vitamin D a day. Magnesium and vitamin D help the body to absorb Calcium. Vitamin B-complex helps nails that are weak, and that have horizontal and vertical ridges. Take one 50 mg B-complex pill (which provides a full range of B vitamins) each morning with food. This pill, available from health food stores, should supply 50 mcg of vitamin B12 and biotin, 400 mcg of folic acid, and 50 mg of all other B vitamins. Vitamin C builds keratin and other proteins needed for healthy nails. Take 3,000 mg a day for 8–12 weeks. High dosages of vitamin C may soften your stool to the point of diarrhea. For most people 3,000 mg is tolerable, but if your stool softens, cut back to 1,000 mg.

**Herbs:** Horsetail is a good sources of silica, a mineral known to strengthen brittle nails. Take 1 g three times a day. Be cautious or avoid using horsetail if you have heart or kidney problems.

**General recommendations:** Do not expose your nails to too much soap and water. Water causes the nails to swell and to become loose from the nail bed, resulting in brittle nails. Do not cut cuticles as this may cause an infection. Instead use a gentle oil or cream to push them back. Do not repeatedly immerse your hands in harsh detergents as this results in split nails. Wear cotton-lined rubber gloves when doing housework.

## HOMEOPATHY

As with hair and skin, the strength, texture, and appearance of the nails can reveal a great deal about a person's general health to a complementary practitioner. If weak or brittle nails occur now and again, especially after a highly stressful time when healthy lifestyle choices such as good nutrition have suffered, taking one of the following homeopathic remedies can help the body to get back on track. However, complaints that include a long-term, deep-seated tendency to develop brittle, discolored, or mis-shapen nails indicate a chronic problem. This kind of condition will respond best to what is called "constitutional" prescribing that is aimed at improving the quality of health and vitality at all levels by getting the body, mind, and emotions into optimum balance.

**Prevention:** Avoid exposing the hands to strong detergents on a regular basis as this can dry out skin and nails. If nails are going through a weak period where they seem to be snapping regularly, massage a nourishing oil into the base of the nail and the cuticle before going to bed. Excellent choices include sweet almond oil or a specially formulated oil that has been designed for this purpose. These are often based on avocado or vitamin E oil.

**Silica:** Consider this remedy to treat nails that show recent signs of developing white flecks, and those that have become weak, yellowed, or mis-shapen. The nails may feel rough to the touch rather than smooth, and there may be a tendency to develop infections around the sides of the nails due to skin that is quick to become infected and slow to heal.

**Antimonium crudum:** Use this remedy for nails that are prone to slow growth, thickening, and splitting. There may also be a thickening of the skin underneath the affected nails. Problems with cracked skin and nails may be combined with symptoms of poor digestion and lack of appetite, with lots of bloating and burping.

**Belladonna:** This is useful where the first signs of swelling or infection have developed around the base of the nail and cuticle. The affected area is likely to look bright red and feel hot, sore, and throbbing. Taken at the first twinge, Belladonna will either resolve the situation, or move it on to the next stage of pus formation, where the remedy Hepar sulph will be helpful in resolving the problem.

**Hepar sulph:** This remedy is appropriate when pus-formation needs to be re-absorbed or dispersed. Pains around the edge or base of the nail are likely to feel sharp, sticking, and sore, and the affected area is hypersensitive.

## HERBALISM

Since nail problems can be the product of a variety of underlying conditions, it is important to understand the cause of your current nail problem in order to effectively treat it.

**Nettles:** For nails that are cracked, brittle, or weak, try drinking a tea of nettle leaf two to three times a day. Add 25–30 g of dried nettle leaf to 4 cups of hot water. Let the tea steep for 10 minutes before straining. Drink 1 cup of this tea two to three times daily. Nettle is generally considered as safe, but may cause a mild upset stomach. If adding horsetail as well, be sure to drink adequate amounts of water. Do not add horsetail if you have kidney or heart problems.

**Burdock root:** Many skin disorders can affect the nails and burdock root is an excellent choice under these circumstances. It can be taken internally as a tea or tincture, or it can be applied directly to the affected area as an essential oil, in an ointment, or in a poultice. There are no reported adverse reactions to burdock, however, burdock, as with all the other topically applied herbs, can potentially aggravate symptoms. If this does occur, discontinue use immediately.

**Garlic:** Often nail problems result from a fungus growing under the nail bed. As a result, many of the herbs mentioned as possible remedies for fungal infections may be useful for nail problems as well. Garlic is a powerful antifungal and general immune booster. It is an excellent first choice for the treatment of fungal infections. Crushed raw garlic can be applied directly to the affected area two to three times a day for one to two weeks, although the odor can be a deterrent. A more effective and tolerable method of delivery is a garlic gel, which can be purchased from your local health food stores. Ajoene, an organosulfur compound found in garlic, is known to have powerful antifungal properties and has been shown to work just as well as over-the-counter antifungal medications. Look for a gel containing 1% ajoene if possible, and apply it twice a day for one week to 10 days. Garlic can also be taken orally in capsule form. Take 500 mg twice a day. Garlic has virtually no side effects when used topically, although minor irritation of area where it is applied is sometimes reported. When taken internally at high, therapeutic doses, garlic may interfere with certain antithrombotic (bloodclotting) drugs.

**Tea tree oil:** This oil can be used topically as an antifungal and antibacterial agent. Apply it to the affected area either as a 5–15% tea tree oil solution, or as a 5–15% tea tree oil cream. This concentration has been shown to be effective in keeping the fungus from spreading and relieving any itchiness or associated skin irritation. A much stronger dose of either solution or cream is needed to produce a cure. Recommendations range from 25–100% strength two to three times a day. Dermatitis is the only significant side effect associated with the prolonged and repeated topical use of tea tree oil. Side effects such as nausea are associated with taking tea tree oil internally.

# PLANTAR WARTS

## DIAGNOSIS

Also known as a verruca, a plantar wart is found on the sole of the foot, and is particularly common in children. It is caused by a viral infection in the skin, which multiplies and spreads. A hard, black, horny swelling is produced, which is pushed under the skin by the pressure of walking. It manifests as a small, brown-black circle on a level with the surface of the skin. Sometimes you can also see tiny black spots. These are caused by bleeding in the plantar wart as a result of standing and walking on it. Plantar warts appear as areas of flat, thicker skin with a harder edge around a softer center. They are seen most commonly where the ball of the foot is exposed to pressure and are often sore to touch and to stand or walk on.

Plantar warts are rarely seen in children under the age of three, but after this age they can become more frequent, particularly if the child swims a lot, as changing rooms and communal pools are a breeding ground for this type of infection. The wart virus is very contagious. The skin cells on the warts contain thousands of viruses, which are released when the wart is touched to infect others. Those with scratches or cuts on the soles of their feet are especially vulnerable. It can take several months for plantar warts to develop after infection. Not everyone is susceptible to the virus. When children share bathrooms that contain wart viruses, some will contract plantar warts, while others seem to be immune. The reason for this variance in susceptibility is unknown.

## SYMPTOMS

- One or more circular lumps, which can be white, flesh-colored, or brown-black, on the sole of the foot, often no bigger than a pin prick
- Occasionally these may appear in clusters, known as a mosaic wart

## TREATMENT GOAL

To clear up the plantar wart and protect against further infections.

## CONVENTIONAL MEDICINE

**Duct tape occlusion:** Plantar warts that are not painful do not need to be treated, but can be removed through duct tape occlusion. Completely cover the area with duct tape for about one week. Remove the tape, soak the foot, and debride the area with a pumice stone. After a day, reapply the duct tape. Continue this treatment until the lesion is gone.

**Topical treatment:** Apply tretinoin cream before bed for several weeks. A 17% salicylic acid, obtained over the counter, can also be applied to a clean, dry foot twice a day. The area should be bandaged after treatment. Flourouracil cream (Efudex®), applied daily for three weeks, can also be applied to treat plantar warts. However, this treatment can lead to a darkening of the skin. If none of these treatments help, liquid nitrogen can be applied, or electrocautery can be performed. If all of these treatments fail, bleomycin, a chemotherapeutic agent, can be injected into the lesion.

**Surgical and laser therapy:** If the lesion is very large or does not respond to the above, the area may be cut off in the doctor's office using a scalpel or other surgical instrument such as a curette or an electrosurgical unit. For plantar warts that are painful, laser therapy can be used. This leaves a wound that takes four to six weeks to heal.

## TRADITIONAL CHINESE MEDICINE

**Herbs:** Although is not generally necessary to take internal Chinese medicine to treat plantar warts, if there are many sores that spread quickly, the following formulas can be used to help the body clean out the virus. The herbs listed below are available from Chinese herbalists or online.

• Herbal decoction: Mix 30 g of Ma Zhi Xian (dried purslane), 10 g of Zi Cao (groom well root), 30 g of Yi Yi Ren (seeds of Job's tears), and 10 g of Da Qin Ye (woad leaf) in a ceramic or glass pot. Add 3 cups of water, bring the mixutre to the boil, and simmer for 30 minutes. Strain the liquid and drink 1 cup three times a day for three to five days.

• Herbal body wash: Boil 15 g of Ma Zhi Xian (dried purslane), 8 g of Chen Pi (citrus peel), 15 g of She Chuang Zi (cnidium seed), 10 g of Ku Shen (sophora root), and 12 g of Bai Zhi (Chinese angelica root) in 5 cups of water. Strain the liquid and allow it to cook. Use the decoction to wash the body, or add it to bath water.

**Moxibustion:** An experienced acupuncturist may burn a small cone of Moxa (an herb) to force the plantar wart corn to come loose and be detached from the skin immediately. Only a trained practitioner should perform this technique.

**Acupressure:** Press and push the plantar wart from its root to remove it. Only an experienced practitioner should perform this treatment.

**Diet:** A healthy diet is recommended to avoid infection.

## NATUROPATHY

**Diet:** Eat a diet based on whole foods to support your immune system. Avoid processed foods that are high in simple carbohydrates as they can weaken your immune system and reduce your body's effectiveness in fighting the virus that causes warts.

**Supplements:** The following nutritional supplements will support immune function and healing, which will help combat the viral infections that cause plantar warts. Take 500 mg of vitamin C twice a day. Take 100,000 IU of beta carotene and 400 IU of vitamin E a day. B complex vitamins (50–100 mg a day) will help to reduce the effects of stress, which can weaken your immune system. Taking 200 mcg of selenium and 15–30 mg of zinc a day is also recommended.

**Herbs:** Thuja has a caustic effect on warts as well as antiviral properties. Apply one drop of thuja tincture, available from health food stores, two to four times a day. Take 500 mg of olive leaf extract orally twice a day for its antiviral properties. Garlic also has antiviral properties, and 1 drop can be applied to the plantar wart two to four times a day. You can also use a raw garlic patch by covering the wart and surrounding skin with a thin layer of castor oil or olive oil and then taping a thin slice of fresh garlic in place. This patch should be left on overnight. To maximize the benefit, place 2–4 drops of greater celandine tincture on the wart before covering it with garlic. This application may need to be repeated nightly for up to three weeks. The wart will turn black as it begins to die.

## HOMEOPATHY

For the best results in treating a well-established case of veruccas (especially if they are widespread and/or severe), you will need treatment from a homeopathic practitioner. Practitioners will aim to treat the underlying imbalance in the constitution that allows the verucca to develop. When this is successful, the current verucca should slowly be eradicated, while the development of any future episodes should be discouraged. However, if a small verucca is showing early signs of emergence and there is no established tendency to this problem, one of the following remedies may encourage it to resolve itself.

**Thuja:** Use Thuja to treat a verucca that is uncomfortable when in contact with cold water. Skin quality may be poor with a greasy texture and a tendency to look sallow and dull. Burning and itchy sensations will be experienced in the verucca.

**Causticum:** To treat an itchy, painful plantar wart that has jagged edges and bleeds very readily, use Causticum. Skin may be cracked and sore, especially where there are folds of skin. Plantar warts are most likely to develop when stressed and/or rundown.

**Antimonium crudum:** This is a possible choice of remedy where veruccas emerge on soles of feet that have a marked tendency to produce calluses and hard skin. The feet may feel generally very tender, with the soles being especially sensitive when walking.

**Silica:** If the emergence of a verucca coincides with poor-quality nails and/or the development of soft corns between the toes, this remedy is worth considering. The soles of the feet may also itch, especially in the evenings.

## HERBALISM

**Oatmeal:** Prepare the oatmeal as if you were going to eat it, let it cool, and spread the paste over the affected area. Cover it with seran wrap and leave it on overnight. Reapply each evening until the wart resolves. Plantar warts are very stubborn and are often resistant even to strong conventional medicine. If there is no change after two weeks, discontinue use and try another form of treatment.

**American mayapple:** Applied topically as an ointment or poultice, this herb may help reduce plantar warts. American mayapple contains a compound called podophyllin that is believed to be effective in treating warts. However, it can injure the surrounding skin, causing irritation and ulcers, and should therefore be administered by an experienced herbal therapist.

**Bittersweet nightshade:** The topical application of this plant as an ointment, available from health food stores, has been shown to be effective in the removal of plantar warts.

**Spurges:** The milky juice that is exuded just after the fresh plant is cut is commonly applied to plantar warts. Caution must be taken as this sap is often a powerful irritant and easily ulcerates the skin. Furthermore, it is a poison and should not be taken internally; immediate medical attention is needed if ingestion occurs.

# PRICKLY HEAT

## DIAGNOSIS

Also known as heat rash, prickly heat is a very common condition, especially in babies and young children, but it can also affect adults, particularly when on vacation in a hot climate. Known medically as miliaria rubra, prickly heat is caused by an overreaction by the body to heat when it is unable to cool down efficiently and sweat ducts become blocked. This leads to a red rash and skin that feels hot and prickly. It is most commonly triggered by hot weather, and is aggravated by sweat, so it is important to keep cool and away from direct sunlight if a rash develops. Wearing cotton clothing will also help the rash to resolve. Also bear in mind that fair-skinned people are more likely to be affected by prickly heat.

The rash normally settles down once the body has become acclimatized to the warmer environment, but if it persists and is still clearly visible several hours after the body has cooled down, contact a doctor. If the rash is still evident and any other symptoms develop, such as vomiting or headaches, or you feel under the weather, seek medical help as you could have heatstroke.

## SYMPTOMS

- A rash of red or pink bumps
- The rash affects the parts of the body that sweat the most and are exposed to sunlight, such as the face, neck, and shoulders
- Prickling and itching sensation
- Occasionally spots fill with fluid and turn into small blisters
- Restlessness and irritability

## TREATMENT GOAL

This can be a distressing condition, particularly for young children. Treatment aims to bring rapid relief for oversensitive skin.

## CONVENTIONAL MEDICINE

**Cool baths:** Prickly heat is generally caused by blocked sweat glands and an overgrowth of the bacterium Staphylococcus epidermidis. Prevention is the best treatment. This involves avoiding overdressing for the ambient temperature and steering clear of thick ointments that can block the sweat glands. At the first sign of a rash, cool the skin. Taking cool baths (without soap) every three to four hours and letting your body air-dry can take the heat out of skin. Alternatively, a cool, wet washcloth applied to the affected area as a compress for 5–10 minutes every three to four hours can be helpful for smaller rashes. Monitor the temperature of your living space and avoid overheating.

**Topical creams:** If the rash does not clear up in two to three days, use a low-strength over-the-counter hydrocortisone cream. Do not use the ointment as it will clog the pores. Calamine lotion is another excellent choice. Calamine oil should be avoided as it can clog the pores. Undiluted tea tree oil can be used topically twice a day as well as aloe vera gel.

**Antihistamines:** An antihistamine such as diphenhydramine (Benadryl®) can be used as directed before bed to calm severe itchiness. Benadryl® does have sedative effects.

**Antibiotics:** Generally, if the rash lasts longer than three days, see your doctor. Although heat rash is not infectious, it can spread to the hair follicles and require antibiotic treatment. Treatment is aimed at eliminating the common skin organisms staph and strep and sometimes antibiotics from the penicillin family or erythromycin are prescribed.

## TRADITIONAL CHINESE MEDICINE

**Herbs:** The herbs listed in the formulas below are available from Chinese herbalists or online.
• Jin Yin Hua tea: Combine 5 g of Jin Yin Hua (honeysuckle flower) and 3 g of Bo He (field mint) in a teapot. Add water, boil, and drink the tea throughout the day for 10–30 days. If you have trouble with prickly heat every summer, drink the tea before the rash occurs for preventive purposes.
• Herbal decoction: This decoction is helpful in treating rashes that are dense, red, and itchy due to dampness and heat. Add 10 g of Huo Xiang (agastache), 10 g of Pei Lan (eupatorium), 12 g of Zhi Zi (Cape Jasmine fruit), 10 g of Jin Yin Hua (honeysuckle flower), and 8 g of Zhu Ye (bamboo leaves) to 3 cups of water in a ceramic or glass pot. Bring the mixture to the boil and let it simmer for 30 minutes. Strain the liquid and drink 1 cup three times a day for three to five days.

**Herbal bath:** Add 15 g of Jin Yin Hua (honeysuckle flower) and 15 g of Jing Jie (schizonepeta bud and stem) to 5 cups of water and boil for five minutes. Strain the liquid and add it to your bath water. It will treat and also prevent prickly heat. Take this herbal bath once a day as long as the condition persists.

**Acupuncture:** To treat prickly heat the principle behind acupuncture is to clear the summer heat and pimples from the skin. Stimulating certain meridian points can help the condition. Regulating a person's circulation, and helping maintain skin health is also the goal of the treatment.

**Acupressure:** Press the Tai Yang point at the temple in the depression between the lateral end of the eyebrow and eyelid. Press the Hegu points located on the back of the hands between the thumb and first finger. Also press the Feng Chi point at the base of the skull, 2 inches left of the center point. Each point should be pressed gently for about one minute once a day.

**Diet:** Some food can remove heat and thus help reduce pimples. Such foods include mung beans, red beans, flat beans, coix seeds, watermelon, and cucumber. Avoid any food that has warm properties, such as beef, mutton, and coriander, as they increase body heat. Also avoid eating deep-fried and baked food during the summer.

## NATUROPATHY

**Diet:** Keep your body cool by drinking eight to 10 glasses of water a day. Essential fatty acids can speed up the healing process of a rash. Fish rich in fatty acids, such as salmon, mackerel, or herring, should be eaten two to three times a week. Other sources of fatty acids include dark green, leafy vegetables and flaxseed oil. Avoid eating meat, spicy foods, and known food allergens such as milk. These foods exacerbate heat symptoms and promote inflammation. Instead, eat plenty of lightly steamed vegetables and salads, which are cooling and nourishing for the skin.

**Supplements:** Vitamin C with bioflavonoids promotes skin healing and raises immunity. Take 1,000 mg three times a day. The gamma linoleic oil (GLA) found in evening primrose oil is an essential anti-inflammatory for the skin. Adults should take 3,000 mg of the oil and children should take 1,000 mg. Vitamin E is invaluable for preventing oxidation of the essential oils and for its skin-healing properties. Adults should take 400 IU and children should take 100 IU. Take 10 g of high-quality omega-3 fish oils a day; its anti-inflammatory properties will soothe the skin.

**Herbs:** Apply aloe vera gel two to three times daily to the affected area to soothe and cool the skin. You can also try drinking a cup of aloe vera juice for a similar effect. Apply neem oil once or twice a day to the affected area to heal inflamed, red skin. Sarsaparilla is a skin tonic with many healing properties; take 500 mg in capsule form or 4 ml of tincture three times a day.

**Hydrotherapy:** Soak for 30–60 minutes in a tub filled with lukewarm water containing 1 cup of baking soda. This will cool the skin and make it alkaline. A paste made up of corn starch and cool water has also been found to help alleviate the prickly heat by soothing the skin and keeping it cool.

**TIP:** PREVENTION
Wear loose-fitting clothing and limit outdoor activities to the mornings and evenings during hot weather. Wherever possible stay in an air-conditioned environment during hot weather.

## HOMEOPATHY

Any of the following remedies can help ease the irritation and itchiness of a mild episode of prickly heat, especially if it is a recent onset. However, as with almost any other skin condition discussed in this book, long-term, recurring, and/or severe episodes of prickly heat suggest a deep-seated problem. Such cases require the attention and treatment from an experienced homeopathic practitioner to allow the problem to be gently, but effectively dealt with at a constitutional level. If successful, flare-ups should weaken in severity and frequency until symptoms are eradicated, or so mild that they are no longer a problem.

**Apis:** Use this remedy to treat rashes that cause stinging sensations as well as profound itchiness. When apis is well indicated there is an unmistakable relief from applying cool compresses, bathing in cool water, and uncovering the skin in order to allow cool air to come into contact with the affected areas. Conversely, becoming warm or hot makes discomfort and prickling much worse.

**TIP:** PREVENTION
Avoid the temptation to take very hot baths and/or showers, and make a point of avoiding highly perfumed soaps or body washes that include a harsh detergent.

**Staphysagria:** Consider this as a possible remedy when itchiness and prickling sensations are especially distressing in bed at night. Staphysagria is helpful if scratching the itchy area gives very brief relief, but the irritation only moves to another site. The mental state associated with this remedy is one of irritability and hypersensitivity.

**Urtica urens:** If itchy, prickling, and stinging sensations are made more distressing by contact with damp, cool air or cool bathing, and if affected areas burn and itch, use Urtica urens.

**Sulphur:** This is the most common remedy for skin problems, especially when they are accompanied with localized itching that is worse at night or after bathing.

## HERBALISM

It is important to keep the skin clean, cool, and dry. This, above all else, will promote healing. Do not apply oils or ointments to the affected area. Prickly heat is caused by blocked sweat ducts and adding these types of products will only worsen the condition. However, there are several herbal therapies that can be employed to speed recovery and help to control symptoms.

**Ginger:** Ginger lessens the body's inflammatory response and boosts circulation, helping to soothe prickly heat. Steep freshly grated ginger in a large pot of boiling water, let it cool, and then sponge it over the affected area.

**Oatmeal:** Along with burdock and chickweed, oatmeal can help greatly to alleviate itchiness. Oatmeal is inexpensive, widely available, and can be used without worry, as there are virtually no known side effects. To treat itchiness, run a cool bath and add approximately 1 cup of finely milled oats.

**Burdock root:** Apply burdock topically to the infected area in the same manner as that described for ginger, or add a small amount to an oatmeal bath.

**Chickweed:** Present in many gardens and flower beds, and often considered unsightly, chickweed possesses interesting medicinal properties, and is useful for many common skin conditions. If itchiness due to prickly heat is widespread, try a strong infusion of chickweed in bath water. Adding oatmeal and burdock to the bath can be therapeutic.

# PRURITUS

## DIAGNOSIS

Pruritus is the medical name for inflammation of the skin associated with itchiness or irritation. It can be triggered by a variety of causes. It can be mild and affect just a small area or be so extreme as to affect the whole body, which can be very distressing. However, pruritus is usually localized, affecting a specific part of the body, particularly the eyes, ears, nose, anus, and vagina.

It can occur as a result of fungal infections such as athlete's foot (see p. 27) and ringworm (see p. 140). Insect bites and stings can also trigger the condition, with head lice (see p. 111) being one cause. Irritation around the nose and eyes is associated with hay fever (see p. 261) and allergic rhinitis (see p. 232). A lack of essential fatty acids can also cause pruritus, especially if the skin on the shins is dry and flaky. Itchiness all over the body is generally an indication of another medical condition, such as chickenpox or severe jaundice. Pruritus can also affect some women badly during pregnancy. It can also be an indication of a severe allergic reaction to food or medicine, and can lead to the white wheals (hives) indicative of urticaria (see p. 159).

## SYMPTOMS

- Persistent itchiness and irritation of the skin
- A rash, either widespread or localized

## TREATMENT GOAL

To identify and treat the underlying condition that has triggered pruritus. When it comes to localized pruritus, the cause must be diagnosed so that the condition can be treated appropriately.

## CONVENTIONAL MEDICINE

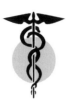

**Antihistamines and topical creams:** Pruritus can be caused by perfumes, detergents, clothes, soaps, or lotions. If such causes are suspected, treating symptoms with antihistamines such as Benadryl®, low-potency steroid creams (hydrocortisone 1%), aloe vera, or calamine lotion is reasonable. If the itchiness resolves within three to five days no further investigation is necessary.

**If lesions are present:** The causes of itchy skin are extensive and sometimes a more serious illness coexists. Treatment is dependent on the cause. A doctor will first determine whether or not skin lesions are present along with the itchiness to decide what kind of treatment is necessary. Some of the causes of itchy skin accompanied by skin lesions are: dry skin, atopic dermatitis or eczema, scabies, drug eruption, herpes, urticaria, contact dermatitis, and fungal infection. If the cause of the lesions is not immediately obvious, the doctor may take a skin biopsy, or carry out allergy testing or scabies testing to determine whether these conditions could be the cause.

**If itchiness exists without a rash:** Itchiness without a rash can be seen frequently in problems of the liver, gallbladder, kidney, certain blood diseases, diabetes, thyroid disorders, chronic drug reactions, and in a syndrome known as psychogenic pruritus. Laboratory testing,including a complete metabolic profile and complete blood count, is the first step to determining the cause of chronic non-rash itchiness. Treatment for each of these conditions needs to be monitored by a doctor.

## TRADITIONAL CHINESE MEDICINE

In traditional Chinese medicine, the seasons, which could complicate pruritus symptoms, are usually taken into consideration.

**Herbs:** These are available from Chinese herbalists or online.
• Summer herbal tea: If pruritus occurs in summer and fall with body sweats, strong thirst, and severe itching, it belongs to the head-wind type of condition. Combine 10 g of Jin Yin Hua (honeysuckle flowers) and 15 g of Lian Qiao (forsythia fruit) in a teapot and add 2–3 cups of water of boiling water. Let the herbs steep for five minutes. Drink this tea three times a day for one to two weeks.
• Winter herbal decoction: If itchy skin occurs during the winter months, combine  10 g of Jing Jie (schizonepeta stem and bud), 15 g of Fang Fen (ledebouriella root), 15 g of Shan Shen (mountain root), 18 g of Xuan Shen (ningpo figwort root), and 15 g of Bai Xian Pi

(dictamnus root bark) in a ceramic or glass pot. Add 4 cups of water, bring the mixture to a boil, and simmer for 30 minutes. Strain the liquid and drink 1 cup twice a day for two to four weeks. If the condition does not improve after two weeks, stop taking it, and consult with your TCM practitioner.

• Herbal wash: Add 20 g of Bai Xian Pi (dictamnus root bark), 20 g of Bai Ji Li (caltrop fruit), and 18 g of Cang Er Zi (cocklebur) to 4 cups of water and bring to the boil. Wash the skin with the liquid twice a day.

• Topical herbs: Add three pieces of ripe green onion to 4 cups of water. Bring the mixture to the boil and simmer for 30 minutes. Strain the liquid, let it cool, and apply to itchy skin.

**Acupuncture:** Acupuncture treatment calms itchy skin and prevents pruritus from recurring. Your acupuncture practitioner may advise you to have treatments one to three times a week.

**Acupressure:** Press the Hegu points, located on the back of the hands between the thumb and the first finger. With the elbow flexed, press the Qu Chi point, located on the outside in the depression at the bend (the lateral end of the traverse cubital crease). Also press the San Yin Jiao point located on the inside of the leg about 3 inches above the anklebone. Taking a sitting position, use your thumb to apply strong pressure to these points for about one minute each two or three times a day.

**Diet:** Eat food that that tastes mild and cool, such as purslane, mung beans, lettuce, mango, cucumber, aubergine, spinach, strawberries, and pears. Avoid shrimp and other seafood, and spicy food.

## NATUROPATHY

If the itchiness is caused by scabies, lice, or hives refer to pp. 155, 111, or 159 respectively.

**Diet:** A high-fiber diet will help eliminate toxins through your bowels, rather than through your skin, which can cause pruritus. Eat plenty of unsweetened cultured foods such as kefir, yogurt, and raw cabbage. These foods have friendly bacteria that live in your digestive tract and are important for the inhibition of candidiasis and other conditions that may cause pruritus. Drink 8–10 glasses of water a day to flush out impurities. Make sure you eat a well-balanced diet that includes fresh fruits and vegetables, wholegrains, legumes, and quality protein such as fish, lean chicken, and beans every day. Eat plenty of green leafy vegetables for their high nutrient content, which boosts the immune system. Avoid foods to which you may be allergic or intolerant, such as shellfish, dairy, eggs, cured meats, peanuts, and citrus foods. Avoid all types of processed junk food as they will depress your immune system, diminish your body's natural defenses, and can eventually cause skin conditions. Decrease the amount of food colorants, preservatives, and flavorings you digest. Some of these chemicals include butylated hydroxytoluene (BHT), butylated hydorxyanisol (BHA), sulfites, dyes, and salicylates. They may contribute to itchy skin.

**Supplements:** Vitamin C can treat hives by lowering histamine released by the body; histamine increases inflammation and may cause pruritus. Take 2,000 mg of vitamin C daily along with citrus bioflavonoids, hesperidin, rutin, and/or rose hips. Quercitin also reduces the effects of histamine; take 1,000 mg three times a day.

**Herbs:** Take 300 mg of freeze-dried nettle leaf in pill form, available from health stores, three times a day as it serves as a natural antihistamine. Burdock root has been traditionally used for all sorts of skin conditions. Take 300 mg in capsule form three times a day or 8 ml of tincture a day. Chamomile may reduce itchiness when used as a cream, and relieves stress when drunk as a tea. Aloe vera gel can be used topically on the affected area for its cooling, soothing, and anti-inflammatory effects. A cool oatmeal bath may help relieve itchiness. Put 1 cup of oatmeal into a piece of cheese cloth or muslin and tie it with a string and hang it under the tap or float it in the bath tub. Soak in warm water for 20–30 minutes.

## HOMEOPATHY

Any of the following measures can be used to relieve the itchiness of a recent, mild bout of pruritus, but more established symptoms will require professional homeopathic attention. If the condition persists, seek conventional medical attention.

**Prevention:** Women who are subject to itchy vulvas and irritation should avoid highly perfumed bubble baths, and wearing clothing that creates a warm, moist environment around the genital area. Common offenders are thongs, tights, leggings, and very tight jeans. Wear underwear made from natural cotton fibers that allow the skin around this area to remain as cool as possible. If problems with hemorrhoids are leading to anal itchiness, bathe the area with warm or cool water (depending on which is more comfortable), and make sure that constipation isn't aggravating the problem by causing straining.

**Sulphur:** To relieve itchiness that affects the anus and/or the vulva, use Sulphur. Symptoms that indicate this remedy include redness and inflammation of the affected tissues, with itchiness that is made much more intense by warm bathing, getting warm in bed, or becoming generally overheated.

**Rhus tox:** Use Rhus tox if itchiness and burning sensations cause great restlessness and distress at night, leading to lots of frustrated tossing and turning. The itchiness may be temporarily eased by warm bathing.

**Calc carb:** If itchiness is especially noticeable and severe in women before and after a period, and/or approaching or following menopause, use Calc carb. It is effective if itchiness and irritation is combined with clamminess, sweatiness, fatigue, and weight gain.

**Teucrium:** This is a potential remedy if itchiness of the anus is related to the presence of threadworms. Signature features include constant irritation and itchiness in this region, with a crawling sensation that is especially noticeable after passing a stool. Symptoms cause great restlessness and distress in bed.

## HERBALISM

 **Oatmeal:** Along with burdock, oatmeal is a first choice among herbalists to treat many skin conditions, including pruritus. Oatmeal is inexpensive, widely available and can be used without worry, as there are virtually no known side effects. For use in the treatment of pruritus, prepare the oatmeal as if you were going to eat it, let it cool, and spread the paste over the affected area. Cover it with plastic wrap and leave it on overnight.

**Burdock root:** Burdock can be taken internally as a tea or tincture, or it can be applied directly to the affected area as an essential oil, in an ointment, or in a poultice. There are no reported adverse reactions to burdock, but there is always the potential for any topically applied herb to aggravate skin symptoms. If you experience an allergic reaction, stop treatment.

**Chickweed:** To treat pruritus, chickweed is best used topically as an ointment or poultice. A strong infusion of chickweed in bath water can soothe widespread itchiness. Adding oatmeal and burdock to the bath can also be therapeutic.

**Peppermint:** To treat mild itchiness add several drops of peppermint oil to a bowl of warm water. Soak a clean washcloth in the mixture, wring out the excess liquid, and place it on the affected area for 5–10 minutes once or twice a day. Bear in mind that some people find peppermint to be heating, and as such, it can make rashes and itching worse.

**Camphor:** The bark and wood of the camphor tree is indicated for a variety of skin disorders, including pruritus. Camphor is best used as an ointment containing anywhere from 3–11% camphor. Apply it directly to the affected area two to three times a day for 7–10 days. Do not take camphor internally.

# PSORIASIS

## DIAGNOSIS

Psoriasis is a chronic, recurring skin disease. It can vary from mild outbreaks, where the person may not even be aware that he or she has psoriasis, to severe cases, which can be very distressing. The condition tends to run in families, although it is by no means certain that it will ever develop in those with a genetic predisposition. The condition can also be triggered by stress, emotional upsets, and exposure to certain stimuli such as medicines. The main type of psoriasis is discoid psoriasis, which manifests as plaques of affected skin on the elbows and knees. Pustular psoriasis generally affects the hands and soles of feet.

## SYMPTOMS

- Red- or pink-colored spots or patches
- Patches grow bigger and become covered with silver-colored scales
- Shedding of silvery scales to expose red patches beneath
- Small spots of blood can be seen underneath
- Psoriasis of the nail often manifests itself as small pits in the nails. The outbreak can be so severe that the nail thickens and crumbles away
- Flexural psoriasis occurs in skin folds (flexures). Red, itchy plaques appear in the armpits, under the breasts, on the stomach, in the groin, or on the buttocks. The plaques are often infected by the yeast-like fungus Candida albicans
- The scalp is usually affected, with loss of scales and matting of hair

## TREATMENT GOAL

Psoriasis is not contagious but it is a chronic condition characterized by intense flare-ups followed by periods of remission. There is no cure for the disease, but treatments aims to control the condition.

## CONVENTIONAL MEDICINE

Drugs are generally prescribed to treat initial outbreaks of psoriasis and to treat any exacerbations of the condition. Non-pharmaceutical treatment is often effective to keep the condition in remission.

**Eliminate triggers:** Stress can trigger psoriasis. Daily meditation as well as other stress reduction techniques, in conjunction with other therapy, can improve the condition. Certain medications are known to make psoriasis worse and should be avoided. These are commonly beta blockers used for hypertension, lithium used for bipolar disease, and antimalarials. Eliminate dairy and gluten from your diet as a trial to see if this is effective. Use probiotics and prebiotics to optimize intestinal health and relieve symptoms. Check vitamin D3 levels (25 hydroxy D), as vitamin D3 therapy leads to improvement in some patients; recent studies correlate psoriasis with a low vitamin D3 level. Amounts of 1,000 IU daily are often used initially.

**Sun exposure:** Sunbathing generally leads to an improvement in psoriasis but sun protection must be used. UVB exposure three times weekly along with oral PUVA (psoralen plus ultraviolet A) given two to three times weekly is effective.

**Topical treatments:** Bathing daily in tepid water with non-detergent soap, and applying lotion such as Cetaphil® immediately after bathing leads to improvement. Topical steroids can provide a brief remission, but they decrease in effect with continued use. They do not help the arthritis that can accompany psoriasis. Salicyclic acid at a strength of 2–10% can decrease scaling. Do not use salicyclic acid at the same time as Dovonex®.

**For severe conditions:** Systemic methotrexate taken at 25 mg a week can be used, as can cyclosporine, to treat severe psoriasis. Side effects of these drugs are extensive. Consult a specialist if the extent of the disease requires this type of medication.

## TRADITIONAL CHINESE MEDICINE

Traditional Chinese medicine suggests that psoriasis is related to dampness, heat, or blood stagnation. The treatment principles are to remove toxins and dispel the pathogenic heat and dampness.

**Herbs:** These are available from Chinese herbal stores or online.
• To treat highly-inflamed psoriasis: If the skin is red, itchy, warm, and damp, make a decoction from 15 g of Huang Qin (baical skullcap root), 12 g of Jin Yin Hua (honeysuckle flower), 18 g of Bai Xian Pi (dictamnus root bark), 15 g of Cang Zhu (atractylodes rhizome),

and 5 g of Gan Cao (licorice). Boil these herbs in 3 cups of water and drink 1 cup of the liquid twice a day for one to four weeks.

• To treat patches of psoriasis: If the skin is dry and the psoriasis patches are thick and dull-colored with white flakes, make a decoction from 18 g of Xuan Shen (ningpo figwort root), 15 g of Dan Shen (salvia root), 18 g of Huang Jing (Siberian Solomon seal rhizome), and 5 g of Gan Cao (licorice). Boil the herbs in 3 cups of water and drink 1 cup of the liquid twice a day for one to four weeks. Consult a TCM practitioner for long-term treatment if the condition persists.

• Herbal bath: Add 18 g of Ma Zhi Xian (dried purslane), 15 g of Jing Jie (schizonepeta stem and bud), 20 g of Tao Ren (peach kennel), 15 g of Huang Bai (phellodendron), and 15 g of Ku Shen (sophora root) to 5–6 cups of water. Boil for 20 minutes, strain the liquid and add it to warm bath water. Soak your body for 20–30 minutes once a day. If the skin becomes irritated, stop the treatment and consult a TCM practitioner.

• Poultice: Pound 50 g of garlic and 50 g of chives together and warm them over heat. Rub the poultice into inflamed skin one to two times a day for several days.

**Acupuncture:** An experienced acupuncturist will perform a traditional Chinese medicine differentiation diagnosis, finding the cause of the problem by gathering information on your overall health. For example, if the patient with psoriasis is also suffering anxiety and/or high stress, the treatment will involve treating anxiety and stress in addition to treating the skin itself. Usually 12 acupuncture sessions makes up one course of treatment. It takes one to three courses to treat chronic psoriasis. Patients may experience improvement as the treatment progresses, but in most cases, long-term treatment is essential.

**Acupressure:** Press the Feng Chi point, located at the base of the skull, 2 inches left of the center point, with your thumb. Begin with gentle pressure and gradually increase, pressing and releasing about 20 times. Press the Hegu points, located on the back of the hands between the thumb and first finger. Also press the Tai Chong point, found on the instep of the foot in the depression between the first and second toe at the base of the big toe. While sitting, press these points for one minute, repeating the treatment two to three times a day.

**Diet:** Eat foods that dispel dampness and heat, such as mung beans, watermelon peel, lotus root, purslane, wax gourd, red beans, banana, and grapefruit. Avoid foods that promote heat and dampness in the body, such as pepper, dried garlic, cloves, dried ginger, green peppers, leeks, green onion, and liver.

**TIP: COMBINE TREATMENTS**
For more severe and complicated cases of psoriasis, a combination of treatments that includes Chinese herbal medicine, acupuncture, and dietary therapy is recommended. Getting enough sleep is also important.

## NATUROPATHY

 **Diet:** Cut alcohol out of your diet as it worsens the condition by impairing function of the liver and gut tissues, increasing the amount of toxins that are absorbed by the body. Also eliminate gluten, found in wheat, barley, and rye; psoriasis patients have been clinically proven to benefit from abstaining from gluten products. Eat a hypoallergenic diet. Stay away from corn, dairy and dairy products, and any other foods to which you may be allergic. Fresh fruits, vegetables, whole grains, and beans are high in fiber and will eliminate many gut-derived toxins, a process which is beneficial to those suffering from psoriasis.

**Topical herbs:** Cayenne contains a resinous and pungent substance known as capsaicin. This chemical relieves pain and itchiness by depleting certain neurotransmitters from sensory nerves. Creams containing 0.025–0.075% capsaicin are generally helpful. The first application may give a slight burning sensation, but this should subside with each application. Ointments containing a 10% concentration of Oregon grape have been shown to be mildly effective against mild psoriasis in clinical trials. Apply the ointments three times a day.

**Herbs:** Polyamines, metabolites of proteins, have been found in high amounts in patients with psoriasis. Berberine, the active ingredient in goldenseal, has been shown to inhibit the formation of polyamines. Take 250–500 mg of a standardized berberine extract 250–500 mg three times a day, or 2–4 ml of a fluid extract three times a day. Smilax sarsaparilla has been used traditionally as a skin tonic and reduces the effects of the bacterial toxins that aggravate psoriasis; take 500 mg in capsule form or 4 ml of tincture three times a day. Milk thistle has an active ingredient, silymarin, that is reportedly useful in relieving psoriasis. Milk thistle seed contains at least eight anti-inflammatory compounds that may act on the skin. Take 70–210 mg of an 80–85% silymarin extract three times a day. Fumitory contains fumaric acid, a compound that has been shown in studies to be useful for treating psoriasis. Topical and oral forms can be taken, but studies have shown some side effects such as flushing, pain, and mild liver and kidney disturbances. Use this substance only under the supervision of a doctor. However, you can brew a strong fumitory tea and apply it directly to the affected area with a cotton ball or clean cloth two to three times a day. The herbs listed here are all available from health food stores.

**Supplements:** Fish oils, which are anti-inflammatory and nourishing for the skin, have been found to improve skin lesions associated with psoriasis. Take 10–12 g a day. This dosage is safe as long as other anticoagulants, such as Coumadin®, are not taken in conjunction. Some studies have shown that some patients with skin conditions have both low amounts of stomach acid and the pancreatic enzyme lipase. Take 2–4 pills containing this digestive enzyme with each meal. Betaine hydrochloride improves stomach acidity and digestion, especially of proteins. Take 1–3 capsules with each meal, but reduce the dose if you experience a warming or burning sensation. Vitamin B12 injections have been shown to improve psoriasis after six weeks of treatment. Ask your doctor to inject 1cc of B12 daily for 10 days. Sublingual B12 may also be used at 400–800 mcg a day. Folic acid is helpful, especially if you are taking methotextrate for psoriasis. Take 400 mcg a day.

## HOMEOPATHY

 This type of condition should be treated by an experienced homeopathic practitioner. The homeopathic suggestions listed below give an idea of the sort of remedies that a practitioner might consider when treating a patient with this condition. On occasion, it may be possible to use an obviously well-indicated remedy to calm down a very mild, limited flare-up of psoriasis. But in the main this is not to be encouraged as there is a risk that taking a homeopathic remedy that works only superficially over an extended period of time may suppress the underlying problem. There is also a risk of unwittingly aggravating symptoms by taking a remedy for too long. Although this is not a permanent problem, since the symptoms will improve once the remedy is stopped, it can be avoided by consulting an experienced homeopathic practitioner.

**Prevention:** Soaking in an oatmeal bath can feel soothing to taut, scaly areas of skin. Suspend a small muslin bag that has been filled (but not stuffed) with oats under the hot tap as the water is running. If stress is noticeably aggravating psoriasis symptoms, investigate stress-reduction and relaxation techniques that can be built in to your daily routine. Choices to consider include meditation, progressive muscular relaxation, yoga, T'ai chi, and/or pilates.

**Arsenicum album:** This remedy can ease the soreness of rough, scaly skin that is so dry it looks like paper. Signature features include burning sensations and soreness as a result of scratching, symptoms that are eased by contact with warmth. Stress and anxiety noticeably aggravate skin problems, and skin eruptions may alternate with asthma.

**Lycopodium:** If dry, raw skin is combined with urinary or gastric problems when feeling physically rundown, use Lycopodium. Anticipatory anxiety (especially anxiety about being the focus of attention when, for example, giving a presentation) aggravate skin symptoms. Skin tends to feel sore and raw in areas of folds (for instance around the ears and/or the nose), while the skin on the hands and the soles of the feet can be especially dry.

**Calc carb:** Consider this remedy if skin is rough and scaly and becomes very readily cracked and chapped, especially in cold winter weather. The skin has a generally pale, unhealthy look to it with a tendency to become sweaty and clammy after the least physical effort, and is also slow to heal.

**Graphites:** This remedy is called for when areas of skin affected by psoriasis become very easily cracked, weepy, and bleed after scratching. Thickened, scaly skin weeps a yellowish-colored discharge that dries to a crust.

## HERBALISM

**Aloe vera:** To treat psoriasis, take the gel from a fresh cut aloe leaf and apply directly to the affected area. If fresh leaves are not available, there are a variety of gels and lotions containing aloe vera that can be purchased at your local health store.

**Burdock root:** Burdock can be taken internally as a tea or tincture, or it can be applied directly to the affected area as an essential oil, an ointment, or a poultice. Although there are few reported adverse reactions to burdock, there is the potential for burdock, as with herbs used topically, to aggravate symptoms. If this happens, discontinue use immediately.

**Cleavers:** Cleavers is thought to have many healing properties and is a wonderful adjunct in the treatment of psoriasis. It can be utilized as a tea or tincture, and can also be prepared for use as an ointment or in a poultice. It is recommended that cleavers be combined with burdock for the most effective treatment. Do not take for an extended period of time.

**Barberry:** Barberry contains a compound called berberine, which is responsible for many of its medicinal properties. Topical application is the best way to administer barberry. Work a small amount of essential oil into the affected area or apply it as a poultice. Barberry has been known to cause skin irritation and allergic reactions when applied topically, so be aware of any adverse reactions.

**Calendula:** Calendula can be applied topically as an ointment or tincture and has very few contraindications or adverse reactions when used topically. There is a small potential for an allergic reaction on the skin, especially in those who react to plants in the daisy family.

**Oil of anise:** This can be applied directly to the affected area 2–3 times a day. Most common side effects are irritation and dermatitis at the site of application. The anise essential oil can be combined with a high-quality oil used in skin care, such as coconut oil, to provide more beneficial effects. More serious side effects may occur if anise is taken internally, so only use this herb topically.

# RINGWORM

## DIAGNOSIS

Ringworm is a fairly common skin disease caused by the infectious fungus tinea. It looks rather like a bull's eye, a ring-shaped mark with a paler area in the center. The name is misleading, as the condition has nothing to do with worms. It is caught by coming into contact with the fungus, by either touching infected skin directly or by coming into contact with items used by those infected with ringworm, for example, washcloths and towels, hats, or brushes.

Ringworm particularly affects children, and can spread quickly around schools and nurseries. It is most common in children between the ages of two and 10. Children often catch ringworm from pets, as dogs and cats can carry the spores in their fur. Warm, moist environments such as bathrooms and swimming pools are an ideal breeding ground for the fungus.

## SYMPTOMS

- Round or oval-shaped patches of reddish-pink skin, starting with a small irritation and then spreading
- Marks are paler in the center, growing redder and slightly raised towards the outside
- Sometimes patches are dry and scaly
- Most commonly found on the face, although they can appear elsewhere on the body, particularly the groin, arms, legs, and scalp
- Sores can be itchy and become inflamed if scratched
- Sores can also appear on the scalp, causing hair to break off, leaving bald patches
- Fingernails may become infected too, as a result of scratching an infected area

## TREATMENT GOAL

Ringworm is not a serious condition but is very contagious and an infected person should avoid contact with others. Treatment aims to clear up the rash, and prevent the fungus from spreading.

## CONVENTIONAL MEDICINE

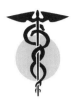

Treating ringworm requires an accurate diagnosis. The rash can be confused with psoriasis (p. 134), seborrheic dermatitis, and candidiasis. Fungal skin conditions such as ringworm can be diagnosed by sending a scraping of skin cells to a hospital laboratory for examination under a microscope. Cultures are usually not needed.

**Prevention:** Identify the source of the fungus to avoid it spreading. Keep the area clean and dry. Many people mistakenly think they have a dry spot and apply ointments and emollients, which can make the lesion grow. Applying tea tree oil three times daily in the initial stages of the rash can also help; continue to apply the oil for a two-week period. Tight clothing or bandages should be avoided, as should hydrocortisone cream.

**Antifungal agents:** Topical antifungal agents such as lotrimin, lamisil, and lotrisone can be applied twice a day for two to three weeks. If these don't work, oral antifungal agents, for example 100 mg of itraconazole or 200 mg of diflucan a day, can be used. These drugs can be harsh on the liver and liver enzyme testing is sometimes done. Taking milk thistle together with these drugs can protect the liver and does not reduce their effect nor cause significant interactions. Using undiluted tea tree oil topically in conjunction with these medications is also appropriate. If there is no resolution within two to three weeks, or if infection recurs, see your doctor.

## TRADITIONAL CHINESE MEDICINE

**Herbs:** External herbal medicines are the primary methods for treating ringworm in traditional Chinese medicine.
• Herbal formula: Soak 9 g of Din Xiang (clove flower bud), and 15 g of Da Huang (rhubarb root and rhizome) in 90 ml of rice vinegar for seven days. Apply an adequate amount of this formula to affected skin twice a day.
• Herbal paste: Combine 30 g of garlic and 30 g of fresh Chinese chives. Pound the garlic and chives together to make a paste and apply it to the inflamed skin, repeating once or twice a day for several days.

**Acupuncture:** Treatment can improve the immune system and reduce itchiness of the skin. You should receive treatment twice a week for three to four weeks.

**Diet:** Eat foods that help clear heat in the blood, remove damp, and moisten dryness such as mustard greens, water spinach, mung beans, and honey.

141

Ringworm is a fungal infection and is often associated with other infections. Once a person has multiple fungal infections they may develop systemic candidiasis. A naturopathic treatment for ringworm should include a plan to rid systemic candidiasis, if this is suspected.

**Diet:** The following dietary measures are part of the standard diet to control candida. Eat chicken, eggs, fish, yogurt, vegetables, nuts, seeds, oils, and lots of raw garlic. Eliminate refined and simple sugars, including white or brown sugar, raw sugar, honey, molasses, or sweeteners. Stevia is a sugar substitute that is allowed. Avoid alcohol, milk, fruit or dried fruit, and mushrooms. Avoid foods that contain yeast or mold, including all breads, muffins, cakes, baked goods, cheese, dried fruits, melons, and peanuts. Increase your fiber intake; take 1 tsp to 1 tbsp of soluble fiber containing guar gum, psyllium husks, flaxseeds, or pectin mixed in an 8 oz glass of water twice a day on an empty stomach.

**Environmental considerations:** Ringworm spores can live in the environment for over a year. Because of this, it is prudent to clean the house as well as possible to rid it of the fungus. Vacuum rugs and carpets frequently and clean all smooth surfaces (floors, counters, windowsills, and so on) with a 5% bleach solution for several weeks. Ringworm fungi collect in tubs, on bathroom floors, and in hampers and dresser drawers. Regularly clean these breeding grounds with a mixture of tree tea oil, thyme, and rosemary oil. Use 10–20 drops of each in a bucket of water. Wash all exposed textiles (clothing, bedding, pillows, and so on) in a 5% bleach solution and hot water. Dry everything in a hot dryer, as high temperatures kill the fungus. Combs and hats should also be thoroughly cleaned and disinfected. Keep your pets free of fungi. If you suspect the ringworm is coming from a pet, take the animal to the vet for a thorough examination and professional treatment. Thoroughly wash any pet bedding.

**Herbs:** Oregano oil has strong antifungal effects. Take 5 drops of liquid under the tongue or mixed with a glass of water. Undiluted drops may be too strong for some people. You can also take 500 mg a day in capsule form. Garlic fights fungus and boost the immune system; take 500 mg twice a day. Take 200 mg of grapefruit seed extract twice a day for its antifungal properties. Undecylenic acid, a derivative from the castor bean oil, has been shown to have strong antifungal activity. Take 200 mg three times a day. Pau d'Arco has strong antifungal properties. Take two cups of the tea a day. Take 200–500 mg of barberry a day for its antimicrobial and antifungal properties.

**Supplements:** Caprylic acid is a fatty acid shown to have antifungal properties. Take 1,000 mg three times a day. Taking 1,000 mg of vitamin C a day helps enhance immune function. Take a high-potency multivitamin for the many nutrients it provides to support immune function. Take probiotics with about four billion micro-organisms twice daily 30 minutes before each meal. These micro-organisms provide acidophilus and bifidus, which are friendly bacteria that prevent yeast overgrowth and fights candida.

**General considerations:** You can't wash away ringworm, but a daily bath or shower may hinder its spread and provide some relief from itchiness. No astringent, gritty, or germ-fighting soaps are needed, just use a plain, gentle soap to keep the area clean. Avoid harsh scrubbing; it will only aggravate the lesions. Ringworm fungi thrive in moisture. After bathing, thoroughly pat the affected area dry and then sprinkle on some absorbent powder. (Do not use cornstarch; fungi will use it as food.) You'll also see improvement if you air out problem areas with an electric hair dryer set on cool.

## HOMEOPATHY

Any of the following homeopathic remedies can be used in a complementary way with conventional treatment in order to speed up recovery from a ringworm infection.

**Prevention:** After washing make sure that affected areas are dried gently, but thoroughly, since warm, damp conditions are an ideal environment for fungal infections to thrive in. Since ringworm is highly contagious, destroy any items that may have been in contact with the infection, such as combs, brushes, and/or hairbands. Also check pets for symptoms, since they may need separate treatment.

**Sepia:** This remedy may be helpful where the classic circular patches particularly affect the skin of the scalp on the crown and/or back of the head. As a result, the growth, fullness, and quality of the hair might be adversely affected.

**Sulphur:** If symptoms of ringworm set in within the context of a history of poor-quality skin and hair, with a tendency to spots, boils, and easily infected skin, use Sulphur. Symptoms include skin that feels very uncomfortable for washing, showering, and getting over-heated (especially in bed).

## HERBALISM

**Bitter orange oil:** There is evidence that suggests the essential oil from this plant may be helpful for ringworm and other fungal infections when applied topically. Take a few drops of the essential oil and place it directly on the affected area two to three times a day. There have been reports of allergic skin reactions to bitter orange oil; discontinue use of this treatment if application site worsens or new symptoms develop. Do not use bitter orange for more than 10 days. Bitter orange oil should not be taken internally as potentially serious side effects can occur, including cardiotoxicity, leading to arrhythmias or heart attacks in some people.

**Garlic:** Garlic has antiseptic and antifungal properties and generally boosts the immune system. Crushed raw garlic can be applied directly to the affected area two to three times a day for one to two weeks. A more effective and tolerable method of delivery is a garlic gel, which can be purchased from your local health food store. Ajoene, an organosulfur compound in garlic, is known to have powerful antifungal properties and has been shown to work just as well as over-the-counter antifungal medications. Look for a gel containing 1% ajoene if possible and apply twice daily for 7–10 days. Garlic can also be taken orally; take 500 mg twice daily or two crushed cloves a day to address fungal infections like ringworm. Garlic has virtually no side effects when used topically, although minor irritation of the application site can sometimes occur. When taken internally at high, therapeutic doses, garlic may interfere with certain antithrombotic drugs.

**Tea tree oil:** Tea tree oil can be used topically as an antifungal and antibacterial agent. Apply it to the infected area either as a 5–15% tea tree oil solution, or as a 5–15% tea tree oil cream, a concentration that has been shown to relieve symptoms effectively. Dermatitis is the only significant side effect associated with the prolonged and repeated topical use of tea tree oil.

**Calendula:** Calendula can be applied topically as an ointment or tincture to treat fungal infections. Dosing recommendations are highly varied, and consultation with a medical herbalist is a good idea. Calendula has very few contraindications or adverse reactions when used topically, although there is a small potential for an allergic reaction.

**Oregano oil:** Know for its strong antifungal properties, oregano oil is best taken orally. Dilute 3–5 drops of oil in a glass of water and drink two to three times a day. Do not take oregano oil if you have an allergic reaction to plants in the mint family. In large doses, it may promote nausea and has the potential to decrease iron absorption.

**Cloves:** When applied topically, cloves have known antifungal properties. Use them as an oil or salve several times daily. Potential adverse reactions with topical application include dermatitis and mucous membrane irritation. Do not take internally for fungal infection.

**Echinacea:** There is evidence that suggests taking echinacea orally, in combination with a topical antifungal herb or medication, may be effective against fungal infections such as ringworm. Do not use echinacea if the fungal infection is due to an underlying autoimmune disease, or if you are pregnant. Discontinue use after three weeks.

# ROSACEA

## DIAGNOSIS

Rosacea is a distressing condition that affects mostly middle-aged adults of both sexes. It looks very similar to acne. Dilated, spidery red blood vessels appear on the face, which assumes an angry, flushed appearance that is very noticeable. It can trigger conjunctivitis and cause the growth of blood vessels into the corners of the eyes. It particularly affects the nose, changing the texture of the skin there, which can eventually become thickened and pitted. There is a tendency for the afflicted person to blush and the affected area gradually becomes redder over a period of time as the blood vessels dilate. The cause is unknown but it is not thought to be hereditary. The main triggers are extreme temperatures, sunlight, spicy food, alcohol, and hot drinks, all of which should be avoided to try to moderate the condition.

## SYMPTOMS

- Flushed appearance
- Dilated, spidery blood vessels on the face
- Persistent redness of the face
- Pimples on the forehead, cheeks, nose, and chin
- Pustules sometimes form
- Occasionally, the condition causes a bulbous nose
- Occasionally, the condition spreads and causes inflammation of the eye

## TREATMENT GOAL

Treatment aims to minimize flushing and improve the appearance of the skin without resorting to laser treatment or surgery. It can take several months for the condition to improve.

## CONVENTIONAL MEDICINE

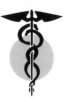

Rosacea must be differentiated from other similarly presenting conditions. Contact dermatitis, facial sarcoidosis, photodermatitis, seborrheic dermatitis, and idiopathic facial flushing all look like rosacea, but have different treatments.

**Prevention:** Use non-drying, non-detergent soap and avoid anything that irritates the skin. Hot drinks, especially coffee, often cause flare-ups. Alcohol and sunbathing are common triggers that worsen the flushing associated with rosacea. Stress reduction techniques can benefit the condition as can adhering to an anti-inflammatory diet that excludes processed foods, dairy, and sugar.

**Topical treatments:** Azelaic acid is based on a natural plant and can be very helpful when applied topically as a cream at a 20% strength. Topical metronidazole (known as MetroGel®) is a mild treatment that can be applied once daily at a strength of 1%. This is used by itself or after a course of antibiotics. Clindamycin (Cleocin) is another ointment that is often used. Oral tetracycline is often prescribed, as is oral metronidazole. Low doses of clonidine can sometimes successfully treat redness and flushing.

## TRADITIONAL CHINESE MEDICINE

**Herbs:** The herbs below are all available from Chinese herbalists.
• To treat acute rosacea: To treat very red skin, where there are no further complications such as yellow urine and constipation, the treatment principle is to clear heat. Combine 10 g of Huang Qin (baical skullcap root), 12 g of Pi Pa Ye (loquat leaf), 10 g of Da Qin Ye (woad leaf), 10 g of Jin Yin Hua (honeysuckle flower), 10 g of Lian Qiao (forsythia fruit), 12 g of Zhi Mu (anemarrhena rhizome), and 5 g of Gan Cao (licorice) in a ceramic or glass pot. Add 4 cups of water, bring the liquid to the boil, and simmer for 30 minutes. Strain the liquid and drink 1 cup of the decoction twice a day. Take this formula for 7–10 days. If the condition hasn't improved, consult a TCM practitioner.
• To treat chronic rosacea: If there is an accompanying menstrual disorder, the traditional Chinese medicine diagnosis will possibly be blood stagnation. Combine 12 g of Chi Shao (red peony root), 12 g of Dan Shen (salvia root), 12 g of Dang Gui (Chinese angelica root), 6 g of Huang Hua (*flos carthami tinctorii*), 10 g Chuan Xiong (Szechuan lovage root), and 5 g of fresh ginger in a ceramic or glass pot. Add 4 cups of water, bring the liquid to the boil, and simmer for 30 minutes. Strain the liquid and drink 1 cup twice a day.

• Herbal cream: If infected pimples accompany the rosacea, use Si Huang Gao, a patent Chinese medicinal cream that you should be able to find in a Chinese herbalist store or online. Apply this cream to the affected area twice a day for one week, which is one course of treatment. Use the cream sparingly at first, and if your skin is highly sensitive or you have an allergic reaction, stop using it immediately and consult your doctor.

**Acupuncture:** This is an effective treatment for rosacea. The acupuncturist will insert needles in your face and other parts of your body to reduce the heat and to remove stagnated blood and energy. The treatment will take one to three months on a twice weekly basis. You may notice a change after a couple of treatments. Your acupuncturist may advise you to stop using antibacterial medication and cream.

**Acupressure:** Pressing the Yin Tang, Ying Xiang, Quan Liao, Di Cang, Hegu points can be effective. The Yin Tang point is located in the depression midway between the eyebrows. Look for the Ying Xiang point to the side and slightly above the lower border of the nostril. The Quan Liao point is about 3 inches away from the nostril, in the depression just below the cheekbone. The Di Cang point is directly below the pupil of the eye beside the mouth angle. The Hegu point is located on the back of the hand between the thumb and first finger.

**Diet:** Eat foods that have cooling properties such as celery, spinach, lettuce, mung beans, and string beans. If you are constipated, foods that helps bowel movement include castor bean, sesame oil, bananas, Chinese cabbage, apricots, and pears.

## NATUROPATHY

**Diet:** Those with rosacea have been shown to have a compromised digestive system. Having freshly squeezed vegetable juices every day is a good way of making sure you get essential nutrients directly into your system. Skin eruptions occur if your body has no other way of eliminating toxins from the system. Eat plenty of fiber, especially from whole grains, vegetables, and fruits, to keep your digestive system clean and free of toxins. Cold-water fish are high in essential fatty acids, which have anti-inflammatory properties. Eat salmon, herring, and mackerel two to three times a week. Avoid foods that may make you flush, such as spicy food, caffeine, and alcoholic drinks. Avoid food allergens that may mimic the symptoms of rosacea and cause inflammation. The most common food allergens are dairy, wheat, corn, soy, and citrus foods.

**Supplements:** Take 100 mg of B-complex (especially riboflavin) a day to compensate for a deficiency in B vitamins that is commonly found in people with rosacea. Vitamin B12 helps to reduce flare-ups of rosacea. Take 400–800 mcg a day, taking into account the amount contained in your B-complex. Vitamin C and flavonoids are well-known nutritional necessities for optimal performance of blood vessels, capillaries, and connective tissue. Take 1,000 mg of vitamin C and 500–650 mg flavonoids twice a day. Probiotics help improve digestion and skin health. Take about 4 billion micro-organisms twice a day, in capsule form or in powder form mixed with juice, 30 minutes before a meal. These micro-organisms provide acidophilus and bifidus, friendly bacteria that promote good health in your gut. Studies show that the digestive system in some patients with rosacea has low amounts of both stomach acid and of the pancreatic enzyme lipase. Take 2–4 pills containing these digestive enzymes with each meal. Betaine hydrochloride improves stomach acidity and digestion, especially of proteins. Take 1–3 capsules with each meal, but reduce the dose if you experience a warming or burning sensation.

**Herbs:** Yellow dock has a long history of use for conditions affecting the gastrointestinal tract and liver. As a result, it is thought to treat skin conditions attributed to toxic metabolites from poor digestion and poor liver function. A tincture of yellow dock, ½–¼ tsp three times a day can be used. Alternatively, a tea can be made by boiling 1–2 tsp (5–10 g) of the root in 2 cups of water for 10 minutes. Drink three cups of the tea a day.

**General considerations:** To minimize stress, which can cause flare-ups, take five deep breaths two to three times a day. You can also take deep breaths when you feel an anxiety attack coming on. Avoid sunbathing, hot baths, and saunas.

## HOMEOPATHY

The remedies suggested below can be used to relieve the symptoms of a recent, fairly mild episode of rosacea. However, if your skin is subject to repeated flare-ups of symptoms over an extended period of time, it will be necessary to be treated by a homeopathic practitioner to treat the underlying weakness in the system that is giving rise to the symptoms.

**Prevention:** Although not the cause, certain foods and drinks can aggravate this condition and are best avoided, or consumed only infrequently. The most common triggers include alcohol, tea, coffee, and spicy foods.

**Belladonna:** Use Belladonna if affected areas of skin feel hot and dry, and look bright red. Belladonna has a reputation for reducing inflammation and should be used at first sign of an outbreak of spots. Belladonna will either disperse the inflammation, or move it on to the next stage of pus production. At this point, a different remedy will need to be selected.

**Nux vomica:** If an acute outbreak of spots results from a highly stressful period of time, where your intake of alcohol, caffeine, and junk food may have increased, use Nux vomica. This is useful if the function of the immune system has been adversely affected by lack of sleep, and if you are consequently strained mentally and emotionally during the day.

**Lachesis:** If the inflamed patches of skin have a dark-red, purplish look, and if the skin has a mottled appearance, use Lachesis. When this remedy is well indicated, symptoms are especially noticeable first thing in the morning.

**Rhus tox:** This is the remedy to consider if spots are especially itchy and/or painful, and react very badly to contact with cold and damp. They may also show a tendency to be limited to, or worse, on the left cheek. The lips may also be noticeably dry and cracked with a tendency to develop cold sores.

**Sulphur:** This is the most common remedy for skin problems, especially when they are accompanied with localized itchiness that is worse at night or after bathing.

## HERBALISM

 Some herbalists consider a chronic skin condition like rosacea to be indicative of an underlying dysfunction of the whole body. As such, one approach is to prescribe general body cleansers or alternatives to detoxify and increase the body's processing and elimination functions.

**Burdock root:** The use of burdock root tincture or tea on a daily basis can help to detoxify the body, especially when it is paired with approaches that promote regular bowel movements in order to improve elimination. Other alternative herbs that occasionally come up in this context are red clover flowers, nettle leaf, and fumitory. To decide upon the most appropriate alterative for a specific case of rosacea, as well as other body system treatments, you should discuss your case with a medical herbalist.

**Oregano oil:** There are many volatile oils in oregano with a variety of antibacterial and antifungal effects, which may account for its ability to improve symptoms of rosacea. A drop or two of the oil can be massaged into the affected skin once or twice daily. However, given that the skin of the face is often delicate and sensitive, it may be more tolerable to apply a cream or ointment that incorporates oregano oil. Any topically applied essential oil has the potential to cause dermatitis, so discontinue use if any redness, swelling, itchiness, or pain develops. People that are sensitive to other plants in the mint family may also react to oregano.

# ROSEOLA

## DIAGNOSIS

Also known as "sixth disease," roseola is a fairly common condition that affects toddlers. It affects children only between the ages of six months to three years, and around one in three children develops the condition at some point. It manifests itself as a rash and fever. The cause of the disease is unknown, but it is thought to be a virus that is transferred through the respiratory tract. There is a fairly long incubation period between infection and the first symptoms appearing, usually around 10–15 days. The fever needs to be treated carefully to avoid the possibility of a convulsion, by administering children's acetaminophen and plenty of water, and by making sure the child is cool but covered with a sheet. Take your child to the doctor to be sure that he/she is not suffering from measles or rubella.

## SYMPTOMS

- Sudden high temperature and fever that last for about three days
- In some cases the child has convulsions as a result of the sudden rise in temperature.
- General feeling of being unwell
- Loss of appetite
- Glands swell in the neck
- Sore throat
- After the fever resolves a patchy pink rash appears, usually beginning on the chest and stomach, and spreading to the arms and legs. It is very rare on the face
- The rash consists of pale, reddish spots, often with small heads. It lasts for a very short time—usually less than a day—and looks like rubella or measles

## TREATMENT GOAL

Roseola is a harmless condition and the child will recover very quickly. Treatment aims to relieve the symptoms and avoid complications such as dehydration and seizures.

## CONVENTIONAL MEDICINE

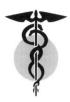

It is important to distinguish roseola from more serious diseases that manifest in similar ways, such as measles, German measles, meningitis, and other bacterial causes of high fever. If the physician is unclear about the diagnosis of roseola, blood tests and cultures will sometimes be carried out to rule out more dangerous infections.

**Keep hydrated:** Avoid dehydration by administering clear fluids in frequent, small amounts to the afflicted child. To ensure that the amount of water given is adequate, monitor the child's urine output (six wet diapers a day is normal).

**Reduce fever:** Fever can be lowered by giving the child lukewarm sponge baths and administering non-steroidal anti-inflammatory medications such as acetaminophen (Tylenol®) or ibuprofen (Motrin®), both made in liquid pediatric formulas and sold over the counter. The directions on the label should be followed for dosage. If the fever does not respond and is over 102°F, medical care should be sought.

**For persistent symptoms:** The illness should not last for more than a week. If symptoms persist or if complications such as febrile seizure, changes in mental status, dehydration, or severe cough develop, seek urgent medical help.

## TRADITIONAL CHINESE MEDICINE

**Herbs:** Traditional Chinese medicine considers wind and heat to be the main contributors to roseola. The following formulas are designed to dispel heat and wind. The herbs used are available from Chinese herbalists.
- Herbal tea: Combine 30 g of Zi Cao (groom well root), 12 g of Da Qing Ye (woad leaf), 15 g of Ci Ji Li (caltrop fruit), 12 g of Jing Jie (schizonepeta stem and bud), and 15 g of Fang Fen (ledebouriella root) in a ceramic pot. Add 3 cups of water, bring the liquid to the boil, and simmer for 30 minutes. Strain the liquid and drink 1 cup three times a day for three to five days. The amounts given are for a one-day dose.
- Herbal bath: Small rashes do not generally require external treatment. To treat extensive rashes, combine 30 g of Jing Jie (schizonepeta stem and bud), 20 g of She Chuang Zi (cnidium seed), 30 g of Di Fu Zi (broom cypress), and 18 g of Zi Cao (groom well root). Boil the herbs in 4–5 cups of water for 20 minutes, strain the liquid and add it to warm bath water. Soak the child in the bath for 20–30 minutes once a day.

**Acupuncture:** Acupuncture treatment can be given at the acute stage of roseola, or if the rash lasts more than four weeks. Acupuncture may shorten the course of the roseola and reduce itchiness and other symptoms.

**Acupressure:** Press the Qu Chi, Hegu, and Feng Chi points with thumbs for one to two minutes each twice a day. This will dispel the pathogenic factors and help the circulation. The Hegu points are located on the back of the hands between the thumb and first finger. When the elbow is flexed, the Qu Chi point is located in the outside depression at the bend (the lateral end of the traverse cubital crease). The Feng Chi point is located at the base of the skull 2 inches left of the center point.

**Diet:** Eat foods that are cooling, such as celery, spinach, lettuce, mung beans, tangerines, and string beans. During the illness, patients should avoid seafood and hot and spicy food, such as pepper, dried ginger, green and red peppers, and chilies.

## NATUROPATHY

**Diet:** Make sure you give the child plenty of fluids to avoid dehydration. If breastfeeding, continue to do so.

**Supplements:** Scientific data shows that cod liver oil is beneficial for those with roseola. Cod liver oil contains vitamin A, vitamin D and essential omega-3 fatty acids, which stimulate immunity among other benefits. Take ½ oz of cod liver oil twice a day; children should take 1 tsp twice a day. Take 250–500 mg of vitamin C two times a day to help stimulate the immune system.

**Herbs:** Catnip lowers fever and reduces spasms. Peppermint has historically been used to treat colds and fevers. Elder will calm your child and its antiviral properties will reduce fever. Fennel will calm an upset stomach and upper respiratory irritation. Yarrow reduces fever and helps restore appetite. Chamomile will stimulate the immune system and will relax your child before bed. Mix 1 tsp of a glycerine extract of every herb in 1½ cups of hot water. Your child should drink ½ cup three to four times per day, or take 30 drops as a tincture three to four times per day. The tincture can be mixed with apple juice or pear juice to make it more palatable for children. In addition, a strong tea (2 tbsp herb) can be added to bath water to keep fever down. If breastfeeding, drink a cup of the tea two to three times a day. You can also make a tea using one to three cloves of garlic and one to three slices of fresh ginger in 2 cups of hot water. This will stimulate the immune system and prevent upper respiratory infections. Lemon and a sweetener, such as honey, may be added for flavor. Do not give honey to children under two years old.

**Hydrotherapy:** Soak cotton socks in cold water, wring them out, and put them on the child's feet, with dry wool socks on over the cotton socks, before bed. This treatment, while uncomfortable at first, will help disperse a fever and allow for a good night's sleep. You can also soak a cotton sheet in cold water, wring it out, and use it to wrap the child. Then wrap the child in another blanket. This will disperse a fever and allow a restful sleep, particularly in infants.

**General considerations:** Make sure your child gets enough rest and lots of fluids. Keep your child from coming into contact with any other child with a known case of roseola. Some children may have febrile seizures as a result of this condition. If your child gets such seizures seek medical help immediately.

## HOMEOPATHY

Any of the following homeopathic remedies can be helpful, when well indicated, in easing discomfort and speeding up recovery from an acute episode of roseola.

**Belladonna:** Use this remedy to treat the first, feverish stage of the illness if a raised temperature has developed very rapidly and dramatically. Belladonna is appropriate if the skin is flushed, dry, bright red, and radiates heat. Confirmatory signs include swollen, aching glands that may be limited to, or be worse on, the right side.

**Pulsatilla:** This remedy tends to be more suited to the established stage of any illness rather than its initial onset. Glands will be swollen and tender and the child is likely to feel very uncomfortable and distressed when in overly hot and stuffy conditions, even though feeling chilly. Signature features include uncharacteristic clinginess and weepiness with a need for sympathy and attention.

**Phytolacca:** Use this remedy for any acute illness that involves extremely tender, swollen glands. Areas especially affected include the glands around the jaw and the throat. When this remedy is indicated the ears are likely to feel painful when swallowing. Cool drinks will feel soothing and warm drinks uncomfortable.

## HERBALISM

There is a long list of herbs that are beneficial in helping to reduce fever, a measure that may help with the roseola rash. Below are some herbs that show the most promise in treating fever and that are considered safe for use by children.

**Garlic:** Thought to have antiviral properties, garlic will generally boost the immune system. Take garlic capsules, which can be found at your local health food store, or simply ingest diced garlic raw or lightly cooked. The probable effective dosage for a child is unknown, but many experts will use half of the adult dosage or course depending on the child's age and weight; 500 mg two to three times a day may be appropriate.

**Yarrow:** This is readily available in health food stores as a dried herb or tincture. Make a batch of a herbal infusion by boiling 28 g of dried herb in a pint of water. Drink ½ cup of this infusion three times a day. This dosage is suitable for children 2–3 years old and above. The infusion can be sweetened with sugar to encourage children to drink it. There is a slight potential for an allergic reaction and yarrow should not be taken if there is a known allergy to plants in the daisy family.

**Boneset:** Dosage recommendations for boneset are consistent with those for yarrow: make a batch by boiling 25–30 g of dried herb in a pint of boiling water and drink ½ cup three times a day. Again, do not take this remedy if there is a known allergy to plants in the daisy family. There is a slight potential for nausea and vomiting when boneset is ingested.

**Meadowsweet:** This has components that are similar to aspirin and is therefore effective at reducing fever. Drink as a tea two to three times a day. Do not take meadowsweet if there is a known sensitivity to aspirin or if you have asthma. Potential, but rare, side effects include an allergic reaction and constriction of the airways.

# SCABIES

## DIAGNOSIS

Scabies is a contagious disease caused by a parasitic mite that feeds off dead skin cells. It appears as an itchy rash, usually starting off on the hands. It spreads from person to person via close skin-to-skin contact, such as occurs when sharing a bed. When there is an outbreak of scabies, it is important that everyone in the family is treated at the same time even if they do not have symptoms. If this is not done, the mites may return after a couple of weeks because they have survived on the skin of some members of the family, who have re-infected others.

Scabies is transferred when fertilized female mites tunnel their way through the top layer of skin and lay their eggs. This tunnelling produces tiny lines on the skin that are sometimes visible. Approximately three weeks later the eggs hatch and a new generation of mites are ready to reproduce and lay more eggs. After a few weeks the body develops an allergic response to the insects' excrement, which manifests itself as an itchy rash. Scratching can cause the skin to form a crust, which looks like psoriasis (see p. 134).

## SYMPTOMS

- Intense itchiness, especially at night
- The mites prefer certain areas of the body, such as the web spaces of the fingers and toes, palms of the hands and soles of the feet, wrists, armpits, skin around the navel, nipples, and scrotum
- The tunnelling shows up as a telltale dark red line
- Itchy red spots and blotches appear
- Intense scratching, particularly at night if you are overheated
- Sore, bleeding areas of skin
- Clear blisters

## TREATMENT GOAL

It is difficult for a doctor to diagnose scabies with 100% certainty unless a mite can be found and examined under a microscope. Treatment aims to relieve itchiness and other symptoms, and rid the body of the parasites and their eggs.

## CONVENTIONAL MEDICINE

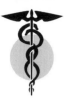

The mite that causes scabies is *Sarcoptes scabiei*. Treatment depends on an accurate diagnosis, which is made by the pattern of the rash that scabies causes. The mites, eggs, and mite feces can be microscopically observed after obtaining a sample from the skin using mineral oil on top of a lesion.

**Prevention:** If scabies is suspected, remove all bed linen, clothes, and towels used by the infected person within the past two days and launder them in hot water with detergent. Good hygiene—especially in crowded institutional settings—is a must in prevention.

**Lindane (Kwell®) lotion:** Apply lindane lotion to the entire body, below the neck, after bathing. If scabies is on the face, lindane can be carefully applied there, taking care to avoid the eyes. Leave the lotion on for about 12 hours before washing it off in the shower with soap. Repeat this treatment one week later. Generally, treatment is recommended for the whole family, as well as for those in close contact, such as care givers. Lindane should not be used on infants or pregnant women as it is potentially neurotoxic. Permethrin cream is a better choice for these patients, massaged into the skin from head to toe and left on for 12 hours. Only one treatment is needed.

## TRADITIONAL CHINESE MEDICINE

**Herbs:** Combine 30 g of She Chuang Zi (cnidium seed), 30 g of Di Fu Zi (broom cypress), 20 g of Tu Fu Ling (glabrous greenbrier rhizome), and 20 g of Ku Shen (sophora root), available from Chinese herbalists. Boil the herbs in 4 cups of water for 30 minutes. Strain the liquid and wait until it has cooled to a tolerable temperature. Soak the affected skin in the liquid for about 20 minutes. Discard the liquid after use. The herbs can be re-boiled one more time to repeat the process twice a day (mornings and evenings), for five to seven days. Itchiness should lessen immediately after soaking, but to prevent it from returning continued treatment is needed.

**Acupuncture:** This will help reduce itchiness and is beneficial for healing and preventing scabies from reoccurring. You should consult a practitioner about the necessity and frequency of treatment.

**Acupressure:** Acupressure is not recommended for scabies.

**Diet:** Food that helps clear heat in the blood, remove damp, and moisten dryness are recommended. This includes mustard greens, water spinach, towel gourd (found in

Chinese groceries), mung beans, and honey. Avoid food that tends to dry the blood and agitate wind, increase damp, and cause infection, such as chilies, pepper, fish, and shrimp.

## NATUROPATHY

**Diet:** Feed your child foods that are high in zinc to boost immunity. Such foods include eggs, turkey, fish, milk, wheat germ, and black strap molasses. Eliminate any foods to which you are allergic.

**Herbs:** Tea tree oil is a powerful herbal disinfectant. Apply undiluted tea tree oil to the affected area twice a day. Comfrey also makes an excellent topical salve and can be applied twice a day. Calendula ointment is healing and soothing to the skin. Add some goldenseal tincture, or purchase the calendula ointment mixed with goldenseal, for its antimicrobial properties.

**Hydrotherapy:** A cool oatmeal bath may help relieve itchiness. Put 1 cup of oatmeal into a cheese cloth and tie it with a string. Hang it under the faucet or float it in the tub. Soak in warm water, immersing in the tub for 20–30 minutes.

**TIP:** WASH ALL LINEN
Wash all bed linen, towels, and clothes in water that is as hot as possible.

## HOMEOPATHY

The following homeopathic advice can be used in a complementary way alongside any conventional medical steps that may need to be taken (such as using an insecticide lotion to destroy the mites that cause the intense itching on the areas of skin affected).

**Prevention:** If scabies is diagnosed, wash all bedding thoroughly and air it to eliminate the mites. If this is not done there is a risk that the cycle of infection will continue.

**Sulphur:** This remedy has a strong reputation for treating scabies. However, it needs to be taken with great caution by anyone who has suffered from a pre-existing skin condition (such as eczema or psoriasis) before developing scabies. In this case, it would be most helpful to consult a homeopathic practitioner in order to manage the progress of the condition most smoothly. Common symptoms that call for this remedy include maddening itchiness of the skin that is at its most intense at night in bed, after washing, and after scratching. The skin burns when scratched and feels intensely sensitive to contact with fresh air. Skin becomes infected easily while also healing very slowly.

## HERBALISM

It is important to exterminate the parasitic mite that causes scabies as opposed to simply treating the symptoms. If proper measures are taken to treat the scabies infestation, herbal remedies can be employed to help deal with the unpleasant symptoms. See the entry on pruritus (p. 129) for recommendations on how to control itchiness and skin irritation.

**Chrysanthemum:** Along with other plants in the daisy family, chrysanthemum produces natural insecticides called pyrethrins. While it is known that pyrethrins are effective in treating head lice (see p. 111), there is limited evidence that pyrethrin extracts are useful in treating scabies. Be cautious when dealing with pyrethrins: these compounds can be toxic when ingested or inhaled. Do not use chrysanthemum if you have asthma or if you are allergic to plants in the daisy family. If you choose to use this course of treatment, consult a medical herbalist. Although there is the potential for serious side effects, these can be avoided with proper administration.

**Anise:** Oil of anise can be used topically to treat scabies. Apply it directly to the affected area two to three times a day. The most common side effects are irritation and dermatitis. Combining a small amount of the anise essential oil with a high-quality oil used in skin care (for example, olive oil or almond oil) may help lessen these effects. Side effects may occur if anise is taken internally.

**Henna:** This is rich in certain chemicals that may be effective in treating scabies. Make a paste with the leaves, fruit, and bark of the plant and apply it directly to the affected area. There are no recorded side effects with the topical application of henna, except for transient discoloration of the skin.

**Black pepper:** This has been used externally to treat scabies. Apply an ointment that incorporates black pepper topically. Such products are available at health food stores.

# URTICARIA

## DIAGNOSIS

Also known as hives, urticaria is an allergic skin reaction that results in unpleasant, itchy red wheals with white, edematous caps. Wheals appear suddenly and then usually fade after a couple of hours. If you know what is causing the urticaria, make sure you avoid coming into contact with that particular substance. Generally, antihistamine drugs are prescribed to reduce itchiness.

**DANGER:** If the rash is making your face, mouth, or tongue swell—even slightly—contact your doctor immediately or go to the nearest hospital emergency room.

## SYMPTOMS

- Small or large patches or spots of raised pink or red skin with clear red edges that are usually circular in appearance, and with a white or yellow raised area or lump in the center
- The wheals are usually very itchy
- Swelling around the rash, particularly if it is on the face
- Eyes can become sore if rubbed
- Either a series of spots or a continuous area of inflamed skin
- The rash can affect any part of the body, but if it affects the mouth, throat, or tongue it can cause serious breathing difficulties
- Wheals fade after a couple of hours but may flare up again, sometimes elsewhere on the body
- Headache, listlessness, joint pains, and a general feeling of being unwell

## TREATMENT GOAL

It is important to determine the cause of the reaction and take action so you do not expose yourself to the allergen. Treatment aims to soothe skin and bring relief as quickly as possible.

## CONVENTIONAL MEDICINE

Urticaria can look like several other rashes, so it is important to obtain an accurate diagnosis for proper treatment. It can be confused with erythema multiforme, herpes, multiple insect bites, and a skin condition called bullous pemphigoid. The doctor will generally carry out blood tests to determine if any of these conditions are present. Once the diagnosis is established, avoidance of the trigger is key. A case of urticaria generally lasts six weeks before resolving itself.

**Prevention:** Urticaria occurs in about 80% of the population at some point in their life. Treatment involves prevention wherever possible and to facilitate this individual triggers need to be identified. The most common are certain foods; drugs, especially penicillin; viral infections, chronic illness such as lupus and thyroid disease; and sometimes environmental stimuli such as the sun and exercise. Different chemicals and food additives can also trigger an episode. Stress is a big trigger of urticaria and treatment involves modifying stress response through meditation, breathing, and exercise. Creative visualization techniques can also be helpful.

**Diet:** An elimination diet excluding dairy, eggs, nightshade plants such as tomatoes, tobacco, white potatoes, and eggplant, nuts, and shellfish can be helpful. Yeast can also exacerbate urticaria.

**Oral drugs:** Oral antihistamines such as cetirizine (Zyrtec®) can be used to relieve itchiness. Occasionally, H2 receptor agonists such as cimetidine, usually used as an antacid, can be added to help the antihistamine work. Oral steroids such as prednisone should be reserved for short-term use and severe cases that do not respond to antihistamines. Doxepin, usually used as an antidepressant, has some beneficial effect on chronic urticaria.

## TRADITIONAL CHINESE MEDICINE

According to traditional Chinese medicine, urticaria is caused by wind with heat, cold, or dampness.

**Herbs:** These are available from Chinese herbal stores.
• Herbal decoction one: Combine 15 g of Jing Jie (schizonepeta stem and bud), 15 g of Fang Fen (ledebouriella root), 12 g of Jin Yin Hua (honeysuckle flower), 15 g of Ci Ji Li (caltrop fruit), 10 g of Huang Qin (baical skullcap root), and 10 g of Fu Ping (spirodela) in a ceramic pot. Add 3 cups of water, bring to the boil, and simmer for 30 minutes. Strain the liquid and drink 1 cup two to three times a day.

• Herbal decoction two: Add 50 g of grated ginger and 100 g of brown sugar to ⅔ cup of vinegar and boil for 10 minutes. Strain the liquid, add a small cup of this decoction to warm water and drink two to three times a day. This recipe can relieve stagnant blood, toxicity, and reduce itchiness.

• Herbal tea: Mix 5 g of Jin Yin Hua (honeysuckle flower), 5 g of Bo He (field mint), and 5 g of Zhu Ye (bamboo leaves) in a teapot and add boiling water. Let the tea steep for five minutes. Drink the tea to reduce itchiness and other common symptoms. If the condition persists, see your TCM practitioner for a more specific formula or treatment.

• Herbal bath: Boil 15 g of Bai Bu (stemona root), 18 g of Ku Shen (sophora root), 18 g of Tu Fu Ling (glabrous greenbrier rhizome), and 18 g of She Chuang Zi (cnidium seed) in 5 cups of water. Strain the liquid and allow it to cool to a tolerable temperature. Add the liquid to bath water and soak the affected skin for about 20 minutes.

**Acupuncture:** To treat urticaria, you may have acupuncture treatment once or twice a week to help reduce itchiness. Research shows that acupuncture has an effect on regulating the body's immune system, and there is the possibility that it also has an antihistamine effect.

**Acupressure:** Press the Qu Chi, Feng Chi, and Xue Hai points. With the elbow flexed, the Qu Chi point is located in the outside depression at the elbow's bend (the lateral end of the traverse cubital crease). The Feng Chi point is located at the base of the skull, 2 inches left of the center point. The Xue Hai point is found on the inside of the leg at the depression just above the knee.

**Diet:** In general, eating fresh vegetables and fruit is recommended. During the acute stage, the patient should avoid seafood and spicy food.

## NATUROPATHY

**Diet:** Urticaria can be caused by toxins that are excreted through the skin. A high-fiber diet that includes two to four servings of wholegrains, fresh vegetables and fruits, and beans a day will help you eliminate toxins through your bowels rather than your skin. If hives are caused by UV rays from the sun, eat plenty of bright-colored vegetables and two to three avocadoes a week, as these foods have components that can improve your skin's resistance to the sun. Eat plenty of unsweetened cultured foods such as kefir, yogurt, and raw cabbage. These foods have friendly bacteria that reside in your digestive tract that are important for the inhibition of candidiasis, a major contributor of urticaria. Drink eight to 10 glasses of water a day to flush out impurities from your system. Avoid foods to which you may be allergic or intolerant, such as shellfish, dairy, eggs, cured meats, peanuts, and citrus fruit. Avoid all types of processed junk food as they will depress your immune system and diminish your body's defenses. Try to decrease the amount of food colorants, preservatives, and flavorings in your diet.

**Supplements:** Vitamin C can help relieve hives by lowering histamine, a chemical that is released by the body during an allergic reaction. Take 2,000 mg of vitamin C a day with the one of the bioflavanoids such as citrus bioflavonoids, hesperidin, rutin, and/or rose hips. Vitamin B12 has been reported to reduce the severity of acute hives as well as to reduce the frequency and severity of outbreaks in chronic cases. Have your doctor inject 1,000 mcg or take 400 mcg by mouth, although the oral form is not as effective. Quercitin also reduces the effects of histamine; take 1,000 mg three times a day.

**Herbs:** Freeze-dried nettle leaves are a natural antihistamine; take 300 mg three times a day. Burdock root has been historically used to treat skin conditions. Take 300 mg in capsule form three times a day or 8 ml amounts of tincture per day. Chamomile may reduce itchiness when used as a cream and relieve stress when drunk as tea. Aloe vera gel can be used topically on the affected area for its cooling, soothing, and anti-inflammatory properties.

> **TIP:** OATMEAL BATH
>
> A cool oatmeal bath may help soothe the itchiness caused by urticaria. Put 1 cup of oatmeal into a cheese cloth, tie it with a string, and hang it under the warm tap or float it in the tub. Soak your body in the tub for 20–30 minutes.

## HOMEOPATHY

Any of the following homeopathic remedies can help ease the itchiness and irritation of a mild or acute episode of urticaria. However, a tendency to develop severe and/or frequent flare ups of this condition requires professional homeopathic attention. A practitioner will address the underlying imbalance in the system that leaves the patient vulnerable to ongoing episodes.

**Urtica:** Bathe itchy, stinging, irritated areas in a solution of diluted Urtica tincture (one part of tincture to 10 parts of water). Urtica cream, available from herbal stores, can also be applied as a salve to reduce irritation, itchiness, and inflammation.

**Rhus tox:** If maddening irritation develops after exposure to cold, damp conditions, consider using Rhus tox. Sensitive skin is noticeably uncomfortable when exposed to cold drafts of air, and sufferers feel worse for getting wet or overworked. Itchiness causes great distress and restlessness in bed at night, triggering feelings of depression and despondency.

**Apis:** This is a possible choice for a blotchy, pinkish raised rash that is sensitive to warmth in any form and is soothed by contact with cold air. The skin eruptions sting and itch, and look waterlogged. There may also be signs of puffiness and swelling of the itchy parts (if this occurs, seek a swift medical opinion, since an allergic response involving swelling of the lips and face can be a medical emergency).

**Hepar sulph:** Symptoms of urticaria that are well-established, with a tendency for the skin to develop infections very readily, may respond well to this remedy. Use Hepar sulph if the skin is very sensitive to the slightest draught of cold air. The patient becomes irritable in response to itchy skin.

**Arsenicum album:** If irritated, itchy, burning areas are noticeably soothed by contact with warmth (in the form of warm bathing or applying compresses), Arsenicum album is a possible remedy. Symptoms lead to distress and feelings of mental and emotional restlessness and anxiety. Symptoms are also likely to be at their worst around 2 a.m., actually waking the patient from sleep.

## HERBALISM

 Caution is advised with the topical use of some plants for this and other skin conditions; if you use any of the herbs mentioned, try a small amount first. If no irritation develops gradually increase the dose. See the entry for pruritis (p. 129) for recommendations to specifically control itchiness.

**Burdock root:** Apply burdock root directly to the affected area as an essential oil, in an ointment, or in a poultice. While there are no reported adverse reactions to burdock, there is the potential for it, as with all other herbs applied topically, to aggravate symptoms. If this happens, stop using it immediately.

**Elderberry:** This can be very useful in controlling allergic inflammation. To make a tea, steep 2–4 g of the dried, above-ground parts of the herb in 150 ml of hot water. Strain the liquid and drink it two to three times a day. Elder flower can also be applied topically as an ointment to the affected area.

**Eyebright:** Like elderberry, eyebright can reduce inflammation. To make a tea, steep 2–4 g of the dried flowers in 150 ml of hot water. Strain the liquid and drink it two to three times a day, or apply eyebright externally in a poultice.

# VARICOSE VEINS

## DIAGNOSIS

Varicose veins are permanently dilated, twisted veins. Although they can occur in any part of the body, they usually develop in the legs. They appear as enlarged, snake-like, blue veins and are most noticeable when standing. They are most commonly seen in the back of the calf or on the inside of the leg, anywhere between the ankle and the groin.

While they are unsightly, which can of course cause distress, they do not usually cause any significant problems unless they are particularly severe. Varicose veins are caused by incomplete blood circulation: veins contain one-way valves every few inches to help the blood return to the heart against gravity. If these valves leak, then the increased pressure prevents the blood from draining properly.

The risk of developing varicose veins increases with pregnancy, a family history of the condition, an occupation that involves prolonged periods of standing (such as hairdressing), and menstruation, with symptoms worsening just before and during menstruation. If the varicose veins are allowed to worsen there is a risk of developing phlebitis (inflammation of the wall of the vein), eczema, leg ulcers, and deep vein thrombosis (DVT). To avoid these complications, an operation may be required. An operation may also be necessary if varicose veins cause pain.

## SYMPTOMS

- Heaviness and tiredness in the legs, particularly after periods of standing
- A creeping sensation across the skin
- Night-time cramps in the legs
- Swollen, sore, and painful legs

## TREATMENT GOAL

Help should be sought when varicose veins cause irritation during the day; if fluid accumulates in the legs; if working while standing up causes discomfort; or if legs become agitated at night, interrupting sleep. Treatment aims to prevent the condition from worsening, and easing any discomfort or distress caused by varicose veins.

## CONVENTIONAL MEDICINE

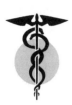

**Prevention:** A good starting place for the treatment of varicose veins involves prevention. Generally, prolonged standing, pregnancy, and obesity all increase the risk of developing varicose veins. The condition is also hereditary. If any of these conditions exist, special support stockings can be used from early morning to bedtime. Elevation of the legs as much as possible is also beneficial, as is weight loss if appropriate.

**For acute varicose veins:** Treatment generally involves the application of topical corticosteroids, as dermatitis can sometimes occur with varicose veins. Avoidance and treatment of any secondary infections is also important.

**For chronic varicose veins:** A technique called sclerotherapy is available in which sodium sulfate is injected to destroy the vein. If the above fails to correct varicose veins, surgery is an option. Several surgical techniques are available including ligation, vein stripping, and laser treatment.

## TRADITIONAL CHINESE MEDICINE

Blood stagnation is a typical cause of varicose veins in traditional Chinese medicine. Herbs proven to remove blood stagnation are generally used to treat this condition. Consult with a practitioner of traditional Chinese medicine for advice on using herbs.

**Herbs:** The herbs used to make the following decoction are available online or from a Chinese herbalist or pharmacy. Combine 12 g of Chi Shao (red peony root), 12 g of Haui Niu Xi (achyranthes root), 12 g of Dan Shen (salvia root), and 15 g of Ji Xue Teng (millettia root) in a ceramic pot. Add 3 cups of water and bring to the boil. After simmering the mixture for 30 minutes, strain the liquid and drink 1 cup two to three times a day. **Caution:** If you also have heart disease or blood disorder, you should not use this formula.

**Acupuncture:** This type of treatment is used to promote circulation in the body. It helps reduce the pain caused by swollen veins, and in some cases, reduces the size of the varicose veins. Usually, long-term and regular treatment are recommended in order to achieve the best results.

**Acupressure:** Press the Xue Hai, Feng Shi, Susanli, and San Yin Jiao acupressure points. The Xue Hai point is found on the inside of the leg at the depression just above the knee. Locate the Feng Shi point along the outside of the leg at the end of the fingers when the arm is hanging straight down at the side. The Susanli point is found on the lower leg, 1 inch to the outside and 3 inches below the kneecap. The San Yin Jiao point is on the inside of the leg, in the center about 3 inches above the anklebone.

## NATUROPATHY

**Diet:** A high-fiber diet can help by decreasing constipation, and therefore causing less of the straining that can lead to varicose veins over time. Build your meals around wholegrains, legumes, fruits and vegetables. Ground flax seeds, 1–2 tbsp a day sprinkled on your breakfast cereal, can also give you plenty of healthy fiber. Consume one or two servings of bright colored fruits and vegetables, such as berries, cherries, and carrots, every day. These contain powerful antioxidants that will strengthen the walls of the veins and improve their elasticity. Try eating pancakes mades with buckwheat, which naturally contains a flavonoid called rutin that will increase the strength of blood vessels. Cook with anti-inflammatory spices such as garlic, onions, ginger, and cayenne pepper to help increase circulation. Avoid hydrogenated oils and saturated fats to prevent sluggish circulation and inflammation.

**Supplements:** Take 25,000 IU of vitamin A in the form of beta carotene for skin integrity and to speed varicose ulcer healing. To aid circulation, promote the healing of sores, and strengthen vein walls to prevent dilation, take 1,000–5,000 mg of vitamin C and 100–1,000 mg of bioflavonoids divided into daily doses. A mixed complex of vitamin E at 400 IU daily will promote blood flow, improve circulation, reduce susceptibility to varicose veins, and sometimes relieve pain. Topical applications of vitamin oil often relieves localized irritation and speeds the healing of varicose ulcers. Taking 50 mg of zinc a day can assist with healing and collagen formation.

**Herbs:** Apply witch hazel ointment or gel on varicose veins for its astringent properties at least three times a day. You should see results after two or more weeks. Witch hazel is not recommended for internal use and may cause minor skin irritation in some people when applied topically. Bilberries support the normal formation of connective tissue and strengthen capillaries in the body, and in this way help prevent varicose veins. Take 160 mg of a standardized extract containing 25% anthocyanosides twice a day. Butcher's broom will help to reduce vein inflammation. Take a standardized extract that gives you 200–300 mg of ruscogenins a day, or prepare the herb as a tea. Take 120 mg of ginkgo biloba twice a day to strengthen blood vessels and improve peripheral circulation. Taking 500 mg of bromelain three times a day, between meals, can reduce inflammation of the veins and may help prevent blood clots.

**Hydrotherapy:** Alternating between hot and cold baths is believed to stimulate circulation in the legs. Fill two buckets or plastic wastebaskets, tall enough to submerge the legs up to the knees, with water—one with hot (but not so hot as to burn the skin) and the other with cool. Add 2 tbsp of epsom salts per quart of water, or add an aromatherapy oil or witch hazel. Soak your feet and legs in the hot water for about three minutes, then immerse them in the cool water for about 30 seconds. Repeat this three times, finishing with the cool soak. Perform this treatment once a day for at least one month to see results. If you have diabetes, use warm (not hot) water.

**General considerations:** Exercise regularly. Staying fit is the best way to keep your leg muscles toned, your blood flowing, and your weight under control. If your job requires you to be on your feet constantly, stretch and exercise your legs as often as possible to increase circulation and reduce build-up of pressure. If you are pregnant, sleep on your left side rather than on your back. This minimizes pressure from the uterus on the veins in your pelvic area and improves blood flow to the fetus.

## HOMEOPATHY

 This condition can vary in severity from a minor cosmetic nuisance to a major problem that causes a great deal of distress in the form of irritation and aching, and homeopathic support needs to be appropriate to the needs of the situation. The following advice is geared towards alleviating the discomfort of varicose veins that only surface infrequently, and are mild in nature. Alternatively, choosing an appropriate remedy from any of the following can be used as a stopgap to relieve pain and distress, while waiting for surgical intervention to provide a more radical solution. To treat varicose veins that appear to be escalating from a moderate nuisance to a more major condition, seek advice and treatment from an experienced homeopathic practitioner.

**Prevention:** The best way to prevent varicose veins from appearing in the legs is to avoid putting undue pressure on vulnerable areas. To achieve this, cross the legs at the ankle rather than the knee. Avoid standing for long periods at a time, but walk as much as possible to stimulate circulation in the legs. If veins in the legs are sore and aching after a long day, make a point of resting with your feet raised slightly on a stool.

**Arnica:** Use this remedy to ease soreness and aching that come on after physical exertion. Legs tend to feel restless and feet feel stiff and achy. There will also be a noticeable sensitivity of the veins to even light touch.

**Hamamelis:** If differentiating symptoms seem to be absent, Hamamelis can be used as an all-purpose remedy to relieve the pain, soreness, and aching of varicose veins. There may be a prickling, constricted sensation as well as a tendency to develop chilblains as a result of poor circulation.

**Lachesis:** This is an appropriate remedy for distended veins with a visible purplish tinge that are worse on, or restricted to, the left side. The affected leg or legs will be noticeably heat sensitive, with pounding, bursting pains that are temporarily eased by taking some exercise. Aching may be especially noticeable on waking from sleep, and eased by contact with cool air, cool water, and cooling compresses.

**Pulsatilla:** Use this remedy to treat aching varicose veins with shifting, changeable pains that are more severe on the right side. There will be a likely tendency to poor circulation with a noticeable general sense of coldness in the hands and feet.

## HERBALISM

 **Horse chestnut:** This is perhaps the best remedy for varicose veins. Look for a standardized extract of horse chestnut seed, as this limits the potential for adverse reactions. The unprocessed seed, bark, and especially flowers carry a risk of significant toxicity. The suggested dosage of horse chestnut seed extract is 200–300 mg one to three times a day. Do not exceed 600 mg in one day. Long-term use may increase the chances of adverse effects. **Caution:** Those who have liver or kidney problems, are pregnant, or have diabetes are advised not to use horse chestnut. It may also interact with certain anti-thrombotic drugs.

**Gotu kola:** Make a tea of gotu kola using 0.5–1 g of the dried herb and drink 1 cup three times a day. The herb can also be taken in extract form (30–60 mg three times a day) or in capsule form (300–500 mg once or twice a day). Gotu kola is a fairly safe herb with minimal side effects, though there are some reports of nausea and cramping. It can also cause drowsiness.

**Bilberry:** The fruits of this plant, besides being a rich source of vitamin C and other powerful antioxidants, show promise in treating varicose veins. The probable effective dosage is 50–200 mg of bilberry extract three times a day. There have been very few reported side effects, with diarrhea being the most common. As with horse chestnut, do not take bilberry if you are on anti-thrombotic drugs.

# VITILIGO

## DIAGNOSIS

This condition causes depigmentation, where the skin loses its color and becomes lighter in patches. Healthy skin contains melanin, a brown pigment produced from the amino acid tyrosine by pigment cells (melanocytes) in the skin, which is responsible for skin becoming tanned. If skin affected by vitiligo is examined under a microscope, melanin is absent and there are signs of inflammation in the deeper layer of the skin. This results in white patches of skin. It affects all races but is most obvious in people with darker skins. It affects approximately one person in every 200.

## SYMPTOMS

- Initially the pigment loss is often patchy
- The areas of depigmentation are usually seen first on skin that is exposed to light, particularly the face or back of the hands. It also appears in the armpits and groin area
- Frequently appears as "halo nevi," in which areas of depigmentation surround small, pigmented nevi (a nevus is any clearly defined skin abnormality present at birth)
- Often vitiligo is symmetrical, with both halves of the body equally affected, but occasionally only one particular area of skin will be affected
- Some sufferers will develop eczema or psoriasis at the site of the depigmentation
- The hairs in areas of vitiligo can turn white. Occasionally premature graying of hair can occur

## TREATMENT GOAL

To ease any associated symptoms and provide psychological help to learn to live with this condition.

## CONVENTIONAL MEDICINE

This is a benign skin condition and once it has been diagnosed, no treatment is necessary. It may be confused with several more harmful depigmenting diseases and so an accurate diagnosis is essential. The most common misdiagnosis is tinea versicolor, or ringworm (see p. 140).

There is also a condition called Vogt-Koyanagi syndrome, which involves deafness and eye problems along with vitiligo. Pityriasis alba also may appear similar to vitiligo.

**Cosmetic products:** Treatment is necessary only if emotional or social stress is debilitating. There are some cosmetic products that conceal vitiligo well, such as Dermablend™, which can be applied to lighter areas of skin to blend them with darker areas. Some covering agents, such as Dy O Derm™, actually stain the skin. Psoralen phototherapy (PUVA), taken orally or applied topically with subsequent UVA therapy for one to two years, is effective. There is also a repigmentation technique that involves the activation and migration of skin cells containing melanin from hair follicles. This is only effective on areas of vitiligo that have hair.

**Steroid creams:** Triamcinolone, which is mid potency, can be used daily for three months.

## TRADITIONAL CHINESE MEDICINE

Traditional Chinese medicine explains that vitiligo is related to a patient's mental stress, emotional health, liver and kidney energy deficiency, and blood stagnation. In many cases, it is possible to regain the normal skin color back, but persistent treatment is needed.

**Herbs:** These can be obtained from Chinese herbalists or online.
• To treat stress-related vitiligo: Mix 10 g of Chai Hu (hare's ear root), 10 g of Dang Gui (Chinese angelica root), 10 g of Yu Jin (turmeric tuber), 12 g of Bai Shao (white peony root), 6 g of Chuan Xiong (Szechuan lovage root), 15 g of Dan Shen (salvia root), and 10 g of Xiang Fu (nut-grass rhizome) in a ceramic or glass pot. Make a decoction by adding 3 cups of water, bringing to the boil, and simmering for 30 minutes. Strain the liquid and drink 1 cup three times a day for three to five days.
• To treat liver and kidney deficiency vitiligo: With this type of vitiligo, the patient could have fatigue, baldness, or graying hair. Herbs that help tonifying liver and kidney energy are suitable for this type of condition. Add 15 g of Guo Ji Zi (wolfberry), 12 g of Tu Si Zi  (Chinese dodder seed), 15 g of Shu Di Huang (Chinese foxglove root cooked in wine), 12 g of Han Lian Cao (eclipta), 12 g of Wu

Wei Zi (schisandra fruit), and 15 g of He Shou Wu (fleece flower root) to 3 cups of water in a ceramic or glass pot. Bring liquid to the boil and simmer for 30 minutes. Strain liquid and drink 1 cup of the decoction three times a day for three to five days.

• To treat vitiligo with blood stagnation: With this type of vitiligo, the border around the area lacking color has dark and distinguished edges. To treat this condition, mix 10 g of Tao Ren (peach kernel), 12 g of Chi Shao (red peony root), 10 g of Chuan Xiong (Szechuan lovage root), 12 g of Dan Shen (salvia root), and 8 g of Huang Hua (*flos carthami tinctorii*). Make a decoction by combining the herbs with 3 cups of water in a ceramic pot. Bring the liquid to the boil and simmer for 30 minutes. Strain the liquid and drink 1 cup three times a day for three to five days.

• External herbal formula: Place 30 g each of Bu Gu Zhi (psoralea fruit), Jiang Huang (turmeric rhizome), and Zi Cao (groomwell root) in a sealable container. Add 500 ml of rice wine, seal, and let the herbs soak for seven days. Apply the liquid to the areas of skin that lack color.

**Acupuncture:** Acupuncture is effective for all types of vitiligo conditions. A long-term treatment is usually required, once a week for three to six months. Treatment can be combined with herbal formulas.

**Acupressure:** The Qu Chi, Hegu, Xue Hai, and San Yin Jiao points should be pressed two or three times a day for one to two minutes each. With the elbow flexed, the Qu Chi point is located in the outside depression at the elbow's bend (the lateral end of the traverse cubital crease). The Hegu point is located on the back of the hand between the thumb and first finger. The Xue Hai point is on the inside of the leg in the depression just above the knee. The San Yin Jiao point is located on the inside of the leg about 3 inches above the ankle bone.

**Diet:** Take food that helps the blood, such as peaches, sweet basil, and chives.

## NATUROPATHY

There is barely any research into herbal treatments for vitiligo. This is due to the unknown causes of the disease and its strong hereditary component. However, some general suggestions follow.

**Diet:** In most traditional medicines, as in herbal medicine, the gut is the root of most skin disorders. Basic nutritional guidelines should be followed. Choose a hypoallergenic diet that eliminates peanuts, dairy, wheat, citrus fruits and juices, eggs, and corn. Reintroduce these foods to your diet one by one every week and note any changes in your skin.

**Supplements:** Data shows certain nutrient deficiencies in people with vitiligo and the following supplements should be taken. Take 10 mg of folic acid a day; 1,000 mcg of vitamin B12 intramuscular injections every two weeks; and 1 g of vitamin C a day.

**Herbs:** St. John's Wort has been shown to be useful for vitiligo as it has properties that make the skin more sensitive to light. Take 2–4 g a day or 1 tsp twice a day. Sarsaparilla is a skin tonic with many healing properties. Take 500 mg in capsule form or 4 ml of tincture three times a day. Taking burdock root, at 300 mg in capsule form three times a day or 8 ml amounts of tincture per day, can also be helpful.

## HOMEOPATHY

Since this condition falls into a chronic rather than acute category (vitiligo is subject to recurrent flare-ups that do not resolve themselves and is a progressive problem), it is more appropriate to seek treatment from a homeopathic practitioner rather than attempting to manage the situation yourself with homeopathic self-help measures. Your practitioner will be able to prescribe at what is called a constitutional level, which involves much more than simply treating your skin condition in isolation. Your health and vitality on mental, emotional, and physical levels should show signs of improvement as the self-regulating and self-healing mechanism your body possesses is given a boost.

## HERBALISM

**Carrot:** This vegetable has several healing and medicinal qualities. It is thought that carrot may be good for pigment anomalies. In addition to regular dietary consumption, drink 1–2 glasses of fresh carrot juice every day.

**Ginkgo:** There are reports that ginkgo may help to slow the progression of vitiligo and in some cases promote repigmentation of affected areas. Due to its increasing popularity, ginkgo is now readily available at local health food stores in pill or capsule form; the most studied form is a standardized extract that will list on the bottle the percentage of phytochemicals in the ginkgo preparation. Ginkgo has few reported side effects, although care should be exercised by those who are also taking anticoagulant and antithrombotic drugs, as there may be an added risk of bleeding.

**Bishop's weed:** Ancient Egyptians used this plant to treat vitiligo, though there are no modern clinical trials to support it. 4–6 g of this plant in powdered form were prescribed per day, though it is also possible to prepare a fluid extract or tincture for topical use.

# WARTS

## DIAGNOSIS

Warts are benign tumors caused by the human papilloma virus (HPV). Common warts on the hands and feet are caused by viruses that only affect humans. More than 60 different viruses that cause warts are known. They are very common, occurring mostly in children and teenagers, and are often spread by close physical contact. The frequency of developing warts drops drastically on reaching adulthood.

Plantar warts (or verrucas, see p. 120) are generally found on the soles of the feet. Genital warts can affect both men and women. They are sexually transmitted but are still caused by HPV. The virus can stay in the body for life, periodically flaring up.

Some types of genital wart virus (particularly HPV types 16 and 18) are linked with an increased risk of developing cervical cancer. These high-risk wart viruses do not cause visible warts, however, and the types of wart virus that do cause visible genital warts do not appear to increase the risk of cervical cancer.

## SYMPTOMS

- Warts on the hands are found most frequently around the nails and on the fingers
- Usually light brown in color
- They appear singly or in cauliflower-shaped clusters
- They may itch and bleed

## TREATMENT GOALS

To clear up any warts, ease painful symptoms, and prevent a recurrence.

## CONVENTIONAL MEDICINE

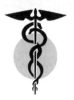

Genital warts should always be treated by a healthcare professional.

**Duct tape occlusion:** Warts that are not painful do not need to be treated, but can be removed through duct tape occlusion. The area surrounding the wart is completely covered with duct tape and left for about a week. The tape is removed and the area is soaked and debrided with a pumice stone. After a day, the duct tape is reapplied. This treatment is continued until the wart is gone.

**Topical treatments:** A 17% salicylic acid, obtained over the counter, can be applied to a wart twice a day for 12 weeks. The area should be clean and dry before application and bandaged after treatment. Liquid nitrogen is sometimes used successfully if other treatments fail, as is electrocautery. If the wart is very large or does not respond to any of the above, the wart may be cut off in a doctor's office. If all of these treatments fail, bleomycin, a chemotherapeutic agent, can be injected into the wart to remove it.

**Laser therapy:** For warts that are painful, laser therapy can be used. This results in a wound that takes four to six weeks to heal.

## TRADITIONAL CHINESE MEDICINE

**Herbs:** In general internal herbal medicines are not used to treat warts. However, if the condition is severe, or warts grow quickly in a short period of time, use the internal formula suggested for plantar warts (see p. 120).

**Moxibustion:** Performed by a trained practitioner, this treatment can successfully remove warts. The practitioner will burn a small cone of Moxa (a herb) to force the wart to become loose and be detached from skin immediately.

**Acupressure:** Press and push the wart from its root to remove it. This treatment should always be performed by a trained practitioner.

## NATUROPATHY

**Diet:** Eat a diet based on whole foods to support your immune system. Avoid processed foods that are high in simple carbohydrates, which can weaken your immune system and reduce the ability to fight viruses that cause warts.

**Supplements:** The following nutritional supplements will support immune function and healing, which will help combat the viral infections that cause warts. Take 500 mg of vitamin C two times a day; 100,000 IU of beta carotene a day; 400 IU of vitamin E a day; 200 mcg of selenium a day; and 15–20 g of zinc a day. Taking 50–100 mg a day of B-complex helps to reduce the effects of stress, which can weaken your immune system.

**Herbs:** Thuja has a caustic effect on the wart and also has antiviral properties. Apply one drop twice to four times a day. Take 500 mg of olive leaf extract twice a day for its antiviral properties. Garlic also has antiviral properties. Apply 1 drop of tincture two to four times a day. You can also use a raw garlic patch. Cover the wart and surrounding skin with a thin layer of castor oil or olive oil. Apply a thin slice of fresh garlic and tape it in place, leaving it on overnight. To maximize the benefit, place 2–4 drops of greater celandine on the wart before covering it with peel or garlic. This application may need to be repeated nightly for up to three weeks. The wart will turn black as it begins to die.

## HOMEOPATHY

Any established tendency to develop warts should be treated by an experienced homeopathic practitioner, who will aim to eradicate the tendency from inside. A minor, recently developed wart can benefit from the following treatments. Also refer to the advice given to treat plantar warts (p. 120).

**Nitric ac:** This is a suitable remedy for warts that are cauliflower-shaped and have a dry texture. Warts may produce sharp, sticking pains, be very sensitive to the touch, and bleed readily after touching or washing.

**Dulcamara:** Consider this remedy if warts are fleshy in texture and appear on the hands and fingers. Warts look smooth and flat and may be combined with a tendency for the palms of the hands to become moist and sweaty.

### TIP: BOOST YOUR IMMUNE SYSTEM
The appearance of warts is thought to be associated with the presence of a virus in the system, so it can be helpful to take practical steps to boost immune function. Simple helpful steps include avoiding alcohol, tea and coffee, and convenience foods that are packed with chemical additives. Eat immunity-boosting foods that are a rich source of antioxidant nutrients, such as tomatoes, strawberries, peppers, citrus fruit, blueberries, and broccoli.

**Natrum mur:** If warts have a tendency to develop on the palms of the hands, this remedy may be a possible choice. Additional symptoms include a tendency to develop very dry, sensitive skin that cracks easily in cold weather. Alternatively, greasy patches of skin and blackheads can also be present, with breakouts of acne or cold sores being a common occurrence, especially when emotionally stressed and/or run down.

**Thuja:** This is one of the leading remedies used for warts, especially if they appear after vaccinations. The condition feels worse when exposed to cold and dampness, and is soothed by exposure to warmth.

## HERBALISM

The herbalist approach for the treatment of warts is often very similar to that for plantar warts (see pp. 120–23).

**Oatmeal:** For use in the treatment of warts, prepare the oatmeal as if you were going to eat it, let it cool, and spread the paste over the affected area. Remember that warts can be stubborn and are often resistant even to strong conventional medical treatments. As a result, many doses of oatmeal may be required to produce results.

**American mayapple:** Applied topically as an ointment or poultice, this may help reduce common warts. This herb contains a compound called podophyllin, which is believed to be effective in treating warts. However, it can injure the surrounding skin, causing irritation and ulcers, and should therefore be administered by an experienced herbal therapist.

**Bittersweet nightshade:** The topical application of this plant as an ointment, available from health food stores, has been shown to be effective in the removal of warts.

**Spurges:** The milky juice that is exuded from a fresh spurges plant just after it is cut can be applied to warts. Caution must be taken as this sap is often a powerful irritant and easily ulcerates the skin. Furthermore, it is a poison and should not be taken internally; immediate medical attention is needed if ingestion occurs. Consult a medical herbalist if you choose this method of treatment.

# EYES
# AND
# MOUTH

# CONJUNCTIVITIS

## DIAGNOSIS

Conjunctivitis is a common eye condition involving an inflammation of the thin membrane that covers the eyeball. It is not serious but can be very uncomfortable and irritating. It usually affects both eyes at the same time, although it may start in one eye then eventually spread to the other. If the whole eye is affected, the condition has probably been triggered by a bacterial or viral infection, which is the most common cause of conjunctivitis. It is a very contagious condition and stringent hand washing is required to prevent it from spreading. Newborn babies are also prone to this condition. If you have recurrent attacks, it is important to isolate the trigger. Triggers and irritants can include a foreign body in the eye, such as a piece of grit, dirt, or dust, an allergy or hayfever, an intolerance to dairy products or other food, or chlorine in swimming pools. Antibiotic drops or ointment, or antihistamines if the conjunctivitis is an allergic reaction, are usually prescribed.

## SYMPTOMS

- Sore, irritated eyes that feel gritty or sandy
- The white of the eye becomes pink or red and bloodshot
- Swollen eyelids
- Weepy eyes
- A thin, watery discharge
- A thick, yellow discharge that is sticky and causes crustiness and gumming together of the eyelashes
- Difficulty opening eyes in the morning as eyelids may be stuck together with pus
- Eye rubbing
- Impaired vision

## TREATMENT GOAL

Always seek medical advice if you develop conjunctivits. Treatment aims to make the eyes comfortable, reduce inflammation, and eradicate any infection.

## CONVENTIONAL MEDICINE

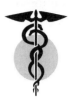

It should not be assumed that "red eye" is conjunctivitis. Treatment depends on whether the cause is viral, bacterial, allergic, traumatic, or chlamydial. If any pain or eyesight changes occur, see your doctor as this indicates a more serious problem than conjunctivitis.

**Artificial tears:** Dry eyes are more prone to conjunctivitis. Artificial tears can be used to remedy this and protect against the condition.

**Compresses:** To help alleviate conjunctivitis at its onset, hold a moist, warm compress to the eye for about 20 minutes three times a day.

**Antibiotic drops:** Two drops of tobramycin, gentamicin, or a floxin ophthalmic solution can be applied to the eye every four hours for about a week. Sometimes betadine eye drops are prescribed. Avoid using eye drops that contain steroids (some antibiotic drops have a steroid in them) if an infection is present, as they will exacerbate the condition.

**For allergic conjunctivitis:** Chronic allergic conjunctivitis is treated with mast cell stabilizing medication such as Patanol, which is like an antihistamine for the eyes.

## TRADITIONAL CHINESE MEDICINE

**Herbs:** The herbs needed for these formulas are available from Chinese herbalists or online.
• Ginger compress: Take one piece of fresh ginger, make a small hole in the middle, and place 1.5 g of Huang Lian (coptis root) inside. Bake the ginger and place it, while warm, on the Tai Yang acupoint. This point is located in the depression midway between the outer edge of the eyebrow and outer corner of the eye.
• Herbal tea: Mix 30 g of Ren Dong Teng (honeysuckle stem), 30 g Xia Ku Cao (common selfheal fruit-spike), 15 g of Pu Gong Ying (dandelion), and 15 g of Xuan Shen (ningpo figwort root) in a ceramic or glass pot. Add 3 cups of water, boil the mixture, and let it simmer for 30 minutes. Strain  and drink 1 cup of tea three times a day for three to five days.

**Acupuncture:** Acupuncture treatment is effective for conjunctivitis. An experienced acupuncturist will insert needles into some points around your eyes, and possibly on your arms and legs. You may be advised by your acupuncturist to have treatment twice a week for three to four weeks.

**Acupressure:** Press the Hegu, Tai Chong, Tai Yang, and Cuan Zhu points. The Hegu point is located on the back of the hand between the thumb and index finger. The Tai Chong point is found on the top of the foot in the depression between the first and second toes, at the base of the foot bones. The Tai Yang point is located at the temple, midway between the outer edge of the eyebrow and the outer corner of the eye. The Cuan Zhu point is found on the inside end of the eyebrow. In a sitting position, close your eyes and place your index finger gently on the Cuan Zhu point. Press with medium pressure for one minute and then press the Tai Yang point for one minute with your thumb. Press each point in turn for one minute. **Caution:** Wash your hands with soap and running water before and after acupressure.

**Diet:** Eat foods with plain flavor, such as Chinese cabbage, celery, fresh lotus rhizome, mung bean sprouts, balsam pears, shepherd's purse, tomatoes, water chestnuts, and pears. Avoid wine, spring onions, garlic, pepper, and chilies.

## NATUROPATHY

**Diet:** Maintain a diet that will strengthen the immune system so that your body is able to fight infections that can cause conjunctivitis. Eat fresh fruits and vegetables, whole grains, legumes, and quality protein such as fish, lean chicken, and beans every day. Eat plenty of green leafy vegetables for their high nutrient content, which will provide a base of nutrients required for a healthy immune system. Avoid foods that weaken your immune system, including processed foods that contain sugar and hydrogenated vegetable oils, store-bought baked goods, and all beverages other than tea, water, and freshly squeezed juices.

**Supplements:** A vitamin A deficiency has been reported in people that suffer from chronic conjunctivitis; take 10,000 IU of vitamin A a day. Take 250–500 mg of vitamin C a day to expedite the healing process and strengthen your immune system to fight toxins. Zinc also strengthens your immune system and helps you heal faster. Take 30–50 mg of zinc a day.

**Herbs:** The following herbs may be used as dried extracts (in the form of capsules, powders, or teas), glycerites (glycerine extracts), or tinctures (alcohol extracts). Compresses and eye washes are external treatments. A compress is made with a clean cloth, gauze pad, or cotton balls soaked in a solution and then applied over the eyes. Eye washes can be administered with an eye cup or a sterile dropper. Chamomile, fennel seed, marigold, and plantain help fight infection, soothe irritation, and have astringent and soothing properties. The fresh leaves are the most effective plant part. Make a soothing poultice with 28 g of bruised flaxseed steeped for 15 minutes in 4 oz of water. Strain the herbs, wrap them in a cheesecloth, and apply them directly to the affected eye. Grated fresh potato has astringent properties and can also be wrapped in cheesecloth and used as a poultice.

**Hydrotherapy:** Alternate using hot and cold compresses on the eye (three to four minutes hot, followed by 20–30 seconds cold). Use the compresses one to three times a day either by themselves or as part of a treatment program that includes an eyewash.

> **TIP:** HERBAL EYEWASH
> Mix 10 drops of goldenseal tincture with 1 tsp of boric acid in 1 cup of water. Use this mixture to wash the infected eyes.

## HOMEOPATHY

 The following homeopathic options can be helpful in easing the symptoms of a mild, recently developed bout of allergic or infected conjunctivitis. If you use the correct remedy, it should speed up the healing process, shortening the duration of an acute episode. However, since eye conditions can be tricky for the layman to diagnose, it is sensible to get a diagnosis that confirms the problem is actually conjunctivitis before beginning a course of homeopathic self-prescribing. Confirmation or otherwise of the condition can be made by your family doctor or opthalmologist. A more established tendency to recurrent bouts of moderate to severe conjunctivitis will require treatment from a trained homeopathic practitioner.

**Prevention:** Avoid spreading the infection by keeping your wash cloth, towel, and make-up separate. Also make a point of washing your hands every time you touch your eyes.

**Belladonna:** Use this remedy at the first sign of inflammation, heat, and redness. When this remedy is appropriate, symptoms always develop quickly and dramatically. Pains feel throbbing and pounding, while the affected eye feels hot and dry. Discomfort is worse for jarring movement and exposure to bright light, while resting propped-up in a darkened room feels soothing.

**Aconite:** This is an alternative choice to treat early symptoms, especially if problems have developed shortly after exposure to dry, cold, windy conditions. This is also the remedy to consider if conjunctivitis has set in after a foreign body has been removed from the eye. The eyes feel dry and gritty, making the sufferer feel restless and fearful due to hypersensitivity to pain and discomfort.

**Apis:** If the distress and discomfort of conjunctivitis is noticeably increased by exposure to warmth, plus signs of pinkish puffiness and swelling around the eyes, consider this remedy. Symptoms include stinging, shooting pains, baggy swelling under the affected eyes and great fussiness and fidgetiness when uncomfortable. Use this remedy for rapidly developing symptoms of allergic conjunctivitis.

**Pulsatilla:** For more established symptoms, especially those that develop as a complication of the later stages of a head cold, use Pulsatilla. Symptoms include an irritating feeling of a film covering the surface of the affected eye or eyes, which makes you want to constantly rub or wipe the eyes. A thick, yellowish-green discharge may also be present, which becomes crusty and sticks the eyelids together in the morning, and you may feel weepy and tearful when in discomfort.

## HERBALISM

**Eyebright:** This plant is only recommended for topical application. Soak a clean piece of gauze or cotton in an infusion of eyebright and dab it on the infected area. Be aware of the possibility of introducing infection if tools are not kept sterile. Use a clean piece of gauze or cotton ball for each application and a fresh infusion of eyebright each time if possible. If you notice the conjunctivitis worsening, or if it has not resolved after a few days, discontinue use and seek professional help.

**Calendula:** The flowers of this plant can be applied topically in the same manner as described for eyebright. Although there are very few contraindications or adverse reactions when used topically, applying calendula to the eye could cause more irritation. Discontinue use if this occurs. There is a small potential for an allergic reaction, but usually only in those who have had reactions to other plants in the daisy family.

**Goldenseal:** While it may be useful for the treatment of conjunctivitis, goldenseal is recommended with reservation due to environmental concerns. Goldenseal is a popular remedy and its depleting numbers in the wild has made it an unsustainable resource. Usually, an infusion or decoction of the roots is used as an eyewash to free powerful alkaloids, berberine and hydrastine, to rid the eye of infection. Check with your herbal therapist to see if goldenseal would help, or if there are other plants that would work.

**TIP:** PREVENTION
Viral and bacterial conjunctivitis are both very contagious. Family members should use separate towels and wash their hands often. Children with this condition should generally be kept home from school and nursery. If you wear contact lenses, keep them clean to avoid further irritation and any future infections. Do not wear lenses until your eyes have healed. People with allergy-related conjunctivitis sometimes develop a severe form with a stringy greenish or yellow discharge, swollen eyelids, scaly skin, vision changes, and significant discomfort. This needs aggressive medical treatment to prevent scarring of the cornea and further damage.

# GINGIVITIS

## DIAGNOSIS

Gingivitis is an inflammatory condition of the gums that, if left unchecked, can eventually lead to the loss of teeth. It is primarily caused by a build-up of dental plaque in the mouth. This tends to accumulate mainly in the space between the teeth and gum. Plaque is comprised of a damaging mix of food debris and bacteria, which causes the gums to become inflamed and pull away from the teeth. This frees up areas for yet more plaque to accumulate. Women can be particularly prone to gingivitis, as hormonal changes during pregnancy and menopause can trigger the condition. The first sign of this condition is usually bleeding gums. Taking some types of medication can destroy protective bacteria in the mouth, leaving gums vulnerable. If left untreated, gingivitis can progress to periodontitis (see p. 196). The bad habits that lead to gum disease often start during childhood, so it is important to get children into a good dental hygiene routine from an early age.

## SYMPTOMS

- Gums become red
- Gums become soft, shiny, and swollen
- Gums feel tender and sore
- Pain experienced when brushing teeth
- Bleeding gums, especially when brushing teeth
- Halitosis
- Painful to chew

## TREATMENT GOAL

If caught early, gingivitis is a reversible stage of gum disease. Treatment involves good dental hygiene, including regular brushing and flossing, plus frequent check-ups to prevent gingivitis from developing.

## CONVENTIONAL MEDICINE

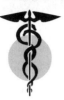

**Prevention:** Gingivitis can occur mildly or as a more severe ulcerative form, known as trench mouth. It occurs more commonly with the hormonal shifts associated with conditions such as pregnancy. It is also associated with excessive use of alcohol and tobacco, a poor dental hygiene routine, and ill-fitting dentures. Treatment involves prevention by looking at and addressing any one of these situations. Regular flossing is the most important factor in good hygiene. Some drugs cause a condition known as hyperplasia of the gums, the symptoms of which are very similar to gingivitis. The most common of these drugs are phenytoin, an antiseizure medication, and nifedipine, which is a blood pressure medication. If you suspect any of these causes, see your doctor.

**Dental treatment:** Regular teeth cleaning together with professional plaque removal are essential. X-rays are usually taken to make sure the disease is not affecting the bones. Changing your toothbrush every three months is also important as worn brushes do not remove plaque well.

**Antibiotics:** These are sometimes used to treat gingivitis in addition to plaque removal. Penicillin or clindamycin is the usual treatment.

**Supplements:** Make sure you take the recommended daily amount of vitamin C and D. 500 mg of vitamin C and 400–1,000 IU of vitamin D can help adults to improve gingivitis.

## TRADITIONAL CHINESE MEDICINE

To treat gingivitis effectively, a traditional Chinese medicine diagnosis is important, with reference to the patient's general physical condition. If a patient with gingivitis also has an elevated temperature, bad breath, severely infected gums, and is thirsty, the pathogen is excessive heat. Treatment for this type of gingivitis will focus on clearing the heat toxin from the body.

**Herbs:** These are available from Chinese pharmacies.
• Herbal decoction: Combine 10 g of Jing Jie (schizonepeta stem and bud), 12 g of Lian Qiao (forsythia fruit), 12 g of Tian Hua Fen (trichosanthes root), 12 g of Fang Fen (ledebouriella root), and 10 g of Jin Yin Hua (honeysuckle flower) in a ceramic pot with 3 cups of water. Bring this mixture to a boil and simmer for 30 minutes. Strain the liquid and drink 1 cup two to three times a day for 10–15 days.
• Herbal decoction: To make this decoction, use the same method described above, but substitute the following herbs: 10 g of Huang Qin (baical skullcap root), 6 g Huang Lian

(coptis root), 12 g Dan Pi (cortex of tree peony root), 10 g Zhi Zi (Cape Jasmine fruit), and 12 g of Niu Bang Zi (great burdock fruit).

• Herbal decoction to treat chronic gingivitis: If the infection in the gums is persistent and the patient is experiencing chronic bad breath, or yellowish-colored urine, this formula will clear the heat and dampness, improve the immune system, and help the body to fight off the chronic infection. Use the same method described above, but substitute the following herbs: 5 g of Huang Lian (coptis root), 12 g of Shu Di Huang (Chinese foxglove root cooked in wine), 12 g of Huang Bai (phellodendron), 15 g of Mu Gua (Chinese quince fruit), and 10 g of Zhi Zi (Cape Jasmine fruit).

• Herbal tea: Add 8 g of Jin Yin Hua (honeysuckle flower) and 6 g of Gan Cao (licorice) to a teapot and add boiling water. Sip the tea throughout the day, but before swallowing swish the tea around and let it remain in your mouth for a few seconds to let the herbs clean the bacteria. Jin Yin Hua and Gan Cao both have proven antibacterial effects.

**Acupressure:** Pressing the Hegu and Di Chang points can be helpful as they are beneficial for dispelling heat and promoting local circulation. The Hegu points are located on the back of the hands between the thumb and first finger. The Di Chang point is found directly below the pupil of the eye beside the mouth. Press each point for one to two minutes twice a day.

**Diet:** Eat food that is cooling such as purslane, mung beans, lotus, lettuce, and mango.

## NATUROPATHY

**Diet:** Avoid sugar and all refined carbohydrates. Sugar is known to contribute to gingivitis while weakening the immune system by decreasing white blood cell function. White blood cells are part of your body's "military" that defends against foreign substances. Eat a well-balanced diet that includes fresh fruits and vegetables, wholegrains, legumes, and quality protein such as fish, lean chicken, or beans everyday. Eat plenty of green leafy vegetables for their high nutrient content, which will provide the nutrients required for a healthy immune system.

**Supplements:** Vitamin C with bioflavonoids can help check bleeding gums by contributing to the build up of collagen, a protein in the formation of gum tissue. In one study, administration of vitamin C plus flavonoids improved oral health in a group of people with gingivitis; there was less improvement, however, when vitamin C was given without flavonoids. Take 1,000 mg of vitamin C and 500 mg of flavonoids twice a day. Coenzyme Q10 (CoQ10) deficiency has been found in people that suffer from gingivitis. Some researchers believe this deficiency could interfere with the body's ability to repair damaged gum tissue. Take 60–100 mg of CoQ10 a day for at least eight weeks. Some studies have shown that a 0.1% solution of folic acid mouth rinse can reduce gum inflammation and bleeding caused by gingivitis. Use 5 ml of solution twice a day for 30–60 days, holding the solution in the mouth for one to five minutes before spitting it out. Zinc benefits oral health by stabilizing the gum membrane, increasing antioxidant activity, promoting collagen synthesis, inhibiting plaque growth, and numerous other immune activities. Take 15–30 mg of zinc in the picolinate form.

**Herbs:** Bloodroot contains properties that inhibit bacteria that breed in the mouth. Toothpastes and mouth rinses containing bloodroot should be used according to manufacturer's directions. A mouthwash combination that includes sage oil, peppermint oil, menthol, chamomile and myrrh tincture, clove oil, and caraway oil has been successfully used to treat gingivitis. Add 10 drops of some or all of the above to 1 cup of water to use as a mouth rinse two times in succession two to three times a day. Keep the solution in your mouth for 30 seconds when rinsing. Blueberries, hawthorn berries, and grapes are all rich sources of flavonoids and help repair gum tissue. Eat these as frequently as possible to supplement your diet.

## HOMEOPATHY

The following homeopathic remedies can ease recently developed, mild, and/or infrequent symptoms of bleeding gums. However, for the best outcome, the use of a homeopathic remedy must be combined with dental treatment. When neglected, gum disease can have serious consequences, eventually leading to the loss of teeth.

**Prevention:** Avoid sugary, sticky foods that can aggravate dental problems. Eat a minimum of five portions of fresh fruit and vegetables every day. Unlike white sugar (which is thought to sabotage the immune system), fresh, raw fruit and vegetables include antioxidant-rich nutrients that support the immune system in fighting infection. Take the time to brush teeth carefully and thoroughly (for advice on the best technique see the entry on sensitive teeth p. 208). Also make a point of flossing regularly after cleaning your teeth. If you find dental floss difficult to master, try using slightly wider dental tape.

**Lycopodium:** If gums are sensitive and there is a persistent unpleasant taste in the mouth that may be bitter, musty, or sour, try using Lycopodium. The patient may experience cravings for sugary foods and drinks, and gums may bleed easily when touched or when teeth are brushed.

**Kreosotum:** This is a suitable remedy for treating spongy-looking, inflamed gums that have a bluish tinge. When this remedy is indicated the teeth are also likely to be of poor quality and breath may be sour. In addition, the lips may look inflamed and have a tendency to bleed very easily.

**Nitric ac:** This remedy is helpful if the gums have taken on a swollen, flabby-looking appearance, while the teeth may be yellow-tinged and develop cavities easily. The tongue may also look furry and generally discolored, while the gums are subject to sharp, splintering pains.

**Carbo veg:** This is a possible choice if blood oozes slowly from the gums when the teeth are brushed. The action of chewing may also trigger pain, sensitivity and discomfort in the affected areas, and this may be accompanied by a nasty taste in the mouth and bad breath. Teeth may also be sensitive to contact with hot and cold food or drinks.

## HERBALISM

 **Eucalyptus oil:** This contains a compound called eucalyptol that possesses antimicrobial properties. Eucalyptol is present in many commercially available mouthwashes. To make your own mouthwash use several drops of eucalyptus oil diluted in water. You can also prepare an infusion by boiling 2–3 g of eucalyptus leaf in 150 ml of water. Do not swallow eucalyptus oil, as ingestion can cause severe side effects, including depression of the central nervous system, nausea, and vomiting. Eucalyptus oil is not recommended for use by small children.

**Tea tree oil:** Since gingivitis is an inflammation usually caused by bacteria in the mouth, it is thought that tea tree oil, with its antibacterial and antifungal properties, is an effective treatment. Use several drops of tea tree oil diluted in water as a mouthwash two to three times a day. As with eucalyptus oil, severe side effects have been reported with tea tree oil ingestion, so avoid swallowing the mouthwash.

**Chamomile:** Prepare a strong infusion, using approximately 3–6 g of dried chamomile in 200 ml of water, and use this as a mouthwash two to three times a day.

**Green tea:** Use 3–6 g of green tea steeped in 200 ml of water as a mouthwash two to three times a day. Taken in this manner there are virtually no side effects, although excessive use may stain your teeth and cause gum irritation. Green tea does contain caffeine and other stimulants and if ingested could lead to agitation, restlessness, and insomni, though the caffeine content is still much less than a cup of coffee.

# GLAUCOMA

## DIAGNOSIS

Glaucoma is one of the most common causes of blindness in the world today, and the likelihood of developing it increases with age. It is an umbrella term for a range of conditions affecting the eye, where the pressure inside the eye becomes too high and the optic nerve at the back of the eye becomes damaged, which can lead to the loss of vision if left untreated. There are two main types of glaucoma. The most common form is chronic simple glaucoma, where loss of vision occurs slowly and is often irreversible, as people do not notice any problem until their vision has already been damaged. This type of glaucoma is rare in people under 40 years old. The second form is acute glaucoma, which comes on suddenly and causes painful red eyes and blurred vision. This condition is very rare in patients under the age of 50.

## SYMPTOMS

### CHRONIC
- Peripheral vision tends to be affected first and, therefore, to begin with, eyesight does not noticeably alter
- The loss of peripheral areas of visual field increases until eventually the central vision is damaged, which can lead to blindness

### ACUTE
- Eye suddenly becomes very painful
- Eye is usually red
- Vision becomes blurred
- You may notice a "halo" effect around lights
- Pupils become dilated
- Headaches
- Feelings of being unwell
- Nausea

## TREATMENT GOAL

Glaucoma is a serious condition that can result in loss of sight. Acute glaucoma is a medical emergency and treatment should be sought immediately. Treatment of chronic glaucoma aims to slow the deterioration of eyesight and relieve any discomfort.

## CONVENTIONAL MEDICINE

Glaucoma can be confused with allergies and with irritation from contact lenses, along with other more rare eye diseases, so treatment requires an accurate diagnosis. A diagnosis is made by using visual field examination and GDx nerve fiber analysis tests. The latter test measures the thickness of the retinal nerve fiber layer as those with glaucoma have been found to have thicker retinal layers. Blood tests are sometimes performed to rule out associated diseases.

**Relieving pressure:** Treatment aims to lower the pressure in the eye and to keep the pressure down. How this is carried out depends on how high the pressure in the eye is. Intravenous mannitol is sometimes given to bring down the pressure. An emergency treatment is an anterior chamber paracentesis, which is rarely necessary.

**Medication:** Eye drops containing pilocarpine, or a course of oral pilocarpine, beta-blockers, and Diamox® all lower intraocular pressure and they are sometimes prescribed for acute conditions to immediately lower the pressure.

**Laser therapy:** For chronic or long-term conditions there are new laser procedures that are effective. Iridotomy and trabeculectomy are traditional surgical procedures, which generally totally cure the elevated pressure so that no further treatment or medication is needed. Filter valves are sometimes placed surgically to prevent the recurrence of glaucoma after acute treatment is given. All of these procedures are done by an ophthalmologist. If your doctor diagnoses glaucoma, he or she will refer you to an ophthalmologist for treatment.

## TRADITIONAL CHINESE MEDICINE

**Herbs:** These are available from Chinese herbalists.
• Herbal decoction: Combine 12 g of Di Huang (Chinese foxglove), 12 g of Bai Shao (white peony root), 10 g of Ye Ju Hua (wild chrysanthemum flower), 12 g of Gou Ji Zi (wolfberry), and 12 g of Gou Teng (stem and thorns of gambir vine) with 3 cups of water in a ceramic or glass pot. Bring the mixture to a boil and simmer for 30 minutes. Strain the liquid and drink 1 cup three times a day for three to five days. This formula nourishes the liver and kidneys, helping to promote energy flow in the eyes.
• Herbal tea: Add 3 g of Ye Ju Hua (wild chrysanthemum flower), 3 g of Bo He (field mint), 8 g of Gou Ji Zi (wolfberry), and 5 g of Cang Er Zi (cocklebur fruit) to a teapot of boiling water. Let the tea steep for five minutes before drinking. This formula has the gentle function of reducing the heat, and nourishing the eyes.

**Acupuncture:** Treatment will help reduce the high pressure in the eyes, but must be performed by a highly trained and experienced practitioner because of the complexity of the particular points and techniques involved. You should have acupuncture treatment once or twice a week. Regular treatments over a period of three to nine months, or even longer in some cases, may be necessary in order to achieve the best possible results.

**Acupressure:** Wash your hands before this treatment. In a sitting position, close your eyes and place your index finger on the Cuan Zhu point (located on the inside end of the eyebrow) using medium pressure for one minute. Next press the Tai Yang point (located at the temple, midway between the outer edge of the eyebrow and the outer corner of the eye) for one minute with your thumb. Press the Chen Xi point (directly below the pupil between the eyeball and orbital ridge) for one minute. When you have finished open your eyes slowly. Perform this procedure twice a day to help circulation to the eyes.

> **TIP: EXERCISE REGULARLY**
> Studies indicate that glaucoma patients who exercise regularly (at least three times a week) can reduce their intraocular pressure by an average of 20%. If they stop exercising for more than two weeks, pressure increases again. Talk to your doctor to determine an appropriate exercise program.

## NATUROPATHY

**Diet:** Eat a wholesome balanced diet based on whole grains and fresh fruit and vegetables. Include as many orange, yellow, and green leafy vegetables as possible. These contain pigments called carotenoids, which are essential for optimum eye health. Eat plenty of fruits such as blueberries and dark cherries, which contain anthocyanidin, a chemical that is also important for good eye health. Foods rich in magnesium and chromium, such as brewer's yeast, kelp, leafy greens, and apples, have beneficial effects on glaucoma.

**Supplements:** Some studies have shown that magnesium can dilate blood vessels and improve vision; take 250 mg twice a day. Taking 1,000 mg of vitamin C two to four times a day can significantly reduce elevated intraocular pressure in cases of glaucoma. Taking 150 mg of alpha lipoic acid a day for a month improves visual function in people with some types of glaucoma. Vitamin A may also have benefits for the eyes; take ½ tbsp twice a day. Chromium, zinc, and the B complex of vitamins, particularly thiamine, also appear to play a role in preventing and treating glaucoma. Those with elevated eye pressure have been found deficient in these elements. Anyone at risk should consider taking the following supplements: 100 mcg of trivalent chromium twice a day; 30 mg of zinc a day; and 50 mg of B complex a day.

**Herbs:** Bilberry contains flavonoids that support eye structure and function. Take 160 mg twice a day for 25% anthocyanosides (the active ingredient of the herb). Rutin has been found useful in restoring normal collagen metabolism and normalizing eye tissue, which helpful in the prevention and treatment of glaucoma. Take 20 mg three times a day.

## HOMEOPATHY

Due to its potential seriousness unless managed by medical assessment and treatment, this condition is best left in the hands of conventional and complementary health professionals. An integrated approach to medical treatment is recommended rather than attempting to deal with the problem through self-prescribing.

**TIP:** USE SUNGLASSES

Glaucoma can cause the eyes to be very sensitive to light and glare and medications can aggravate the situation. Sunglasses solve this problem and are important in preventing cataracts. Protective sunglasses do not have to be expensive. Choose ones that block both UVA and UVB.

## HERBALISM

**Ginkgo:** Ginkgo can be taken as a tea or tincture two to three times a day; most scientific studies use standardized extracts once or twice a day. Ginkgo has few reported side effects, although care should be exercised for those who are also taking anticoagulant and antithrombotic drugs as there may be an added risk of bleeding.

**Coleus:** Coleus contains a compound called forskolin that may be helpful in lowering the pressure inside the eye, which is of primary importance when treating glaucoma. Coleus is not easily available, and standardized extracts may be even harder to find. It is best used topically by applying 50 mcl of forskolin suspension eye drops (1%). There are few reported side effects with topical application, but be aware that allergic reaction to this formula is possible, and may manifest as eye redness, burning, or tearing.

# MACULAR DEGENERATION

## DIAGNOSIS

One of the most common problems associated with eyes is the slow progressive loss of vision, known as age-related macular degeneration. This condition begins with the deterioration of the retina, gradually resulting in blurred vision and a difficulty reading, and eventually leading to a blind spot in the center of the visual field. It is the leading cause of eye problems in people over 60 years old. Risk factors include smoking and not protecting the eyes adequately from bright sunlight. The condition usually starts in one eye and then eventually affects the second eye as well. In the preliminary stages, the "healthy" eye compensates for the deterioration in the affected eye. Those with macular degeneration do not go totally blind as they retain their peripheral vision. The disease progresses very slowly and affected people often manage to go about their normal business without the condition affecting their daily routine. There are two main types of macular degeneration. The dry type, which affects the majority of sufferers, causes the retina to thin and generally affects one eye first. The wet type is more severe and progresses at a faster rate, distorting vision quickly.

## SYMPTOMS

- Gradual distortion of vision
- Blurring of central sight
- Difficulty reading
- Colors seem faded

## TREATMENT GOAL

There is currently no treatment for dry macular degeneration, but laser techniques can be effective for some cases of wet macular degeneration. The condition is diagnosed by an eye examination.

## CONVENTIONAL MEDICINE

All cases of macular degeneration should be followed by an ophthalmologist. Any sudden decline in vision is a medical emergency.

**Diet:** Berries, especially blueberries, have a high antioxidant content and are helpful in treating macular degeneration. Bilberry is also useful.

**Exercise:** Regular moderate-intensity exercise and relaxation techniques, particularly yoga and meditation, may be valuable in preventing degeneration as they increase the blood flow to the eyes.

**Anti-aging protocols:** High-dose antioxidants such as vitamin A, E, and C, as well as the minerals zinc and selenium and the nutrients alpha lipoic acid, N-acetyl cysteine, coenzyme Q10, and glutathione, are all very powerful, free radical scavenging agents.

**Steroids:** To treat acute macular degeneration, intravitreous steroids are used, which involves injecting steroids into a chamber of the eye.

**Laser treatment:** Argon laser treatments can be performed to destroy any abnormal blood vessels.

## TRADITIONAL CHINESE MEDICINE

**Herbs:** The herbs listed inthe formula below are available from Chinese herbalists or online.
• Herbal tea: Add 12 g of Gou Ji Zi (wolfberry), 12 g of Sang Shen Zi (mulberry fruit-spike), 15 g of Di Huang (Chinese foxglove), 15 g of Fuling (poria), 15 g of Shan Yao (Chinese yam), and 10 g of Ju Hua (chrysanthemum flower) to 3–4 cups of water in a ceramic pot. Bring the liquid to the boil and simmer for 30 minutes. Strain the liquid and drink 1 cup twice a day. This formula is good for strengthening the liver, kidneys, and blood, which, according to traditional Chinese medicine, are all directly related to eye health.

**Acupuncture:** Treatment involves inserting needles into points around eyes and should only be performed by an experienced acupuncture practitioner. Treatment once a week for at least six months is necessary to see results. Acupuncture can slow down the degeneration process by working on the liver, kidneys, and blood and by improving circulation around eyes.

**Acupressure:** To treat this degenerative condition, self-help is important. Press the Jing Ming point on the face between the bridge of the nose and inner corner of the eye. Also press the Feng Chi point in the depression at the base of the skull, 2 inches from the center point. To treat headaches, press the Tai Yang point, located at the temple, midway between the outer edge of the eyebrow and the outer corner of the eye. For nausea and vomiting, press the Nei Guan point 1 inch above the center of the wrist on the palm side. To reduce intraocular pressure, press the Xing Jian point, on the instep of the foot just behind and between the first and second toe, and the San Yin Jiao point, in the center on the inside of the leg about 3 inches above the anklebone. Press these points using gentle pressure once or twice a day.

**Diet:** Foods that are good for the liver and blood, such as loquat, persimmon, pineapple, chives, duck, grapes, lotus, yam, tangerine celery, and chicken liver, are recommended. Foods that nourish the kidneys are also recommended. These include chicken liver, black sesame seed, and string beans. Avoid food that is warm and pungent, such as wine, spring onions, garlic, pepper and chilies, and dried ginger.

## NATUROPATHY

**Diet:** Eat a wholesome diet based on whole grains and fresh fruits and vegetables. Consume as many orange, yellow, and green leafy vegetables as possible. These contain pigments called carotenoids that are essential for optimum eye health. Fruits such as blueberries and dark cherries contain anthocyanidin, a chemical that is also important for good eye health. Vitamin C is also found in these foods, which is helpful for building up the structures around the eye. Avoid any foods that can cause or contain free radicals. These include saturated fats, hydrogenated fats and oils or partially hydrogenated fats and oils, sugar, alcohol, and charred or grilled meats.

**Supplements:** Take 15 mg of lutein with a meal. Lutein is an antioxidant in the carotenoid family, which can benefit the part of the retina where macular degeneration occurs. It also helps prevent oxidative damage. Zeaxanthin also prevents oxidative damage of the macula; take 3 mg with food. Taking 30 mg of zinc has been shown in some studies to be helpful for macular degeneration. Fish oils contain DHA, a substance concentrated in the retina of the eye, and the consumption of fish oils has been shown to reduce the risk of macular degeneration. Take a product that can give you 1,000 mg of DHA a day. Vitamin E complex acts as an antioxidant and has been shown to improve vision in people with age-related macular degeneration. Take 400 IU a day. Macular degeneration is a common ailment among the elderly, who often have low levels of gastric acid and digestive juices, fluids that are important for the metabolism of protein and absorption of nutrients. Protein and a variety of nutrients are important for eye health. The supplement betaine hydrochloride improves stomach acidity and digestion, especially of proteins. Take 1–3 capsules with each meal, but reduce the dose if you experience a warming or burning sensation.

**Herbs:** Bilberry is recommended in treating macular degeneration. Take 160 mg twice a day standardized for 25% anthocyanosides. Ginkgo biloba improves blood flow and contains flavonoids that support eye structure. Take 60 mg three times a day with 24% flavone glycoside extract. Rutin restores normal collagen metabolism and normalizes eye tissue. Take 20 mg three times a day.

> **TIP:** TAKE PREVENTIVE MEASURES
> Smoking has been linked to macular degeneration. Giving up may reduce your risk of developing the condition. Regular moderate exercise will help keep your blood flowing properly to the eyes. Wear sunglasses that filter out 98% of the ultraviolet spectrum.

## HOMEOPATHY

Due to the potential seriousness of this condition, unless it is managed by medical assessment and treatment, macular degeneration is best left in the hands of conventional and complementary health professionals. An integrated approach to medical treatment rather than self-prescribing is ideal.

## HERBALISM

**Ginkgo biloba:** Most of ginkgo's beneficial effects are derived from the herb's purported ability to increase blood flow. By improving blood flow to the eye, gingko may lessen any degenerative changes. Due to its overwhelming popularity, ginkgo is readily available at local health food stores in pill or capsule form. Most studies have used 120–240 mg daily with 60–80 mg tablets taken two to three times daily. Ginkgo can also be taken as a tea or tincture two to three times daily. There have been few reported side effects, although care should be exercised for those who are also taking anticoagulant and antithrombotic drugs, as there is an increased risk of bleeding.

**Bilberry:** This treatment is recommended without reservation due to its lack of side effects and the fact that bilberry has many positive qualities, such as being packed with antioxidants. The suggested dose is 50–120 g of berries two to three times a day. If it is difficult to find fresh or dried berries so look for the extract; 80–160 mg diluted in juice or water is recommended.

# PERIODONTITIS

## DIAGNOSIS

Periodontitis is a serious form of gum disease where severe inflammation of the gums is accompanied by erosion of the bone and ligaments that support the teeth. This can eventually lead to a tooth becoming loose in its socket and falling out. How quickly the disease progresses largely depends on the type of bacteria present and how well your body's natural defenses work against it. The main trigger for this condition is the build-up of plaque on teeth, so practicing good dental hygiene is the best way to avoid this particular type of gum disease. This includes cleaning your teeth regularly, flossing, and frequent check-ups at the dentist. It is also a good idea to see a dental hygienist regularly to help further prevent the build-up of plaque on the teeth.

## SYMPTOMS

- Gums become red
- Gums become soft, shiny, and swollen
- Gums feel tender and sore
- Pain experienced when brushing teeth
- Persistent bleeding from the gums, especially during brushing teeth
- Halitosis
- Painful to chew
- Toothache triggered by hot or cold foods or drinks
- Offensive taste in the mouth
- Wobbly, loose teeth

## TREATMENT GOAL

This condition is not easily cured. The aim of treatment is to prevent the disease from progressing further. Surgery may be required if the condition is advanced.

## CONVENTIONAL MEDICINE

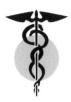

**Prevention:** Good oral hygiene and a non-processed, sugar-free, relatively alkaline diet are essential in protecting against periodontitis. Adequate and high-quality dental work on a regular basis is also important. Keeping stress at bay by regular stress reduction techniques, such as meditation, lowers cortisol and enhances immune function; both of these are key in the prevention of periodontitis. Hormonal balance is also important, as periodontal disease is exacerbated during the premenstrual time. Smoking of any kind encourages periodontal disease. The severity and risk of the disease goes up in direct proportion with the number of cigarettes smoked. Poor antioxidant levels, particularly of vitamin C, is associated with the disease. At the first sign of disease, vitamin C should be supplemented in amounts of 500 mg a day. Coenzyme Q10 in amounts of 100 mg a day can slow periodontal disease, as does eating soy and avocado.

**Treatment:** Treatment depends on the progression of the disease. A focus on the bacteria that cause the problem is needed. For example, certain herpes viruses and varicella (chickenpox virus) are known causes of gingivitis, which precedes periodontitis. Treatment involves the removal of plaque in a dentist's office and a low dose of oral or topical antibiotics. Fluoride treatments discourage formation of plaque forming bacteria. Sometimes surgery is needed, which is done by a periodontist.

## TRADITIONAL CHINESE MEDICINE

**Herbs:** The following herbs are available from Chinese herbalists or online.
- Herbal decoction: Mix 12 g of Huang Qin (baical skullcap root), 10 g of Jin Yin Hua (honeysuckle flower), 10 g of Da Qin Ye (woad leaf), 10 g of Chuang Xin Lian (green chiretta), 8 g of Lian Zi Xin (lotus flower), 10 g of Pu Gong Ying (dried dandelion), and 5 g of Gan Cao (licorice) in 3–4 cups of water. Boil the combination in a ceramic pot for 30 minutes and then strain. Drink 1 cup of the liquid two to three times a day.
- Herbal powder: Grind 6 g of dried ginger, 6 g of hard red dates, and 6 g of dried alum into a powder and apply over the affected area.
- Qin Dai powder: This patent formula, available from Chinese pharmacies, reduces infection. Apply it to the inflammation area as indicated on the package, or consult the pharmacist about the usage.

**Acupuncture:** Treatment can reduce inflammation, and reduce pain. If you have chronic periodontitis, your acupuncturist may suggest that you have treatment regularly. Once a week for 10 weeks is the average length of a course of treatment. For an acute condition, you should consult your dentist and acupuncturist.

**Acupressure:** Press the Hegu points, located on the back of the hands between the thumb and first finger. Press the Di Chang point, directly below the pupil of the eye beside the nostril. Also press the Feng Chi point at the base of the skull 2 inches below the center point. Press each of these points for one to two minutes.

**Diet:** Foods that are good for this condition include purslane, mung beans, lotus, lettuce, mango, aubergine, spinach, strawberries, pears, red beans, flat beans, and coix.

## NATUROPATHY

**Diet:** Avoiding sugar and all refined carbohydrates is extremely important. Sugar is known to contribute to dental problems, while weakening the immune system by decreasing white cell function. White blood cells help defend the body against foreign substances, such as bacteria. Eat a well-balanced diet that includes fresh fruits and vegetables, whole grains, legumes, and quality protein (such as fish, lean chicken, and beans) every day. Eat plenty of green leafy vegetables for their high nutrient content, which provides the foundation required for a healthy immune system. Blueberries, hawthorn berries, and grapes are all rich sources of flavonoids and help in repairing gum tissue. Eat these as frequently as possible.

**Supplements:** Vitamin C with bioflavonoids can help check bleeding gums by contributing in the build up of collagen, a protein involved in the formation of gum tissue. Take 1,000 mg of vitamin C and 500 mg of flavonoids twice a day. Some researchers believe that a deficiency in coenzyme Q10 (CoQ10) could interfere with the body's ability to repair damaged gum tissue. Take 60–100 mg a day for at least eight weeks. A 0.1% solution of folic acid in a mouth rinse is thought to reduce gum inflammation and bleeding. Use 5 ml twice a day for 30–60 days, rinsing the mouth with the solution for one to five minutes before spitting it out. Zinc stabilizes the gum membrane, increases antioxidant activity and collagen synthesis, and inhibits plaque growth; take 15–30 mg of the picolinate form.

**Herbs:** Bloodroot contains properties that inhibit oral bacteria. Use a toothpaste and mouthwash that contain bloodroot according to the manufacturer's directions. Make a mouthwash by combining 10 drops of some or all of the following: sage oil, peppermint oil, menthol, chamomile and myrrh tincture, clove oil, and caraway oil. Dilute these oils in 1 cup of water and rinse the mouth for 30 seconds twice in succession two to three times a day.

## TIP: PRACTICE GOOD HYGIENE

Floss your teeth thoroughly twice a day. Studies show that an electric toothbrush can remove 98.2% of plaque; only 48.6% is removed through conventional brushing. Make a mouth rinse with hydrogen peroxide ($H_2O_2$) in a 3% solution, mixed half-and-half with water, and swish it around your mouth for 30 seconds. Use this wash three times a week to inhibit bacteria, but do not swallow.

## HOMEOPATHY

Due to the nature of this condition, this is a problem that needs to be addressed by consultation with an experienced homeopath in combination with treatment from your dental specialist.

## HERBALISM

Due to the advanced nature of this disease, and the risk of permanent damage resulting in teeth removal, herbal therapy is not recommended as a first option for treatment. The suggestions listed below are beneficial as adjuncts to therapy provided by your dentist.

**Eucalyptus oil:** Eucalyptol, a compound found in eucalyptus oil, possesses antimicrobial properties and is present in many commercially available mouthwashes. To make your own mouthwash dilute several drops of eucalyptus oil in water. You can also prepare an infusion by boiling 2–3 g of eucalyptus leaf in 150 ml of water. Do not swallow eucalyptus oil; ingestion can cause severe side effects, including depression of the central nervous system, nausea, and vomiting.

**Tea tree oil:** Periodontitis is an inflammation usually caused by bacteria in the mouth, and tea tree oil, with its antibacterial properties, can be an effective treatment. Dilute several drops of tea tree oil in water and use it as a mouthwash two to three times a day. As with eucalyptus oil, severe side effects have been reported from ingesting tea tree oil, so avoid swallowing the mouthwash.

**Green tea:** To treat periodontitis, prepare a strong infusion and use it as a mouthwash. Used in this manner there are virtually no side effects to green tea, although it does have the potential to further irritate the gums and can stain the teeth. Green tea does contain caffeine and other stimulants that, in excessive quantities, can lead to agitation, restlessness, and insomnia.

# PUFFY EYES

## DIAGNOSIS

Puffy eyes are usually caused by an unhealthy lifestyle, but they can also be symptomatic of a more serious condition. The eyes are supported by soft pads of fat and muscle. When you are tired, your facial muscles aren't as animated and fluid can collect in the eye socket area. As the muscles get weaker, they bulge out, creating a bag effect. This can result from too many late nights, which leads to fatigue, over-indulging in alcohol, and poor nutrition. Puffy eyes can also be aggravated by over-exposure to the sun, menstruation, and pregnancy. Occasionally bags under the eyes are accompanied by dark circles, which are usually caused by higher-than-average amounts of melanin (which gives the skin its pigment). Rubbing your eyes can cause folds that darken the color of the skin, creating the appearance of bags under the eye.

Puffy eye bags are usually passed on genetically and tend to become more prominent as you get older. In winter, nasal congestion associated with conditions such as sinusitis (p. 286) and catarrh (p. 237) can lead to puffy eyes. In the summer, if you suffer from hay fever you may get puffy eyes during the season, whereas if you are prone to allergic rhinitis it can be a year-round problem.

Occasionally, puffy eyes can be a sign of a more serious condition. If your eyelids are swollen you may have an inflammation of the eye and will need to see your doctor for a diagnosis. Puffy eyes can be linked to conditions such as conjunctivitis (p. 178) or blepharitis (inflammation of the eyelids). It can also be an indication of a thyroid disorder. There is also an infection of the eye socket tissues called orbital cellulitis that produces pain and swelling of the eyelid and surrounding area. This is a serious condition and needs immediate medical treatment.

## SYMPTOMS

- Puffy bags under the eyes
- Dark circles under the eyes

## TREATMENT GOAL

To improve the look of your eyes and establish the cause of the condition, whether it is connected to lifestyle or related to a medical problem.

## CONVENTIONAL MEDICINE

If you seek conventional medical treatment for puffy eyes, your doctor will not be able to prescribe medication to make the puffy eyes go away. He or she is obligated to determine the cause of the puffy eyes, whether it results from an illness or otherwise. This is not always conclusive, but it is important that any dangerous causes are ruled out. The focus of the examination will be on ruling out hypothyroidism, which is common and is associated with puffy eyes among many other symptoms, but which can also occur without puffy eyes. Other less common causes are lupus and other autoimmune connective tissue or eye disorders. In women, hormone imbalances causing water retention, such as estrogen dominance or progesterone imbalance, can cause puffy eyes.

**Eye exam:** The doctor will also do a thorough examination to determine whether there is an infection, corneal abrasion, conjunctivitis, or tear duct abnormalities.

**Home treatments:** Treatment is based on what is causing the puffy eyes. Puffy eyes can be treated at home with cold compresses, green tea bags on the eyes for 15 minutes, or a cold eye mask. If there is no resolution, or if the puffy eyes are associated with other symptoms, see an ophthalmologist or general physician.

## TRADITIONAL CHINESE MEDICINE

Traditional Chinese medicine views puffy eyes as a symptom of an internal disorder or deficiency, particularly conditions relating to spleen and kidney health.

**Herbs:** To help relieve puffy eyes, combine 15 g of Bai Zhu (atractylodes rhizome), 18 g of Fuling (poria), 15 g of Mu Gua (Chinese quince fruit), 15 g of Shan Yao (Chinese yam), 12 g of Ji Shen (jilin root), and 12 g of Dan Zhu Ye (lophatherum stem and leaves) in a ceramic pot. Add 3–4 cups of water, bring the mixture to a boil, and let it simmer for 30 minutes. Strain the liquid and drink 1 cup three times a day. The herbs listed here are available from Chinese herbalists or online.

**Acupuncture:** Treatment will aim to relieve the underlying problem that is causing the puffy eyes. If puffy eyes are due to spleen and/or kidney deficiency, the treatment principle will be to disperse water retention, enhancing spleen and kidney energy. Treatment causes are determined by the individual patient's condition.

**Acupressure:** Wash your hands before pressing the following points. In a sitting position, close your eyes and use medium pressure to press the Cuan Zhu point (on the inside of the end of the eyebrow) with your index finger for one minute. Then press your temple for one minute with your thumb. Press the Si Bai point directly under the pupil in the depression below the eye socket bone. Press the Tai Yang point at the temple, in the depression one finger's width between the lateral end of the eyebrow and eyelid. Also press the Tong Zi Liao point, which is about a ½ inch from the outside corner of the eye.

**Diet:** Eat foods that disperse dampness such as mustard greens, water spinach, towel gourd (found in Chinese groceries), mung beans, and honey. Foods that are good for the spleen and kidneys are ham, potatoes, sweet potatoes, and string beans.

## NATUROPATHY

**Diet:** Reduce your consumption of alcohol and salt, especially at night. These substances can cause fluid to build up around the eyes, causing puffiness. Drink 2–3 cups of black or green tea every day. These teas have chemicals called tannins that have astringent properties, absorbing water and helping to tighten the skin.

**Black tea compress:** Add two black tea bags to boiling water and let them brew for five minutes. Remove the tea bags, wring them out, and place them in the freezer for 10–15 minutes. Place the tea bags over your eyelids for 10–15 minutes. The polyphenols and tannin in the tea are astringents and mild stimulants, and the treatment also has a slight tightening effect to reduce puffiness.

**Witch hazel:** Add a drop of witch hazel to a few egg whites, stiffly beaten. Apply the mixture under the eyes with a brush to make the skin feel tighter and look less puffy.

**Cold compress:** Dunk a washcloth in cool water (or wrap it around some ice cubes), lie down, and place the cloth over your closed eyes. When the cloth gets warm, wring it out and repeat three or four times.

**TIP:** USE A POTATO OR CUCUMBER EYE COMPRESS
Lie down, preferably in a quiet room, for 15 minutes with either a slice of raw potato or cucumber over each eye, or cotton wool pads soaked in witch hazel. All of these substances contain properties that reduce eye swelling.

## HOMEOPATHY

The possible self-help strategies for this condition vary depending on the cause of the problem. For example, puffy eyes that result from an allergic reaction or conjunctivitis are likely to respond well to medical attention, while puffy eyes that are caused by too many late nights can be dealt with cosmetically. With this in mind, any of the following strategies can be useful in easing the symptoms and speeding the recovery of a recently developed, mild bout of puffy eyes that have an obvious cause or trigger. As always, a more established, recurring, or severe condition requires professional homeopathic attention and treatment.

**TIP:** USE A EUPHRASIA TINCTURE EYE COMPRESS
Soak two cotton wool pads in diluted euphrasia tincture, squeeze them out, and place them over puffy, tired eyes for 10 minutes as you rest (ideally with your feet up).

**Apis:** This remedy can reduce the puffiness and swelling that can develop around the eyes as a result of an allergic reaction. When this remedy is appropriate, the puffy areas look pink and fluid filled, and swelling comes up quickly and dramatically. Applying cool compresses to the affected areas feels soothing, while exposure to warmth feels very uncomfortable.

**Kali carb:** Puffy eyes that are related to a mild or recently occurring bout of fluid retention may benefit from this remedy. Signature symptoms are puffiness and swelling of the inner angle of the eyelid, or between the upper eyelid and the eyebrow. The eyelids may also feel cold.

**Arsenicum album:** This remedy can be helpful in reducing puffiness and swelling around the eyes with redness and inflammation of the eyelids. There may also be a burning sensation in the eyes, which may produce excessive amounts of tears. Burning sensations in and around the eyes are unusually temporarily soothed by warm compresses.

**TIP:** MAINTAIN A HEALTHY DIET
If you have puffy eyes after a night of over-indulgence and lack of sleep, drink plenty of still, filtered water to flush out the system, eat generous portions of vitamin C-rich fresh fruit and vegetables, and avoid alcohol or caffeinated drinks.

## HERBALISM

Puffy eyes can often result from allergies. The treatments given below may help relieve the puffiness, but do not address the underlying cause. If you have symptoms of allergies (i.e., a runny nose, watery eyes, sinus pressure, or congestion) in addition to puffy eyes, it may be wise to treat those as well. Please refer to the section on allergies (p. 22) and allergic rhinitis (p. 232) for treatment options.

**Chamomile:** Arguably the best herb to revitalize tired puffy eyes is chamomile, which has calming properties and anti-inflammatory effects. As with most treatments for eyes, a compress is perhaps the most effective method of treatment. To make the compress steep approximately 2–5 g of dried chamomile flowers in 200 ml of boiling water for 20 minutes. Strain the mixture and allow it to cool. Soak two cotton wool balls or a washcloth in the liquid, wring out the excess, and place them over your closed eyes for as long as you can tolerate (up to 10 minutes) once or twice a day. Another option is to steep two chamomile tea bags in boiling water, allow them to cool, and place them directly on your eyelids for 10–15 minutes once or twice a day. Be aware that this may cause more irritation than the previous method. If you begin to notice redness or irritation, stop the treatment. Do not use chamomile if you are allergic to plants in the daisy family.

**Green tea:** Prepare a compress of green tea in the same manner as chamomile to treat puffy eyes.

**Cucumber:** Cucumber is a classic home remedy for tired puffy eyes, due to its cooling and tonifying effects, and seems to work quite well, although there is a lack of any real scientific evidence to support this. Place slices of fresh, cool cucumber on your closed eyes for 15–20 minutes once or twice a day, or as long as you have time for (even a few minutes can make a difference). There is the potential for an allergic reaction to occur. If you notice any redness, itchiness, or irritation, discontinue use.

# SENSITIVE TEETH

## DIAGNOSIS

Sensitive teeth are a common problem, and if you suffer on a daily basis it can be very uncomfortable. Teeth are covered by a protective layer of enamel. When this is eroded the cavities underneath become exposed and sensitive. Tooth decay, an abscess, or gum disease—including conditions such as gingivitis (see p. 183) and periodontitis (see p. 196)—can leave the roots of teeth exposed, leading to pain and sensitivity. Another trigger could be a cavity that needs filling, or a filling that needs repairing. More general sensitivity is often triggered by everyday substances, such as hot and cold food or drinks. Aching teeth can also be caused by poor brushing technique. Using a toothbrush with bristles that are too hard or brushing too vigorously are two of the most common problems. Toothpastes designed for those with sensitive teeth can help relieve symptoms. If your teeth are causing you pain and discomfort, make an appointment to see your dentist to get checked out for any underlying disease that could be causing you problems.

## SYMPTOMS

- Sudden shooting pains in teeth when eating hot or cold food or drinking hot or cold drinks
- A dull aching sensation in teeth or gums

## TREATMENT GOAL

To determine the underlying causes of the pain and resolve them to bring relief from the discomfort.

## CONVENTIONAL MEDICINE

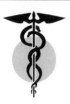 Sensitive teeth is not a disease in itself but a symptom of a larger problem. Conventional medicine aims to diagnose and treat the cause. For immediate alleviation of pain while the cause is being sought, non-steroidal anti-inflammatory drugs are prescribed, which can be obtained over the counter.

**If an infection is present:** The doctor will carry out a history, examination, and laboratory tests to determine whether the tooth pain is infectious and what is most likely to be the cause. Infections of the sinuses, inner ear, and teeth can all cause sensitivity in teeth. A sinus infection is treated with a 14-day course of antibiotics. An ear infection is treated with a seven-day course of antibiotics. A tooth infection should be treated by a dentist.

**If headaches are present:** Headaches can cause teeth pain, particularly migraines. Generally the migraine would have other symptoms as well, with head pain being the most obvious. To relieve pain in the teeth, treat the migraine (see p. 658).

**If hypothyroidism is present:** Hypothyroidism is another illness that can include among its symptoms generalized sensitivity of the teeth, although this is an unusual cause of dental pain. To treat sensitive teeth, treatment of the thyroid hormone deficiency is needed.

**Treating children:** Normal growth and development in children includes a stage of teeth eruption, which causes pain. This can be treated with symptomatic pain relievers, such as children's Tylenol® or Motrin®.

## TRADITIONAL CHINESE MEDICINE

 Traditional Chinese medicine is based on an ancient system in which, historically, "dentistry" did not exist. However, many classic TCM books have mentioned treatment for problems with the teeth. Traditional Chinese medicine approaches sensitive teeth from the perspective of treating pathogenic heat and wind. The condition is caused by excess stomach heat in the majority of cases due to the special relationship between the stomach and teeth.

**Herbs:** The following herbs are available from Chinese pharmacies or online.
• Internal decoction: Add 15 g of Shi Gao (gypsum), 15 g of Shen Di Huang (Chinese foxglove root), 6 g of Shen Ma (bugbane rhizome), 10 g of Huang Qin (baical skullcap root), 10 g of Dan Pi (cortex of tree peony root), and 5 g of Huang Lian (coptis root) to 3–4 cups of water in a ceramic pot. Bring the mixture to the boil, simmer the herbs for 30 minutes, and then strain the liquid. Drink 1 cup two to three times a day.

• Herbal tea: Combine 10 g of Bai Zhi (Chinese angelica root), and 10 g of Wu Zhu Yu (evodia fruit) in a ceramic pot. Add 3 cups of water and boil for 20 minutes. Drink the tea throughout the day, but before swallowing it, swish the tea around your mouth for a while to allow the herbs have the maximum effect.

• Watermelon frost: This patent herbal medicine is available from traditional Chinese medicine stores and is safe to use in the mouth. Watermelon frost cleans out the heat in the teeth and calms the sensitivity. Spray the fine powder on the surface of the sensitive area.

**Acupuncture:** This treatment is helpful in healing chronic infection and reducing pain. You may choose acupuncture treatment to complement dental care. Individual patients may require a different treatment plan. Consult with your dentist and your acupuncture practitioner for the best treatment plan to reduce teeth sensitivity and pain, and to reduce or avoid over-reliance on antibacterial drugs.

**Acupressure:** Press the Xia Guan point, located in front of the ear in the depression above the jawbone, the Jie Che point, found on the cheek in the depression in front of where the jawbone turns at the back, and the Di Cang point, which is directly below the pupil of the eye beside the mouth angle, for one minute. Repeat two to three times a day, washing your hands before each treatment.

**Diet:** Eat foods that are cooling, such as mung beans, lotus, lettuce, mango, cucumber, aubergine, spinach, strawberries, and pears. Avoid foods that are hot and spicy.

**TIP:** EAT RICE PORRIDGE
If your teeth are highly sensitive to cold and hot, try eating rice porridge, which contains cooling properties and has a mild taste. Add 100 g of rice to 1,000 ml of water. Cook the rice in plain water until it is soft. Eat the porridge as part of a meal.

## NATUROPATHY

**Diet:** Good dietary habits are the first step towards overall healthy teeth and treating sensitive teeth naturopathically. Avoiding sugar and all refined carbohydrates is important. Sugar is known to contribute to teeth and gum problems by feeding bacteria surrounding your teeth, which decrease white blood cell function. White blood cells are part of your body's "military" that defends you against foreign substances. Eat a balanced diet that includes fresh fruits and vegetables, whole grains, legumes, and quality protein (such as fish, lean chicken, and beans) every day. Eat plenty of green leafy vegetables for their high nutrient content to provide a base of nutrients required for a healthy immune system. Do not eat acidic foods or sweets. Lemons, tomatoes, and other foods with a high acid content can eat away at your tooth enamel and hinder your teeth's natural healing process. For some people, eating sweets causes a flare-up of pain. Serve hot or cold foods at temperatures close to room temperature, and try to avoid biting into foods of different temperature extremes at the same sitting.

**Supplements:** Nutritional supplements that help with periodontal problems can be helpful in treating sensitive teeth. Vitamin C with bioflavonoids can help treat gum disease by contributing to the building of collagen, a protein that is important in the formation of gum tissue. Take 1,000 mg of vitamin C and 500 mg of flavonoids twice a day. Coenzyme Q10 (CoQ10) deficiency has been found in people with gum disease. Some researchers believe this deficiency could interfere with the body's ability to repair damaged gum tissue. Take 60–100 mg of CoQ10 a day for at least eight weeks. Some studies show that folic acid in a 0.1% solution used as a mouth rinse has reduced gum inflammation and bleeding. Rinse the mouth with 5 ml of solution, available from health food stores, twice a day for one to five minutes for 30–60 days. Zinc stabilizes the gum membrane, increases antioxidant activity, promotes collagen synthesis, inhibits plaque growth, and performs numerous immune activities. Take 15–30 mg of the picolinate form a day.

---

**TIP:** ADOPT A GOOD BRUSHING TECHNIQUE

Brush your teeth using a gentle up and down motion, and be careful when brushing close to the gum line, which is where most sensitivity occurs. Bad brushing can not only cause hypersensitivity, it can undo all of nature's repair work. Use a soft-bristle brush, as stiff, hard brushes can scrape and strip away enamel and cause gums to recede, especially in those who use excessive pressure when brushing. Softer bristles are less likely to irritate sensitive teeth and will not expose underlying nerves.

---

## HOMEOPATHY

Your dentist should be able to identify the reason for undue sensitivity in your teeth (usually due to extremes of hot and cold) so that you can have the best chance of remedying the problem. Your brushing technique may be part of the problem. Once you have established the cause of the problem, one of the following homeopathic remedies may be helpful in easing pain and sensitivity when used in the short-term.

**Chamomilla:** If teeth become sensitive to warm food and drinks, or when breathing in the cold night air, consider using Chamomilla. Pain and discomfort may cause a tantrum-like reaction, to the point of using abusive language to vent feelings.

**Staphysagria:** For poor-quality, sensitive teeth that show signs of decay very readily, this remedy may be used. It is well indicated if hypersensitivity of the teeth is aggravated or brought on by eating or during a menstrual period. Applying heat and pressure helps to ease the pain.

**Pulsatilla:** This may be a helpful remedy if hot food and drinks make sensitivity more intense, and if pain is relieved by contact with cool things. Symptoms include a dry mouth without thirst and a white-coated tongue. Another key symptom is a tendency to burst into floods of tears when in pain and discomfort, with a need for sympathy and attention.

**Coffea:** Use this remedy if there is a huge intolerance to pain that feels insupportable. Sensitive teeth are soothed by the cooling sensation of ice water in the mouth.

**TIP:** USE A TOOTHPASTE FOR SENSITIVE TEETH
If you know your teeth have a tendency to become sensitive, use a toothpaste that has been specially formulated with this problem in mind. However, you will need to use it on a regular basis in order to reap the cumulative benefits.

## HERBALISM

**Cloves:** These can be processed to extract an oil called eugenol, which can be used as a pain reliever and local anesthetic. Traditional therapies for teething babies have often included clove oil due to these properties. To treat sensitive teeth apply 1–2 drops of clove oil directly on the sensitive tooth four to six times a day. If the oil causes a burning sensation, discontinue use. There is also the potential for an allergic reaction inside the mouth.

**Chamomile:** There is some suggestion that a chamomile tea gargle may work well to relieve sensitive teeth. Prepare a strong infusion by adding approximately 1 tbsp of dried chamomile to 1 cup of water. Use this as a mouthwash two to three times a day.

# STYE

## DIAGNOSIS

A stye is a bacterial infection that develops at the root of an eyelash, causing an inflamed lump to form that resembles a small boil. The hair follicle becomes stretched as it fills with pus. It causes redness and swelling of the eyelid, so the eye looks slightly closed. After approximately seven days the stye will usually come to a head and burst. Styes can spread easily from eye to eye, and they are often recurrent. It is also common to get several styes at once because of cross infection. If you develop a stye it is important not to touch your eyes, especially if you haven't washed your hands, as there is a risk of spreading the condition. There is no obvious reason for people to get styes, but triggers include being rundown and having a depressed immune system, which lowers your body's resistance to infection. Some people are more susceptible to styes than others, and repeated flare-ups may sometimes indicate diabetes. See your family doctor if the stye is particularly large, if it seems to have developed on the inside of the eyelid, or if pain persists.

## SYMPTOMS

- Itchiness, soreness, and swelling of the eyelid
- A painful red lump that grows into a yellow head
- Inflammation along the rim of the eyelid
- Feeling that there is something in the eye; a gritty sensation

## TREATMENT GOAL

While irritating and unsightly, styes cause no damage to the eye itself. Treatment aims to relieve the symptoms and keep the immune system strong to prevent recurrent attacks.

## CONVENTIONAL MEDICINE

A stye is known medically as a hordeolum. Treatment depends on the cause of the inflammation. About 80% are caused by the bacterium Staphylococcus aureus. The bacterium streptococcus causes a few and a minority are caused by a mix of both organisms. Before treatment a doctor will determine that the stye is not another type of eye bump, such as an abscess of the eyelid, which must be taken seriously; chalzion (swelling due to a blocked lubrication duct), a contact dermatitis; or cellulitis of the eyelid. A herpes infection of the eye can also look like styes.

**Eye compress:** Good hygiene and warm compresses on the eye sometimes help to prevent and treat styes when they are in the early stages. Ideally the compress should be a sterile gauze pad soaked in water.

**Antibiotics:** Topical erythromycin ophthalmic ointment can be applied two to four times a day to the rim of the eye or the eyelid until the stye has cleared up, which usually takes about a week. If the redness and enlargement of the stye does not begin to resolve within 48 hours, oral antibiotics are used (usually a penicillin or analog to combat staphylococci).

**Surgery:** Very occasionally, surgical intervention is needed to treat repeated and progressive infections. This procedure involves making an incision and draining the stye, and should always be performed by a surgeon. Emergency treatment by an ophthalmologist is needed if there is a problem with eyesight or the movement of the eye.

**Long-term prevention:** If you suffer from chronic styes, an anti-inflammatory diet that excludes processed foods, sugar, dairy, and gluten, and immune-boosting protocol with the right nutrition and supplements should be followed.

## TRADITIONAL CHINESE MEDICINE

**Herbs:**
• Yin Qiao Je Du Pain: This herbal pill is designed for clearing heat and infection. It is commonly used to treat upper respiratory infections, but it is also effective in the treatment of styes. It is available from traditional Chinese medicine stores.

• Herbal decoction: Combine 12 g of Pu Gong Ying (dandelion), 10 g of Jin Yin Hua (honeysuckle flower), 6 g of Bo He (field mint), 8 g of Huang Qin (baical skullcap root), and 10 g of Ye Ju Hua (wild chrysanthemum flower) with 3 cups of water in a glass or ceramic pot. Boil the mixture and let it simmer for 30 minutes before straining it. Drink 1 cup three times a day for three to seven days.

**Acupuncture:** Treatment will be different for acute- and chronic-stage styes. For the acute stage, the main principle of treatment is to disperse heat. For a chronic condition, treatment involves tonifying the body's immune system and promoting blood circulation.

**Acupressure:** If the stye is on the upper eyelid, press the Yu Yao, Tai Yang, and Yang Bai points. The Yu Yao point is on the eybrow, directly above the pupil. The Tai Yang point is at the temple between the lateral end of the eyebrow and eyelid, in the depression one finger behind. The Yang Bai point is also directly above the pupil, but 1 inch above the eyebrow. If the stye is on lower eyelid, press the Si Bai and Tai Yang points. The Si Bai point is directly under the pupil in the depression below the eye socket. Wash your hands thoroughly and, in a sitting position, apply gentle pressure with your index finger to each of these points for one minute two to three times a day.

**Diet:** Eat foods that are cooling, such as celery, spinach, lettuce, mung beans, tangerine, watermelon, and string beans. Avoid hot foods such as black and white pepper, dried ginger, green and red peppers, and chilies, as they increase internal heat.

## NATUROPATHY

**Diet:** The general idea of dietary therapy is to strengthen the immune system so that your body is able to fight infections that can cause styes. Make sure you eat a well-balanced diet that includes fresh fruits and vegetables, whole grains, legumes, and quality protein such as fish, lean chicken, and beans everyday. Eat plenty of green leafy vegetables for their high nutrient content, which will provide a good foundation of the nutrients required for a healthy immune system. Avoid foods that weaken your immune system, such as processed sugar, hydrogenated vegetable oils, baked goods, and all drinks other than tea, water, and freshly squeezed juices.

**Supplements:** Zinc strengthens your immune system and helps you heal faster. Take 30–50 mg per day. Take 25,000–50,000 IU a day of a betacarotene supplement for its antioxidant support. Recurring styes can be a sign of a vitamin A deficiency; take 25,000 IU daily. Pregnant women should not exceed 10,000 IU of vitamin A a day.

**Herbs:** Eyebright helps fight infection and dry up excess fluid; chamomile or fennel seeds also help fight infection; marigold soothes irritation; and plantain is astringent and soothing (the fresh leaves are the most effective plant part). To make a compress from any of these herbs dilute 5 drops of tincture in ¼ cup water, or steep 1 tsp of the herb in 1 cup of hot water for 5–10 minutes before straining. Soak a clean cloth or piece of gauze in the solution and apply it to the eyes for 10 minutes three to four times a day. To make a soothing flaxseed poultice wrap 28 g of bruised flaxseed steeped for 15 minutes in 4 oz of water in cheesecloth and apply it directly to the affected eye. Grated, fresh potato can also be wrapped in cheesecloth and apply to the affected area for its astringent properties. Another compress formula is diluted eyebright, goldenseal, and raspberry leaf. These herbs have antibacterial and antiviral properties and also work to support the immune system to prevent infections. Goldenseal is bright yellow and will stain fingers and worktops, so use it with care. You can also use this mixture as an eyewash to bathe both eyes or use a dropper bottle to place a few drops into each eye. Do this for 10–15 minutes four times a day.

## HOMEOPATHY

Any of the following homeopathic options can be very helpful in easing the inflammation and discomfort of a stye, encouraging it to resolve itself gently, quickly, and efficiently. However, an underlying tendency to develop frequent and/or severe styes would suggest that more professional help is required from a homeopathic practitioner.

**Belladonna:** Think of this as a possible remedy if redness and throbbing sensations develop rapidly at the margin of the eyelid. Belladonna is helpful if the overall area affected is very sensitive, while the eyes feel dry and hot.

**Hepar sulph:** Consider this remedy to treat large, swollen styes that produce a thick, yellowish pus. Signature symptoms include discomfort and sensitivity to contact with the slightest draught of cold air. Pains in the affected area will be characteristically sharp and splinter-like. They are noticeably relieved by applying warm compresses or bathing in warm water.

**Pulsatilla:** If styes affect the lower eyelid and produce a gluey, thick discharge that forms a crust in the morning, sticking the lids together, use Pulsatilla. Pain and sensitivity of the affected part of the eyelid is noticeably more intense for contact with warmth. An itchiness creates a constant desire to rub the eyes.

> **TIP: MAINTAIN A BALANCED DIET**
> If a stye has developed after a period of high stress and pressure, make a deliberate point of taking adequate rest and include foods in your diet that have a reputation for boosting the immune system, such as fresh fruit, vegetables, whole grains, nuts, seeds, garlic, and green and/or white tea. Avoid sugary foods, which lower the immune system while also encouraging bacterial infection to develop.

**Apis:** This remedy is always suitable when puffy, bag-like swellings develop around the eyes very rapidly and dramatically. The affected tissues feel as though they sting, and tears produced also feel painful. The discomfort becomes more intense if the affected area gets hot, while applying cool compresses brings relief.

## HERBALISM

The best treatment method is proper hygiene of the infected area and warm, wet compresses. There are a few herbs that can be added to the compress to augment healing.

**Eyebright:** This herb is only recommended for topical application. Make an infusion of eyebright by steeping a handful of the dried herb in a bowl of boiling water. Allow the infusion to cool to a warm temperature. Soak a clean washcloth in the infusion, wring out the excess liquid, and place it directly on closed eyes to help a stye resolve.

**Chamomile:** This herb has calming properties and anti-inflammatory effects. To treat a stye, make a chamomile compress by steeping approximately 2–5 g of dried flowers in 200 ml of boiling water for 20 minutes. Strain the mixture and allow it to cool. Soak a clean washcloth in the liquid, squeeze out the excess, and place it over your closed eyes for five to 10 minutes several times a day. If you begin to notice redness or irritation around the application site, discontinue use. Do not use chamomile if you are allergic to plants in the daisy family.

# TEETH GRINDING

## DIAGNOSIS

Teeth grinding is a frustrating condition—both for those who suffer from the problem themselves and for those who live with someone who is afflicted. Some people habitually grind their teeth while asleep. Occasionally, the grinding can be so loud that it can actually wake someone up in the next room. Teeth grinding can seriously affect your sleep patterns and those of the people with whom you live, leading to disturbed nights and frayed tempers. If the condition continues over a period of years, the action of repeatedly clenching and then relaxing the jaw can wear away at the protective enamel that coats the teeth, which can eventually weaken teeth to the point that they fall out. It is thought that anxiety, stress, and tension can trigger teeth grinding, so the best way of treating it is to first deal with the underlying psychological problem. If the condition is chronic, it is possible to wear a dental guard at night that helps protect your teeth from damage.

## SYMPTOMS

- Loud grinding of the teeth when asleep
- Wear and tear of tooth enamel
- Loose teeth

## TREATMENT GOAL

To determine what is causing the emotional upset and anxiety that triggers teeth grinding, and find ways of lowering stress levels to prevent further damage to the teeth.

## CONVENTIONAL MEDICINE

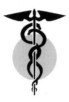

This condition is known medically as bruxism. Teeth grinding tends to occur more in people who drink large amounts of alcohol, experience high stress, smoke, take certain drugs, and have a type A personality. However, it is also thought that those who have malocclusion of the bite and particular facial bone structures are more prone to teeth grinding. If the condition is causing damage to the teeth, an immediate referral to a dentist is needed.

**Prevention:** Adopting a healthier lifestyle by quitting smoking, cutting back on alcohol intake and drug use, as well as practicing stress-reduction techniques such as meditation or counseling, can help prevent teeth grinding from occuring.

**Night guards:** Oral splints such as a night mouthpiece are commonly used. A dental referral for the correction of a bad bite is part of treatment.

**Sleeping agents:** Medications such as gabapentin, and anxiety and sleep agents such as trazodone and benzodiazepines may be prescribed to prevent teeth grinding. Long-term use of these medications is best avoided.

## TRADITIONAL CHINESE MEDICINE

**Herbs:** Several Chinese herbal medicine formulas can help with teeth grinding. The below are available from Chinese pharmacies or online. For each formula, combine the herbs in a ceramic pot and add 3–4 cups of water. Bring the mixture to a boil, let it simmer for 30 minutes, and strain the liquid.

• Herbal decoction: This formula will treat teeth grinding that is due to stomach heat with complications of bad breath, constipation, and yellowish urination. Mix 10 g of Huang Qin (baical skullcap root), 5 g of Da Huang (rhubarb root and rhizome), 12 g of Bai Zhi (Chinese angelica root), 12 g of Bai Zhu (white atractylodes rhizome), and 3 g of Gan Cao (licorice). Drink 1 cup three times a day.

• Herbal tea: If teeth grinding is accompanied by restless sleep, tension and/or anxiety, stress, irritability, or depression use the following formula. Mix 12 g of Chai Hu (hare's ear root), 15 g of Bai Shao (white peony root), 12 g of Yu Jin (turmeric tuber), 8 g of Bo He (field mint), 12 g of Zhao Ren, 12 g of Bai Zhu (white atractylodes rhizome), and 15 g of Ye Jiao Teng (fleeceflower vine). Drink 1 cup two to three times a day.

**Pumpkin seeds:** To treat teeth grinding resulting from indigestion due to parasites in the intestine, chew 15 g of raw pumpkin seeds before going to bed.

**Acupuncture:** An experienced acupuncturist will treat this condition by working on the cause of the teeth grinding (see the herbal formulas above for the various possibilities). Treatment lasts between one and six months.
.

**Acupressure:** Press the Nei Guan point, located in the center of the wrist on the palm side about 1 inch below the crease, and the Shen Men point, located in the depression at the bend of the wrist in line with the little finger, for one minute each two to three times a day.

**Diet:** Eat food that is calming and nourishes Yin and the kidneys, such as tangerines, string beans, grapes, chives, plums, chicken egg yolk, and licorice.

## NATUROPATHY

The following suggestions may help to minimize any pain caused by tooth grinding.

**Diet:** Do not eat sweets four hours before going to bed. Many dentists believe that consuming sugar before bedtime increases the likelihood and intensity of tooth grinding.

**Herbs:** Chamomile helps to relax the nervous system. Drink a cup of chamomile tea before bed to minimize the stress that may lead to tooth grinding. Do not use chamomile if you are allergic to ragweed. Clove oil acts as a general anesthetic. Blend 1 drop of clove oil with 1–2 drops of olive oil. Use your fingers or a cotton swab to massage the mixture on your gums to relieve any pain. The application should be used in moderation, as excessive amounts can cause blistering. Licorice powder can also relieve pain in the gums. Mix 1 tsp with enough water to make a paste and gently apply it to the gums.

## HOMEOPATHY

Teeth grinding can affect children and adults while asleep, resulting in a surprisingly loud sound. It is often a sign of anxiety, stress, or tension and needs professional attention as it can damage teeth if it is allowed to continue for an extended period of time without dental supervision. By its nature this condition tends to fall into a chronic category, particularly if it is stress-related, so it is best to consider consulting a homeopathic practitioner who will take the emotional and physical health of adults or children into account when prescribing. The following homeopathic remedies give an idea of some of the remedies that may be considered.

**Nux vomica:** Use this remedy when symptoms arise that are linked to high levels of stress and tension, especially if caffeine, alcohol, or cigarettes are used as a coping mechanism. Muscle tension and spasms particularly affects the jaw, and there is an associated tendency to clamp the jaw shut tight. When waking, sufferers feel headachy and anxious.

**Arsenicum album:** This is a particularly strong candidate to treat tooth grinding that is related to high anxiety levels that result in poor sleep patterns and a tendency to wake around 2 a.m. Both mental and physical restlessness is pronounced at night, leading to an inability to relax and drift off to sleep easily.

**Zinc:** This remedy can be used in cases of tooth grinding that are combined with very disturbed, twitchy sleep patterns and a tendency to feel low and depressed. The feet in particular are fidgety and restless, with a tendency to jerk when drifting off to sleep.

## HERBALISM

**Valerian root:** If constant tooth grinding is affecting your sleep (or more commonly the sleep of your partner) valerian may be helpful. Valerian is a proven and effective herbal remedy for insomnia and anxiety. The suggested dosage is 1–2 g as a tea or 100–200 mg in capsule form at bedtime. The tea has a very strong, and often unpleasant, taste, so many people opt for a capsule. Driving or operating heavy machinery should be avoided after taking valerian. Be aware that it may also interact with other medications or substances that cause drowsiness, such as alcohol and barbiturates.

**Lavender oil:** This is a wonderful antispasmodic tension reliever when applied topically. Some people find that they sleep better with lavender flowers tucked inside their pillowcases. Lavender oil massaged into the part of the jaw located just in front of the ears can serve as a muscle relaxant that could be useful for tooth grinding, given that the muscles of the jaw are working overtime during this condition. Be careful not to get the oil in your eyes; if you do, wash it out with water immediately.

**Kava kava:** Until recently, one treatment recommended for teeth grinding, especially if it was thought to be due to underlying anxiety or stress, was kava kava root. However, recent well-documented reports of liver toxicity has made many people shy away from this plant. Kava kava has been used on the islands of the South Pacific for over 300 years and is part of the same family as black pepper, sharing some of its spicy, peppery flavor. The plant is traditionally used as an infusion of the root. In the United States and Europe, standardized extracts of different types were popular until liver toxicity became apparent. Even though there may have been a role for kava kava in treating anxiety and tooth grinding, the data accumulating about its adverse effects means that its use can no longer be recommended.

# TEETHING

## DIAGNOSIS

Teething is the process whereby a baby's teeth break through the gums. Children have around 20 milk or primary teeth, and usually have a complete set by the age of two. Babies usually start producing teeth when they are about five months old. Although some lucky babies seem to be untroubled by the teething process, there are many others who suffer greatly and it can be a very painful process. A baby's sleep may be disturbed and there will probably be quite a high level of irritability during the daytime too. As the teeth emerge, your baby will find comfort in gnawing on a cold object, such as a stick of raw carrot from the fridge. Parents often blame a baby's slightest upset on the fact that he or she is teething, and there is the danger that it may become an excuse that is used to explain anything else going on with the baby. Sometimes a fever can occur during teething, but if it lasts for longer than two days consult your doctor as your child may have an unrelated infection.

## SYMPTOMS

- Redness on the cheek on the side the tooth is coming through
- Dribbling
- A rash around the mouth
- Biting on anything
- Putting fist in mouth
- Inflammation of the gums
- Crying and irritability
- Clinginess
- Disturbed sleep
- Fever
- Upset stomach
- Loss of appetite
- Diaper rash

## TREATMENT GOAL

Teething is an inevitable part of a child's development, but there are many things that can be done to help ease the painful symptoms.

## CONVENTIONAL MEDICINE

Teething is a normal process of development that all babies go through. A high fever is not usually a symptom of teething, but a slight temperature elevation can occur.

**Non-pharmaceutical treatment:** Try to comfort and reassure your baby. A cold teething ring can provide relief, as can cool drinks and gels that numb the gums. Do not use a pacifier dipped into honey, sweet drinks, or alcohol. Do not give your baby freezing items to suck on, as they can damage gum tissue, or items that may be choking hazards.

**Over-the-counter medications:** Children's pain relief should always be given in the correct dosage as labeled.

**When should I consult a doctor?** If your baby has a fever of over 100.5°F, severe diarrhea, lethargy, or unremitting screaming, and a complete loss of appetite such that fluids are not consumed for three or more hours during the daytime, speak to your doctor. These symptoms may indicate a more serious condition.

## TRADITIONAL CHINESE MEDICINE

**Herbs:** Chinese herbal medicine is not appropriate for treating teething.

**Acupressure:** Press the Hegu point, located on the back of the hand between the thumb and first finger, for one minute. Press the Xia Guan point, which is found in front of the ear in the depression above the jawbone, for one minute.

**Diet:** Mothers who are breastfeeding should avoid food that is warm and spicy such as ginger, pepper, chilies, cloves, leeks, mussels, beef, mutton, and coriander.

## NATUROPATHY

Teething is a natural process and cannot be prevented, but pain can be minimized by following the remedies below.

**Diet:** Do not allow your child to eat sweets four hours before going to bed. Many dentists believe this increases the likelihood of tooth grinding.

**Herbs:** Chamomile helps relax the child's nervous system before going to bed. Give your child a cup of chamomile tea in the evening before bedtime. Do not use this remedy if your child is allergic to ragweed, the symptoms of which are a skin rash, watery eyes, and excess mucus in the nasal passages. Clove oil acts as a general anesthetic. Blend 1 drop of clove oil with 1–2 drops of olive oil. Using your fingertips or a cotton bud, gently massage the mixture onto your child's gums. This application should be used in moderation as directed above as excessive amounts can cause blistering.

## HOMEOPATHY

The results from treating teething homeopathically can seem miraculous. When an appropriate homeopathic remedy is given, your child should become calmer, less factious, and less distressed very quickly. Since distress with teething tends to be intermittent, make sure you have the remedy that most often works for your child in the medicine cabinet so it can be administered at the first signs of pain. The appropriate remedy should both reduce localized inflammation and pain, and have an emotionally soothing effect.

**Belladonna:** This remedy will help reduce pain and inflammation that occurs rapidly and dramatically, making your child hot and bothered and very irritable. Use Belladonna if there is a general state of feverishness and if your child's skin looks flushed, red, and dry, and feels very hot to the touch. Symptoms are also likely to be restricted to, or be more intense on, the right side, with possible associated earache.

**Chamomilla:** If your child is beside themselves and frantic with pain, and has one flushed and one pale cheek, consider Chamomilla as a possible remedy. Temper tantrums associated with teething pains reach such a crescendo that any toys offered in an effort to pacify the child get hurled to the floor.

## HERBALISM

**Cloves:** Traditional therapies for teething babies have often included clove oil. Apply 1–2 drops of clove oil on a cotton swab and pass the swab under running water to dilute the oil. Apply this to the gums four times a day. There is the potential for an allergic reaction inside the mouth, so watch for any signs of irritation.

**TIP:** USE HAMAMELIS
Give teething babies a towel soaked in hamamelis, commonly known as witch hazel, to help numb the gums.

# THRUSH, ORAL

## DIAGNOSIS

Oral thrush, also know as candidosis or moniliasis, is an infection caused by the yeast fungus candida albicans. It establishes itself in the membranes that line the mouth and the throat. Many people have the candida yeast present in their mouths without necessarily suffering any ill effects. The condition does not manifest itself until there is a change in the delicate internal balance, making the environment ripe for infection. It is particularly likely to be present in those who wear false teeth, take antibiotics, suffer from diabetes, or have immune deficiencies as a consequence of poor nutrition. Newborns are also prone to outbreaks of oral thrush. The symptoms of thrush are similar to many other conditions, so it is important to have a thorough check-up by your doctor if you suspect you have oral thrush. Oral thrush is generally treated by antifungal medicines applied to the mouth. If whatever caused the thrush can be brought under control, the infection is likely to go away after a few days of treatment with a fungicide.

## SYMPTOMS

- Spots in the mouth that are white, cream, or yellow in color
- Occasionally, pale pinks spots on the lips
- A burning sensation in the mouth and throat
- Sensitivity in the mouth

## TREATMENT GOAL

To establish and remove the cause of the thrush to clear up the infection and prevent the condition from reoccurring.

## CONVENTIONAL MEDICINE

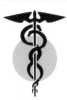

Oral thrush is caused by an overgrowth of the candida yeast, which is found normally on the skin and in the mouth. Certain environmental and physical factors can allow the colonization of the yeast to increase, resulting in an infection. This imbalance often occurs after taking certain antibiotics, as a side effect of using inhaled steroids (to treat asthma or an allergy), or in those with compromised immunity or who have experienced chronic trauma that has disrupted the body's delicate internal balance.

**Prevention:** Enhance your immune system by minimizing your intake of sugar, alcohol, yeasty foods, and high fructose foods such as fruit—substances upon which yeast thrives. Take probiotics (at the billion or trillion colony-forming-unit quantity) and the probiotic sachromyces boullardii (which is found in Florastore) to discourage yeast. These may be taken daily by those prone to oral thrush, but should always be taken with antibiotics to prevent yeast formation.

**To treat an existing infection:** Treat oral thrush with 1 ml of nystatin oral suspension (Mycostatin) four times daily or ketoconazole 2% cream (Nizoral) four times daily as a first step. Take 100 mg of systemic fluconazole (Diflucan) a day for 7–10 days or 200 mg of itraconazole (Sporanox) a day for seven to 10 days if the oral suspension does not work. Liver enzymes should be taken if liver failure or incompetence is present, which is determined by a blood test.

## TRADITIONAL CHINESE MEDICINE

**Herbal tea:** Combine 8 g of Jin Yin Hua (honeysuckle flower), 5 g of Bo He (field mint), and 3 g of Gan Cao (licorice) in a pot and add boiling water. Drink the tea three to four times a day, swishing it around and holding it in your mouth for a few seconds before swallowing. Young babies with oral thrush should drink 1–2 oz of tea twice or three times a day.

**Acupuncture:** This is not appropriate for treating oral thrush.

**Acupressure:** Gently press the Di Chang point, found directly below the pupil of the eye above the cheekbone, and the Xia Guan point, located in front of the ear in the depression above the jawbone.

**Diet:** Mothers who are breastfeeding a baby with this condition should eat food that disperses dampness such as mung beans, red beans, flat beans, coix seeds, watermelon, and cucumber. Food that has a pungent flavor is also recommended, such as spring onions, garlic, pepper, and chilies. Hot and spicy foods should be eaten only in small amounts.

## NATUROPATHY

**Diet:** To help control candida, eat chicken, eggs, fish, yogurt, vegetables, nuts, seeds, oils, and plenty of raw garlic. Increase your fiber intake to 1 tsp–1 tbsp of soluble fiber, containing guar gum, psyllium husks, flaxseeds, or pectin, mixed with 8 oz of water, drunk twice a day on an empty stomach. Eliminate refined and simple sugars, including white or brown sugar, raw sugar, honey, molasses, or grain sweeteners. The sugar substitute stevia is allowed. Avoid milk, alcohol, fruit or dried fruit, and mushrooms. Avoid foods that contain yeast or mold, including all breads, muffins, cakes, baked goods, cheese, dried fruits, melons, and peanuts.

**Supplements:** Take 1,000 mg of caprylic acid, a fatty acid that has been shown to have antifungal properties, three times a day. Vitamin C, taken at a dose of 1,000 mg twice a day, helps to enhance immune function. Take a high-potency multivitamin to obtain many nutrients that will help support immune function. Take probiotics with about four billion micro-organisms twice daily 30 minutes before each meal. These micro-organisms provide acidophilus and bifidus, which are friendly bacteria that prevent yeast overgrowth and fight candida. Take 200 mg of grapefruit seed extract two to three times a day for its anti-candida properties.

**Herbs:** Take 500 mg of garlic twice a day to fight fungus and boost the immune system. Take 200 mg of grapefruit seed extract twice a day for its antifungal properties. Undecylenic acid, a derivative from castor bean oil, has been shown to have strong antifungal activity; take 200 mg three times a day. Drink 2 cups of Pau d'Arco tea a day, which also has strong antifungal properties. Take 250–500 mg of barberry a day for its antimicrobial and antifungal properties. Tea tree oil had anti-yeast properties and can be used as a mouth wash. Mix 15 drops in water and swish it around in your mouth two to three times a day.

---

**TIP:** FOR BREASTFEEDING MOTHERS WITH A CHILD WITH ORAL THRUSH
Keep your nipples clean and dry, as dry, cracked skin can harbor yeast and bacteria and lead to thrush. Rinse your nipples after each feeding with a mixture of 1 cup of water and 1 tbsp of apple cider vinegar.

**TIP:** USE A NEW TOOTHBRUSH

Candida can collect on your toothbrush. Change your toothbrush monthly to avoid reinfecting yourself.

## HOMEOPATHY

 Any of the following homeopathic options can be helpful in speeding up recovery from a recently developing bout of oral thrush. However, if you are dealing with a situation that is not a one-time occurrence, but more of an on-going tendency to develop problems with oral thrush at regular intervals, this suggests that more professional homeopathic support will be appropriate. This will allow the practitioner a chance to prescribe at a level that will be aiming to eradicate the underlying tendency in the system that is leaving it vulnerable to candida overgrowth.

**Natrum mur:** If oral thrush is accompanied by a tendency to develop dry, cracked lips and sore corners of the mouth, consider using Natrum mur. Contact with heat intensifies distress, while cool things are soothing.

**Kali mur:** This is a possible remedy if symptoms of oral thrush are combined with genital thrush. When this remedy is appropriate there is a "mapped," patchy appearance to the tongue, which is coated with a white or gray film. The gums of breastfeeding babies may also take on a whitish tinge. Symptoms are worse during the night and for becoming overheated. Rubbing the affected area and contact with cool things provides temporary relief.

**Mercurius:** If oral thrush leads to noticeably bad breath and increased saliva to the point of drooling (especially on the pillow at night), use Mercurius. Confirmatory symptoms include a flabby-looking tongue that becomes imprinted by the teeth in older children and adults.

**TIP:** AVOID HOT AND ACIDIC FOODS

Since the mouth is likely to be sore and sensitive, especially in babies and toddlers who suffer from oral thrush, avoid giving any foods that are too hot or acidic. Instead give foods and drinks that are cool, bland, and as nutritious as possible. Let your child drink with a straw if possible as this can make drinking feel more comfortable.

## HERBALISM

 **Garlic:** Fresh cloves of garlic are most effective in treating yeast infections. However, a garlic tincture, oil, or capsule with at least 10 mg of the phytochemical allicin can also be used. Crush the clove to activate the allicin, rub it on the affected areas on the mouth, and then swallow. Avoid using garlic in large amounts or when taking blood-thinning medications.

**Thyme:** This is a potent antifungal, antibacterial, and anti-inflammatory herb that also has antioxidant properties. A few drops of the essential oil diluted with in ½ tsp of olive oil can be placed on the patches of thrush daily. Do not use in large amounts if pregnant.

**Oregano oil:** This oil eradicates yeast on the membrane of the mouth. Take a few drops of essential oil diluted in 1 tsp of olive oil and swish the mixture around the mouth for 10 seconds before spitting it out. Repeat three times a day for one week. Parents can "paint" this mixture on the inside of the cheeks and tongue of young children three times a day for one week to try to rid the mouth of the fungal infection. It is safe if some of the mixture is swallowed. Alternatively, you can take up to 200 mg in capsule form three times a day. Oregano and thyme exhibit more potent antifungal activity when taken together. Large doses should be avoided by women who are pregnant or during lactation.

**Goldenseal:** The alkaloids berberine and hydrastine, which are effective against yeast and bacteria, can be found in goldenseal. This bitter herb stimulates digestion, creating a tonifying, healing effect on all mucosal tissues. Boil 1 tsp of the dry herb per 1 cup of water, or take 30 drops of tincture in water three times per day. Swish either form around the mouth before swallowing.

**Pau d'Arco:** This herbal panacea is best known for its treatment of chronic candidiasis, but it also has properties as an immune stimulant and an antibacterial and anti-tumor agent. Simmer 10 g of Pau d'Arco bark in 600 ml of water for 10 minutes. Drink the tea throughout the day, swishing it around in your mouth before swallowing.

# TOOTHACHE

## DIAGNOSIS

Toothache is a very unpleasant condition that can make life miserable. It usually indicates that something is wrong in your mouth, and the first thing to do is visit the dentist. The most common causes of toothache are an abscess, dental decay, inflammation of the tooth pulp, a damaged tooth, an exposed tooth root, or irritation following dental treatment. Other triggers include an ulceration or inflammation of the gum caused by conditions such as gingivitis (see p. 183), periodontitis (see p. 196), and sinusitis (see p. 286). The best way to prevent toothache is to make sure your teeth and gums are healthy. Try to reduce your intake of sugary foods and drinks, brush your teeth regularly using a toothpaste containing fluoride, and make sure you floss as often as is practically possible. Visit your dentist regularly so that any problems that may be developing can be detected early.

## SYMPTOMS

- Continuous or intermittent throbbing pain
- Raised temperature
- Pain above and below the gum level
- Chewing becomes painful
- Swollen gums
- Earache and swelling on one side of the face
- Swelling in the neck
- Pain in the face
- Sinusitis (see p. 286)
- Difficulty eating

## TREATMENT GOAL

To identify the cause of the toothache, relieve any immediate pain, and prevent future problems from developing. Most cases of toothache require the attention of a dentist.

## CONVENTIONAL MEDICINE

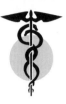

Toothache is not a condition in itself, but a symptom of another disease. Conventional medicine aims at diagnosing the cause of the toothache and treating the underlying problem. In the interim, take pain relief, such as 800 mg of ibuprofen three times a day, as needed (but for a short period of time only).

**Prevention:** Preventing toothache involves rigorous oral hygiene including daily flossing, proper brushing, and avoiding sugar and processed foods in your diet. Maintaining good oral flora with probiotics is also helpful. Look for a product with colony-forming units of bifidus in the billions. Adequate amounts vitamin C (500 mg a day) and CoQ10 (120 mg of an oil-based product a day) can help maintain gum health. To keep your teeth in good condition, regular dental examinations are also crucial, particularly during high-risk times such as childhood and middle age.

**When should I see a dentist?** A dentist should be your first port of call if toothache develops. The most common cause of toothache is tooth decay, which if not addressed can lead to further problems such as a bacterial infection of the tooth pulp and irritation of the nerve of the tooth. Treatment requires dental work. Other common causes are a fracture or crack in the tooth, gum disease, overuse (grinding or gum chewing), or a damaged filling. Ask your dentist for an examination to locate the problem. Generally, you can wait until the next available appointment unless there is an unpleasant-smelling discharge or fever accompanying the toothache, in which case you will need an emergency appointment.

## TRADITIONAL CHINESE MEDICINE

Toothache has various causes and you should always see a dentist for diagnosis and treatment, but using traditional Chinese medicine can help to reduce pain and inflammation, treat the original cause, and aid in prevention.

**Herbs:** The herbs listed below can be bought from Chinese herbalists or online.
• Herbal decoction: Combine 15 g of Shi Gao (gypsum), 15 g of Shen Di Huang (Chinese foxglove root), 6 g Shen Ma (bugbane rhizome), 10 g Huang Qin (baical skullcap root), 10 g of Dan Pi (cortex of tree peony root), and 5 g of Huang Lian (coptis root) in a ceramic or glass pot. Add 3–4 cups of water, bring the liquid to the boil, and simmer for 30 minutes before straining it. Drink 1 cup three times a day to reduce the infection and inflammation of the teeth and relieve the pain.

• Herbal tea: Place 12 g of Bai Zhi (Chinese angelica root) and 10 g of Wu Zhu Yu (evodia fruit) in a teapot and add 3–4 cups of boiling water to make a herbal tea that will cleanse the mouth. Drink the tea throughout the day, but swish it around and hold it in your mouth for a few seconds before swallowing to le t the herbs cleanse the bacteria.

• Ya Tong Shan (toothache powder) or watermelon frost: These two patent formulas are herbal mixtures in powder form. Apply the powder three to four times a day to the area that is causing you pain. If after using the above formulas for one to two days you do not get any relief from the pain or infection, see your dentist.

**Acupuncture:** An experienced acupuncturist will treat toothache from two different perspectives. First to reduce the pain by using local points and points that control pain; and second to treat the related issue according to his or her diagnosis. Treatment may vary in acute and chronic stages.

**Acupressure:** Press the Hegu points, located on the back of the hands between the thumb and first finger, and the Jie Che point, found on the cheek in the depression above the jawbone, with strong pressure for one minute two to three times a day.

**Diet:** Foods that cleanse heat, such as mung beans, red beans, flat beans, coix seeds, watermelon, and cucumber, are recommended. Avoid food that is hot and spicy.

## NATUROPATHY

**Clove oil:** Make a compress of clove oil, which contains eugenol, a natural painkiller and antibacterial. Mix 2–3 drops of pure clove oil with ¼ tsp of olive oil and apply the mixture with a cotton wool bud two to three times a day. You can also saturate a cotton wool ball with the mixture and place it inside the mouth beside the tooth.

## HOMEOPATHY

The following homeopathic remedies can be used in the short term to relieve pain until you can see your dentist.

**Hepar sulph:** Use this remedy if toothache is combined with an excruciating sensitivity to the slightest draught of cold air. Pains are characteristically sharp and splinter-like, especially when associated with abscess formation.

**Belladonna:** This remedy tends to be most helpful when given at the first twinge of discomfort. Signature symptoms are throbbing, shooting, and piercing pains, and inflammation and redness around the affected gum. This remedy is most effective in treating pains that appear suddenly, violently, and dramatically.

**Hypericum:** Consider this remedy to relieve toothache that feels so intense it's intolerable. Pains are characteristically shooting, are made more intense for sudden, jarring movements, and are temporarily eased by lying quietly on the affected side.

**Arnica:** Once dental work has been done, Arnica, which reduces swelling, pain, tenderness, and bruising, can be used to ease traumatized tissues. Do not use Arnica after a wisdom tooth extraction: It has a very powerful potential for promoting re-absorption of blood from damaged tissue and can leave the patient vulnerable to developing a dry socket.

## HERBALISM

 As the causes of toothaches are manifold, a dentist should always be consulted to address any potential infection or medical condition. The herbs recommended below are primarily to decrease swelling and pain, and facilitate healing of the tissue surrounding the tooth.

**Witch hazel:** This soothing antibacterial agent heals inflamed and infected mucous membrane tissue and decreases inflammation, blood flow, and pain. Place 30–60 drops of a tincture in the mouth, swish it around, and let it sit for two minutes before swallowing. As the tannins in witch hazel can be irritating, use this regime for three days on, then three days off.

**Cranesbill and marshmallow:** With its astringent and anti-inflammatory properties, cranesbill will help shrink irritated and swollen mucous membranes surrounding the tooth. Cranesbill works best when taken with a soothing, demulcent herb such as marshmallow. Combine ½ tsp of each dry herb in 1 cup of hot water or take 30–60 drops of tincture.

**Jamaican dogwood:** This herb has analgesic, sedative, anodyne, narcotic, and antispasmodic properties, making it wonderful for toothache relief. Dilute 30–60 drops of tincture in a small amount of water and drink three to four times daily.

**Hops:** This bitter herb has similar sedative and pain-relieving properties to Jamaican dogwood. Many people unknowingly consume this herb in its most common form: beer.

# EARS, NOSE, AND THROAT

# ALLERGIC RHINITIS

## DIAGNOSIS

Rhinitis is the inflammation of the mucous membrane lining the inside of the nose. It can occur either as a seasonal affliction or perennially, meaning you are affected all year round. Triggers and irritants include pollen, pets' fur and dander, the house dust mite, molds, certain foods, and chemicals in household products. Weak digestion, poor nutrition, or poor general health can also trigger attacks, as how your body handles rhinitis is linked to the strength of your immune system. The inhalation of airborne irritants prompts an exaggerated response of the immune system, which forms antibodies to fight against invaders. This triggers the release of histamine, which causes inflammation and mucus production in the nasal passages. Hay fever sufferers (see p. 261) can be affected from spring right through to fall, with tree pollen acting as an irritant in the spring, grass pollen in summer, and weed pollen in the fall, but the condition generally tends to peak in the summer months. Perennial sufferers will experience a reaction throughout the year, and it is often very hard to identify the exact allergen. Rhinitis is a common complaint, and affects around 10% of the population. It runs in families, and is more common in those with a history of asthma or eczema.

## SYMPTOMS

- Constantly runny nose
- Copious clear mucus
- Sneezing, particularly on first waking
- Blocked-up nose
- Breathing through mouth
- Snoring
- Itchy nose
- Stuffy head

## TREATMENT GOAL

To relieve the symptoms and identify the irritants. If you are suffering badly, allergy testing can be carried out to identify the exact trigger for the attacks.

## CONVENTIONAL MEDICINE

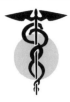

**Avoid allergens:** Avoid outdoor exposure and use HEPA filters indoors during the pollen season. Exposure to dust mites can be minimized by encasing pillows and bedding in plastic and using a dehumidifier. Shampoo pets on a regular basis to reduce pet dander. Humidifiers can be used in a dry climate, as they will help to moisturize the respiratory system. Too much humidity however, can cause more problems. The optimum level is about 35%.

**Nasal washes:** Using saline (saltwater) made from 1 tsp of salt to each pint of distilled warm water is an inexpensive and effective treatment. Sniff a small amount of the saline water into the nostrils one at a time and blow your nose. A syringe can also be used as can a nasal spray.

**Supplements:** Take 1,000 mg of quercetin (eucalyptus flavonoid) three times a day. Take 500 mg –1 g of vitamin C a day, and add zinc and vitamins A and E to your diet. Take 4 g of EPA DHA (an omega-3 fat) fish oil a day in a 3:2 ratio.

**Diet:** Eliminating dairy products from your diet usually decreases the symptoms of the allergic reaction. Other common allergens are spices, yeast products, and gluten.

**Medication:** Topical nasal steroids such as Flonase®, oral antihistamines, topical azelastine, or cromolyn sodium in combination with mucolytics (guaifenesin) and decongestants are usually prescribed. Although they do mask symptoms, they do not alleviate the actual cause.

## TRADITIONAL CHINESE MEDICINE

Traditional Chinese medicine practitioners will classify the particular type of allergic rhinitis to focus treatment. Patients may be diagnosed for lung deficiency, lung and spleen deficiency, or lung and kidney deficiency.

**Herbs:** To bring relief to sinus congestion and a runny nose, use the following decoction. Add 2 g of Niu Bang Zi (great burdock root), 12 g of Chang Er Zi (cocklebur), 12 g of Fang Fen (ledebouriella root), 10 g of Jing Jie (schizonepeta stem and bud), and 5 g of Gan Cao (raw licorice) to 3–4 cups of water in a ceramic pot. Bring to the mixture to a boil, simmer for 30 minutes, and then strain the liquid. Drink 1 cup of the liquid two to three times a day. These raw herbs are available from a Chinese herbalist or online.

**Acupuncture:** Treatment can help reduce the symptoms of acute allergic rhinitis. To address chronic allergic rhinitis and regulate your immune system, you may need to plan for long-term treatment. Six months to one year is the average treatment period, with sessions once or twice a week.

**Acupressure:** The Ying Xiang point is located just to the side of, and slightly above, the lower border of the nostril. The Yin Tang point is in the depression midway between the eyebrows. Use your thumb or fingertip to gently press these points for about one minute.

**Diet:** Eat fresh vegetables such as carrots, squash, kale, Chinese cabbage, and broccoli.

> **TIP:** NASAL WASH
> Pound an adequate amount of green onion stalks and collect the juice. Wash the nasal cavity with a saline solution at night and then apply the green onion juice to both nasal cavities with a cotton wool ball. This will help to open the nasal pathways.

## NATUROPATHY

 **Diet:** Look at your nutrition to work out strategies for mucus reduction, elimination of allergenic pathogens, and immune support. Choose non-mucous-forming foods, including gluten-free whole grains (brown rice, quinoa, and buckwheat), fresh fruit and vegetables, cold-pressed oils, and raw seeds and nuts. Eat a well-balanced diet that includes fresh fruits and vegetables, legumes, and quality protein (fish, lean chicken, and beans) every day. Eat plenty of green leafy vegetables for their high nutrient content. This will provide a good base of the nutrients required for a healthy immune system. Make sure you get enough anti-inflammatory essential fatty acids (omega-3s) in the form of fatty fish, walnuts, flax seeds, cod liver oil, fish oil, and flax seed oil. Also make sure you drink plenty of water—aim for at least eight glasses a day. Identify aggravating substances, including food dyes and colorings, artificial preservatives, and additives, and eliminate them from your diet. Avoid dietary sources of arachidonic acid (found in animal products), which contributes to inflammation.

**Supplements:** Vitamin C has natural antihistamine effects. Take 1,000 mg three to five times a day (reduce the dosage if diarrhea occurs). Take 250 mg of quercetin three times a day to control inflammation by reducing the release of histamine and other mediators of allergic reactions from cells. Quercetin also works by stabilizing cell membranes so they are less reactive to allergens. Take 3 g of fish oils a day to relieve inflammation associated with allergic rhinitis and allergies in general. Probiotics have been shown to be beneficial for allergies. Take a product that contains four billion organisms of Lactobacillus acidophilus and bifidus. Protease enzymes assist in decreasing inflammation; take 2 capsules twice a day on an empty stomach. Digestive enzymes along with Betaine hydrochloride assist in the digestion of food and reduce the chances of food sensitivities. Take 1–2 of each with each meal.

**Herbs:** Take 300–500 mg of freeze-dried stinging nettles. They have been shown to be beneficial for allergic rhinitis and hay fever. Butterbur is a traditional herbal remedy used for seasonal allergies and asthma. Research has shown it to be as effective but less sedating than commonly prescribed antihistamines for treating seasonal allergies over a two-week period. Consult a practitioner regarding an appropriate dosage.

## HOMEOPATHY

This condition falls into the chronic category and is best treated by a homeopathic practitioner who will prescribe at a level that is beyond the scope of anything you can do at home. Treatment will aim to gently but effectively stimulate the body's self-regulating, self-balancing mechanism so that symptoms are less likely to be a problem. Acute remedies can be used in the short term to temporarily relieve severe episodes of allergic rhinitis, but they will not discourage symptoms from recurring. If problems with allergic rhinitis are combined with asthma and/or hay fever, consult a homeopathic practitioner.

**Allium cepa:** Use Allium cepa if there is an acrid nasal discharge that burns the skin of the upper lip. Although the eyes water profusely, the tears feel bland in contrast to the nasal discharge. When this remedy is indicated symptoms tend to be more intense in the evening and in humid weather, and contact with cool, fresh air feels soothing.

**Euphrasia:** When this remedy is well indicated tears feel hot and burning, while the nasal discharge is profuse and bland. As a result, the eyes look red, inflamed, and sore. Symptoms tend to be at their worst when indoors and are relieved by walking in cool, fresh air.

**Apis:** Think of this as a possible remedy if allergic symptoms build rapidly and dramatically, making the eyes look pink, swollen, and puffy. Stinging, itching sensations are marked in the eyes and throat and the eyelids look noticeably swollen. If these symptoms become intense, and/or there is any sign of swelling of the lip, seek emergency medical attention. The eyes are likely to feel light sensitive and produce tears that sting. Contact with heat feels awful, while cool compresses and cool bathing bring temporary relief.

**Nux vomica:** If you are prone to allergic rhinitis symptoms when stress levels are high, especially if this is combined with a lack of sleep, reliance on junk foods and caffeine to keep the pace, and cigarettes and alcohol to unwind, use Nux vomica. Signature symptoms include itchiness and irritation in the ears, throat, and/or roof of the mouth. The nose may be unpleasantly sensitive to strong odors and perfumes, with repeated, violent bouts of sneezing. The nose runs freely by day, especially when in the fresh, open air, and gets very stuffed up at night. There will be a strong general feeling of irritability when unwell.

**Pulsatilla:** Consider using Pulsatilla if mucus discharges are thick, bland, and yellow-green in color. When this remedy is appropriate symptoms are noticeably more distressing when resting in bed at night, and especially uncomfortable if you are in stuffy, over-heated surroundings. Due to a general sense of congestion in the ears, nose, throat, and chest, there is likely to be a reduction in, or complete loss of, hearing, smell, and/or taste. You are also likely to cough up mucus when you first get up in the morning. Because of nasal congestion, you may breathe through the mouth during the night, leading to a dry mouth and tongue in the morning.

---

**TIP:** GENERAL RECOMMENDATIONS

Bathing the eyes with cool water tends to be universally soothing to irritated, itchy eyes, and using a humidifier can soothe nasal passages. Vacuum mattresses and carpets and dust surfaces with a damp cloth regularly to keep house dust mites at bay.

---

## HERBALISM

It is important to begin treatment four to six weeks prior to the time when your symptoms of allergic rhinitis first appear. If you are currently symptomatic, you can begin the herbal therapies mentioned below, but it may take several weeks for your symptoms to improve.

**Butterbur:** This plant and the compounds it contains (called petasins) stop the inflammation associated with allergic rhinitis without causing drowsiness like other anti-allergy medicines. Whole butterbur herb contains compounds called pyrrolizidine alkaloids that are toxic to the liver; only standardized extracts that are free of pyrrolizidine alkaloids should be used and dosage (ranging from 25–75 mg two to three times a day) will depend on the product chosen.

**Nettle leaf:** Take either 10 g of dried nettle, 3–6 ml of a 1:2 liquid extract, or a freeze-dried standardized extract a day to help with allergy symptoms. Some practitioners prefer the standardized extract because they feel it is more effective and because of its use in clinical trials, but also because it is the most convenient form to take. Although there is a lack of scientific evidence for the effectiveness of stinging nettles on allergies or allergic rhinitis, many experts have found it very useful for their patients.

# CATARRH

## DIAGNOSIS

Catarrh results from having too much mucus in the nose and throat. The mucous membrane becomes inflamed and produces excess fluid so that your nose alternates between being blocked up and runny. It is also quite usual to develop a cough and sometimes even earache. Catarrh can be triggered by many things. Most commonly it results from upper respiratory tract infections such as colds, coughs, or flu, allergies such as allergic rhinitis or hay fever, sinusitis, ear infections, measles, and nasal polyps. Some people suffer from the condition permanently, without any obvious cause. Catarrh is very common in children, particularly in toddlers, but as children get older they often grow out of it, usually by the time they go to grade school. One of the complications associated with a bad attack of catarrh is sinusitis (see p. 286), where the condition spreads into the sinuses. If the mucus turns thick and yellow and is accompanied by facial pain and an offensive smell, this can indicate that a bacterial infection has set in. If this is the case, antibiotics may be needed.

## SYMPTOMS

- Excess of thick mucus in the nose
- Blocked-up sensation
- Bad breath
- Muffled breathing through the mouth
- Persistent sore throat
- Troublesome cough
- Coughing up phlegm
- Sensation of having something stuck in the back of your throat

## TREATMENT GOAL

To relieve the discomfort caused by the condition and resolve the symptoms before infection sets in.

## CONVENTIONAL MEDICINE

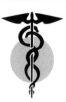

Catarrh is a symptom of an underlying condition. Treating catarrh first involves diagnosing the cause and ruling out any problematic illnesses. It is necessary to assess whether the catarrh is triggered by a viral infection or is an allergic reaction.

**Decongestants:** Over-the-counter decongestants, such as pseudephedrine, and nasal sprays, such as oxymetazoline (afrin), are effective for immediate, short-term alleviation. They can be used to relieve discomfort while searching for the cause of the discharge, but tend to cause rebound congestion if used for longer than three days. When this occurs your body adapts to the drug so that congestion persistently recurs unless the drug is used. People with hypertension should not use them.

**If infection is present:** Usually infection is viral in nature and treatment involves taking rest, fluids, high levels of vitamin C (1 g a day), and zinc (40 mg daily). Preventing infectious catarrh involves enhancing immune function with good nutrition and stress reduction, plus basic good hand-washing techniques. Medical treatment should be sought for catarrh that is accompanied by fever, is foul smelling, or lasts for longer than 10 days. Thick, colored, foul-smelling nasal discharge may indicate a sinus infection, in which case antibiotics are usually prescribed.

## TRADITIONAL CHINESE MEDICINE

**Herbs:** Yin Qiao Je Tu Pian is the pill commonly used for this condition.
• Herbal tea: Place 5 g of Jin Yin Hua (honeysuckle flower), 3 g of Bo He (field mint), and 3 g of Shen Gan Cao (raw licorice) in a teapot, add boiling water, and let the raw herbs steep for three to five minutes. Drink the tea throughout the day. These herbs have no side effects and can be found in your local Chinese herbal store.

**Acupuncture:** Acupuncture has proven to be effective for shortening the catarrh course. You may seek acupuncture treatment right away, as it may help your immune system to fight the inflammation. Generally a few sessions in succession are the most effective way to proceed.

**Acupressure:** The Feng Chi point is located at the back of the head at the base of the skull 2 inches below the center point. Beginning with gentle pressure and gradually increasing, press and release this point with your thumb about 20 times. Use the tip of your thumb to press the Hegu points, located on the back of the hands between the thumb and first finger, with strong pressure for one to two minutes.

**Diet:** Green onions are an important food in Chinese medicine and are frequently used to relieve upper respiratory infection or inflammation at its early stage. Make a tea by crushing 4–6 green onion heads and adding 1 cup of hot water. Drink the tea three times a day.

## NATUROPATHY

**Diet:** Eat light foods such as steamed vegetables, soups, and broth. Drink miso or chicken soup and add garlic, ginger, and onions. These tonifying spices have antimicrobial and warming properties. If you don't have an appetite, do not force yourself to eat. Cut out all milky and mucus-forming foods such as cheese, yogurt, red meat, and simple carbohydrates. Eat lots of fresh fruit and vegetables and freshly made vegetable soups. Drink plenty of water, freshly squeezed juices, and teas. Hydration will help cleanse your body of toxins and keep the respiratory tract from drying out. Herbal teas will also assist your body in healing.

**Supplements:** Take 500–1,000 mg of vitamin C every four hours until symptoms subside. Bioflavonoids work synergistically with vitamin C and have immune-enhancing properties; take 500 mg twice a day, once in the morning and once at night. Zinc supports the immune system and may have antiviral properties; take 25 mg in zinc lozenges every two waking hours for one week.

**Herbs:** Try drinking peppermint, eucalyptus, and chamomile tea three times a day. You can add cayenne to stimulate the circulation, cinnamon for its gentle warming effect, or grated ginger root to induce sweating. Rub lavender, eucalyptus, thyme, or tea tree essential oils gently on the chest to loosen and shift sticky mucus. Always dilute these essential oils in a carrier oil such as olive oil, apricot oil, or almond oil. Elderflower and elderberry is an effective natural antiviral. Adults can take 10 ml and children 5 ml three times daily. Echinacea and goldenseal enhance the immune system and have antiviral properties. Take 2–4 ml of a combined tincture four times a day. Lomatium dissectum has strong antiviral effects. Take 500 mg or 2–4 ml of tincture four times a day. Astragalus is excellent for treating and preventing catarrh. Take 500–1,000 mg or 4–6 ml of tincture three times a day. Garlic is helpful in fighting and preventing infection. Take plenty of raw garlic or 300–500 mg in capsule form a day.

**Aromatherapy:** Steam inhalations work directly on the sinuses to loosen thick mucus and fight infection. Add 5–10 drops of eucalyptus, lavender, peppermint, pine, thyme, or tea tree oil, or a combination of these oils, to a bowl of steaming hot water. Cover your head with a towel, place it over the bowl, and inhale two to three times before uncovering. Repeat this three to four times as one set of treatment. Complete three to four sets a day. The oils will fight the virus, help with congestion, and stimulate circulation.

## HOMEOPATHY

Although it is not a serious problem, catarrh can be an irritating condition if it occurs regularly. The suggestions below may provide some significant relief for recently developing symptoms. If catarrh is chronic, especially if it is combined with a marked tendency to minor infections and recurrent colds, seek treatment from a homeopathic practitioner. If you suck lozenges that include eucalyptus or menthol to try and clear your throat and air passages, do bear in mind that aromatic substances of this kind appear to interfere with the medicinal action of homeopathic remedies.

**Arsenicum iod:** This is a possible remedy if mucus produced by the nose and throat is yellow in color and sticky in texture. Confirmatory symptoms include sneezing set off by a tingling sensation in the nasal passages. Because the nose drips so much, the skin under the nose has a tendency to become sore and sensitive.

**Kali bich:** A classic symptom that calls for this remedy is a pain at the bridge of the nose due to a generally congested state around the nose and sinuses. When this remedy is well indicated, a yellowy-green mucus is produced that is very difficult to shift. Because of post nasal drip there is also likely to be a very unpleasant smell in the nasal passages.

**Natrum mur:** Signature symptoms include mucus secretions that alternate between a clear, jelly-like substance (resembling uncooked egg white), and a thin, very liquid discharge that makes the nose run. Consider Natrum mur if catarrh is associated with hay fever or allergic rhinitis, with the nose feeling alternately dry and blocked or running profusely. Cold sores and dry lips are common additional symptoms.

## HERBALISM

The following remedies help to ease symptoms of catarrh; however, as with similar conditions, the cause of the inflammation must be found and eliminated to result in a long-term cure.

**Mullein:** Primarily used as a soothing upper respiratory decongestant and expectorant, mullein contains several active constituents: iridoids, which act to decrease the amount of discharge; saponins, which encourage mucus movement from the lungs; and mucilages, which soothe the respiratory tract. Infuse 2 g of dry herb in 1 cup of water for 10 minutes. Drink 3 cups a day.

**Elder:** This gentle, wonderful tasting herb, is a popular remedy for children. Elder has long been used as a remedy for any condition where large amounts of mucus are produced. Infuse 2 g of elder flowers in 1 cup of water for 10 minutes. Drink the tea three to five times a day, or take 3 tbsp of elder syrup daily.

**Eyebright:** The iridoids, flavonoids, and lignans in eyebright impart astringent, expectorant, decongestant, and anti-inflammatory properties. Eyebright decreases profuse discharge, especially from the nasal and sinus passages. Infuse 3 g per cup of water, or take 3 ml of tincture three times daily.

**Buckhorn plantain:** This soothes the mucous membranes, while alleviating congestion and inflammation in the respiratory tract. Buckhorn plantain is useful in treating allergic and non-allergic rhinitis, coughs, colds, flu, and fever. Infuse 2 g of herb in 1 cup of water and let it steep for 10 minutes. Drink 2 cups daily.

# COMMON COLD

## DIAGNOSIS

Colds affect everyone at one time or another, especially during the winter months, and it is usual to get at least two a year. A cold, one of the most common ailments, can be caused by over 200 different types of virus. The cold virus is contracted by breathing in infected droplets that have been coughed or sneezed into the atmosphere, or by picking up germs on your hands then transferring them to your nose or mouth. The virus can survive outside the body for three hours, so it is easy to see why it is so virulent. The infection manifests in the mucous membranes in the nose and upper respiratory tract, causing them to swell and produce even more mucus. Older people and those who don't maintain a healthy diet are more at risk. Pre-schoolers with immature immune systems also tend to suffer repeated infections until they have built up a stronger immunity by being exposed to constant infections. Triggers and irritants include lifestyle issues, such as being rundown, tired, or stressed.

## SYMPTOMS

- Feeling under the weather
- Aching joints and feeling shivery
- Sore throat and swollen glands
- Runny nose
- Stuffed-up nose
- Sneezing
- Running watery eyes
- Difficulty breathing
- Tickly cough from mucus running down the throat
- Congestion and popping in the ears
- Slight fever
- Lack of appetite
- Tiredness and irritability

## TREATMENT GOAL

There is no cure for the common cold. Antibiotics are of no use in treatment, nor are there any effective antiviral drugs available yet. Treatment aims to alleviate the symptoms.

## CONVENTIONAL MEDICINE

The medical name for a cold is an upper respiratory tract infection and it is caused by something called a rhinovirus. There are more than 100 types of rhinovirus.

**Prevention:** Frequent hand washing is of paramount importance in preventing the virus from spreading. Vitamin C, zinc, and immune-stimulating plants such as echinacea, larch arabinogalactodes, and reishi mushrooms are good daily supplements to take during the cold season. Stress lowers the immune system's ability to work efficiently so, at the onset of a cold, resolution may occur more quickly if stress reduction techniques such as meditation are introduced.

**Nasal decongestants:** Use a saline nasal spray to prevent the build-up of mucus and nasal obstruction. Using a gentle decongestant such as neo-synephrine or Afrin® for about three days can provide relief, but should be avoided by anyone with a history of cardiac or blood pressure problems, as well as anxiety disorders. You can also place peppermint oil or eucalyptus oil just under the nostrils several times a day to relieve nasal congestion.

**If a cough is present:** Dextromethorphan may be effective for a limited period in both adults and children. This should not be taken by children less than five years of age or by anyone with asthma.

## TRADITIONAL CHINESE MEDICINE

**Herbs:** The herbs below are available from Chinese pharmacies or online.
• Gan Mao Lin: This Chinese patent herbal pill will help deal with the common cold. Take 3–4 pills three times a day.
• Herbal decoction: To treat a severe cold, combine 12 g of Ban La Gen, 12 g of Lian Qiao (forsythia fruit), 12 g of Niu Bang Zi (great burdock fruit), 8 g of Bo He (field mint), 10 g of Huang Qin (baical skullcap root), and 6 g of Gan Cao (licorice) in a ceramic pot. Add 3–4 cups of water, place on the stove, and bring to the boil. Lower the heat and let the mixture simmer for 30 minutes. Strain the liquid and let it cool. Drink 1 cup three times a day for three to five days or until symptoms subside.

**Acupuncture:** To shorten the course of the cold, acupuncture can help the body disperse the pathogen by cleaning out the wind cold or wind heat. If you receive treatment as soon as the cold sets in, it helps you recover quickly. Acupuncture can also prevent the cold from worsening and can stop the infection spreading to the bronchial tubes and lungs. Regular acupuncture sessions can improve the body's defensive energy and internal balance and help prevent future infection.

**Acupressure:** Pressing the Feng Chi, Tai Yang, and Hegu acupressure points when you have a cold will help relieve symptoms such as headaches and congestion. The Feng Chi point is located at the back of the head at the base of the skull 2 inches below the center point. The Tai Yang point is found at the temple in the depression between the lateral end of the eyebrow and eyelid. Press and release these points with your thumb, beginning with gentle pressure and gradually increasing, about 20 times. Use the tip of your thumb to press the Hegu point, located on the back of the hand between the thumb and first finger, with strong pressure for one to two minutes.

**Diet:** Soft and liquid foods such as watery porridge, noodles, lotus rhizome powder, and fresh vegetables are recommended. Mung beans, Chinese cabbage, turnips, and pears can be used to induce perspiration, while ginger and spring onion are useful for clearing heat. Avoid greasy food and seafood.

## NATUROPATHY

**Diet:** It is important to stay hydrated by drinking plenty of water, freshly squeezed juices, and herbal teas to cleanse your body of toxins and keep the respiratory tract from drying out. Include in your diet lots of fresh fruit and vegetables, and light foods consisting of steamed vegetables, freshly made vegetable soups, and broth. Add garlic, ginger, and onions, which are tonifying spices that have antimicrobial and warming properties, to chicken soup. Avoid milky and mucus-forming foods such as cheese, yogurt, red meat, dairy, and simple carbohydrates.

**Supplements:** While symptoms last, take 500–1,000 mg of vitamin C every four hours to support the immune system. Take 1,000 mg of bioflavonoids a day in divided doses. Bioflavonoids work synergistically with vitamin C and have immune-enhancing properties. Take 25 mg of zinc in lozenge form every two waking hours for one week for its antiviral properties.

**Herbs:** Try drinking peppermint, eucalyptus, and chamomile tea three times a day. Add cayenne to stimulate the circulation, cinnamon for its gentle warming effect, or grated ginger root to induce sweating.

**Aromatherapy:** Steam inhalations can loosen thick mucus. Add 5–10 drops of eucalyptus, lavender, peppermint, pine, thyme, or tea tree oil, or a combination of these oils, to a bowl of steaming hot water. Cover your head with a towel, place it over the bowl, and inhale.

## HOMEOPATHY

Although a well-indicated homeopathic remedy is unlikely to stop a cold in its tracks once it's well under way, it can shorten the duration of infection and prevent complications of sinus and/or chest infections. Also see the remedies listed under allergic rhinitis (p. 231), since the symptoms of the common cold and this condition can be very similar.

**Aconite:** This remedy is appropriate for treating cold symptoms that develop in response to exposure to dry, cold winds. If you feel well when going to bed, but wake in the early hours of the morning feeling restless, fearful, and feverish, usually with a hot head and chilly body, try Aconite. The throat is likely to feel hot and dry with a marked thirst. Always bear in mind that this remedy is best used at the first onset of symptoms that arise abruptly and dramatically.

**Belladonna:** Like Aconite, Belladonna is most effective when taken in the earliest stage of a cold. Characteristic symptoms include feeling unwell with a high fever and flushed, dry skin that radiates heat. The throat will also feel hot and inflamed, making it uncomfortable to swallow liquids unless bending forward. Earache may also develop with the cold symptoms, with problems being worse on the right side.

**Ferrum phos:** Symptoms that respond best to this remedy are less intense and severe. The throat and ears are likely to ache, with a sense of swelling in the throat that is very painful when swallowing. Signature symptoms include being alternately flushed then pale when feverish.

**Arsenicum album:** Consider this as an option if there are generalized burning sensations in the nose and throat that are noticeably soothed by contact with warmth. Symptoms also include scanty, clear, nasal discharge that makes the nostrils feel sore and raw, and a dry, tight cough that is much more persistent and irritating while lying flat in bed, and eased a little by lying propped up on two or three pillows. Although exhausted when feeling ill, patients who do well with this remedy are driven crazy with anxiety if their surroundings aren't neat, tidy, and organized.

**Natrum mur:** This remedy can be helpful in treating a cold where the nose alternates between being dry and blocked and running profusely. Nasal discharge is made more intense by sneezing bouts that are especially troublesome when the patient is exposed to bright sunlight. Cold symptoms are often accompanied by cold sores and dry lips.

**Nux vomica:** If cold symptoms make you feel hungover, especially on waking, use Nux vomica. Symptoms include a runny nose during the day and an uncomfortably dry nose at night. Being indoors makes the nose feel uncomfortably stuffed up, while taking a walk in the open air makes it run.

**Pulsatilla:** This can be an immensely helpful remedy for clearing up any residual symptoms that are associated with the last, established stage of a cold. Symptoms that respond well to this remedy include a very stuffed-up sensation in the ears, nose, and sinuses, with a significant production of mucus that is thick and greenish-yellow in color. There may also be a good chance of catarrh in the throat and congestion in the chest, with lots of mucus being raised on first getting up in the morning. The general feeling of being uncomfortably stuffed up and congested is made much more intense when staying in stuffy rooms, while taking a gentle stroll in the fresh air helps clear the head.

## HERBALISM

 **Andrographis:** This bitter antiviral herb is high in antioxidants. Andrographis stimulates the immune system to fight the cold while improving digestion and detoxifying the liver, thus protecting the body from harmful toxins due to infection. Because of its cold, bitter properties, andrographis is best taken with "warm" herbs such as ginger and astragalus. Take up to 6 g in capsule form or up to 12 ml of tincture per day during the infection. Take half the dose for prevention. Do not use during pregnancy.

**Licorice:** Also known as "sweet root," licorice soothes inflammation and throat irritation while acting as a potent antiviral agent, reducing the severity and duration of the cold. Boil and steep 1 tbsp of root per cup of water for 15 minutes. Drink 3–4 cups of the tea or 3–6 ml of tincture daily until the cold resolves. Do not use long term, as licorice may cause high blood pressure.

**Lemon balm:** Effective on a cold that causes restlessness, anxiety, insomnia, and headache associated with stress, lemon balm's sedative, antiviral, antispasmodic, and carminative (soothing and anti-flatulent) qualities ensure healing and relaxation. Dilute 2 tsp in 1 cup of water and drink before bed.

**Osha:** This herb is excellent for respiratory infections with excess mucus congestion. It has strong antiviral and immune-stimulating properties due to volatile oils contained within the root. Boil 1–2 tsp of chopped root in 1 cup of water for 20 minutes. Drink this tea, or take 2 ml of tincture, three times a day.

**Astragalus:** The flavonoids, polysaccharides, and saponins in astragalus enhance immunity by increasing antioxidant activity and the destruction of the offending virus. Boil 2 tsp of root in 1 cup of water for 20 minutes. Drink this tea, or take 3 ml of tincture, once a day.

# EAR INFECTION

## DIAGNOSIS

The ear is a very delicate part of the body, and if it becomes infected it can be incredibly painful. The ear is divided into three areas: the outer ear, the middle ear, and the inner ear. The lining of the ear canal is lubricated by wax, which helps keep the ear clean and free from infection. The middle ear is the most common place for an ear infection to occur, particularly in children, who tend to get ear infections far more often than adults. The infection usually stems from blocked eustachian tubes, which are the drainage canals running from the ear to the nose and throat. These tubes tend to be narrow in children, and problems arise when colds, sinus conditions, and throat infections cause the tubes to become blocked so that the mucus is unable to drain. Infection of the middle ear (otitis media) is an extremely painful condition that can result in intense earache and fever. Occasionally hearing is affected, and sometimes the eardrum will burst, releasing a thick yellow matter. This will eventually heal on its own. Middle ear infections can occur as a primary problem or secondary to other conditions such as tonsillitis, sinusitis, hay fever, sore throat, coughs, or colds. The outer ear can also become inflamed, causing pain, discharge, and loss of hearing. This is referred to as swimmer's ear (otitis externa, see p. 308). Inner ear infections are generally caused by a virus, usually related to a cold or a bout of the flu.

## SYMPTOMS

- Pain in the ear
- Pulling or rubbing at the ears
- May feel dizzy
- Discharge from the ear
- Raised temperature and fever
- Loss of hearing on the affected side
- Swollen glands and tonsils

## TREATMENT GOAL

Treatment is aimed at easing the pain and clearing up any existing infection. It is important to get a proper diagnosis if the pain continues for more than 24 hours or if there is any loss of hearing.

## CONVENTIONAL MEDICINE

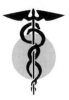

Ear infections primarily affect children between 6–36 months, or four to six years old. But they also affect adults. An adult who has experienced more than one case of ear infection should ask his doctor to refer him for a specialist ears, nose, and throat (ENT) evaluation. Generally, most uncomplicated cases will resolve themselves without antibiotics.

**General recommendations:** Make sure the child drinks plenty of fluids to remain hydrated. Decongestants may be used to encourage the mucus to drain through the eustachian tube. Avoid any substance that may be contributing to the inflammation, such as smoke or specific individual allergens. Feeding babies in an upright position is another prophylactic therapy.

**Antibiotics:** If the infection does not resolve itself within two to three days amoxicillin is prescribed. Some bacteria are resistant to amoxicillin, so if there is no improvement after three days, a broader spectrum antibiotic, such as augmentin, is prescribed. Treatment generally lasts for 10–14 days.

**Myringotomy:** This surgical procedure is used to decompress the middle ear in cases of persistent purulent secretions. If the secretions remain in the middle ear, they may build up to cause pressure pain or become infected. The infection may spread to structures around the ear, which can be dangerous. A ventilation tube (tympanostomy tube) is sometimes inserted into the eardrum for drainage if a child has multiple ear infections in a short period of time.

## TRADITIONAL CHINESE MEDICINE

**Herbs:** The herbs listed in the formulas below are available from Chinese herbalists or online. For each formula, mix the herbs in a ceramic pot and add 3–4 cups of water. Bring the mixture to a boil and simmer for 30 minutes. Strain the liquid and drink 1 cup two to three times a day.

• To treat an acute stage of ear infection: Combine 10 g of Jin Yin Hua (honeysuckle flower), 12 g of Lian Qiao (forsythia flower), 2 g of Jie Geng (ballon flower root), 6 g of Bo He (field mint), 12 g of Niu Bang Zi (great burdock fruit), 12 g of Lu Gen (reed rhizome), 10 g of Jing Jie (schizonepeta stem and bud), and 10 g of Xia Ku Cao (common self heal fruit-spike).

• To treat acute ear infection with a ruptured ear drum: If symptoms such as ear discharge, fever, ear pain, and hearing loss occur, mix 10 g of Jin Yin Hua (honeysuckle flower), 10 g Ye Ju Hua (wild chrysanthemum flower), 10 g of Pu Gong Ying (dried dandelion), 10 g of Zi Hua Di Ding (Yedeon's violet), and 12 g of Zhi Zi (Cape Jasmine fruit).

• To treat a chronic ear infection: If ringing in the ear or loss of hearing occurs, mix 12 g of Jin Yin Hua (honeysuckle flower), 12 g of Zhao Jiao Ci (spine of the Chinese honeylocust fruit), 12 g Dang Gui (Chinese angelica root), 10 g of Chai Hu (hare's ear root), and 10 g of Bai Zhi (angelica root).

**Acupuncture:** Treatment clears pathogenic heat and improves the immune system. The treatment courses vary according to specific symptoms.

**Acupressure:** The Xia Guan point is located in front of the ear in the depression above the jawbone. The Yi Feng point is situated just behind the ear lobe. The Er Men point is found in front of the notch on the forward edge of the ear. Press these points using gentle to medium pressure to reduce the pain in the ear and assist healing.

**Diet:** Food that has clearing heat properties is recommended, such as mung beans, red beans, watermelon, cucumber, grapefruit, and bananas.

## NATUROPATHY

**Diet:** Avoid common food allergens, including wheat, eggs, dairy foods, corn, citrus, and peanuts, especially with chronic cases of ear infection. While suffering from an ear infection, avoid simple carbohydrates such as sugar, honey, biscuits, sweets, ice cream, carbonated beverages, chocolate, dried fruits, and fruit juices. To help prevent babies from developing allergies, breastfeed for as long as possible. Breastfeeding mothers should also avoid food allergens. Introduce new foods carefully to babies, watching to see if a reaction occurs. Wheat, eggs, and dairy foods should not be introduced to babies in the first nine months of life. Babies can drink diluted fruit juices instead of milk or in conjunction with a non-dairy formula.

**Supplements:** Vitamin C supplementation reportedly stimulates immune function; take 500 mg and 1,000 mg a day in separate doses. Reduce the dose if you notice diarrhea. Zinc supplements have also been reported to increase immune function. Adults should take 25 mg per day, and children should take lower amounts. For example, a 30 lb child might be given 5 mg of zinc per day while suffering from an ear infection. Vitamin A supports immunity. Give a child up to six years of age 2,000–5,000 IU of vitamin A a day to support immunity. You should be able to find this in liquid form.

**Herbs:** Larix enhances immune function and also has antimicrobial activity. Dissolve 1–2 tsp in a non-dairy formula, or in water for older children or adults. Echinacea and goldenseal enhance immune function and have antimicrobial properties. Children should take 2 ml four times a day or as directed on the bottle. Thymus extract supports immune function. Take 50 mg per pound of weight a day. Mix St. John's wort oil with garlic oil to relieve ear pain and reduce infection. Place two warm drops of oil in the affected ear twice a day then gently place a cotton ball in the ear. Do not use this treatment if the ear is perforated.

## HOMEOPATHY

 A one-off, mild episode of recently developing ear infection may respond very well to the selection of the most appropriate acute homeopathic remedy, which can be given along with conventional treatment if necessary. Remedies can reduce distress and pain, and encourage the healing process to work to its maximum efficiency. Recurrent ear infections (especially if they are severe in nature) will require treatment from a homeopathic practitioner. A practitioner will prescribe to discourage the infection from developing. He or she can also provide advice with regard to appropriate homeopathic support in the event of an acute infection developing.

**Belladonna:** Use this remedy at the first sign of inflammation. Although it is often used to bring down high temperatures, it is also effective in easing localized inflammation accompanied by throbbing pains. Symptoms may be restricted to or worse on the right side, with the glands becoming inflamed and swollen in sympathy with affected ear.

**Aconite:** Use this at the first sign of inflammation that follows exposure to dry, cold, and windy weather. Pains come on suddenly and dramatically and wake the sufferer from sleep. When this remedy is well indicated there is a hypersensitivity to pain, with a tendency to react by becoming fearful and fractious. There may also be an uncharacteristic sensitivity to noise (music in particular), which feels painful to sensitive ears.

**Hepar sulph:** Use this remedy to treat a later stage of infection, where pains in the ears are characteristically sharp and splinter-like. The glands are also likely to be sensitive and swollen. There is a high sensitivity to cold drafts, which make pain and discomfort much more intense and distressing. Signature symptoms also include a marked tendency to be short-tempered and irritable when in pain.

**Chamomilla:** If ear infection in children is associated with a severe bout of teething, this is a potential remedy. Symptoms include one flushed and one pale cheek (the flushed one usually being on the painful side), and temper tantrums that are not easily comforted. Sharp, sticking pains in the ears are combined with a generally stuffed-up feeling.

**Pulsatilla:** Consider this as a possible remedy if an ear infection has set in as a later complication of a heavy head cold. Characteristic symptoms include swollen glands and a general sense of mucus congestion involving the ears, nose, sinuses, and/or the chest. Mucus is thick, bland, and yellowish-green in color. Signature symptoms include a strong tendency to be clingy, weepy, and in need of a lot of sympathy and attention when in pain or feeling ill. Although chilly, being in stuffy surroundings feels unbearable.

## HERBALISM

Ear infection can be classified in several different categories: acute infection due to a virus or bacteria; chronic inflammation in the middle ear; and inflammation and/or infection in the external ear canal. Consult a doctor to diagnose the condition before beginning treatment.

**Echinacea, Oregon grape, eyebright, and licorice:** The combination of these herbs creates a synergistic healing concoction. Studies have shown that echinacea and Oregon grape root stimulate the immune system and boost tissue healing, while acting as antiviral and antibacterial agents. Eyebright heals internal mucus congestion and licorice reduces swelling. Adults should take 0.5 g of dried herb in a tea, 250 mg in capsule form, or 1 ml as a tincture of each herb three times a day. Give half of the above dose to children under six. The herbs can be safely used by children as young at two years old. Take the herbs until the infection resolves.

**Garlic and mullein:** Garlic oil and mullein oil can be used to decrease pain, infection, and swelling in the ear canal in both acute and chronic infections. Place 3–5 drops of warm oil in the ear and cover with a soothing warm towel. Before using this therapy, please check with your doctor to confirm there are no ruptures to the ear's membrane, which makes this treatment unadvisable.

**Yarrow:** Yarrow is excellent for easing the quick onset of fever, discharge, reddish complexion, hot, dry skin, and restlessness. Infuse 1 tsp per cup or take 30 drops of tincture three times a day. Do not use if pregnant.

**Gallium:** Gallium is a gentle lymph mover, good for dispelling heat, swelling, and stagnation. This assists the body in directing much needed nutrients and immune cells to the affected areas, while stimulating the kidneys and liver to detoxify and remove infectious agents. Take 4–6 g daily.

# EAR WAX

## DIAGNOSIS

The ears produce a protective wax that lines the external canal of the ear to discourange insects from entering and to trap foreign bodies. Wax usually dries up of its own accord and is passed out, as the ears are self-cleansing. Occasionally ears may produce too much wax, which can lead to problems such as impaired hearing due to too much debris remaining in the ears. It is important not to poke inside your ears to try to resolve the problem yourself. The ear canal and eardrum are very delicate, and poking inside your ear could be painful and could push any accumulated wax further inside your ear. Ask your doctor for advice on how to resolve the situation. He or she may decide that your ears need syringing. This works by injecting a stream of warm fluid into the ear canal to loosen the wax, which then comes out of the ear mixed with the fluid.

**DANGER**: Do not poke anything such as a cotton bud into a waxy or itchy ear as this can cause damage. Leave any wax removal up to a medical practitioner.

## SYMPTOMS

- Hearing impairment
- An itching sensation in the ear
- Accumulation of dark brown wax

## TREATMENT GOAL

To remove excess wax safely and restore normal hearing.

## CONVENTIONAL MEDICINE

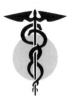

It is healthy to have wax inside the ear as it prevents dust and dirt from entering the ear canal and keeps a proper pH balance in the ear to protect it from infection. The ear usually cleanses itself but sometimes, for unknown reasons, wax can build up, causing pain or hearing loss. Erumen impaction is another name for the blockage of the ear canal by ear wax.

**Ear drops:** Mineral oil or eardrops, available from pharmacies to soften ear wax, can be used as a first step in removing excess ear wax. Add several drops to the ear canal of the affected ear. Within 48 hours, the excess wax should begin to move out of the ear. Olive oil and tea tree oil is available as a herbal preparation that can be used in the same manner. If you have severe pain or have previously had a ruptured eardrum, bypass this step and go straight to the doctor.

**What can my doctor do?** An irrigation kit designed for ear wax removal is a common treatment. Manual removal of ear wax with a curette is also an option. A suction tool may also be used for ear wax removal. Persistent unremitting wax blockages are generally referred to an ear, nose, and throat specialist so that structural integrity is intact and no anatomical blockages occur.

## TRADITIONAL CHINESE MEDICINE

**Herbs:** The following formula may help relieve symptoms and prevent ear wax accumulating in the future. The herbs are available from Chinese herbalists or online.

• Herbal decoction: Mix 12 g Zhi Zi (Cape Jasmine fruit), 10 g Chai Hu (hare's ear root), 12 g of Dang Gui (Chinese angelica root), 10 g of Huang Qin (baical skullcap), 8 g of Huang Lian (coptis root), 12 g of Dan Pi (cortex of tree peony root), 12 g of Niu Bang Zi (great burdock fruit), and 6 g of Gan Cao (licorice) in a ceramic pot. Add 3–4 cups of water, bring the mixture to the boil, let it simmer for 30 minutes, and strain the liquid. Drink 1 cup two to three times a day.

**Acupuncture:** It is not necessary to treat this condition by acupuncture unless the patient has some related issue, such as strong discomfort in the ear. For severe cases of ear wax, consult a practitioner. There is the possibility that acupuncture will be able to help.

**Acupressure:** Use the tip of your finger or thumb to press the Xia Guan point, located in front of the ear in the depression above the jawbone, with gentle pressure. Apply gentle pressure to the Yi Feng point, situated just behind the ear lobe, for one minute. Also press the Er Men point, in front of the notch found on the forward edge of the ear.

---

**TIP:** SESAME OIL DROPS

Apply sesame oil drops in the ear three times a day for three days to soften and loosen ear wax. Take the wax out after it becomes soft and loose.

---

## NATUROPATHY

**Diet:** Eat plenty of cold-water fish such as herring, mackerel, and salmon. These contain essential fatty acids, which are shown to be low in those individuals who produce too much ear wax.

**Supplements:** Fish oils are found in low levels in those who suffer from excess ear wax. Consult a practitioner regarding an appropriate dose.

**Irrigate ear wax:** Gently irrigate your ear with body-temperature water. Use a rubber ear syringe (available at most pharmacies) and a sink full of water. Make sure the water is warm enough so that your hands feel comfortable in it. Hold your head over the sink and very gently squirt the water into your ear, letting the water and wax run out into the sink. Be sure to dry the ear canal after washing. To do this, fill an eyedropper with rubbing alcohol and squeeze the alcohol into the ear. It will absorb moisture and dry the ear. If you're prone to excess wax build-up, irrigate your ears once or twice a month as a precautionary measure. Do not squirt anything in your ear if you have any kind of eardrum damage. Check with your doctor first, and again if you feel any pain.

**Baby oil:** Use baby oil to soften ear wax if it refuses to budge. Warm up the oil to body temperature and place a few drops into the ear twice a day. It will melt or soften the wax and you can then irrigate.

**Hydrogen peroxide:** Fill the ear with hydrogen peroxide using a dropper, and let it bubble and work for five minutes before flushing it away with water. If you need to, put a piece of cotton wool in the opening of the ear canal, so you can sit up while the peroxide goes to work.

**Ear candling:** This ancient technique involves using a hollow candle with the narrow end held gently onto the edge of the ear. The flame creates a relative vacuum in the ear, which draws out wax and other residues.

## HOMEOPATHY

 If over-production of ear wax is a problem on an on-going basis, it will need to be treated constitutionally by a homeopathic practitioner, who will take this symptom into account when assessing which homeopathic remedy is likely to be beneficial to the system as a whole. The excess production of ear wax should improve as part-and-parcel of your overall improved health. For an isolated episode of this problem, the following advice may be helpful.

**Causticum:** If you are going to have the wax removed by your doctor, it can be helpful to prepare the ear in advance by putting a single drop of almond or olive oil into the affected ear for five nights before going to bed. Taking Causticum twice daily for the five days during which the oil is being applied can facilitate the process. Characteristic symptoms that call for this remedy include intermittent bouts of reduced hearing with associated ringing, roaring, and/or pulsating noises. Ear wax that is produced looks dark brown and may have an offensive odor.

**Silica:** This may be more appropriate if the wax that is produced is crusty. Temporary reduction in, or loss of, hearing is eased by blowing the nose and/or coughing. There may be an associated itchiness in the ear, as well as roaring or hissing sounds.

## HERBALISM

 The presence of excessive ear wax is considered a sign of essential fatty acid deficiency. Several over-the-counter products are available to soften ear wax within the canal, allowing for easier extraction by a doctor. Unfortunately, there are not many herbal alternatives for this condition. That said, one herbal approach is to combine garlic oil and olive oil and to place 3–5 drops within the affected ear canal before bedtime. Cover the affected ear with a warm, moist towel to further promote penetration. The oil will soften the wax making it easier to remove. Repeat three to four nights in a row for maximum effect. See the entry on glue ear (p. 256) for other options.

# GLUE EAR

## DIAGNOSIS

Glue ear, also known as serous otitis media, affects the middle ear. It is a long-term condition that begins with the inflammation of the middle ear, which fills up with a thick discharge that has the texture of glue, hence the condition's common name. It arises mainly because secretions are unable to drain away down the eustachian tubes running from the ears down to the nose and throat, rather than from an infection. The condition is aggravated if the adenoids are also swollen. There may also be an accompanying nose or throat infection. Glue ear is prevalent in young children and often starts in early infancy. It is a form of fluctuating deafness that can have quite serious implications in terms of learning difficulties, and it often shows up as delayed speech development in young children. There is also a strong connection between recurrent upper respiratory tract infections and glue ear, and the condition tends to be more common during the winter months.

## SYMPTOMS

- Pain in the ear
- Stuffy feeling in the ear
- Thick discharge
- Muffled hearing, but the child is often unaware anything is wrong
- Poor concentration

## TREATMENT GOAL

To relieve symptoms and remedy the condition. This condition can be easily treated once detected.

## CONVENTIONAL MEDICINE

Conventional medicine diagnoses glue ear by looking into the ear at the tympanic membrane and noting redness, bulging, decreased movement, and an often dull appearance with fluid behind.

**General recommendations:** Make sure you drink plenty of fluids to remain hydrated. Decongestants may be used to encourage the mucus to drain. Allergens may contribute to inflammation, so any known irritants should be avoided.

**Antibiotics:** If the condition does not improve of its own accord within two to three days, see your doctor, who may prescribe amoxicillin. If there is still no improvement after three days, a broader spectrum antibiotic, such as augmentin, may be taken. A 10–14 day course of antibiotics is generally prescribed.

**Myringotomy:** If mucus remains in the middle ear for an extended period of time, it may begin to spread to areas around the ear, which can be dangerous. To avoid this, myringotomy can be performed to decompress the middle ear. A ventilation tube (tympanostomy tube) is sometimes inserted into the eardrum for drainage if multiple ear infections occur over a short period of time.

## TRADITIONAL CHINESE MEDICINE

**Herbs:** Herbs that have been proven to have anti-inflammatory functions may help this condition. Those listed below are available from Chinese medicine clinics and Chinese pharmacies.
- Chuan Xing Lian Pian: This herb is proven to have some effect on anti-infectious diseases, but its function is mild and therefore not ideal for treating a severe infection.
- Niu Huang Shang Qin Wan: This patent herbal pill is also useful in treating glue ear as it helps to clear infection.

**Acupuncture:** Treatment may reduce the pressure from fluid behind the eardrum. It may also reduce the pain, assist healing, and prevent deafness.

**Acupressure:** Apply medium pressure to the Yi Feng point, situated just behind the ear lobe. Also press the Xia Guan point, located in front of the ear in the depression above the jawbone. These points can be pressed a number of times for one minute each time.

**Diet:** Mung beans, red beans, bean sprouts, wax gourd, pears watermelon, and purslane are good choices, since these foods have cooling properties and dispel heat and damp. Also recommended are bananas, cucumber, mango, and mustard greens. Avoid eating fatty and greasy food.

## NATUROPATHY

**Diet:** Avoid common food allergens such as wheat, eggs, dairy foods, corn, citrus, and peanuts, especially with chronic conditions. Avoid simple carbohydrates, including sugar, honey, biscuits, sweets, ice cream, carbonated beverages, chocolate, dried fruits, and fruit juices. Babies can drink diluted fruit juices instead of milk or in conjunction with a non-dairy formula. To help prevent the development of allergies in babies, breastfeed for as long as possible. Breastfeeding mothers should also avoid food allergens. Introduce new foods carefully to babies, watching to see if a reaction occurs. Wheat, eggs, and dairy foods should not be introduced to babies during the first nine months of life.

**Supplements:** Vitamin C supplementation reportedly stimulates immune function. Take 500–1,000 mg a day in separate doses. Reduce the dose if you notice diarrhea. Zinc supplements have also been reported to increase immune function. Adults should take 25 mg per day and children should take lower doses according to weight. For example, a 30 lb child might be given 5 mg of zinc per day while suffering from glue ear. Vitamin A also supports immunity. Give children up to six years old 2,000–5,000 IU a day. Vitamin A is available in liquid form.

**Herbs:** Larix enhances immune function and has antimicrobial properties. Dissolve 1–2 tsp in a non-dairy formula or in water for older children. Echinacea and goldenseal enhances immune function and has antimicrobial properties. Children should take 2 ml four times a day or as directed on the bottle. Thymus extract also supports immune function; take 50 mg per every pound a child weighs a day. You can also mix St. John's wort oil with garlic oil, to relieve ear pain and reduce infection. Place two warm drops of oil in the affected ear two times a day then gently place a cotton wool ball in the ear. Do not use this treatment if the ear is perforated.

## HOMEOPATHY

Due to its chronic nature, homeopathic treatment for this condition needs to be placed in the hands of a trained homeopathic practitioner. This is a worthwhile step to take before considering inserting grommets. The surgical option should not be ruled out, but allow a complementary option time to improve the condition before resorting to more radical measures. Since the repeated use of antibiotics to treat recurrent ear infections may be associated with the development of glue ear, it may be worth considering treatment with cranial osteopathy, shown in research to reduce the incidence of ear infections in children aged six months to six years. The following remedies are given with a view to suggesting the possible treatment options that a practitioner might consider, rather than encouraging self-prescription.

**Kali mur:** This remedy is a positive candidate if problems with recurrent ear infections and swollen, tender glands have followed on from a vaccination. Characteristic symptoms include blockage of the eustachian tube and hearing reduction associated with cracking noises on swallowing or blowing the nose. The eustachian tube may feel sore as well as congested, and there may also be a significant amount of itching in the affected ear or ears.

**Pulsatilla:** If there is an established history of mucus production and congestion that affects the ears, nose, and/or chest, this remedy is well indicated. The mucus produced is characteristically thick and yellowish-green in color. The affected ears feel constantly stuffed up, with the sensation being mildly relieved only when traveling in a car. The external ear may also become swollen and inflamed, with a sense of pressure, as though something were pushing itself out of the ear.

**Lycopodium:** If there is a tendency for ear problems to be combined with snuffles and a constantly stuffed-up nose that leads to forced breathing through the mouth, use Lycopodium. Noises in the ear include humming and roaring sounds, and hearing may become poor. There may also be an associated echoing sound in response to any noise. The ears feel generally hot and inflamed, and may develop patches of eczema (see p. 73).

## HERBALISM

 **Eucalyptus, thyme, and rosemary:** The inability of the eustachian tube, the tube which connects the inner ear to the throat, to drain is one of the main contributors to the development of ear inflammation and infection. Studies show that more discharge was observed in people in low-humidity environments. Therefore, using a humidifier can improve drainage from the eustachian tube. Add antimicrobial and antispasmodic effects by placing 3–5 drops each of eucalyptus, thyme, and rosemary oil into a humidifier. These essential oils should not be used to treat children; they can be too strong and even cause breathing problems.

**Bitter orange:** Another excellent way to encourage drainage from the eustachian tube is to place bitter orange oil onto the drainage site of the throat, allowing movement of stagnant material. Bitter orange has astringent and sedative qualities that allow it to tonify and open the tissue around the eustachian tube opening. Place 3 drops on a gloved finger, find the "bump" on the side of the throat behind the tonsils, and place the oil over the bump while pulling downward. This treatment may not be suitable for someone with a strong gag reflex; however, it is quite effective at encouraging drainage.

**Garlic and mullein:** Garlic oil and mullein oil can be combined with olive oil to create a soothing, healing blend for the ear canal. The antimicrobial properties of garlic inhibit infection, while mullein heals inflamed tissue, thereby decreasing discharge and pain. Place 3–5 drops of warm oil in the ear and cover with a warm towel. Before using this therapy, please check with your doctor to confirm there are no ruptures to the ear's membrane, which makes this treatment inadvisable.

# HAY FEVER

## DIAGNOSIS

Hay fever is a type of seasonal rhinitis typified by an allergic reaction to pollen. The mucous membrane that lines the nose, plus the eyes and the air passages become inflamed due to pollen and other airborne allergens. This causes the body to release histamine, which leads to inflammation and swelling. The most obvious symptoms of hay fever include a runny nose, sneezing, itchy eyes that are often red and watery, an irritated throat, and a general feeling of being under the weather. Some people find they are only slightly affected, while others are debilitated by the condition if it affects them severely. Hay fever symptoms become worse during hot, dry weather, when the pollen count rises.

Although hay fever often flares up for the first time during the teenage years, it is now becoming more common among young children as well. There is often a link between hay fever and conditions such as asthma, eczema, and psoriasis. It often occurs in those with a tendency to catarrh or frequent upper respiratory tract infections. Sometimes those with weak digestion, who don't have good nutrition, or who suffer from poor general health are more susceptible to pollen as their immune system is weak.

**DANGER**: If breathing becomes difficult, any asthma symptoms worsen, or there is any swelling of the lips or throat, seek immediate medical attention.

## SYMPTOMS

- Frequent sneezing
- Blocked-up nose
- Congestion with cold-like symptoms
- Prolific clear mucus
- Difficulty in breathing properly
- Wheezing
- Red, sore, gritty eyes
- Watery and itchy eyes
- Feeling of being stuffed-up
- Generally being under the weather

## TREATMENT GOAL

There is no cure for hay fever. Treatment aims to ease symptoms as far as possible. Allergy tests can be arranged to identify the exact trigger for the hay fever attacks.

## CONVENTIONAL MEDICINE

**Avoid allergens:** Avoid outdoor exposure and use HEPA filters indoors during the pollen season. Humidifiers can be used in a dry climate, as they will help to moisturize the respiratory system. Too much humidity however, can cause more problems. The optimum level is about 35%.

**Nasal washes:** Using saline (saltwater) made from 1 tsp of salt to each pint of distilled warm water is an inexpensive and effective treatment. Sniff a small amount of the saline water into the nostrils one at a time and blow your nose. A syringe can also be used, as can a nasal spray.

**Supplements:** Take 1,000 mg of quercetin (eucalyptus flavonoid) three times a day. Take 500 mg–1 g of vitamin C a day, and add zinc and vitamins A and E to your diet. Take 4 g of EPA DHA (an omega-3 fat) fish oil a day in a 3:2 ratio.

**Medication:** Topical nasal steroids such as Flonase®, oral antihistamines, topical azelastine, or cromolyn sodium in combination with mucolytics (guaifenesin) and decongestants are usually prescribed. Although they do mask symptoms, they do not alleviate the actual cause.

## TRADITIONAL CHINESE MEDICINE

**Herbs:** The herbs listed in the formulas below are available from Chinese pharmacies and online.
• Herbal decoction: Combine 10 g of Jin Yin Hua (honeysuckle flower), 12 g of Fang Fen (ledebouriella root), 12 g of Niu Bang Zi (great burdock fruit), 8 g of Gui Zhi (cinnamon), 12 g Bai Shao (white peony root), and 6 g Raw Gan Cao (licorice) in a ceramic pot. Add 3 cups of water, bring the mixture to the boil, and let it simmer for 30 minutes. Strain the liquid and drink 1 cup twice a day.
• Herbal tea: Mix 8 g of Ye Jiu Hua (chrysanthemum flower), 3 g of Bo He (field mint), and 5 g of Jing Jie (schizonepeta stem and bud) in a teapot and add boiling water. Let the mixture steep for five minutes. Drink the tea throughout the day.

**Acupuncture:** This is very effective in treating hay fever as it works on regulating the body's immune system to reduce the reoccurrence rate, as well as treating symptoms. Consult a practitioner of traditional Chinese medicine regarding treatment possibilities. A twice-weekly treatment session during the hay fever season is normally recommended.

**Acupressure:** For hay fever the Feng Chi, Tai Yang, and Yin Tang acupressure points are recommended. The Feng Chi point is found at the back of the head at the base of the skull 2 inches below the center point. The Tai Yang point is located at the temple in the depression between the lateral end of the eyebrow and eyelid. The Yin Tang point is in the depression midway between the eyebrows. Press and release these points with your thumb about 20 times. Start with gentle pressure, then gradually increase it.

**Diet:** Varieties of fresh vegetables that are light and easy to digest are suggested, such as Chinese cabbage, kale, napa cabbage, celery, and cooked cucumber. Use light and gentle cooking methods such as steaming, boiling, and sautéing.

**TIP: TAKE PREVENTIVE MEASURES**

To avoid suffering from hay fever seasonally, ask a TCM practitioner for help before the symptoms occur. When you can get treatment for prevention, regular and earlier treatment is better.

## NATUROPATHY

**Diet:** Eat a well-balanced diet that includes fresh fruit and vegetables, whole grains, legumes, and quality protein such as fish, lean chicken, and beans every day. Eat plenty of green leafy vegetables for their high nutrient content that will provide a good base of nutrients required for a healthy immune system. Eat non-mucus forming foods such as non-gluten wholegrains (brown rice, quinoa, and buckwheat). Consume anti-inflammatory essential fatty acids (omega-3s) in the form of fatty fish, walnuts, flax seeds, cod liver oil, fish oil, and flax seed oil. Eat plenty of raw seeds and nuts. Avoid mucus-forming foods such as fried and processed foods, refined flours, eggs, and dairy products. Make sure you drink plenty of water. Identify and eliminate aggravating substances, including food dyes, food colorings, preservatives, and additives. Avoid dietary sources of arachidonic acid (found in animal products), which contribute to inflammation.

**Supplements:** Take 1,000 mg of vitamin C for its natural antihistamine effects (reduce the dosage if diarrhea occurs). Take 250 mg of quercetin three times a day to control inflammation by reducing the release from cells of histamine and other mediators of allergic reactions. Quercetin also stabilizes cell membranes so they are less reactive to allergens. Take 250 mg three times a day. Probiotics are also proven to be beneficial for treating allergies; take a product that contains four billion organisms of lactobacillus acidophilus and bifidus. Protease enzymes assist in decreasing inflammation. Take two capsules twice a day on an empty stomach.

**Herbs:** Take 300–500 mg of the freeze-dried stinging nettles, which are beneficial for allergic rhinitis and hay fever. Butterbur is a traditional herbal remedy used to treat seasonal allergies and asthma. Research has shown it is as effective and less sedating than a commonly prescribed antihistamine. Take 8 mg two to four times a day.

## HOMEOPATHY

 There is a great deal of homeopathic support available to hay fever sufferers. Help is provided on two levels: the acute stage is treated in the summer months to relieve immediate symptoms, while treating the chronic condition continues over the fall and winter months. During the winter, a homeopathic practitioner will prescribe with a view to strengthening the patient's overall health. By doing so consistently over a few years, symptoms should gradually fade away as acute bouts become shorter-lived and less severe. The remedies listed below can be used to reduce the misery of acute symptoms. However, for more lasting relief, treatment should be sought from a trained practitioner. Also see the entry on allergic rhinitis (p. 232).

**Sabadilla:** If you are sensitivite to the smell of flowers, which provokes repeated bouts of sneezing with profuse nasal discharge, use Sabadilla. Symptoms include one nostril becoming blocked at a time, while tickling sensations in the nose feel as though they are spreading all over the body.

**Pulsatilla:** This is a potential remedy for stubborn hay fever symptoms that produce a characteristic, thick, bland discharge that is yellowish-green in color. Signature symptoms include feeling distressed, uncomfortable, and stuffed up at night, and a runny nose during the day. Hot, stuffy conditions make everything feel worse, while contact with fresh, cool air gives temporary relief.

**Nux vomica:** Think of this remedy if hay fever symptoms are noticeably more troublesome after a period of living in the fast lane with high stress levels. Common symptoms include a rough, raw sensation in the throat that feels as though it has been scraped. The nose is oversensitive to odors and violent, abortive bouts of sneezing are preceded by an unpleasant crawling sensation in the nostrils that may be worse on the left side. Congestion in the eustachian tube leads to itchiness and irritation in the ears, while the roof of the mouth may also feel itchy.

**Arsenicum album:** This is a potential remedy for burning sensations in the eyes, nose, and/or throat that are soothed by contact with warmth. The eyes and nose water and run, with an unpleasant stuffed-up sensation persisting in the nose. Sneezing is frequent, but does not bring relief. The chest may also feel tight and wheezy with a dry, irritating cough making it difficult to sleep soundly at night. All symptoms tend to be more severe during the night, and/or the early hours of the morning, causing lots of anxiety and physical, mental, and emotional restlessness.

> **TIP:** EYE MASK
>
> To soothe very itchy and irritated eyes, soak a couple of eyepads in diluted, cool Euphrasia tincture and rest them over the eyelids. To make the dilution, add 4 drops of tincture to 150 ml of boiled, cooled water.

## HERBALISM

 To treat hay fever, a herbalist will recommend plants that mediate the allergic reaction and fight the inflammation in the upper respiratory tract, thereby alleviating symptoms. Some of these herbal medicines will work best when started several weeks prior to the time when the plants or flowers you react to are blooming, and the herbs should be taken on a daily basis in order to prevent the symptoms from occurring or from becoming severe. Some herbs can also be used as treatments in addition to prevention. It is important to begin treatment four to six weeks prior to the time when your symptoms of hay fever generally first appear. If you are currently symptomatic, you can also begin the herbal therapies mentioned below, bearing in mind that it may take several weeks for your symptoms to improve.

**Butterbur:** Butterbur and the compounds it contains (called petasins) stop the inflammation associated with hay fever and allergies, thereby improving the symptoms. Butterbur has the advantage of not causing the drowsiness that most anti-allergy medications do do. Whole butterbur herb contains compounds called pyrrolizidine alkaloids that are toxic to the liver; only standardized extracts that are free of pyrrolizidine alkaloids should be used and the specific dose (ranging from 25–75 mg two to three times daily) will depend on the product chosen.

**Nettle leaf:** Take either 10 g of the dried herb, 3–6 ml of a 1:2 liquid extract, or a freeze-dried standardized extract of nettle leaf. Although there is limited scientific evidence for the effectiveness of stinging nettles on allergies or hay fever, many experts have found it very useful for their patients.

**Gumweed:** Taking 30–60 drops of tincture of this plant three times daily can help settle the symptoms of hay fever, especially the cough that results from overactive sinuses, leading to phlegm and a runny nose.

# HEARING LOSS

## DIAGNOSIS

Hearing loss is a very distressing condition. Total hearing loss is very rare and usually present from birth. Partial hearing loss comes on more suddenly and generally stems from infection, injury, or deterioration as you get older. There are two kinds of deafness: conductive and nerve deafness. Conductive deafness results from a defect in the mechanical part of your hearing. It can result from a blockage of wax, or damage to the eardrum, which can become perforated. Nerve deafness results from a defect in or damage to the delicate inner ear, from where sound vibrations are carried to the brain. This can stem from prolonged exposure to loud music, or sudden, very loud bangs, or simply the effects of aging. A side effect of this condition is often tinnitus, which is ringing in the ears. As we get older our hearing becomes less acute and less sensitive to high-frequency sounds. Age-related hearing loss occurs in around one-third of people over 65, but hearing can start to deteriorate from the age of 40 onwards.

## SYMPTOMS

- Difficulty understanding people on the phone
- Confusion as to where sounds are coming from
- Misunderstanding what people are saying
- Ringing or rustling noises in the ear
- Earache
- Discharge from the ear
- Dizziness
- Nausea

## TREATMENT GOAL

Once your doctor has determined the cause of your hearing loss, you may be referred to a specialist for a series of tests. Age-related hearing loss is permanent, but hearing loss that results from other causes can potentially be treated.

## CONVENTIONAL MEDICINE

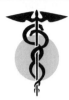

Treating hearing loss depends to some extent on the cause. Hearing loss can occur in those with diabetes, or during pregnancy. It can be a consequence of mumps, measles, herpes, syphilis, or mononucleosis. It is also seen in some autoimmune vascular diseases, which are relatively rare. Some common causes are obstruction of the ear canal and swimmer's ear. Some more rare and serious causes are a tumor, such as an acoustic neuroma. Certain medications, particularly of the antibiotic class aminoglycosides, as well as aspirin, can cause hearing loss. Conventional medical treatment begins with an evaluation of the hearing loss to determine its cause.

**Hearing tests:** An audiogram is performed to determine if the loss is sensorineural, that is, to do with the nerves and surrounding anatomy, or if it is conductive, that is, related to some middle or external ear condition. Generally an MRI or CT scan is carried out to rule out brain or ear abnormalities such as tumors and to rule out other causes such as multiple sclerosis.

**Conductive hearing loss:** Causes of conductive hearing loss include otitis media, Eustachian tube dysfunction, a perforated eardrum, a foreign body in the ear canal, or problems with the small bones of the ear.

**Sensorineural hearing loss:** Causes of sensorineural hearing loss include, most commonly, presbyacusis (hearing loss in old age), Meniere's disease, multiple sclerosis, loss due to hereditary causes, diabetes, or acoustic neuroma.

**Hearing aids:** For hearing loss due to old age, a hearing aid can be used. For all others, the cause of the hearing loss must be addressed.

## TRADITIONAL CHINESE MEDICINE

Traditional Chinese medicine recognizes three types of hearing loss: excess syndrome, deficiency syndrome, and stagnant energy. With excess syndrome, hearing is lost suddenly and accompanied by intensified dizziness and/or headache, with or without emotional trauma. With deficiency syndrome, hearing decreases over time (due to ageing) and is accompanied by a low, dull noise in the ear, insomnia, or depression. With stagnant energy, there is a ringing in the ear that comes and goes and hearing loss is accompanied by the sense that the ear is blocked. To treat all types of hearing loss, an experienced practitioner of Chinese medicine will first identify the cause of the condition.

**Herbs:** Take Chai Hu Shu Gan Wan to treat excess syndrome; take Zhi Bai Di Huang Wan, or Er Ming Zhu Hi Wan to treat deficiency syndrome; or take Long Dan Xie Gan Wan to treat stagnant energy. These patent herbal pills can all be found in Chinese medicine clinics, Chinese pharmacies, or online. Follow the directions on the label for dosage.

**Acupuncture:** This is one of the most effective treatments for some cases of hearing loss. An experienced practitioner will be able to assess your condition, find the primary cause, and decide on the treatment plan. After a few sessions, the practitioner may be able to make a prognosis.

**Acupressure:** Use your finger tip or thumb to apply gentle to medium pressure to the Ting Hui point, located on the face just in front of the ear. You can also press the Xia Guan point, found in front of the ear in the depression above the jawbone. Another helpful point is the Yi Feng point, which is situated just behind the ear lobe. Apply gentle pressure to these points for one minute at a time.

**Diet:** Foods that are good for strengthening the kidneys and nourishing the blood, such as chicken liver, black sesame seed, string bean, sword bean, spinach, beef, oysters, grapes, and tangerines, are recommended.

## NATUROPATHY

**Diet:** Avoid cow's milk. Researchers found high amounts of a protein molecule identical to one in cow's milk in the hearing organs of 89% of patients with age-related hearing loss, while people with normal hearing had none.

**Supplements:** Take 15–30 mg of zinc a day to produce superoxide dismutase, an antioxidant your body makes that may prevent noise-related hearing damage. Deficiency in copper, which also helps in making superoxide dismutase, has been associated with the auditory system. Taking 2 mg of copper every other day, with zinc, is suggested. You can also take 15 mg of manganese a day to help produce superoxide dismutase. Magnesium has been shown to have protective benefits against noise-induced hearing loss. Take 500–1,000 mg of elemental magnesium a day. Vitamin A deficiency has been shown to be a factor in hearing loss, including noise-induced hearing loss. A supplement that supplies 10,000 IU of vitamin A a day is suggested—but pregnant women should not take more than 10,000 IU of vitamin. The B vitamins have shown positive benefits for persons with hearing loss. A high-potency complete B-complex is recommended. Alternatives are to take 500 mg of vitamin B1, 250 mg of B6, and 500 mcg of vitamin B12. Vitamin D deficiency has been found in people with chronic hearing loss, so take 400 IU daily. Vitamin C is crucial for its anti-oxidant properties. Take 2,000 mg a day.

**Herbs:** Ginkgo biloba may also help to stabilize hearing loss; take 80–120 mg of ginkgo daily.

## HOMEOPATHY

 If hearing loss follows an infection the remedies below can be used. Also see Ear Infection (p. 248) and Glue Ear (p. 256) for additional recommendations.

**Aconite:** Use this remedy at the first sign of ear inflammation that follows exposure to dry, cold, and windy weather. When Aconite is well indicated there is a hypersensitivity to pain, with a tendency to react by becoming fearful and fractious. There may also be an uncharacteristic sensitivity to noise (music in particular), which feels painful to sensitive ears.

**Kali mur:** This remedy is a potential candidate if problems with recurrent ear infections and swollen, tender glands have followed on from a vaccination. Characteristic symptoms include blockage of the eustachian tube and hearing reduction associated with cracking noises on swallowing or blowing the nose. The eustachian tube may feel sore as well as congested, and there may also be a significant amount of itching in the affected ear or ears.

**Lycopodium:** If there is a tendency for ear problems to be combined with snuffles and a constantly stuffed-up nose that leads to forced breathing through the mouth, use Lycopodium. Noises in the ear include humming and roaring sounds, and hearing may become poor. There may also be an associated echoing sound in response to any noise. The ears feel generally hot and inflamed, and may develop patches of eczema (see p. 73).

### TIP: PROTECT YOUR EARS
Wear headphones or ear plugs whenever you may be exposed to more than 85 decibels of noise, such as when you use a lawn mower or a chain saw, or attend a concert where music is likely to be played at an exceptionally loud volume.

## HERBALISM

The herbal medicines recommended below promote healing of the hearing apparatus by encouraging circulation to the area, improving antioxidant availability, and decreasing toxins that may be to blame for chronic hearing loss over time.

**Asian and Siberian ginseng:** Both of these herbs are known to increase and improve circulation in the brain. Studies have shown that increasing circulation to the hearing organ and the surrounding neural tissue improves hearing in some cases. Boil 1 tsp of root in a cup of water to drink, or take 40 drops of tincture, twice daily.

**Ginkgo:** Studies show ginkgo improves flow to the brain. Do not use this herb with blood-thinning medications.

**Stinging nettles, bitter orange, bromelain, and perilla:** In a review of over 100 cases, it was found that allergies were related to an average of 50% of ear conditions that contribute to hearing loss. These herbs demonstrate significant anti-allergy activity. Combine equal parts in tincture form and take 5 ml in water daily.

**Grape seed, green tea, and pomegranate:** New research has shown that many of the toxins found in cigarettes are directly related to hearing loss. Studies indicate that protection from hazardous chemicals in the environment that may damage the vascular and neural integrity of the hearing organ will decrease hearing loss progression. Herbs that contain high levels of proanthocyanidins, found in grape seed, and catechins, found in green tea, protect blood vessels from toxin damage while improving the structural integrity of the vessels to withstand damage. Pomegranate, high in antioxidant polyphenols, is possibly even stronger than grape seed and green tea. Take 150–300 mg of grape seed, up to 240 ml of pomegranate juice, or drink 3–5 cups of green tea daily.

# LARYNGITIS

## DIAGNOSIS

Laryngitis is a painful condition that results in inflammation of the voice box, or larynx. The larynx becomes inflamed and swollen, vibrates less easily, and therefore produces less sound, in effect distorting the voice apparatus. This causes hoarseness and the distinctive croaky voice associated with laryngitis. Often, people with this condition temporarily lose their voices altogether. In the acute form, this condition appears suddenly and is usually caused by an infection, such as a cold, flu, or bronchitis. This type usually clears up of its own accord in a couple of weeks and antibiotics are rarely needed. The chronic type of laryngitis recurs on a regular basis. It can be triggered by shouting, loud singing or excessive use of the voice, or smoking, activities which should be avoided if you want to break the pattern of recurrent attacks. Your throat may need investigating to see if there are polyps on the larynx, which could be causing problems.

Laryngitis is a painful condition but it is not dangerous. It usually clears up once the voice has been given a complete rest. If the hoarseness continues for more than two weeks, you lose your voice after a head or neck injury, or your voice disappears suddenly for no apparent reason, see your doctor.

## SYMPTOMS

- Difficulty speaking
- Sore throat
- Hoarse and throaty, or whispering, voice
- Dry coughing
- Occasionally, loss of voice completely
- Painful and tender larynx
- Sometimes, fever and a feeling of being generally under the weather

## TREATMENT GOAL

To ease symptoms of pain and discomfort in the throat and to encourage the voice to return to normal.

## CONVENTIONAL MEDICINE

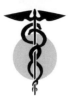

Treatment of laryngitis depends on whether it is in an acute or chronic stage. Acute laryngitis usually develops after an upper respiratory tract infection. If the laryngitis does not resolve in three weeks, it is considered chronic. Chronic laryngitis may be due to a lesion present on the larynx, chronic sinusitis, or hypothyroidism.

**Rest and hydrate your voice:** Drink plenty of water, maintain a healthy diet, and completely rest your voice. Using a humidifier may also help the laryngitis to resolve.

**Mucolytic:** A mucolytic, such as guaifenesin, can be used to provide lubrication and encourage any thick mucus stuck on the larynx, which exacerbates an irritation, to resolve.

**Antibiotics:** Occasionally, laryngitis results from a bacterial infection. If this is the case penicillin or erythromycin is prescribed to resolve the condition.

**To treat chronic laryngitis:** An ear, nose and throat (ENT) specialist may do a scope to identify any potential lesions on the larynx. These will need to be surgically removed. Speech therapy is sometimes helpful after a prolonged bout of chronic laryngitis.

## TRADITIONAL CHINESE MEDICINE

**Herbs:** The herbs listed below are available from Chinese herbalists or online.

• Herbal decoction: To treat wind and heat, combine 10 g of Jin Yin Hua (honeysuckle flower), 8 g of Jing Jie (schizonepeta stem and bud), 12 g of Jie Geng (balloon flower root), 12 g of Niu Bang Zi (great burdock fruit), 8 g of Bo He (field mint), 10 g of Zhu Ye (bamboo leaves), 6 g of Gan Cao (licorice), and 12 g of Lian Qiao (forsythia fruit) in a ceramic pot. Add 2–4 cups of water, bring the liquid to the boil, and simmer for 30 minutes. Strain the liquid and drink 1 cup twice a day.

• Herbal decoction: To treat cold wind, running nose, and chills, mix 12 g of Fang Fen (ledebouriella root), 6 g of Bo He (field mint), 10 g of Jing Jie (schizonepeta stem and bud), 10 g of Zi Su Ye (perilla leaf), 12 g of Jie Geng (balloon flower root), 5 g of fresh ginger, and 3 g of Gan Cao (licorice). Follow the directions above to make a decoction.

• Herbal tea: To treat yin deficiency, place 5 g of Mai Men Dong (ophiopogon tuber), 3 g of Gan Cao (licorice), and 3 g of Bo He (field mint) in a teapot and add boiling water. Let the herbs steep for five minutes before drinking. This tea can be sipped throughout the day.

**Acupuncture:** Consult a practitioner of traditional Chinese medicine for acupuncture treatment. Herbal medicine may be more appropriate in some cases.

**Acupressure:** Use the tip of your thumb and press the Hegu point, located on the back of the hand between the thumb and first finger, with strong pressure for one to two minutes. Apply similar pressure to the Nei Guan point, which is found in the center of the wrist on the palm side, about 2 inches below the crease. These acupressure points can be pressed a couple of times during the day as needed.

**Diet:** Eat foods that are juicy and mild such as lettuce, bok choy, Chinese broccoli (found in Chinese groceries), daikon radish, strawberries, pears, mango, grapes, cantaloupe melon, and watermelon. Hot, spicy foods, such as chilies, red and green peppers, and pepper, should be avoided.

## NATUROPATHY

 **Diet:** Eat light foods consisting of steamed vegetables, freshly made soups, and broths. Add garlic, ginger, and onions to soup for their tonifying, antimicrobial, and warming properties. Cut out all milky and mucus-forming foods such as cheese, yogurt, red meat, dairy, and simple carbohydrates. Drink plenty of water, freshly squeezed juices, and teas to cleanse your body of toxins. Herbal teas will assist your body's ability to heal itself. The most beneficial kinds of herbal teas are listed in the herbal section of this entry. Take 1 tbsp of honey and lemon juice with a pinch of cayenne pepper twice a day. The mixture helps coat your larynx, which can relieve laryngitis.

**Supplements:** Take 500 mg–1,000 mg of vitamin C every four hours until symptoms subside to support the immune system. Bioflavonoids work synergistically with vitamin C and have immune-enhancing properties of their own. Take 1,000 mg a day in divided doses. Zinc supports the immune system and may have antiviral properties. Take 25 mg of zinc in lozenges several times a day for one week.

**Herbs:** Drink a tea made from peppermint, eucalyptus, and chamomile three times a day. Add cayenne to the tea to stimulate the circulation, or cinnamon for its gentle, warming effect. Grated ginger root can also be added to induce sweating. Elderflower and elderberry is an effective, natural antiviral that can be used to ease symptoms of laryngitis. Adults can take 10 ml of tincture and children 5 ml three times a day. Echinacea and goldenseal enhance the immune system and have antiviral properties. Take 2–4 ml of a tincture that combines the two, four times a day. Lomatium dissectum has strong antiviral effects; take 500 mg in capsule form or 2–4 ml of tincture four times a day. Take plenty of raw garlic or 300–500 mg in capsule form a day to fight and prevent infection.

**Hydrotherapy:** Try applying compresses to help speed up the healing process. Use a piece of an old sheet that's long and wide enough to wrap around your throat, and a similar-sized piece of cloth. Soak the sheet in cold water, wring it out, and wrap it once around your throat. Cover the sheet with the dry cloth and secure it with a safety pin. As your body heat warms and dries the compress, circulation will increase. Change the compresses every six to eight hours.

**Aromatherapy:** Carefully pour about 4–6 cups of boiling water into a large bowl and add 3 drops of eucalyptus oil. Hold your head over the bowl and cover both with a towel, making sure that you do not put your face too close to the hot water. Close your eyes and breathe slowly and deeply, continuing the treatment for about 15 minutes. If you start to feel overheated or uncomfortable, remove the towel. Repeat the steam inhalation for 5–10 minutes every hour over the course of a day. Inhaling eucalyptus oil presents an extremely low level of risk to most people. However, prolonged exposure (perhaps an hour or more) to relatively high levels of essential oil vapor (undiluted oil directly inhaled from the bottle) could lead to headache, vertigo, nausea, and lethargy. In certain cases, serious side effects such as incoherence or double vision may be experienced. **Warning:** Those with serious heart problems and nervous disorders such as epilepsy, and pregnant women, infants, children, and the elderly may not be able to respond appropriately to this type of heat treatment.

## HOMEOPATHY

The remedies below can be helpful in speeding up recovery from a recently developed, acute episode of laryngitis. They will be most effective if used in combination with practical measures such as avoiding over-using the voice and smoky atmospheres, and drinking plenty of soothing fluids. A history of repeated episodes of severe laryngitis is best treated by a homeopathic practitioner.

**Aconite:** If symptoms come on very rapidly and dramatically, consider using Aconite. Over-exposure to dry, cold winds trigger sensitivity to pain and restlessness. Symptoms tend to emerge most strongly when waking from sleep in the early hours.

### TIP: TAKE SUPPLEMENTS
If laryngitis has developed as a consequence of being infected with a nasty cold, boost your immune system's functioning by taking 1 g of vitamin C daily split into two doses of 500 mg taken morning and evening. Also take zinc, garlic, and echinacea as directed.

**Phosphorus:** Use this remedy to treat hoarseness and complete loss of voice that is accompanied by a furry, raw sensation in the larynx and pain that is worse for speaking. If the voice has not been lost altogether, it is likely to sound very low. Symptoms are the most intense and distressing in the evening.

**Causticum:** Think of this as a possibility if the throat feels burning, raw, scraped, and constricted so that there is a need to swallow continuously. Efforts to cough up mucus are ineffectual, which prompts more swallowing. There is also a tendency to swallow the wrong way because of sensitivity and inflammation in the throat.

---

**TIP:** USE THROAT LOZENGES

If your throat feels dry and raspy, sucking throat lozenges can provide temporary, soothing relief by providing lubrication. Avoid lozenges that contain substances that may interfere with homeopathic remedies, such as eucalyptus, menthol, or peppermint.

---

## HERBALISM

**Queen's root:** This remedy is effective for laryngeal inflammation and irritation, combined with swollen lymph nodes in the neck and throat. As a potent lymphagogue and alterative, it promotes mucus secretion and the removal of infectious and metabolic waste. Boil 1 tsp of root per cup of water for 15 minutes, or take 30 drops of tincture, and drink three times per day. The fresh plant can be toxic. Do not use during pregnancy.

**Yerba santa:** A warming, aromatic, sweet herb, yerba santa fights infection while opening the bronchioles in the lungs and encouraging mucus expectoration. Infuse 1 tsp of leaves in 1 cup of hot water, or take 30 drops of tincture, and drink three times daily.

**Stone root:** Originating from the mint family, stone root is cooling and astringent. These properties soothe and tonify inflamed mucous membranes and decrease mucus production and pain. Stone root is best indicated when there is a feeling of constriction or tickling in the throat. Infuse 1–2 tsp of herb per cup of hot water, or take 30–60 drops, and drink three to four times a day. Do not use the aerial parts, as they may cause vomiting.

# MENIERE'S DISEASE

## DIAGNOSIS

Meniere's disease is a disorder of the inner ear caused by a change in pressure, which leads to an accumulation of fluid. It can strike quite suddenly without any warning, and an attack can last from a few minutes up to several hours. It causes a person to experience a spinning sensation, dizziness, and nausea. The dizziness can come out of the blue and be so severe that sufferers need to hold on to someone or something to avoid falling over. The excess fluid in the eardrum causes the balance center of the inner ear to malfunction, sending chaotic signals to the brain that result in dizzy spells. A sense of imbalance that can last for days follows an attack. Meniere's can also cause fluctuating hearing loss and a sensation of ringing in the ears (see Tinnitus, p. 312). The hearing loss can remain even after the attack has subsided, or can come and go. The exact cause of the condition is not known, although stress is thought to be one of the main triggers. Unfortunately, there tends to be a pattern of repetition, either regular or irregular, to the attacks. However, in time they do become less frequent and less severe, and can disappear entirely for years. There is no cure for Meniere's disease. If you are diagnosed with this condition it is important to rest and adopt a low-stress lifestyle.

## SYMPTOMS

- Dizziness and a sense of vertigo with "spinning" vision
- Nausea
- Vomiting
- Impaired hearing or loss of hearing with noises in the ears (tinnitus)

## TREATMENT GOAL

Although there is no cure, treatment will aim to relieve immediate symptoms and address long-term prevention.

## CONVENTIONAL MEDICINE

Treating Meniere's disease effectively depends on its correct diagnosis. Meniere's can sometimes be confused with ear infection, viral labrinthitis, acoustic neuroma, migraines, and multiple sclerosis. Diagnosis usually involves an MRI scan, which involves taking a picture of the brain to make sure there is not a tumor present. It may also involve an electronystagmograph and an electrocochleograph, which are tests performed by an ear, nose, and throat (ENT) specialist.

**Prevention:** Avoid atypical food allergens, processed foods, caffeine, and alcohol. Maintaining good nutrition and general health, and taking anti-inflammatory supplements, can help to improve the condition at times by maximizing your immune status. Stress reduction and meditation techniques can also be helpful.

**Medication:** Prochlorperazine at a dose of 5–10 mg four times a day, or promethazine at a dose of 25 mg every six hours, may be prescribed. Meclozine and scopolamine patches are also used. Diazepam at a dose of 10 mg is prescribed for acute attacks. These treatments work for about 90% of patients; surgery is an option for those who do not respond to any of the above.

## TRADITIONAL CHINESE MEDICINE

**Herbs:** The herbs and herbal pills listed below are available from Chinese pharmacies.
• To treat Meniere's disease due to deficiency of kidney yin: Symptoms will include dizziness, feeling off-balance with ringing in the ears, insomnia, and fatigue. To treat this condition, take herbs that are tonifying to kidney yin, such as the patent herbal pill Qi Ju Di Huang Wan. Follow the dosage directions listed on the package.
• To treat Meniere's disease due to deficiency of kidney yang: Symptoms will include dizzy spells when changing body position, feeling cold, and water retention. Make a tea using 5 g of Gui Zhi (cinnamon), 3 g of dried ginger, and 3 g of Gan Cao (licorice). Boil the herbs for five minutes before straining. Drink the tea once or twice a day.
• To treat Meniere's disease due to liver Qi stagnation: Symptoms will include severe dizziness, ringing in the ears, and irritability. Use the patent herbal pill Long Dan Xie Gan Wan to reduce the liver "fire" that is caused by stagnant energy. Follow the dosage directions on the package.

• To treat Meniere's disease due to internal phlegm (stagnated body fluids in the internal system): Symptoms will include dizziness, poor appetite, ringing in the ears, heaviness in the ears and chest, and fatigue. Mix 6 g of Chen Pi (tangerine peel), 12 g of Fa Ban Xia (pinellia rhizome), 10 g of Tian Ma (gastrodia rhizome), 12 g of Guo Teng (stem and thorns of gambir vine), 12 g of Shi Chang Pu (sweetflag rhizome), and 6 g of fresh ginger in a ceramic pot. Add 3 cups of water, bring the mixture to a boil, and simmer for 30 minutes. Strain the liquid and drink 1 cup twice a day.

**Acupuncture:** Treatment will dispel the pathogenic factors listed above, and work on strengthening the internal systems. Sessions two or three times a week are necessary. You can have acupuncture to both relieve and prevent symptoms.

**Acupressure:** The Tai Yang point is found on the temple in the depression between the lateral end of the eyebrow and eyelid. The Feng Chi point is located at the back of the head at the base of the skull 2 inches below the center point. The Nei Guan point is in the center of the wrist on the palm side, about 1 inch below the crease. Beginning with gentle pressure and gradually increasing the force, press and release these points with your thumb about 20 times.

**Diet:** Eat foods that are fresh and fragrant such as celery with leaves, orange squash, pineapple, peas, and Chinese chives. Avoid fatty and greasy food.

## NATUROPATHY

**Diet:** Treatment attempts to decrease pressure of fluid in the inner ear. This is done by restricting your daily intake of sodium to 6 g or less. This is sometimes done in combination with taking a diuretic (water pill). It is important not to decrease salt intake too much, as sodium is an essential mineral. Do not add salt to your food and inspect all food labels to see how much salt the contents contain. Avoid salty snacks such as potato chips, pretzels, salted nuts, and processed and convenience foods. Remember that bread, breakfast cereals, and tinned vegetables can also contain a lot of salt.

**Supplements:** Magnesium supplements, taken at 1,000 mg a day, may relieve the tinnitus associated with Meniere's disease and protect the ears from resulting damage. The B vitamins may be beneficial to those with hearing loss. A high-potency complete B-complex vitamin is recommended. Alternatively, take 500 mg of vitamin B1, 250 mg of B6, and 500 mcg of B12. Vitamin C has been shown to relieve Meniere's disease symptoms in some patients. Take 1,000 mg three times a day. Make sure you take a formula that contains at least 250 mg of bioflavonoids.

**Herbs:** Studies have shown ginkgo biloba extract to be useful in treating Meniere's disease; take 80–120 mg a day. Fenugreek tea (fenugreek steeped in cold water) stops cricket noises and ringing in the ears. Chamomile tea promotes relaxation and may help the patient to sleep.

**TIP:** ADDITIONAL THERAPY
Chiropractors, osteopaths, or naturopaths may adjust the head, jaw, and neck to relieve movement restrictions that could affect the inner ear. Craniosacral therapists may gently move the bones of the skull to relieve pressure on the head.

## HOMEOPATHY

In treating Meniere's disease, homeopathic practitioners will focus on resolving the chronic condition with a deep-acting remedy to steer the patient towards improvement and recovery. When treatment is successful, acute episodes of dizziness, loss of balance, and/or vomiting should become less frequent, less severe, and eventually subside altogether. Your practitioner can also provide support on an acute level to decrease the intensity of attacks when they happen. The suggestions below give an idea of some of the acute remedies available.

**Tabacum:** If you experience severe vertigo on opening the eyes, and feel very sweaty and clammy, try Tabacum. Symptoms include severe nausea with a feeling of pressure, like a tight band around the head, and lots of saliva secreted into the mouth before vomiting. Motion of any kind makes symptoms much worse, while there is a brief feeling of relief after vomiting.

**Cocculus:** This remedy can provide relief if symptoms of dizziness and vomiting are made much more intense by lifting the head. Nausea is accompanied by sensations of anxiety and palpitations, which tend to be worse in the mornings. Signature symptoms include feeling prostrated and weak when ill and also loss of hearing. Sleep makes the symptoms worse, while sitting still helps to some degree.

**Nux vomica:** Use this remedy if you feel hung over during an acute episode of nausea and dizziness, which may have been triggered by too much coffee, alcohol, cigarettes, or loss of sleep due to stress. Feeling hemmed in or being in a crowded place aggravates symptoms, as does exposure to very bright lights. Symptoms tend to be worse first thing in the morning and progressively improve as the day goes on.

## HERBALISM

 **Dandelion:** One approach to managing Meniere's disease is to decrease the amount of fluid present in the inner ear by lowering the amount of fluid within the body by taking diuretics. Diuretics can prevent attacks, but do not treat an active attack. Dandelion is a bitter, cooling plant that acts as a gentle diuretic. The whole plant can be taken, but the leaves have the strongest diuretic action. Dandelion also has laxative effects and encourages the liver to remove toxins. Boil 1 tsp of root or infuse 2 tsp of leaves in a cup of water and drink twice a day. Dandelion can also be taken in tincture form at 30 drops twice a day.

**Burdock:** This is a strong diuretic, encouraging the release of excess fluid from the body, as well as being an anti-inflammatory, a mild laxative, and a lymph and blood circulatory stimulant. Due to its circulatory and diuretic properties, it is excellent at removing toxins from the body. It is currently being studied as another possible approach to treating Meniere's disease. Boil 1 tbsp of root or seeds in cup of water, or take 30 drops of tincture, and drink twice a day.

**Licorice:** This herb demonstrates potent anti-inflammatory effects by encouraging the breakdown of endogenous cortisol (our own natural steroid). Licorice is high in flavonoids, which are also a natural anti-inflammatory. Boil 1 tsp of root in a cup of water, or take 60 drops of tincture, and drink twice a day. **Warning:** Licorice may cause high blood pressure. Do not take it if you are diagnosed with hypertension or heart or kidney failure.

# NOSEBLEEDS

## DIAGNOSIS

Nosebleeds are a very common condition, and can occur at any age. They can be worrying, especially for children, but often look worse than they are. Causes include a direct blow, bump, or other injury to the area; an infection of the mucus membrane that lines the nose, such as sinusitis; or the drying out of the nose due to cold weather. Nosebleeds tend to be more frequent during the winter months because of the dry air produced by central heating. When the membranes inside the nose dry out they bleed more easily. Other triggers include upper respiratory tract infections such as colds, flu, or coughs, allergic rhinitis or hay fever, abscesses, and nasal polyps. If you have a cold or are congested and blow your nose too hard, the delicate lining to the nose can easily become damaged. If the nosebleed follows a blow to the head or has not stopped after half an hour, always seek medical advice. Frequent nosebleeds can be a symptom of anemia.

## TO STOP A NOSEBLEED

- Sit and lean forward to prevent blood going down your throat
- Using your fingertips, pinch the soft part of your nose just above the nostrils and breathe through your mouth
- Hold this position for 5–15 minutes until the bleeding stops
- If bleeding does not stop, go to your nearest emergency room

## TREATMENT GOAL

To stop the nosebleed, determine the cause, and treat any underlying condition.

## CONVENTIONAL MEDICINE

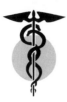

Non-drug-based treatment is usually successful in treating nosebleeds. However, in more serious cases the source of the bleeding is from the lungs, esophagus, or tracheal/larynx area. The doctor can determine the source by examining the patient. If the patient has had many episodes or has unstable vital signs such as low blood pressure, the doctor may carry out tests to determine if the red cells and clotting cells are adequate.

**Stop the bleeding:** Leaning forward and breathing through the mouth, pinch the lower part of the nose for 10–15 minutes, or stay the blood with a cotton ball or tissue. Apply an ice pack to the bridge of the nose to try to constrict the blood vessels and stop the bleeding.

**Pharmaceuticals:** If these treatments fail, the doctor will apply a lidocaine and epinephrine cotton swab to the nostril, or a lidocaine and Afrin™ plug. This helps to constrict the blood vessels and stop the bleeding. Failing this, cocaine 4% is applied to a nasal tampon and inserted in the nostril by a physician. Cauterizing, or sealing the blood vessels, with silver nitrate is also an option.

**Nasal packing:** If the above options fail, gauze is layered into the nostril from the front nasal cavity to the back of the nose, or anterior chamber. This is done under local anesthetic, as pressure must be applied to pack the gauze. A catheter balloon or a nasal sponge can also be packed into the back of the nose.

**To treat chronic nosebleeds:** A procedure can be carried out to cauterize the vessels, a simple procedure that involves sealing them using heat.

**Warning:** Caution should be taken to prevent high blood loss during a nosebleed as this is life threatening. Also, blood loss can be so rapid as to cause cardiac instability.

## TRADITIONAL CHINESE MEDICINE

If nosebleeds do not stop by using the self-help methods recommended here, go to the hospital immediately. Some women experience nosebleeds during menstruation. If this is the case see the entry for menstrual disorder (p. 799).

**Herbs:** The following herbs are available from Chinese herbalists or online.

• To treat all kinds of nosebleeds: Place 10 g of Bei Mao Gen (wooly grass rhizome) and 5 g of Jin Yin Hua (honeysuckle flower) in a teapot and add boiling water. Let the herbs steep for five minutes before drinking.

• To treat chronic nosebleeds: Make a decoction using 12 g Han Lian Cao (eclipta), 15 g of Xiun Shen (ningpo figwort root), 15 g of Zhi Mu (anemarrhena rhizome), 12 g of Di Gu Pi (cortex of wolfberry root), 12 g of Dan Pi (cortex of tree peony root), and 12 g of Mai Men Dong (ophiopogon tuber). Place these herbs in a ceramic or glass pot and add 3–4 cups of water. Bring the mixture to the boil, simmer for 30 minutes, and strain. Drink 1 cup two to three times a day. If you have loose bowel movements or diarrhea, do not use this decoction.

**Acupuncture:** An experienced acupuncturist will diagnose the condition. Nosebleeds are usually due to severe heat in the lung meridian, stomach heat, and liver stagnation. Spleen or kidney deficiency is also found in some cases. Treatment is dependent upon the diagnosis, but will aim to stop the nosebleed and prevent them from recurring.

**Acupressure:** Apply an ice bag to the Yin Tang point, located in the depression midway between the eyebrows. You can also press the Yin Tang point with your index finger very gently while in a sitting position with your head tilted back.

**Diet:** Eat foods that are cooling such as purslane, mung beans, lotus, lettuce, mango, aubergine, spinach, pears, and cucumber. Avoid foods that assist heat such as mutton, chicken, black pepper, chives, clove, fennel, ginger, red pepper, and sword bean.

## NATUROPATHY

**Diet:** Eat two to three servings of green leafy vegetables a day. These have many of the nutrients that help your blood to clot.

**Supplements:** Vitamin C deficiency is associated with nosebleeds. Adults should take 2,000 mg with 500–1,000 mg of bioflavonoids; children should take 250–500 mg with 100–200 mg of bioflavonoids. Bleeding problems can occur because of a vitamin K deficiency. Take 15 mcg of vitamin K a day to help the blood to clot. Apply vitamin E, squeezed from a gel capsule, to the inside of the nose to lubricate dry airways. Vitamin E may increase the risk of bleeding in some patients and you should not take to more than 200 IU a day. Zinc is a natural wound healer and low levels can improve healing; take 15–30 mg a day.

**Herbs:** Agrimony, yarrow, and witch hazel are astringent herbs that can be used topically to decrease or eliminate bleeding. Bilberry decreases the fragility of small blood vessels. Take 120–240 mg of an extract standardized to contain 25% anthocyanosides, the herb's active ingredient, twice a day. Nettle tea contains vitamins A and C, both of which work to strengthen the mucous membrane in the nose. The tea also provides an easily absorbed form of iron. It has a strong "planty" taste, so you can add it to orange or apple juice to encourage children to drink it. Adults should drink 2–3 cups of tea a day. Do not use ginkgo biloba if you are experiencing nosebleeds as it can increase the risk of bleeding.

**TIP:** KEEP YOUR NOSE LUBRICATED

Use a humidifier in the dry, winter months, or year round if you live in a dry climate (especially at night time while you are sleeping). Using a saline (saltwater) spray for your nose three to four times a day also prevents nosebleeds by keeping the mucous membranes in your nose from drying out.

## HOMEOPATHY

Any of the following suggestions can be helpful in stopping a mild nosebleed. Persistent, regular nosebleeds are best treated by a homeopathic practitioner, who will prescribe to treat the underlying problem.

**Arnica:** Use this remedy if a nosebleed has been triggered by a minor accident. It will relieve the physical trauma, and encourage the body to recover from the psychological shock of an accident.

**Ipecac:** If nosebleeds tend to gush bright red blood, and the bleeding is accompanied by nausea and cold sweats, use Ipecac. There is also a profound queasiness made unbearably intense by movement of any kind.

**Phosphorus:** This remedy is especially helpful in stopping nosebleeds that result from blowing the nose repeatedly and violently during a cold. Characteristic symptoms also include noticeable anxiety and a need for reassurance when bleeding.

**Carbo veg:** This as a potential candidate for nosebleeds that result in steady, oozing blood loss (unlike the gushing blood loss that calls for Ipecac). Symptoms include a marked sensation of faintness and dizziness during a nosebleed. Burning sensations are common with a noticeable craving for contact with cool, fresh air, or a strong desire to be fanned if indoors.

Chronic bleeding typically reflects a lack of blood vessel strength and nasal mucosa irritation. The goal of treatment is to improve integrity of the blood vessels and to reduce inflammation and irritation in the nasal passages.

**Cinnamon:** This herb can be used to stop bleeding, whether applied locally or taken internally. It also relieves pain and tonifies tissue. Place 1–2 drops of tincture on a cotton swab and place against the bleeding area within the nose, or drink a tea made from 1 tsp of bark steeped for 30 minutes in 1 cup of hot water.

**Calendula:** Antiseptic, anti-inflammatory, and demulcent, calendula is ideal for healing traumatized tissue, especially wounds and skin conditions that are slow to heal. Infuse 2 tbsp of calendula flowers in 1 cup of hot water. Apply it directly to the nasal tissue until bleeding resolves.

**Canada fleabane:** This herb has astringent and hemostatic properties. To stop bleeding, infuse 2 tsp of herb in 1 cup of hot water. Dip a cotton swab into the solution and apply it to the affected site.

**Cranesbill:** Cranesbill can be used to treat an acute nosebleed, or to tonify tissues irritated by chronic mucus proliferation. Combine with a demulcent herb (such as marshmallow, corn silk, or oat) to balance its vigorous astringent effect. Take 2 ml of tincture in water twice a day.

**Grape seed:** Studies on grape seed extract have shown its ability to increase blood vessel integrity and to prevent damage by toxins and chemical and environmental irritants. Take 300 mg daily for three weeks, then decrease the dosage to 75 mg a day to prevent future nosebleeds.

**Blueberries, bilberry, and huckleberries:** These all contain high levels of antioxidant flavanoids and phenolic acids, which promote and ensure vessel strength. Eat one cup of the mixed berries a day.

# SINUSITIS

## DIAGNOSIS

Sinusitis is a condition that can suddenly flare up (known as acute sinusitis) or recur for months or even years (chronic sinusitis). Acute sinusitis is much more common than chronic, but both types can be very painful. The sinuses, small air-filled cavities located at the front of the skull in the cheeks and forehead, and between the eyes and nose, are lined with a membrane that is lubricated with mucus. Infection results when the tube that runs from the nose to the sinus becomes blocked and the lining of the sinuses becomes inflamed. Infection can also spread to the sinuses in the cheek from an abscess on the root of a tooth. Symptoms include pain in the cheeks, forehead, or the bridge of the nose. There may be partial nasal blockage and a lot of green mucus. Acute sinusitis can be triggered by a number of factors, but is usually the result of a cold or other tract infection. If acute sinusitis fails to clear up completely it may develop into chronic sinusitis, but chronic sinusitis can also develop without any preceding illness. Chronic sinusitis can only really be diagnosed by taking an X-ray or carrying out a CT scan of the sinuses, so it is very difficult for a physician to make a definite diagnosis of chronic sinusitis.

## SYMPTOMS

- Blocked or runny nose
- Bad breath
- Loss of sense of smell
- Swelling and pain around the eyes
- Headaches and the sensation of a build-up of pressure in the head
- Abscess

## TREATMENT GOAL

Sinusitis often resolves itself. Treatment involves preventing fluid from accumulating in the sinuses, and clearing up an existing infection.

## CONVENTIONAL MEDICINE

**Identify allergens:** Environmental and dietary allergens can trigger sinusitis. Dairy products commonly cause mild, chronic respiratory congestion in individuals who are susceptible to sinusitis. Try eliminating dairy from your diet for 21 days and see if there is any improvement.

**Enhance your immune system:** Good nutrition, especially making sure you get enough zinc and vitamin C, can help you avoid infection. Exercising regularly and keeping stress levels low are also vital to a healthy immune system.

**Clear your sinus passages:** Peppermint oil, Afrin™ nasal spray and steam inhalation can all reduce inflammation and encourage mucus to drain from your sinuses.

**Antibiotics:** Amoxicillin, Septra™, erythromycin, or ceftin can be used to treat sinusitis. If there is no improvement after one week, try a more potent antibiotic such as augmentin or levofloxin. Antibiotics should be used for at least 14 days. A four- to eight-week course is sometimes prescribed in chronic cases.

**Warning:** A complication of sinusitis called periorbital cellulitis requires immediate medical attention. Infection can sometimes spread to the brain, and this condition requires immediate hospitalization for treatment. Medical attention is also needed if the infection spreads to the bone.

## TRADITIONAL CHINESE MEDICINE

**Herbs:** There are two types of acute sinusitis that can be treated by herbal remedies. The first is due to wind cold attacking the sinuses, which leads to nasal congestion, sneezing, chills, a runny nose, and headache. The second type is caused by wind with heat, resulting in nasal congestion with yellow mucus, fever, and a dry mouth.

• To treat type one: Combine 12 g of Chuan Xiong (Szechuan lovage root), 10 g of Jing Jie (schizonepeta stem and bud), 6 g of Bo He (field mint), 10 g of Bei Zhi (Chinese angelica root), 6 g of Gan Cao (licorice), 10 g Xin Yi Hua (magnolia flower), and 12 g of Fang Fen (ledebouriella root) in a ceramic pot. Add 3–4 cups of water, bring to the boil, simmer for 30 minutes, and strain the liquid. Drink 1 cup two to three times a day.

• To treat type two: Take the patent herbal pill Yin Qiao Pian. This is available from Chinese pharmacies or online.

**Acupuncture:** Treatment can be effective for any stage of sinusitis, chronic or acute, to quickly relieve nasal congestion.

**Acupressure:** Press the Yin Xiang point, located to the side of and slightly above the border of the nostril, and the Yin Tang point, found in the depression between the eyebrows. This will relieve congestion relief and help open the nasal pathways.

**Diet:** Patients with sinusitis should eat foods that clear away heat such as balsam pear, mung bean sprouts, eggplant, persimmon, loquat, pears, banana, and Chinese chives. To help treat spleen deficiency and lung Qi use foods that can reinforce spleen and lungs, such as coix seeds, Chinese yams, carrots, and duck. Avoid fatty, pungent, or irritating foods and do not drink wine.

## NATUROPATHY

 **Diet:** Avoid dairy, oranges, white sugar, and foods containing white flour because they promote the formation of mucus. Sugar inhibits the immune system from clearing bacteria. Eliminate wheat, soya, fermented foods, and eggs from your diet for a couple of weeks to see if sinus symptoms improve, and then re-introduce them to see if symptoms temporarily worsen. In general, a diet that is rich in vegetables, whole grains, and beans, and low in saturated fat (meat and dairy), sugar, mucus-forming, and allergenic foods will be beneficial to the sinuses. Adding cayenne, garlic, ginger, horseradish, and onions to dishes will aid mucus drainage and ease the pressure in your sinuses. Drink plenty of fluids, six to eight glasses of water a day, particularly during a cold or times of stress. If you are taking antibiotics, consume plenty of non-dairy sources of probiotics such as yogurt, sauerkraut, or kefir.

**Supplements:** Vitamin A and vitamin C can help with a sinus infection. Vitamin A thins the mucus, promotes the growth of healthy mucus-promoting cells, and strengthens the immune system. Take 10,000 IU of vitamin A and 1,000–2,000 mg of vitamin C a day. Take 500 mg of bioflavonoids a day with the vitamin C to improve its benefits.

**Aromatherapy:** Steam inhalations work directly on the sinuses, loosening thick mucus and fighting infection. Pour 5–10 drops of eucalyptus, lavender, peppermint, pine, thyme, or tea tree oil, or use a combination of some or all of these, in a bowl of hot, steaming water. Lean over the bowl with a towel over your head and inhale two to three times to complete one set. Complete three to four sets three times a day. The oils will fight the virus, ease congestion, and stimulate circulation.

**TIP:** PLACE PRESSURE ON YOUR NOSE
Pressure on the sides of your nose can relieve pain. Press the top of your nose on either side between two fingers for a few minutes and release.

**Herbs:** Take ½–1 tsp of a liquid extract of echinacea every three to four hours to stimulate the immune system and fight against bacteria. Echinacea can also be taken in capsule form (500–1,000 mg every three to four hours) or as a standardized extract 3.5% echinacoside (150–300 mg every three to four hours). Goldenseal has broad antibacterial activity and can stimulate the immune system against infections of the mucous membrane. Take ½–1 tsp of a liquid extract, 500–1,000 mg in capsule form, or as a standardized extract (8–12% alkaloid content) every three to four hours. Grapefruit seed extract can be used in a nasal spray four times a day.

**TIP:** USE A HUMIDIFIER

Use a cool-mist humidifier. Moist air can help clear the mucus in your nasal passages. Also try resting a towel or washcloth that has been wrung out with hot water over your face for a few minutes. It can stimulate blood circulation, loosen mucus, and relieve pain.

## HOMEOPATHY

Any of the following homeopathic remedies can help ease the pain of recently developed bouts of sinusitis and encourage the condition to resolve itself speedily. If the condition is chronic, consult a homeopathic practitioner for treatment.

**Kali bich:** Use this remedy if sinus pain and pressure is lodged at the bridge of the nose and accompanied by an unpleasant, offensive smell in the nasal passages. Pain and congestion affect the sinuses above the eyes, and the mucus produced is stringy, sticky, and greenish in color. Discomfort and pressure are aggravated by stooping and bending forward, while applying warmth and firm pressure brings temporary relief.

**Hepar sulph:** If there is a marked sensitivity to cold drafts of air and a tendency to swollen glands, and if a thick yellowish mucus and sharp, splinter-like pains are present, consider this remedy. When it is well indicated there is sneezing and nasal obstruction, with pains and discomfort radiating to the bones of the face. Symptoms tend to be worse at night and are relieved by warm, humid conditions.

**Phosphorus:** This remedy is helpful in treating sinus pains that tend to be one-sided. The yellowish mucus produced is often streaked with blood when the nose is blown. The eyes may be especially affected, feeling heavy and tired, and the eye sockets may also feel very tender. The nasal passages feel generally swollen and congested and the sense of smell is strong.

**Pulsatilla:** If sinusitis develops at the end of a very heavy head cold, if a yellowish-green, thick mucus is produced, and if there is a marked aversion to rooms that are over-heated and stuffy, consider using Pulsatilla. The nose feels uncomfortably stuffed-up at night and flows more freely during the day. Pains and discomfort lead to weepiness and a noticeable need for sympathy and attention.

## HERBALISM

**Neti pot and goldenseal:** Try using a neti pot, a small porcelain pot with a spout, containing a small amount of infused goldenseal herb. Goldenseal is a potent antimicrobial that will tonify the tissues and decrease inflammation and discharge. Infuse ½ tsp of goldenseal herb in 1 cup of hot water for 10 minutes and strain thoroughly. Allow infusion to cool to room temperature and place it in the neti pot. Put the spout in one nostril, tilt the head and allow the liquid to run through your sinuses out through the other nostril. Repeat two to three times a day on each nostril.

**Echinacea and goldenseal:** To treat a bacterial sinus infection, combine echinacea and goldenseal for a powerful antimicrobial effect. Take 500 mg of echinacea and goldenseal root each, or 3 ml of a combined tincture, every four hours. Choose cultivated goldenseal.

**Cleavers:** Cleavers can be used during an acute sinus infection, but is best for treating stagnation most often found in chronic conditions. Take 30–60 drops of tincture per day.

**Osha:** Osha is helpful in treating upper respiratory conditions, especially for increased mucus production and congestion. Boil 1 tsp of root per cup of water for 20 minutes, or take 30 drops of tincture, and drink four times daily.

**Sinus oil blend:** Create a cooling decongestant for the sinuses using antimicrobial and anti-inflammatory oils. Blend 3–5 drops each of wintergreen, peppermint, tea tree, and eucalyptus essential oils into 70 ml of glycerin, 25 ml of water, and 5 ml of alcohol. Place oils into slightly steaming water and breathe in deeply, or rub over the sinuses. Do not take internally.

# SNEEZING

## DIAGNOSIS

A sneeze, which occurs when the nasal lining becomes irritated, is a violent reflex and contraction of the body that propels air out of the lungs and through the nasal passageways at over 400 miles an hour. Because of this, sneezing is a very effective way of transmitting different infections. It is the body's way of clearing out the breathing passages. It is often the most obvious symptom of infections such as the common cold and pneumonia, or of allergies such as allergic rhinitis and hay fever. Some people are troubled by persistent bouts of sneezing and it is helpful to try to locate the cause.

## SYMPTOMS

- Itchy nasal passages
- Repeated sneezing

## TREATMENT GOAL

To isolate the cause of the sneezing and treat the condition accordingly.

## CONVENTIONAL MEDICINE

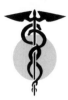

Sneezing is not a medical disease, but a symptom of nasal congestion and a reflexive attempt to clear the nasal passages. Generally it indicates an infection such as a cold (see p. 242), or allergies (p. 232). A foreign object will cause a similar reaction as will chemical irritation of the nasal passages.

**Nasal washes:** Using saline (saltwater) made from 1 tsp of salt to each pint of distilled warm water is an inexpensive and effective treatment. Sniff a small amount of the saline water into the nostrils one at a time and blow your nose. A syringe can also be used, as can a nasal spray.

**Nasal sprays:** Over-the-counter treatments include products such as Afrin™ nasal spray, which should be used for no more than three days to prevent rebound rinorrhea.

**Decongestants:** Pseudoephedrine is an effective decongestant but should not be used by people with hypertension or anxiety.

**Antihistamines:** To treat sneezing due to allergies, take an antihistamine such as Benadryl™ at bedtime and Claritin™ during the day to suppress the sneezing. Quercetin is a natural supplement that also treats sneezing caused by allergies; take 1 g twice a day.

## TRADITIONAL CHINESE MEDICINE

**Herbs:** If sneezing persists, try some tea formulas that are convenient and effective for reducing this condition. If you have an allergic reaction to any herb, stop drinking the tea.
• Winter herbal tea: Place 5 g of Jing Jie (schizonepeta stem and bud), 3 g of Gui Zhi (cinnamon), 3 g of Bo He (field mint), and 3 g of Gan Cao (licorice) in a teapot and add boiling water. Let the herbs steep for six minutes before drinking.
• Summer herbal tea: Mix 5 g of Huo Xiang (agastache), 5 g of Jin Yin Hua (honeysuckle flower), and 3 g of Bo He (field mint). Make the tea as described above.

**Acupuncture:** Treatment can relieve sneezing by regulating body defensive energy. You can seek treatment if you have sneezing that is severe or seasonal.

**Acupressure:** Use the tip of your thumb to press the Hegu points, located on the back of the hands between the thumb and first finger, with strong pressure for one to two minutes. Beginning with gentle pressure and gradually increasing, press the Feng Chi point, located at the back of the head at the base of the skull 2 inches below the center point, with your thumb. Press and release about 20 times.

**Diet:** Avoid spicy food and dishes that contain chilies, black or white pepper, dried ginger, and horseradish.

## NATUROPATHY

Excessive sneezing is most often caused by seasonal allergies. The following treatments focus on relieving allergy symptoms, including sneezing. To treat sneezing that is not caused by an allergy, you must identify and treat the underlying problem. Some possibilities are listed below.

**Diet:** Eat non-mucus-forming foods such as fresh vegetables and fruits, healthy cold-pressed oils, raw seeds, and nuts. Peanuts are legumes and should be avoided along with any other foods to which you might be allergic. Eat lean proteins such as antibiotic- and hormone-free chicken and grass-fed meats, tofu, and seafood. Avoid mucus-forming food, including processed sugars, dairy products, and flours. Foods that decrease immunity, such as hydrogenated oils and trans-fatty acids, should also be avoided. Drink one green freshly squeezed drink a day to raise immunity and flush toxins from the body.

**Supplements:** Take 50 mg of zinc picolinate a day for its ability to enhance the immune system and nourish the skin. Take 4 g of fish oil a day for its ability to reduce skin inflammation. Taking 1,000 mcg of vitamin C a day will help to raise the immune system. (If stools soften cut back 1,000 mg a day.) Quercitin is a natural antihistamine and anti-inflammatory that has been shown to help with seasonal allergies. Take 1,000 mg three times a day. Thymus extract has been shown to subdue the immune system during an acute allergic attack. Take as directed on the label.

**Herbs:** Ginkgo contains several unique substances (ginkgolides) that interfere with a chemical the body produces that plays a key role in triggering allergies, asthma, and inflammation. Take 60–240 mg of standardized extract a day, but no higher dose.

**General recommendations:** Avoiding exposure to an offending allergen is the best way to control sneezing caused by allergies. Remove pets from the home to eliminate animal dander and change furnace filters regularly. Use a high energy particulate air (HEPA) filter in rooms in which you spend the most time. Dust-proof your bedroom by eliminating wall-to-wall carpets, down-filled blankets, feather pillows, and other dust catchers. Substitute window shades for venetian blinds to reduce dust traps; be sure to wash curtains regularly in hot water to kill dust mites. Encase your mattress in an airtight, dust-proof plastic cover, dust your furniture with a damp cloth, and damp-mop floors regularly to pick up dust.

## HOMEOPATHY

Sneezing is generally a symptom of an underlying condition, and treatment involves first determining the cause. The remedies listed below can be used to reduce symptoms, but also see the entries on allergic rhinitis (p. 232) and hay fever (p. 261).

**Nux vomica:** If the nose is oversensitive to strong odors and violent, abortive bouts of sneezing are preceded by an unpleasant crawling sensation in the nostrils, use Nux vomica.

**Arsenicum album:** If sneezing is frequent, but does not bring relief, try using Arsenicum album. The chest may also feel tight and wheezy with a dry, irritating cough, making it difficult to sleep soundly at night. All symptoms tend to be more severe during the night, and/or the early hours of the morning, causing lots of anxiety and physical, mental, and emotional restlessness.

## HERBALISM

The following herbal recommendations will soothe the mucous membranes, support the immune system, and eliminate infectious or chemical irritants.

**Peppermint oil:** Place a few drops of essential oil diluted in a small amount of olive oil onto a cotton swab and place it in the nasal passages. Peppermint oil has a mild cooling and anesthetizing effect on irritated membranes.

**Antiviral tea:** Sneezing due to cold and flu viruses is best addressed by eliminating the virus. Support your immune system with rest, fluids, and a relaxing, antiviral tea. Valerian root and hops leaf help your body relax; osha and desert parsley decrease the viral presence in the body; elder and yarrow have astringent qualities that reduce inflammation and induce a mild sweat to rally the body's natural defenses. Combine equal parts of these herbs and infuse 1 tbsp of the mixture in 1 cup of hot water. Drink 3–4 cups of the infusion a day until the sneezing resolves.

**Anti-allergy blend:** Nettle and bromelain inhibit histamine release; bupleurum and astragalus are traditional Chinese herbs used to energize Qi, the internal vital force, by stimulating the immune system and encouraging the release of anti-inflammatory components; mullein and corn silk are soothing demulcents. Combine equal parts of each herb in tincture form. Take 4–6 ml a day diluted in water to prevent allergic reactions.

# SNORING

## DIAGNOSIS

Approximately one-quarter of adults snore regularly; and one-quarter of adults snore occasionally. It is most common in men, especially those who are older or middle-aged, and overweight. When we sleep, the throat muscles relax and the throat gets narrower as we breathe in. If the throat is narrowed to a slit, the airflow is disturbed and creates an audible vibration. If the throat becomes so narrow that it is partially or completely blocked, the sleeper will fight for breath, which will eventually wake him up. This condition is known as sleep apnea.

If your nasal passages are inflamed, because of a cold or allergy, for example, you may find that you snore more than usual. Drinking alcohol relaxes the throat opening muscles, making snoring worse. Certain types of allergy tablets, such as antihistamines, and sleeping pills can worsen the condition. Obesity, especially if there is excess fat in the neck area, can also trigger snoring as fatty tissue presses on the upper respiratory tract, causing it to narrow. Snoring is also associated with pregnancy and post menopause.

Simple self-help measures include: losing weight, exercising regularly, avoiding alcohol for three hours before going to bed, giving up smoking, and avoiding sleeping pills, sedatives, and antihistamines before going to bed. Sometimes changing your sleeping position, from your back to your side, can decrease snoring.

## SYMPTOMS

- Snoring
- Breaks in breathing during the night
- Sleepiness during the day

## TREATMENT GOAL

Snoring is rarely a life-threatening condition, but nevertheless sleep specialists take it seriously, and will usually carry out an examination to try to establish what is causing it. There are no medicines to treat this condition, and it seldom goes away on its own. It is important to identify what is causing the snoring and treat accordingly.

## CONVENTIONAL MEDICINE

Treating snoring depends on whether there is a partially or completely obstructed airway (known as sleep apnea). Diagnosis involves sleep studies where a patient's sleep is observed and episodes of obstruction are recorded.

**To treat partially obstructed airways:** Non-obstructive snoring is a nuisance, but does not have long-term effects. A respiratory infection or allergies can cause inflammation of the nasal passages and airways, triggering snoring. Try eliminating dairy and gluten, two of the most common food allergens, from your diet, but seek nutritional advice to ensure you do not develop dietary deficiencies. Taking herbs that reduce inflammation in the nasal passages, such as peppermint oil, may also be useful, as may saline solution washes. If obesity is a factor, begin a weight-reduction program. Avoid muscle relaxants and sedatives, including alcohol, as these relax the palate. Oral devices, that prop the palate open, lessening obstruction, are available and often helpful. Surgical procedures to eliminate snoring also sometimes indicated. These must be done through an ear, nose, and throat (ENT) specialist.

**To treat sleep apnea:** As above, treatment involves weight reduction where applicable and avoiding sedatives. The mainstay of treatment in this case, however, is a device that provides continuous positive airway pressure (CPAP). This is worn at night to prevent airways from becoming obstructed. If snoring is associated with sleep apnea, treatment should be sought immediately. Studies have shown that untreated sleep apnea can result in pulmonary and systemic hypertension and neurocognitive problems.

## TRADITIONAL CHINESE MEDICINE

To use traditional Chinese medicine to treat cases of snoring, it is best to consult a practitioner. The primary cause of snoring is the focus for prescribing medicinal formulas.

**Acupuncture:** Treatment can be used to address the underlying problem causing the snoring. Targeting the local points around nasal passages and throat is very beneficial. Treatment once a week is normal, but the frequency depends on an individual's condition. You may experience relief immediately, but regular treatments are needed to achieve long-term results.

**Acupressure:** The Yin Tang point is located in the depression midway between the eyebrows. The Ying Xiang point is just to the side of, and slightly above, the lower border of the nostril. The Yang Bai point is on the forehead, directly above the pupil, about 1 inch above the eyebrow. The Nei Guan point is in the center of the wrist on the palm side, about

2 inches below the crease. Use the tip of your finger or thumb to press these points with gentle to medium pressure for one minute and release. Repeat a couple of times.

**Diet:** Eat foods that disperse and remove dampness. These include mung beans, lotus root, wax gourd, red beans, banana, grapefruit, mustard greens, water spinach, towel gourd (found in Chinese groceries), and honey.

## NATUROPATHY

There are various lifestyle changes and natural remedies that can help you stop snoring, particularly if it is a result of obesity or allergies. To treat snoring that results from other causes, you may have to go to a sleep clinic and be evaluated.

**Diet:** Stick to a healthy weight-loss program that will help you lose 10% of your body weight. Overweight people tend have bulky neck tissue, which can lead to snoring. Losing just modest amount of weight—even just 10% of your body weight—can make a difference. Avoid alcohol and other sedatives, such as sleeping pills. Anything that causes sedation can also cause snoring because it tends to suppress your breathing drive.

> **TIP: CHANGE YOUR SLEEPING POSITION**
> Sleep on your side, rather than your back. You may also want to try raising the head of your bed 4 inches so you are sleeping in an elevated position. To do this, place blocks or wedges under the head of the mattress.

## HOMEOPATHY

The advice given below can ease snoring that has developed as a result of congestion of the nasal passages due to an acute infection such as a cold. Established and frequent problems with snoring will require more professional medical attention, especially if snoring is combined with sleep apnea (a condition that is closely related to snoring and causes you to hold your breath during sleep). Those who suffer from sleep apnea are potentially more vulnerable to health problems such as strokes.

**Calc carb:** This is a potential remedy if colds and ear infections frequently occur during the fall and winter months, leading to lingering catarrh and swollen glands, which can cause snoring. Being overweight may also make snoring more likely.

**Pulsatilla:** Use this remedy in the established or final phase of a heavy cold, when you are likely to breathe through the mouth at night because nasal passages become severely stuffed up when lying down. As a result, the mouth and tongue feel extremely dry and coated on waking, and there may be a tendency to wake during the night to take a sip of water to ease the unpleasant, dry sensation in the mouth.

**TIP:** MAINTAIN A HEALTHY DIET

If snoring has developed following a cold, avoid sweets or dairy products since these may encourage and prolong problems with mucus congestion. Also consider using a high-potency garlic supplement, which encourages the breakdown of mucous deposits, and appears to have therapeutic properties and act as an antibacterial and antiviral agent.

## HERBALISM

**Rhodiola:** Rhodiola may help to increase the ability to exercise, addressing snoring that may be due to obesity. It improves mild mood depression and increases vitality. Studies have demonstrated rhodiola's capacity to improve exercise performance by increasing the availability of oxygen to the muscles, heart, and brain. It is best to take a standardized extract of roseroot to guarantee a consistent level of active compounds. Begin taking 50 mg twice daily. Increase your intake up to 250 mg per day if necessary.

**Ashwagandha root:** This herb is thought to convey vitality and strength. Many studies of its adaptogenic constituents demonstrate an improvement in endurance and exercise performance. The effects are greatest in people who are debilitated and exhausted. Make a decoction by boiling 1 tbsp of root for 20 minutes, or take 2 ml of tincture, and drink three times a day in combination with an exercise plan. Do not take ashwagandha root during pregnancy.

**Cayenne:** A member of the nightshade or solanaceae family, cayenne is used as an antiseptic, neural, and circulatory stimulant, and an anti-inflammatory. This pungent herb is indicated for individuals who are sluggish and cold with circulatory stagnation. Studies show it is the long-term ingestion of capsaicin, the active constituent of cayenne, that is most effective at decreasing inflammation and reducing mucus production due to allergies. Take 1–5 drops of tincture in water twice daily. Do not use this herb if you have digestive ulcers or nightshade allergies.

# SORE THROAT

## DIAGNOSIS

A sore throat, also known as pharyngitis or tonsillitis, occurs when the pharynx or tonsils become inflamed. Sore throats are common all year round, not just during the winter months, and generally last for around two to three days. The infection is passed on through airborne droplets, which are breathed in, or by physical contact, particularly with hands, with a person carrying the infection. Sore throats can be caused by both a virus or a bacteria. Among the bacteria that cause sore throats, the streptococcus group A is the most common. With this type of sore throat the patient has swollen, coated tonsils, runs a temperature, has sour breath, and may feel quite ill (see Strep Throat, p. 304). If the cause is bacterial the condition can be treated with antibiotics. A sore throat can also be a side effect of other conditions, such as flu, glandular fever, and earache, and often clears up as soon as the underlying illness resolves. Usually a sore throat causes no trouble, but the following complications may arise: a secondary infection in the middle ear or sinuses, occasionally a throat abscess, and in very rare cases diseases such as rheumatic fever or kidney disease.

**DANGER**: Always call your doctor if you have any type of throat discomfort that lasts for more than two weeks.

## SYMPTOMS

- Fever
- Bad breath
- Generally feeling unwell
- White spots on the tonsils
- Painful throat
- Difficulty swallowing
- Swollen tonsils
- Pain may spread to the ears
- The throat is red, and may be coated
- Possibly a high temperature
- Swollen lymph nodes

## TREATMENT GOAL

To establish the cause of the sore throat, whether it is viral or bacterial, and bring relief.

## CONVENTIONAL MEDICINE

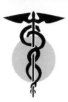

Treating a sore throat depends on an accurate diagnosis. It can be caused by a viral or bacterial infection, by a chemical inflammation, or as a side effect of medications, and is known as pharyngitis in conventional medicine. The remedies below aim to alleviate pain, stop the infection, and prevent the secondary complications associated with bacterial infections.

**To treat viral infections:** Acetaminophen (Tylenol®), or ibuprofen (Motrin®) may be used as directed to alleviate pain. Saltwater gargles (1 tsp of salt mixed in 2 cups of distilled water) may also be helpful. Eating cool fruit that feels good to the throat for a couple of days may be more comfortable. Some plants, such as larch taken at 1 g twice a day in powder form, may boost the immune system and decrease the length of the viral infection.

**To treat bacterial infections:** Streptococcus A (see Strep Throat, p. 304) is the most common bacterial infection and is primarily treated with antibiotics. A course of antibiotics can be started before results of throat cultures are received. The use of a five-minute, in-office "rapid-strep" test is now common practice. If a patient has a history of rheumatic heart disease, treatment is started immediately even before the doctors' evaluation. Penicillin and its derivatives are prescribed to treat strep throat. Erythromycin is used if a patient is allergic to penicillin. Some strains of the bacteria have become resistant to penicillin and erythromycin. If no improvement occurs after 48 hours, or if the culture indicates a resistance, an alternative such as clarithromycin (Biaxin®) is used.

**Other causes:** More rarely, yeast infections, herpes, diphtheria, gonococcus, syphilis, and chlamydia, as well as tuberculosis, can cause a sore throat. Treatment is specific to the organism causing the infection.

## TRADITIONAL CHINESE MEDICINE

**Herbs:**
• To treat an acute sore throat: In the acute stage, chills, fever, and a cough often accompanies a sore throat. To treat this stage of a sore throat, take the patent herbal pill Yin Qiao Jie Du Pian or make the following herbal tea. Combine 10 g of Jin Yin Hua (honeysuckle flower), 10 g of Ye Ju Hua (wild chrysanthemum flower), 8 g of Shen Gan Cao (raw licorice), 10 g of Ge Geng (kudzu root), and 8 g of Huang Qin (baical skullcap root) with 3 cups of water. Bring the mixture to the boil, simmer for 30 minutes, and strain the liquid. Drink 1 cup twice a day.

• To treat a chronic condition: If you develop a sore throat regularly, which is usually due to yin deficiency, make the following herbal tea: Place Mai Men Dong (ophiopogon tuber), 3 g of Gan Cao (licorice), 6 g of Da Zhao (Chinese jujube), and 3 g Bo He (field mint) in a teapot. Add boiling water and let the herbs steep for five to six minutes. Drink the tea throughout the day. This tea is safe for long-term use.

**Acupuncture:** Treatment can clear the pathogenic factors and nourish body yin and the throat. You may have treatment regularly if you suffer from chronic sore throats.

**Acupressure:** The Shao Shang point is on the corner of the thumb, a ½ inch from the outside of the fingernail. The Chi Ze point is found on the inside bend of the arm, just off center. The Hegu points are located on the back of the hands between the thumb and first finger. The Qu Chi point is about 3 inches from the nostrils in the depression just below the cheekbone. Press these points with medium pressure for one minute at a time.

**Diet:** For acute sore throats eat foods that are light and mild in flavor, such as persimmons, olives, figs, turnips, peppermint, and honeysuckle. For chronic sore throats, pears and water chestnut are helpful. Avoid pungent and spicy foods.

## NATUROPATHY

**Diet:** Allicin, the compound responsible for garlic's pungent odor, has antibiotic and antifungal properties that can heal many types of sore throat. Take two or more cloves, crushed or whole, at the first sign of a sore throat and continue eating two cloves a day until your symptoms clear up. An ice cold fruit juice popsicle can be an effective temporary anesthetic for a sore throat. Reduce your intake of dairy and simple carbohydrates, such as fruit, and stick to a diet that consists primarily of vegetables and whole grains. Drink fluids through the day consisting of water, teas, and soups. Chicken soup and miso soup are great for this condition.

**Supplements:** Vitamin C supports the immune system. Take 500–1,000 mg every four hours, until symptoms subside. Bioflavonoids work synergistically with vitamin C and have immune-enhancing properties of their own. Take 1,000 mg in two 500 mg doses a day. Take 25 mg of zinc a day in lozenges for one week. Zinc supports the immune system and may have some antiviral properties.

**Herbs:** Rub lavender, eucalyptus, thyme, or tea tree essential oil gently on the chest and around the front side of the neck. Only use the oils externally, and always dilute them in a carrier oil such as olive, apricot, or almond oil. This serves as an anti-infective and helps to loosen and shift sticky mucus. Elderflower and elderberry are effective natural antivirals and have been effectively used to treat sore throat symptoms. Adults can take 10 ml and children 5 ml three times daily. Take a combination of echinacea and goldenseal tincture, using 2–4 ml of each, four times a day for their immune-enhancing and antiviral properties. Lomatium dissectum also has strong antiviral effects; take 500 mg in capsule form or 2–4 ml of tincture four times a day.

## HOMEOPATHY

The homeopathic remedies suggested below can be helpful in shortening the duration, easing the pain, and speeding up recovery from a recently developed sore throat. However, recurrent, severe sore throats are best treated by a homeopathic practitioner who will aim to prescribe in order to strengthen the body's defenses against infection.

**Aconite:** Consider this remedy if a sore throat develops dramatically and abruptly after exposure to dry, cold winds. Aconite can ease a sore throat that emerges early in the morning when you wake feeling fearful, restless, and agitated. The throat feels dry, tingly, and/or numb with a sensation of acute pain and constriction when swallowing.

**Belladonna:** Opt for this remedy at the first twinge of a sore throat, especially if it is accompanied by a sense of being feverish with hot, flushed, dry skin. Signature symptoms include a nasty dry sensation in the throat with burning and throbbing pains that make it very difficult to swallow even liquids.

**Lachesis:** Use Lachesis to treat sore throats that are left-sided or worse on the left than the right side. Symptoms are at their most distressing when waking, or when trying to swallow warm liquids. Swallowing cool drinks and food feels temporarily soothing.

**Hepar sulph:** If there is a sharp pain that feels as though a splinter were sticking into the sore throat (which is often worse on the right), try Hepar sulph. Glands may also be swollen and painful, while any mucus present is likely to be thick and yellowish. Contact with the slightest draft of cold air intensifies pain, distress, and irritability. Warmth feels comforting.

**Apis:** This is a potentially helpful remedy for treating sore throats that result from an allergic reaction. The throat looks bright red, shiny, and swollen and the uvula (the little lump of tissue at the back of the throat) looks inflamed and glossy. There are also likely to be stinging pains in the throat that are sensitive to heat and temporarily soothed by cool things.

**Phosphorus:** Consider this remedy to relieve a sore throat that is combined with hoarseness. Signature symptoms include dryness and constriction of the throat with noticeable swelling of the tonsils and uvula and possible glandular tenderness. All symptoms tend to be more severe, or develop, in the evening. A sore throat may also be brought on by stress and over-excitement, and the anxiety that accompanies most symptoms is eased by reassurance, care, and attention.

**TIP:** SAGE, CIDER VINEGAR, AND HONEY GARGLE
Infuse sage by adding 1 tsp of the dried herb to a large cup of hot water. Let it steep for one minute before straining the liquid and adding 1 tsp each of cider vinegar and honey. Let the mixture cool to a comfortable temperature and gargle in the morning and evening.

## HERBALISM

**Yerba mansa:** Used to treat pale and irritated tissues, yerba mansa is a warming, astringent, and slightly pungent pain-relieving herb. Boil 1 tsp of root in 1 cup of water, or take 20–40 drops of tincture, and drink three to four times per day.

**Sage:** Taken internally, this herb is pungent and tonifying, and has a strong antimicrobial effect. It reduces throat irritation upon contact, but should not be used long-term due to its thujone content. Infuse 1 tsp of the herb in 1 cup of water, or take 20–30 drops of tincture, and drink three to four times daily for five to seven days. Gargle and swallow. Do not use during pregnancy.

**Myrrh:** Studies show that myrrh stimulates immune cell activity, encouraging the body to eradicate infection. Gargle with and swallow 30 drops of tincture in water two to four times per day. Do not use during pregnancy. Large doses may cause diarrhea.

**TIP:** SOOTHING GARGLE
Herbal combinations typically have a stronger medicinal effect than one herb alone. This synergistic formula soothes and heals the throat, relieves discomfort and swelling, and actively treats infection. Combine peppermint, calendula, barberry, burdock, and licorice in equal parts. Use 2 tsp of herbs per cup of water to make a tea, or use 5 ml at a time of tincture diluted in water. Gargle for 30 seconds before swallowing, four to six times a day.

# STREP THROAT

## DIAGNOSIS

This is a common bacterial infection of the throat caused by group A streptococcus, which gives the condition its common name. It can be quite serious if not treated, and can lead to rheumatic fever, kidney disorders, ear infections, and sinusitis. Strep throat can spread quickly and easily, and is especially prolific during late winter and early spring. A strep infection also has the potential to spread within the body, resulting in pockets of pus in the tonsils and abcesses in the soft tissue around the throat.

**DANGER**: Call your doctor immediately if you have a sore throat that prevents you from drinking or is accompanied by pain when swallowing, labored breathing, excessive drooling, or a temperature above 100°F.

## SYMPTOMS

- Throat pain
- Fever
- Coating on the tonsils and tongue
- Pain on swallowing
- Loss of appetite
- Hoarseness and coughing
- Runny nose
- Swollen glands
- Headache
- Generally feeling unwell
- Children can also experience nausea, vomiting, and abdominal pain

## TREATMENT GOAL

To identify if strep is the causitive organism of the sore throat and treat with antibiotics; also to alleviate painful symptoms associated with the infection.

## CONVENTIONAL MEDICINE

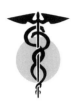

Strep throat is differentiated from other sore throat conditions by the presence of swollen lymph glands around the neck, thick exudate of pus on the tonsils, absence of cough, and a fever of greater than 100°F. When all these symptoms are present, antibiotics may be taken without first taking a bacteria culture. It is important to start antibiotics immediately if you have a history of rheumatic heart disease.

**Antibiotics:** Penicillin V is the first choice for treating strep throat. An intramuscular shot of penicillin G may be prescribed if it is suspected that the full course of antibiotics may not be taken, for more rapid response to symptoms, or if the patient prefers a single-dose treatment. Medications related to penicillin such as amoxicillin are generally used to treat cases of strep throat in children as they taste better. Erythromycin can be used by those who are allergic to penicillin. If there is no improvement after 24–48 hours, the strep bacteria may be resistant to the type of antibiotic and a different one may be prescribed. Cephalosporins and newer macrolides, which are alternative antibiotics, are reserved for treating unresponsive cases.

**Complications:** It is important to treat strep throat with antibiotics as it can lead to complications such as muscle infections, toxic shock syndrome, and rheumatic fever. Other less common complications include serious kidney conditions, sinusitis, mastoiditis, meningitis, infection of the blood stream, and pneumonia.

## TRADITIONAL CHINESE MEDICINE

**Herbs:**
• Patent herbal pills: Yin Qiao Jie Tu Pian and Chuan Xin Lian Pian are patent Chinese medicines available from Chinese pharmacies or groceries. Take both pills three times a day for one week (refer to the dosage as indicated on the package).
• Herbal decoction: Combine 10 g of Jin Yin Hua (honeysuckle flower), 15 g of Ban Lan Gen (isatis root), 10 g of Da Qin Ye (woad leaf), 5 g of Shen Gan Cao (raw licorice), and 10 g of She Gan (belamcanda rhizome) in a ceramic or glass container. Bring to the boil and simmer for 30 minutes. Strain the liquid and drink 1 cup twice a day. If you have a severe case of strep throat, you can take this decoction together with one of the pills mentioned above.

**Acupuncture:** An experienced practitioner should perform acupuncture for strep throat, focusing on some points on the lung meridian in the local throat area.

**Acupressure:** Use the tip of your thumb to press the Hegu point, located on the back of the hand between the thumb and the first finger, with strong pressure for one to two minutes. Beginning with gentle pressure and gradually increasing, use your thumb to press the Feng Chi point, which is located at the back of the head, at the base of the skull, about 2 inches from the center. Press and release about 20 times.

**Diet:** Eat foods that are mild and cooling, such as cucumber, mango, aubergine, spinach, strawberry, pears, and lettuce. Avoid hot, spicy foods.

## NATUROPATHY

**Diet:** Take two or more cloves of garlic, crushed or whole, at the first sign of a sore throat and continue eating two cloves a day until your symptoms clear up. Garlic contains allicin, which has antibiotic and antifungal properties. Your diet should consist primarily of vegetables, whole grains, lots of soups (particularly chicken and miso soup), and water. Dairy products and simple carbohydrates, such as fruit, should be avoided. An ice cold fruit juice popsicle can be an effective temporary anesthetic.

**Supplements:** Take 500–1,000 mg of vitamin C every four hours until symptoms subside to support the immune system. Take 1,000 mg of bioflavonoids in two 500 mg doses a day. Bioflavonoids work synergistically with vitamin C and have immune-enhancing properties. Zinc also supports the immune system and may have some antiviral properties. Take 25 mg in lozenges every day for one week.

**Herbs:** Dilute lavender, eucalyptus, thyme, or tea tree essential oil in olive, apricot, or almond oil and rub it gently on the chest and the front of the neck. These should only be used topically. These oils are anti-infective and will help to loosen and shift sticky mucus.

## HOMEOPATHY

If you have a severe sore throat (especially if there is marked difficulty in opening the mouth or swallowing) your doctor will want to take a swab in order to establish whether a streptococcal infection is present. If this is the case, conventional treatment will be prescribed to treat the infection. However, homeopathic treatment can be used in a complementary fashion to ease pain, general distress, and feelings of being unwell. Once the immediate problem has been dealt with, consider more long-term homeopathic treatment from an experienced practitioner in order to discourage recurrence. (Also see Sore Throat, p. 299.)

**Gelsemium:** If there is an overwhelming feeling of exhaustion and weariness when feeling ill, Gelsemium may help. Symptoms that respond well to this remedy characteristically come on slowly and progressively over a few days, rather than appearing abruptly. There may be a very nasty taste in the mouth, with severe pain in the throat and ears that is made worse when swallowing. As a result, the patient may be unwilling to drink.

**Mercurius:** When a severe sore throat is combined with swollen, tender glands, increased amounts of saliva, and an unpleasant sweetish or metallic taste in the mouth, use Mercurius.

**Phytolacca:** Try this remedy if there is a characteristic pain at the root of the tongue, which becomes more severe when sticking the tongue out when being examined.

---

**TIP:** DRINK FLUIDS
Keep your fluid intake up to encourage the body to flush out infection and to keep the body temperature down. Avoid acidic, citrus drinks that can make glandular tenderness worse, especially if the salivary glands are affected.

---

## HERBALISM

The following herbs may be used in addition to antibiotics to relieve the symptoms of strep throat and treat infection.

**Meadowsweet:** Water and alcohol extracts of all parts of this plant have demonstrated antimicrobial activity against streptococcus. Meadowsweet also exhibits anti-inflammatory, anticoagulant, astringent, and diuretic properties. Take 4 g of the herb or 6 ml of tincture a day. Do not use with anticoagulant medications.

**Ginger:** This pungent, hot herb is used to treat cold conditions. Normally regarded as a soothing digestive remedy, it may also have antimicrobial activity against streptococcus. Take 500 mg of fresh or dried root, or 3 ml of tincture, three times a day.

**Goldenseal root:** This herb may inhibit the streptococcus bacteria, as well as other types of bacteria, fungi, and protozoa. Boil 2 g of dried root per cup of water, or take 3–5 ml of tincture in water, and drink three to four times daily.

# SWIMMER'S EAR

## DIAGNOSIS

Swimmer's ear is the common name for the condition otitis externa. It is an infection of the ear canal caused by bacteria or fungi, and is associated with any pastime that involves repeatedly immersing the ear canal in water, such as swimming. It may also occur if water is trapped in the ear after bathing or showering, particularly if there is a significant amount of ear wax or the climate is very humid. Swimmer's ear is most common during the summer months, as humidity also increases the possibility of infection, but the condition can occur year round. Symptoms include swelling or redness of the skin of the external ear canal, fluid draining into the ear canal, and tender lymph nodes near the ears.

To help prevent this condition, try to keep your ear canal dry. After a swim thoroughly dry your ears with a hair dryer set on a low heat. When swimming, try to limit your time exposed to water and use a cotton wool ball covered with a layer of petroleum jelly to keep water out of your ears.

**DANGER**: Some people can develop a severe form of this condition known as malignant otitis externa that requires immediate hospitalization for treatment with intravenous antibiotics. If you have diabetes or another condition that makes you more susceptible to infections, contact your doctor immediately if you develop symptoms of swimmer's ear.

## SYMPTOMS

- Itchiness in the ear canal
- Redness of the skin in the ear canal
- Discharge from the ear canal that is often yellow or green
- Pain, when touching the ear or moving the jaw while talking or eating
- Hearing is affected

## TREATMENT GOAL

To relieve symptoms and resolve the infection. It is also important to identify the cause of the infection to prevent the condition from recurring. Call your doctor if the symptoms worsen, and fever or any other new symptoms develop, or there is no improvement after two to three days of treatment.

## CONVENTIONAL MEDICINE

Swimmer's ear has many different names, including otomycosis, acute diffuse otitis externa, furunculosis, and eczematious otitis externa.

**Prevention:** Practise good hygiene and use a topical acetic acid (such as white vinegar) or isoprpyl alcohol (rubbing alcohol) if you are prone to swimmer's ear.

**Topical treatment:** Generally, a topical corticosteroid along with acetic acid or some other mild acidifying agent is used. If the condition is more severe, a topical antibiotic is also prescribed. Most commonly, ciprofloxin or neomycin mixed with polymixin sulfate is used.

**Antibiotics:** If there is redness that has spread to the skin or enlarged lymph nodes, an oral course of antibiotics geared to treat staphylococcus is prescribed.

**Irrigation:** In some cases, cleaning and debridement (using irrigation or suction) are necessary to remove debris, pus, and other material from the ear canal so that medication can be applied.

## TRADITIONAL CHINESE MEDICINE

**Herbs:** Place 3 g Jin Yin Hua (honeysuckle flower), 3 g of Ye Ju Hua (wild chrysanthemum flower), and 3 g of Bo He (field mint) in a teapot and add boiling water. Let the tea steep for five to six minutes and drink the tea throughout the day. It may help speed up your recovery time.

**Acupuncture:** Treatment may reduce the pain and shorten the duration of the ear infection. You can have treatment once to three times a week, depending on the severity of the condition.

**Acupressure:** The Yi Feng and Ting Hui acupressure points are recommended for this condition. The Yi Feng point is situated just behind the ear lobe. The Ting Hui point is on the face, just in front of the lower notch of the ear. Use your thumbs to apply gentle pressure to these, and gradually increase the pressure. Press and release about 20 times.

**Diet:** Avoid hot and spicy food, including dried ginger, chilies, hot radishes, and mustard. Eat plenty of fresh fruit and vegetables.

**TIP:** USE SESAME OIL

One traditional remedy to help prevent swimmer's ear is to put 1 drop of sesame oil into the ears before going into the pool.

## NATUROPATHY

**Diet:** Avoid the most common food allergens, including wheat, eggs, dairy foods, corn, citrus fruit, and peanut butter, especially for chronic cases of swimmer's ear. Also avoid simple carbohydrates, including sugar, honey, cookies, candy, ice cream, sodas, chocolate, dried fruits, and fruit juices.

**Supplements:** Zinc gluconate lozenges have both antiviral and immune-stimulating effects. Adults should take 25 mg per day; children should take a lower dosage. For example, a 30 lb child can be given 5 mg of zinc per day while suffering from swimmer's ear. Take 500 mg and 1,000 mg of vitamin C a day in separate doses to stimulate immune function. Reduce the dosage if you notice diarrhea. Vitamin A supports immunity. Give children up to six years old 2,000–5,000 IU of vitamin A a day, usually available in liquid form, to support immunity; adults should take 10,000–25,000 IU a day. Pregnant women should not take more than 10,000 IU of vitamin A a day.

**Herbs:** Mullein oil can be used to treat minor inflammation. To ease the discomfort of swimmer's ear, place 1–3 drops of a mullein preparation in the ear every three hours. Larix enhances immune function and has antimicrobial activity. Dissolve 1–2 tsp in a non-dairy formula or in water for older children or adults. Echinacea and goldenseal also enhance immune function and have antimicrobial properties. Children should take 2 ml four times a day, or as directed on the bottle. Mix St. John's wort oil with garlic oil and place 2 warm drops in the affected ear twice a day to relieve ear pain and kill infection. Do not use this treatment if the eardrum is ruptured.

## HOMEOPATHY

A one-off, mild episode of swimmer's ear may respond well to the homeopathic remedies listed below, which can be given along with conventional treatment if necessary. Remedies can reduce distress and pain, and encourage the healing process to work to its maximum efficiency. Recurrent infections (especially if they are severe in nature) will require treatment from a homeopathic practitioner. A practitioner will prescribe to discourage the infection from developing. (Also see Ear Infection, p. 248, and Glue Ear, p. 256.)

**Belladonna:** Use this remedy at the first sign of inflammation. Although it is often used to bring down high temperatures, it is also effective in easing localized inflammation accompanied by throbbing pains. Symptoms may be restricted to or worse on the right side, with the glands becoming inflamed and swollen in sympathy with affected ear.

**Hepar sulph:** Use this remedy to treat a later stage of infection, where pains in the ears are characteristically sharp and splinter-like. The glands are also likely to be sensitive and swollen. There is a high sensitivity to cold drafts, which make pain and discomfort much more intense and distressing. Signature symptoms also include a marked tendency to be short-tempered and irritable when in pain.

**Pulsatilla:** If there is an established history of mucus production and congestion that affects the ears, nose, and/or chest, this remedy is well indicated. The mucus produced is characteristically thick and yellowish-green in color. The affected ears feel constantly stuffed up, with the sensation being mildly relieved only when traveling in a car. The external ear may also become swollen and inflamed, with a sense of pressure as though something were pushing itself out of the ear.

## HERBALISM

 Most treatment of swimmer's ear is topical. However, only use topical treatments once a ruptured eardrum has been ruled out by your doctor. All of the herbs listed below may be combined to treat swimmer's ear.

**St. John's wort:** Studies show this herb to be effective as an antiviral and antibacterial agent. Its ability to heal wounds is thought to be due to its high flavonoid and procyanidin content. Place 3–5 drops of oil into the affected ear(s). Cover with a warm, moist towel to ease discomfort.

**Calendula:** The flowers of this herb have been shown to be antiviral, anti-inflammatory, antiseptic, and to inhibit the growth of bacteria. Place 3–5 drops of calendula oil into the affected ear to soothe and promote healing of the ear canal.

**Chaparral:** The resins found in chaparral have been found to display antibacterial, anti-inflammatory, and antioxidant properties. Place 1–2 drops of the oil into the affected ear. Do not take this herb internally—it is toxic to the liver.

**Garlic:** Garlic can inhibit the growth of a number of bacteria. The active compound, allicin, has antimicrobial properties. Place 3–4 drops of garlic oil into the affected ear.

# TINNITUS

## DIAGNOSIS

Tinnitus is a condition that causes you to hear noises in your ears, most commonly ringing or buzzing. Sometimes other noises manifest themselves, such as hissing or whistling. Tinnitus can vary in intensity from intermittent to constant noise and it is often linked with hearing loss. It is often caused by exposure to extreme noise, but it can also be triggered by a variety of conditions affecting the ear, including diseases of the inner ear such as age-related hearing loss, or Meniere's disease; an obstruction in the ear canal, such as those caused by a large amount of earwax; a perforated eardrum; and inflammation of the middle ear. Rarely, it can be caused by a benign tumor on the acoustic nerve. Underlying health conditions that can be linked with tinnitus include allergies, heart disease, high blood pressure, and anemia. Sometimes medication, such as aspirin, antibiotics, and sedatives, can trigger the condition.

In some cases, tinnitus disappears without treatment. It can be successfully treated, although there is no cure for tinnitus caused by extreme noise. A hearing specialist will often be able to determine the cause of the tinnitus by examining the ear canal and eardrum and by hearing tests.

## SYMPTOMS

- Buzzing, ringing, hissing, or whistling noises in the ear
- Intensity and loudness of noise can vary
- Noises are constant or intermittent

## TREATMENT GOAL

To identify the cause of the tinnitus and relieve the symptoms where possible.

## CONVENTIONAL MEDICINE

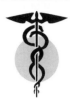

Also known as ringing in the ears, this is a false perception of sound without any acoustic stimulus present. Tinnitus has multiple causes and these must be determined before deciding on a treatment plan. To determine the cause, an audiological evaluation is done. Sometimes brain imaging is carried out and blood tests performed to check for infection and other abnormalities such as tumors on the acoustic nerve.

**Prevention:** Avoid drugs associated with tinnitus, such as non-steroidal anti-inflammatories and asprin. Also make sure you wear ear protection whenever you are likely to be exposed to loud noise to prevent any further hearing impairment.

**Medication:** Several medications have been tried for tinnitus with some success: antiarrhythmic drugs, benzodiazepines, anticonvulsants, and certain antidepressants. The herb ginkgo biloba has also been used.

**Tinnitus retraining programs:** These involve counseling and using broadband noise exposure, a type of wavelength that we are commonly exposed to on a daily basis, to habituate a person to tinnitus.

## TRADITIONAL CHINESE MEDICINE

Traditional Chinese medicine categorizes tinnitus into two common types: the first is due to excess heat in the liver and the second is due to deficiency in the kidney.

**Herbs:** The herbs and patent herbal pills listed below are available from Chinese herbalists.
• To treat excess heat in the liver: The symptoms of this type of tinnitus are ringing in the ear, headaches, flushed face, yellow urine, and constipation. Combine 10 g of Jin Yin Hua (honeysuckle flower), 10 g of Huang Qin (baical skullcap root), 12 g of Zhi Zi (Cape Jasmine fruit), 10 g of Ye Ju Hua (wild chrysanthemum flower), 10 g of Long Dan Cao (Chinese gentian root), 10 g of Xia Ku Cao (common selfheal fruit-spike), and 5 g of Gan Cao (licorice) in a ceramic pot. Add 3 cups of water, bring the mixture to the boil, and simmer for 30 minutes. Strain the liquid into a glass container and drink 1 cup twice a day. You can also purchase Long Dan Xie Gan Wan (patent herb pills) to treat this condition. Take the pills as the package indicates.

• To treat kidney deficiency: Symptoms may include a ringing in the ears that intensifies in the night or during exertion, or dizziness, insomnia, lumbago, and weak knees. To tonify the kidney, add 12 g of Di Huang (Chinese foxglove), 10 g of Shan Zhu Yu (asiatic cornelian cherry fruit), 15 g of Zhi Mu (anemarrhena rhizome), 12 g of Sang Shen Zi (mulberry fruit-spike), 12 g of Ji Shen (jilin root), 15 g of Niu Xi (achyranthes root), and 8 g of Da Zhao (Chinese jujube) to 3 cups of water. Bring to the boil, simmer for 30 minutes, and strain the liquid. Drink 1 cup twice a day. Er Ming Zhu Chi Wan and Zhi Bai Di Huang Wan patent herbal pills may also be helpful.

**Acupressure:** In sitting position, use your index fingers to apply medium pressure to the Er Men, Tin Hui, and Yi Feng points for one minute each twice a day. The Yi Feng point is located just behind the ear lobe. The Er Men point is in front of the notch on the forward edge of the ear. The Ting Hui point is on the face just in front of the ear.

## NATUROPATHY

**Diet:** Eat plenty of foods that contain zinc, as zinc deficiency is associated with tinnitus and certain kinds of hearing loss. Good sources of zinc include spinach (the best), papaya, collards, Brussel sprouts, cucumbers, string beans, endive, cowpeas, prunes, and asparagus. It is difficult to get the recommended daily amount of zinc (60 mg) from diet alone, but make a point of taking more zinc from your food while trying other herbal treatments for tinnitus. You can also take a 60–120 mg zinc supplement a day.

**Supplements:** Magnesium deficiency may cause tinnitus, and magnesium supplements (1,000 mg a day) may relieve tinnitus associated with Meniere's disease and protect the ears from damage. A manganese deficiency may be the cause of some cases of Meniere's disease, so if you have been diagnosed with this condition take 5 mg of manganese a day. The B vitamins have shown positive benefits for those suffering from hearing loss, and taking a high-potency complete B-complex capsule is recommended. Alternatively, take 500 mg of vitamin B1, 250 mg of B6, and 500 mcg of B12. Vitamin C has also been shown to relieve the symptoms in some patients with Meniere's. Take 1,000 mg three times a day. Make sure you take a formula that contains at least 250 mg of bioflavonoids.

**Herbs:** Fenugreek tea (fenugreek steeped in cold water) stops cricket noises and ringing in the ears, while chamomile tea promotes relaxation and may help the patient to sleep. If you suffer from tinnitus, do not take aspirin or aspirin-like herbs, including willow bark, meadowsweet, and wintergreen. High doses of aspirin may cause ringing in the ears. Other herbs, such as cinchona, black haw, and uva ursi, have been linked with tinnitus.

## HOMEOPATHY

As tinnitus tends to be an on-going, chronic problem, it is best managed by consulting a homeopathic practitioner, rather than attempting self-help.

**TIP:** STRESS MANAGEMENT

If you notice that tinnitus increases in intensity when stress levels rise, investigate pro-active ways of stress management. These may include stress counseling, taking up T'ai chi or yoga, or making relaxation techniques a regular part of your daily routine.

## HERBALISM

Tinnitus can be caused by many conditions. The herbs listed below focus on treating tinnitus relating to allergies and decreased circulation.

**Ginkgo biloba:** Research has shown that ginkgo is an effective treatment for tinnitus, especially when the condition is related to poor circulation. It is thought that the active constituents in ginkgo, the ginkgolides, prevent metabolic damage from poor blood flow by increasing small arterial circulation. The ginkgolides also decrease the blood's ability to clot, thereby assisting circulation. Because of this ability, ginkgo should not be used by individuals on blood-thinning medication.

**Dong quai:** One of dong quai's traditional uses is to treat tinnitus by improving circulation. Dong quai is warming and bitter, and displays anti-inflammatory and antiplatelet properties. Boil 3–5 g of root in 1 cup of water, or take 4–6 ml of tincture, and drink once a day. Do not use dong quai during the first trimester of pregnancy or with blood-thinning medications.

**Stinging nettle:** One study of those suffering from tinnitus demonstrated that 33% of people tested had tinnitus related to allergies. Nettle leaf has anti-inflammatory and anti-allergic qualities as its key constituents, which act as antihistamines while significantly decreasing pro-inflammatory chemicals within the body. Take 4 g of dried leaf or 6 ml of tincture a day.

**Butterbur:** Butterbur acts to decrease histamine, one of the main chemicals released by the body in an allergic reaction. To treat tinnitus related to allergies, take 50 mg of an extract certified to be free of pyrrolizidine alkloids twice a day.

# TONSILLITIS

## DIAGNOSIS

The tonsils are situated at the back of the throat and they form part of the body's immune system. They, like the rest of the immune system, contain special cells to trap and kill bacteria and viruses that roam the body. When the main site of infection is within the tonsils they swell, become red and inflamed, and may be coated with white spots. This condition is known as tonsillitis. It manifests with flu-like symptoms, including a sore throat and trouble swallowing. It is an extremely common ailment in children of school age, but can affect anyone. It spreads from person to person by airborne droplets that are breathed in, hand-to-hand contact, or through kissing. Tonsillitis is usually caused by the bacteria streptococcus, but it can also occasionally be caused by a virus. Other triggers include congestion, a cold, flu, laryngitis, or being rundown due to a lack of fresh air, rest, exercise, and a poor diet. If you suffer from recurrent tonsillitis, it is important to start assessing the cause so that it can be resolved. Always seek the advice of your doctor if you have a fever with a sore throat and swollen glands.

## SYMPTOMS

- Sore throat
- Difficulty swallowing
- Red and swollen tonsils
- Swollen glands
- Fever and chills
- The adenoids can also be affected, resulting in snoring
- Poor appetite and lethargy
- Voice loss or changes to the voice
- Cough
- Earache

## TREATMENT GOAL

To treat and relieve symptoms in acute cases, and to determine and remove the cause in chronic cases.

The standard treatment is a course of antibiotics. Tonsillectomy (surgery to remove tonsils) is still used occasionally to treat recurrent and acute tonsillitis, particularly if linked with breathing problems. If three or more attacks per year (documented as due to strep) occur that are sufficiently disabling as to prevent attendance at school or work, a tonsillectomy should be considered.

## CONVENTIONAL MEDICINE

Tonsillitis can be bacterial or viral in origin and should be treated accordingly. (Also see Sore Throat, p. 299, and Strep Throat, p. 304.) A medical emergency exists if there is an abscess surrounding the tonsils. Also if the tonsils remain very enlarged following treatment, referral to an ear, nose, and throat (ENT) specialist is usual.

**To treat viral infections:** Acetaminophen (Tylenol®), or ibuprofen (Motrin®) may be used as directed to alleviate pain. Saltwater gargles (1 tsp of salt mixed in 2 cups of distilled water) may also be helpful. Eating cool foods that feel good to the throat for a couple of days may be more comfortable. Some plants, such as larch taken at 1 g twice a day, may decrease the length of the viral infection.

**To treat bacterial infections:** Penicillin and its derivatives are prescribed to treat tonsillitis. Erythromycin is used if a patient is allergic to penicillin. Some strains of the bacteria have become resistant to penicillin and erythromycin. If there is no improvement after 24–48 hours, the bacteria may be resistant to the antibiotic and an alternative, such as clarythromycin (Biaxin®) or a cephalosporin (Keflex®), is prescribed.

**Recurrent tonsillitis:** This is generally a reason for surgical removal of the tonsils.

## TRADITIONAL CHINESE MEDICINE

Traditional Chinese medicine is effective in treating both acute and chronic tonsillitis. If you have tried antibiotics without success, and before you resort to surgery, try comprehensive traditional Chinese medicine treatment.

**Herbs:** The herbs below are available from Chinese pharmacies, local Chinese medicine clinics, or online.
• To treat acute tonsillitis: The following herbal tea formulas are convenient and effective for easing symptoms. Combine 5 g of Ye Ju Hua (wild chrysanthemum flower), 3 g of Gan Cao (licorice), and 5 g of Jin Yin Hua (honeysuckle flower); or 5 g of Bo He (field mint), 8 g of Ban Lan Geng (isatis root), and 8 g of Jie Geng (balloon flower root); or 5 g of Pu Gong Ying (dried dandelion) and 5 g of Bai Hua She She Cao (heydyotis). Place the raw herbs from one of these combinations in a teapot and add boiling water. Let the tea steep for three to five minutes and drink throughout the day.
• To treat chronic tonsillitis: The following herbal tea formulas are convenient and effective for easing symptoms. Combine 10 g of Pi Pa Ye (loquat leaf), 3 g of Chen Pi

(tangerine peel), 8 g of Wu Mei (mume fruit), and 3 g of Gan Cao (licorice); or 10 g of Xuan Shen (ningpo figwort root), 10 g of Mai Dong (ophiopogon tuber), 10 g Jie Geng (balloon flower root), and 5 g of Gan Cao (licorice). Add 3 cups of water to the herbs from either formula and let them boil for six to 10 minutes. Drink the decoction throughout the day.

**Acupuncture:** The course of treatment for tonsillitis is based upon the stage and history of the condition. In general, it requires 3–10 treatments. Consult your practitioner.

**Acupressure:** Use the tip of your thumb to press the Hegu and Tai Yang points with strong pressure for one to two minutes to help relieve symptoms that accompany tonsillitis. The Hegu points are located on the back of the hands between the thumb and first finger. The Tai Yang point is on the temple in the depression next to the lateral end of the eyebrow and eyelid.

**Diet:** Rice porridge is comforting if you are suffering from tonsillitis. Place 1 cup of washed rice in a pot and add 5 cups of water. Bring the rice to a boil and cook just under the boil until rice is soft and creamy.

## NATUROPATHY

**Diet:** Drink fluids throughout the day consisting of water, teas, and soups, particularly chicken soup and miso soup. Reduce the amount of dairy and simple carbohydrates (found in fruits and processed foods, and in anything with refined sugar added) you are consuming. Your diet should consist primarily of vegetables, whole grains, some fresh fruit and lots of soup and water.

**Supplements:** Take 500–1,000 mg of vitamin C every four hours to support the immune system until symptoms subside. Children should take 250 mg of vitamin C three times a day. Bioflavonoids work synergistically with Vitamin C and have immune-enhancing properties of their own. Take 1,000 mg in divided doses a day; give children 100–200 mg three times a day. Zinc also supports the immune system and may have antiviral properties. An aggressive dose of zinc is needed to treat tonsilitis, so consult a practitioner. Zinc depletes the body's store of copper so also take copper alongside zinc supplements.

**Herbs:** Echinacea and goldenseal enhance the immune system and have antiviral properties. Take 2–4 ml of a combination tincture four times a day. Astragalus is excellent for treating and preventing tonsillitis and infections in general. Take 500–1,000 mg in capsule form or 4–6 ml of tincture three times a day. Take plenty of raw garlic or 300–500 mg in capsule form to fight infection or as a preventive measure. Drink slippery elm and marshmallow root tea two to three times a day. Place 1 oz of slippery elm root and 1 oz of marshmallow root in 5 cups of cold water. Boil the mixture for ½ hour and strain the liquid. Let it cool before drinking. It is very soothing to the tonsils and throat. Shiitake and reishi mushrooms are effective for viral and bacterial tonsillitis. Once fever has resolved, take 2–6 g of the extract a day. Teas and baths prepared with peppermint and thyme assist in reducing fever. Drink peppermint or thyme tea, or use 10 drops of peppermint or thyme oil in a warm bath, as needed.

**TIP:** STAY WELL RESTED

Make rest a priority. A well-rested body has a stronger immune system.

## HOMEOPATHY

Any of the following homeopathic remedies can be helpful in easing pain and inflammation, and speeding up recovery, from an isolated bout of tonsillitis. However, a recurrent condition should be treated by a homeopathic practitioner who will prescribe to treat the problem at a more fundamental level. See the suggestions given for sore throat (p. 209) and strep throat (p. 304) in addition to the following.

**Arsenicum album:** If burning pains are present in the throat that cause great anxiety, distress, and restlessness, especially in the night and/or the early hours of the morning, try Arsenicum album. The body is likely to feel incredibly chilly, while the head feels better from contact with cool, fresh air (ideally while the body is kept very warm). Taking small sips of warm drinks temporarily soothes the burning sensations in the throat.

**Lycopodium:** Consider this remedy if symptoms arise when feeling anxious and stressed. Symptoms characteristically start on the right side and move to the left, or may remain more painful and inflamed on the right side. Pain and distress is made more severe by contact with cold drinks, and eased by warm liquids.

**TIP:** GENERAL HEALTH

Get as much rest as possible, maintain a stable temperature to avoid getting chilly or overheated, and keeping fluid intake up. Stick to food that is easily digestible.

## HERBALISM

The herbal approach to tonsillitis is to support the immune system, while fighting infection.

**Andrographis:** This herb has several active constituents that impart antiviral, immune-stimulating, and antioxidant properties that may successfully treat tonsillitis. Because Andrographis is very bitter, some people may find it easier to take in capsule form. A preventive adult dose is 2–3 g or 4–6 ml of tincture a day. During infection, take up to 6 g or 12 ml of tincture a day. Do not take during pregnancy.

**Astragalus:** Although astragalus has demonstrated a potent ability to enhance immunity, inhibit viral infections, and improve fatigue, it should not be used to treat an acute infection. Astragalus is best taken to treat chronic tonsillitis or as a preventive measure. Boil 10 g of root in 1 cup of water and drink, or take 6 ml of tincture per day.

**Echinacea:** Although several species of echinacea are used medicinally, *Echinacea purpurea* is the most widely cultivated due to the fact it can be easily grown and the whole plant (flower, leaf, seed, and root) can be taken. Studies have shown that echinacea has immune-stimulating, antibacterial, mild antiviral, and anti-inflammatory properties. Take 2–3 g of dried root or 3–5 g of whole plant of E purpurea, or 3–6 ml of tincture a day until the infection resolves.

> **TIP:** THROAT SPRAY
> Combine 6 g each of licorice, sage, echinacea, and osha (a relative of lovage) tincture with 6 g of a 20% vegetable glycerin and 3–5 drops of bitter orange oil to create a soothing, antimicrobial, antiviral, and immune-stimulating blend. Spray this mixture directly into the throat throughout the day as needed.

# DIGESTIVE SYSTEM AND URINARY TRACT

# ACID REFLUX

## DIAGNOSIS

Acid reflux, also known as gastro-esophageal reflux, is a common condition that affects many people. It is the most frequent cause of indigestion and can also trigger heartburn. The condition is caused when the sphincter (ring of muscle at the lower end of the throat or esophagus) becomes abnormally relaxed, allowing the acidic contents of the stomach to flow back or "reflux" into the throat. Acid reflux is typically triggered by lifestyle choices such as eating large or rich meals with a high fat content, drinking alcohol, or smoking. Certain physical positions can also cause a flare-up of reflux symptoms, particularly lying down, bending over, and lifting heavy objects. The reflux tendency increases when the stomach is over-full, leading to increased pressure. Obesity also increases pressure on the stomach, causing the contents of the stomach to travel up into the throat. The same thing happens during pregnancy. Prolonged exposure to refluxed acid results in the serious condition esophagitis (inflammation of the esophagus), which can eventually lead to difficulties swallowing and in some cases a condition called Barrett's esophagus, which may lead to esophageal cancer. Fortunately, this complication is rare, but persistent symptoms require investigation by a scope passed into the esophagus and stomach.

## SYMPTOMS

- Painful burning sensation in the chest
- The acid reflux may reach the throat and mouth
- Sour taste in the mouth
- Occasionally, breathing difficulties occur
- Hoarseness due to irritation of the larynx
- Belching

## TREATMENT GOAL

Conventional and complementary treatments aim to relieve the symptoms and identify the cause of the acid reflux to prevent further problems from occurring. This may involve lifestyle changes as well as medications.

## CONVENTIONAL MEDICINE

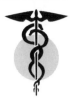

**Antacids:** These can be taken on an intermittent basis according to the instructions on the packet. Antacids can reduce the absorption of certain vitamins, especially B vitamins, so it is a good idea to take a multivitamin with extra B vitamins when on this kind of medication. The multivitamin should be taken at a different time in the day than the antacid.

**Lifestyle modification:** Try raising the head while sleeping by elevating the head of the bed. Avoid alcohol and nicotine, and any foods that aggravate the condition. Spicy foods such as onions, peppers, tomatoes, and peppermint may stimulate reflux. Obesity is a contributing factor, and in these cases weight loss can also help. Stress reduction techniques are important as the hormone released when stressed (cortisol) affects the acid level of the stomach as well as the muscle tone of the stomach, making acid reflux worse.

**H2 blockers:** If the above techniques do not work, medications that block acid receptors in the stomach (H2 blockers) such as cimetidine, ranitidine, famotidine, and nizatidine can be tried. These do bring relief from symptoms, but can also affect the body's absorption of B vitamins. Be sure to take extra B vitamin supplements if you are taking these medications.

**Proton pump inhibitors:** This class of drugs helps by reducing the secretion of acid in the stomach. They are stronger than antacids and acid blockers and are usually reserved for severe diseases.

**Surgery:** If the reflux becomes very severe and the esophagus is damaged, then surgery may be required, some of which may be done through new endoscopic procedures.

## TRADITIONAL CHINESE MEDICINE

**Herbs:** The herbs below are available from Chinese herbalists or online. If your condition worsens, consult your doctor immediately.
• To relieve heartburn and other symptoms caused by acid reflux: Combine 10 g of Mu Xiang (costus root), 5 g of Sha Ren (cardamon), 12 g of Bai Zhu (white atractylodes rhizome), 15 g of Shan Yao (Chinese yam), 12 g of Fa Ban Xia (pinellia rhizome), 30 g of Dai Zhe Shi (hematite), 12 g of Lian Qiao (forsythia fruit), and 3 g of Gan Cao (licorice) in a ceramic pot. Add 3 cups of water, bring to the boil, and simmer for 30 minutes before straining the liquid into a container. Drink 1 cup twice a day for 10 days as one course of treatment. Take three to five courses of treatment.

• To treat a deficient digestive system: Combine 12 g Tai Zi Shen (pseudostellaria), 10 g of Huang Qi (milk-vetch root), 12 g Bai Zhu (white atractylodes rhizome), 8 g of Zhi Ke (bitter orange), 15 g of Fuling (poria), and 3 g of Gan Cao (licorice) in a ceramic pot with 3 cups of water. Bring the mixture to the boil, simmer for 30 minutes, and strain. Drink 1 cup of the liquid twice a day for 10 days as one course of treatment. Take three to five courses of treatment.

**Acupuncture:** Treatment can usually relieve symptoms gradually. You may need regular treatment for a significant length of time to achieve the best results.

**Acupressure:** Apply gentle pressure to the Nei Guan, Susanli, and San Yin Jiao points for one to two minutes. The Nei Guan point is located in the center of the wrist on the palm side about 2 inches below the crease. The Susanli point is on the lower leg, 1 inch to the outside of and 3 inches below the kneecap. The San Yin Jiao point is on the inside of the leg, about 3 inches above the anklebone.

**Diet:** Eat food that is nourishing to the spleen and stomach such as sweet rice, beef, honey, corn, celery, spinach, lettuce, and potatoes. Avoid fruits (especially oranges, lemons, pineapple, and apricots) and acidic food such as tomato and chilies.

## NATUROPATHY

**Diet:** Cut common trigger foods, including coffee, chocolate, fried and fatty foods, alcohol, and spices, out of your diet. Increase the amount of high-fiber foods to help your body absorb excess acid and gas, and rid itself of toxins more quickly. Eat plenty of whole grains and fresh fruit and vegetables. Drink at least eight glasses of water each day to allow your body to expel acid naturally. Herbal teas containing chamomile, ginger, licorice root, and catnip, as well as green tea, help the stomach lining repair itself. Steep these herbs in water overnight and drink 1 cup of tea, diluted to taste, after dinner to reduce acid reflux. Do not drink any kind of mint tea. This may worsen the symptoms.

**Herbs:** Take 500–1,000 mg of slippery elm three times a day to soothe the gastrointestinal (GI) tract. Deglycyrrhizinated licorice (DGL) capsules can also bring quick relief and may help heal the damaged lining in the stomach. Take two DGL licorice tablets (380 mg) three or four times a day between meals as needed. Aloe vera juice is another fast-acting supplement that frequently helps soothe an irritated esophagus. Take ½ cup of aloe vera juice three times a day between meals. Make sure it contains 98% aloe vera and no aloin or aloe-emodin. To treat chronic acid reflux, take 150 mg of gamma-oryzanol three times a day on an empty stomach. This rice bran oil extract can help repair the entire digestive system and also improve the central nervous system's digestive control. Choline, pantothenic acid, and thiamine are B-complex vitamins that can have long-term digestive benefits. If you suffer from chronic acid reflux, try them in combination for a month or so to see if they help.

**Supplements:** Medications used to treat acid reflux deplete the body of vitamin B12, folate, and various minerals. Take a multivitamin/multimineral supplement to compensate for this problem. Take 500 mg of choline, sold as plain choline or phosphatidylcholine, three times a day. To treat chronic acid reflux, take this in combination with 1,000 mg of pantothenic acid twice a day and 500 mg of thiamine first think in the morning for one month to see if symptoms resolve. Digestive enzymes, such as lipases, proteases, and amylases, help to speed the digestive process, often helping eliminate acid reflux altogether. Take two to three capsules with every meal. You can also take papaya enzyme as a chewable capsule after each meal.

## HOMEOPATHY

The remedies listed below may help ease the discomfort of a mild case of acid reflux that is due to a specific cause. Chronic conditions will benefit most from professional homeopathic treatment.

**Arsenicum album:** This remedy can be helpful in easing symptoms that develop in the night or early hours of the morning. Sipping on warm drinks temporarily soothes gastric uneasiness. Any nausea that is present causes a disproportionate amount of anxiety, restlessness, and mental and physical distress. Other symptoms include feeling more comfortable for lying slightly raised on two or three pillows.

**Lycopodium:** If there is a noticeable amount of noisy gurgling and rumbling combined with acid reflux, use Lycopodium. Signature symptoms are noticeably aggravated or triggered by stress. Dietary factors can also trigger the condition, with very high-fiber foods having a noticeably adverse effect on digestion. Appetite is also irregular, with a tendency to sit down to a meal feeling ravenously hungry, but becoming quickly satisfied, leaving most of the meal untouched.

**Bryonia:** Use this remedy if there is a heavy feeling in the stomach that develops almost immediately after eating, and if a bitter-tasting liquid washes up into the mouth. Symptoms are aggravated by moving around, pressure to the stomach (for instance, from clothes that are too tight), and by eating quickly.

**Nux vomica:** This is a leading remedy for heartburn and acid reflux. It is especially useful when used by those who are irritable, impatient, competitive, and prone to anger fits. Symptoms may be worse after eating a large amount of rich or spicy food, or drinking coffee or alcohol.

## HERBALISM

 Herbs can help with reflux in several different ways. Demulcent herbs coat the skin and can soothe and protect the inflamed mucous membranes in the esophagus and stomach that may occur with reflux. Anti-inflammatory herbs can improve acid reflux symptoms and help the damaged tissue to heal. Anti-anxiety herbs are part of an herbalist's overall healing approach to a patient with acid reflux.

**Slippery elm root bark powder:** Stir 1–2 tbsp of this demulcent powder into a glass of water and drink after meals and before bedtime. Begin with a smaller amount of powder until you become accustomed to it; if too much powder is mixed in the water, the preparation can be very thick and difficult to tolerate. To improve the taste, it can be sweetened slightly with honey or sugar. Slippery elm is safe, though some of the compounds contained in it can bind medications that are taken at the same time and decrease their absorption. Do not take slippery elm within one to two hours of taking any other medication.

**Marshmallow:** This demulcent herb can relieve acid reflux symptoms. Make a tea with 5–6 g of marshmallow leaf or root and drink throughout the day. As with slippery elm, medicines taken at the same time may not be absorbed as well.

**Chamomile:** This herb has an anti-spasmodic effect on the intestines and acts as an anti-inflammatory to treat acid reflux. Make a tea from 1–3 g of chamomile flowers and drink three to four times daily. Chamomile is generally well-tolerated, but should not be consumed by those who are allergic to plants in the daisy family.

**Anti-anxiety botanicals:** Anxiety and acid reflux can be linked in some people. Common anti-anxiety plants recommended as part of an acid reflux prescription are valerian and skullcap; see Anxiety (p. 833) for more information.

# BAD BREATH

## DIAGNOSIS

Bad breath, also known as halitosis, is a common problem and is usually triggered by bacterial activity in the mouth. One of the most common causes is poor oral hygiene, which leads to a build-up of plaque and gum disease. Most people have bad breath to a certain degree first thing in the morning, because while you are asleep the amount of saliva that is moved around the mouth decreases. Bacteria then start to work on any particles of food or other debris present in the mouth, creating an unpleasant smell (morning breath). Many illnesses can also lead to bad breath. Infections in the mouth or throat, including nasal congestion, sinusitis, tonsillitis, bronchitis, and swollen adenoids, can all be contributing factors to bad breath. Indigestion caused by acid reflux can also play a role. Other causes of bad breath include smoking, drinking alcohol, or eating certain foods such as onions, garlic, and spicy dishes such as curries. An empty stomach and crash dieting can also result in problems with bad breath due to ketones produced in the fasting state. These are produced when the body is no longer supplied with energy-giving carbohydrates and it begins to break down its fat stores. Bad breath can also be an indication of some more serious health conditions such as diabetes, where the breath smells like acetone (i.e., nail polish remover), and liver or kidney failure, where the breath smells like fish or ammonia.

## SYMPTOMS

- A sour taste in the mouth
- Foul-smelling breath

## TREATMENT GOAL

Bad breath on its own is normally not generally a reason to see the doctor. For persistent cases, make an appointment with your dentist. Treatment is directed towards identifying and then, when possible, removing the cause of bad breath.

## CONVENTIONAL MEDICINE

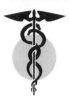

**Prevention:** Oral hygiene is the first line of defense against this condition. Brush your teeth twice a day using fluoride toothpaste. Using an electric toothbrush seems to produce the best results. Brushing along the gum line and over the tongue is important. Remove food from between the teeth with floss once a day. Visit a dentist at least twice a year.

**Diet:** Eat at least seven portions of fresh fruit and vegetables every day. Avoid foods that cause bad breath such as garlic, onions, and curry—unless these are being used for therapeutic purposes to treat another condition. A dry mouth is more prone to bad breath, so keeping the mouth moist with regular amounts of filtered water is important. Avoid tobacco products as these are a common cause of bad breath and also promote gum disease.

**When should I see my doctor?** If bad breath is still occurring after taking the above measures, visit your doctor. Certain gastrointestinal conditions, such as acid reflux, gut dysbiosis (a bacterial imbalance in the intestines), infections, and heavy metal toxicity, can cause bad breath. These unusual causes need to be identified and treated on an individual basis.

## TRADITIONAL CHINESE MEDICINE

Below are some recommendations for freshening your breath. Remember, however, that there can be an underlying disorder causing bad breath that will need to be treated to resolve the condition completely.

**Herbs:** This herbal formula will clean out stomach heat and refresh the lungs and digestive system. Put 5 g of Jin Yin Hua (honeysuckle flower) and 5 g of Bo He (field mint) into a teapot. Add boiling water and let the herbs steep for five minutes. Drink the tea three times a day. It can be used regularly to freshen breath, but consult your doctor if you think bad breath is related to other health concerns.

**Acupuncture:** To treat bad breath, an experienced acupuncturist will try to find and address the cause of the condition, such as stomach heat or a disorder in the digestive system. To achieve results, have treatment once or twice a week for one to three months.

**Acupressure:** The Hegu point is located on the back of the hand between the thumb and first finger. The Nei Guan point is found in the center of the wrist on the palm side about

2 inches below the crease. The Tai Chong point is on the sole of the foot in the depression between the first and second toe, at the base of the big toe. In a sitting position, press each of these points for one minute two to three times a day.

**Diet:** According to Chinese dietary therapy, foods that are cooling and that clear heat and promote smooth bowel movements are appropriate for this condition. Choose coix seed, watermelon, mutton, bitter melon, and coriander. Other good foods to consider include celery, mung beans, spinach, carrots, peach, persimmon, banana, figs, papaya, and sesame oil. Drink at least eight glasses of fresh water a day.

## NATUROPATHY

Some causes of bad breath include constant postnasal drip from sinusitis, alcoholism, kidney failure, diabetes, liver disease, and some medications. These should be dealt with by a doctor. If you have bad breath for more than a few days, your dental practitioner or doctor should be able to help.

**Diet:** Toxins stored in the digestive tract can cause bad breath. Base your meals on a diet of whole grains, raw or lightly cooked fruits and vegetables, beans, nuts, and seeds. These will improve your digestive system and help get rid of toxins. Avoid pungent foods that enter your digestive tract and bloodstream and eventually permeate your whole body so that every breath picks up the offending odor in your lungs and releases it. This is why it can take up to 24 hours to get rid of some offending smells. Such foods include garlic, onions and hot peppers; cheeses such as blue cheese, Camembert, and Roquefort; spicy, oily meats including pastrami, pepperoni, and salami; and anchovies. Drinks that can cause problems with your breath include coffee, beer, wine, and whiskey. Carrots, apples, and celery all help to fight the development of plaque on the teeth and keep breath fresh. Parsley is high in chlorophyll and has agents that neutralize odors in the blood stream and lungs. Green vegetables, watercress, and alfalfa also have high levels of chlorophyll. Eat foods high in vitamin C and vitamin A, such as squash, carrots, sweet potatoes, spinach, red peppers, and citrus fruits, for their good dental health properties.

**Supplements:** Vitamin C supports the immune system and helps to keep teeth and gums healthy. Take 500–1,000 mg every four hours, or up to bowel tolerance; give children 250 mg three times a day. Take 12,000–25,000 IU of vitamin A a day to support the immune system in fighting bacteria. Pregnant women should not take more than 10,000 IU of vitamin A day. Coenzyme Q10 is helpful if you have active gum disease; take 200 mg a day.

**Herbs:** Take 1 tsp of liquid chlorophyll after meals to keep the breath fresh. Alternatively, take 5 drops of parsley extract after each meal. Gentian contains bitter components that improve overall digestion. Take as directed on the container before each meal.

---

**TIP:** PRACTICE GOOD ORAL HYGIENE

Use a soft-bristled brush to gently brush your tongue when cleaning your teeth to wash away microscopic bits of food that become trapped on the surface. Floss at least once a day, preferably just before brushing, to remove food from between the teeth. If you use dentures, don't forget to clean them regularly and thoroughly. Like natural teeth, they harbor food and bacteria that can cause bad breath. Change your toothbrush regularly, about every two months, as bacteria can begin to build up.

---

## HOMEOPATHY

The following advice can help treat bad breath that results from an obvious trigger, such as drinking too much coffee or eating very pungent food. Persistent bad breath can be a symptom of another, more deep-seated condition, such as dental problems or a digestive disorder, and should be investigated by your family physician or dentist.

**Pulsatilla:** This remedy may clear a bout of bad breath triggered by eating too many rich, high-fat foods, or by mucus congestion in the nose, sinuses, and/or throat associated with the later stages of a cold. Signature symptoms include a dry mouth without thirst and a tongue that is likely to be furry and coated with a whitish-colored deposit.

**Mercurius:** This remedy is appropriate for treating bad breath that is combined with a sinus infection and/or mouth ulcers. Symtoms include an excessive amount of saliva in the mouth, accompanied by an unpleasant sweetish or metallic taste.

**Arnica:** This remedy can be helpful when bad breath is triggered by dental work that involves significant bleeding, such as a tooth extraction.

**Nux vomica:** If bad breath follows drinking excessive amounts of alcohol or coffee, or smoking cigarettes, try Nux vomica. Symptoms are likely to be at their worst on waking, when the whole system feels "toxic."

**TIP:** EAT FRESH PARSLEY
Use fresh parsley to flavor your food as it temporarily deodorizes the breath. Avoid foods and drinks that contribute to bad breath, such as strong tea, coffee, alcohol, garlic, and spicy food.

## HERBALISM

 Chronic bad breath is thought to affect approximately 25% of the population and is usually due to pathogenic bacteria in the mouth. However, it can also be related to a range of conditions from chronic dry mucous membranes to poor digestive health.

**Berberis bark:** This herb has a long history of being used as a mouthwash, to astringe and heal inflamed tissues while eliminating trouble-making bacteria. Fresh or dried root bark contains several active antimicrobial constituents. Berberis assists digestion by improving the breakdown of food in the stomach and stimulating the release of enzymes throughout the digestive tract, while acting as a very mild laxative. This allows for better assimilation of nutrients and improved elimination of toxins. Decoct 2 g of the root in 1 cup of water, or take 3 ml of tincture in water, swish the liquid around the mouth for one to two minutes and then swallow.

**Chelidonium:** This herb encourages liver detoxification and repair, allowing toxins to be eliminated from the body and improving food digestion. Less stagnation in the digestive system equals sweeter-smelling breath. Dilute 3–5 drops of a tincture in 1 cup of water and drink twice a day. Swish the liquid around in your mouth for one to two minutes before swallowing.

**Prickly ash:** Use this herb to treat bad breath that is related to dry mucous membranes. Prickly ash stimulates the production of saliva and creates a slight tingling effect when placed on the tongue. It is also slightly antimicrobial and can improve movement in the digestive and circulatory systems. Place 3–5 drops on the tongue to stimulate saliva production a few times daily. Do not use during pregnancy.

# CELIAC DISEASE

## DIAGNOSIS

Celiac disease can affect people in different ways. Common symptoms include bloating, diarrhea, and nausea. It is often mistaken as an allergy, but is in fact an auto-immune disease, which means that it causes the body to produce antibodies that attack its own tissues. These attacks are triggered by a type of protein, gliadin, that form part of the gluten fraction found in wheat, rye, and barley. Some people with celiac disease also react to oats. Symptoms of celiac disease may range in intensity. The first step towards making a diagnosis is to discuss your symptoms with your physician. Do not, at this stage, remove gluten from your diet as any tests needed will not give a true reading. Continue to eat normally. Your physician can take a simple blood test to check for endomysial antibodies (EMA) and/or tissue transglutaminase antibodies (tTGA). Then if necessary your physician will refer you to a gastroenterologist for a biopsy of the gut. This involves inserting a flexible viewing tube, known as an endoscope, into the mouth and down into the small intestine (this can be done using local anesthetic and sedation). A small tissue sample is collected and examined under a microscope to check for abnormalities.

## SYMPTOMS

- Bloating and gas
- Diarrhea or constipation
- Nausea
- Tiredness
- Anemia
- Mouth ulcers
- Headaches
- Weight loss
- Hair loss
- Skin problems
- Infertility, recurrent miscarriages
- Joint/bone pain
- Osteoporosis

## TREATMENT GOAL

There is no cure for celiac disease. Treatment focuses on identifying the cause of the symptoms, and following a gluten-free diet, supplemented with appropriate vitamins and minerals where necessary.

## CONVENTIONAL MEDICINE

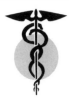

Treatment of celiac disease is very dependent on an accurate diagnosis. However, this is a common and notoriously under-diagnosed condition as there is no one easy test to determine whether a patient has celiac disease or not. A strict gluten-free trial, monitoring symptoms closely, is often utilized. If the condition improves then celiac is a likely diagnosis.

**Diet:** All food substances containing gluten should be avoided. There are many gluten-free guidelines available for exact referencing but all wheat, barley, and rye products are to be strictly avoided. Oats that are pure whole grain, rolled, or steel cut can be eaten, but many oats are mass-produced and contaminated with gluten so these are best avoided.

**Supplements:** Celiac disease can cause chronic diarrhea and inflammation of the digestive tract, which wears out the important absorptive lining in the gut. This decreases the body's ability to absorb certain nutrients, particularly iron, folic acid, the B vitamins (especially B12), calcium, and selenium. Often amino acids are improperly absorbed as well. It is important to restore good bacteria (flora) to the gut. Take a good probiotic that includes Sachromyces boullardii and bifidus species daily. Herbs such as mallow root help improve the intestinal lining. A high dose B vitamin and a multivitamin with minerals should be taken as well. Flax oil and fish oil can help relieve the chronic inflammation associated with celiac disease. Vitamin D is also useful to prevent associated osteoporosis.

**Medication:** To treat severe celiac disease, prednisone is prescribed along with a gluten-free diet.

## TRADITIONAL CHINESE MEDICINE

The spleen is an important organ for digestion in the theory of traditional Chinese medicine. Celiac disease is commonly diagnosed as spleen deficiency and intestinal dysfunction. The herbal formula below promotes spleen function and corrects disorders of the digestive system.

**Herbal decoction:** Combine 12 g of Tai Zi Shen (pseudostellaria), 12 g of Bai Zhu (atractylodes rhizome), 16 g of Fuling (poria), 12 g of Shen Zha (dried hawthorn), 6 g of Chen Pi (tangerine peel), and 10 g of Mu Xiang (costus root) in a ceramic pot. Use half of the above amounts to treat children under 10 years old. Add 3 cups of water, bring to the boil, simmer for 30 minutes, and strain. Drink 1 cup twice a day.

**Acupuncture:** Treatment may help your body regulate spleen Qi and strengthen digestion. You may need long-term treatment to see results as this condition is usually not easy to correct. Consult your acupuncturist regarding a prognosis.

**Acupressure:** The Nei Guan point is located in the center of the wrist on the palm side about 2 inches below the wrist crease. The San Yin Jiao point is about 3 inches above the anklebone on the inside of the leg. The Zhong Wan point is on the upper abdomen about 3 inches above the belly button. Lie on your back or sit and use the tip of your thumb or finger to press these points for one minute, and then release for one minute. Repeat twice. You can perform this treatment on young children, but with gentler pressure.

**Diet:** Eat a variety of fresh vegetables that are light and easy to digest, such as Chinese cabbage, kale, napa cabbage, celery, and cooked cucumber. Avoid food that contains gluten, including cereal grains such as wheat, rye, and glutinous rice.

## NATUROPATHY

**Diet:** A proper diet is the single most important treatment for this condition. Eliminate all foods containing gluten from the diet, including ice cream and ice cream cones, baby cereal, canned meats, biscuits, infant formula, bread, breakfast cereal, pasta, cakes and cake mixes, cookies, milk (malted and powdered), frankfurters, noodles, pudding mix, pancakes and pancake syrup, salad dressings, wheat flour, crackers, whipped cream substitutes, and potato chips. Grains to be avoided include wheat, rye, and barley. While oats contain a substance similar to gluten, modern research suggests that eating moderate amounts of oats does not cause problems for most people with celiac disease. Oats that are pure whole grain, rolled, or steel cut can be eaten, but many oats are mass-produced and contaminated with gluten, so these are best avoided. While symptoms are evident also follow a lactose-free diet. Dairy and lactose are common allergens and can mimic gluten sensitivities in sufferers of celiac disease.

**Supplements:** Celiac patients tend to have a lot of nutritional deficiencies. Rather than taking a supplement to address each deficiency, take a good multivitamin/multimineral, following the dosage directions on the label. Also take two to three digestive enzyme capsules with every meal, less if you feel a warm sensation in your abdomen. Get a high-potency B-complex vitamin injection from your physician, or take 100 mg in capsule form three times a day, as those with celiac disease do not absorb B vitamins easily. You may need extra vitamin B12; get injections of B12 or take it in capsule or sublingual form. Other common deficiencies are essential fatty acids, iron, vitamin D, vitamin K, calcium, magnesium, folic acid, and zinc. Consult a practitioner to identify your nutritional deficiencies and then supplement them in the following dosages:

400 mcg of folic acid a day; 50 mg of zinc twice a day, with 1–2 mg of copper a day; 100 mg of iron a day, continually lowering the dosage until the deficiency is resolved; 1,000 IU of vitamin D a day; 60 mcg of vitamin K a day; 1,000 mg of calcium (citrate or malate) a day with 400 mg of magnesium citrate.

## HOMEOPATHY

It is recommended that you receive constitutional homeopathic treatment from an experienced practitioner for this condition, rather than home prescribing. However, the following acute remedies may give some temporary relief while seeking professional advice and treatment.

**Nux vomica:** If stools are passed frequently but the bowel movement feels incomplete, try Nux vomica. Cramping pains, and associated bloating and gas, are likely to develop an hour or so after eating. Lying or sitting down in tranquil surroundings can provide temporary relief.

**Lycopodium:** If the digestive tract feels disordered as a result of acidity, bloating, and gas, use Lycopodium. Constipation is likely to alternate with diarrhea, and spasm in the rectum makes the stool initially lumpy and then soft and narrow.

**Calc carb:** Try this remedy if there is a general state of sluggishness, especially in the digestive tract, that leads to frequent indigestion and burping, with an unpleasant sour taste in the mouth. You may be constipated, or experience recurrent, watery, offensive-smelling diarrhea that is especially severe in the afternoons.

**Bryonia:** When this remedy is well indicated, sufferers experience indigestion and uneasiness in the stomach. Symptoms also include recurrent constipation, and passing stools that are large, hard, and dry. Low-grade dehydration is often present, and the tongue is likely to be coated with a white or yellow substance.

## HERBALISM

There are no specific herbs that cure someone of celiac disease. The best treatment, of course, is to avoid gluten in all of its forms. A herbalist's approach in treating celiac disease is to relieve symptoms, depending on how someone reacts to gluten, until the gastrointestinal system has recovered and is once again functioning normally in the absence of gluten. Diarrhea (p. 366), constipation (p. 346), and colitis (p. 341) may all result from celiac disease; the most useful herbs for these symptoms can be determined by consulting the appropriate sections.

# COLIC

## DIAGNOSIS

Colic is a common condition in babies, affecting around one in five newborns. It is characterized by a gripping pain in the abdomen, thought to be caused by trapped gas or intestinal spasms. It affects both breast- and bottle-fed babies. The baby becomes very uncomfortable and will cry continually unless rocked, walked, carried in a baby sling, or otherwise comforted. Symptoms may occur at roughly the same time every day. Some babies feel comforted when wrapped in a blanket or held tightly. Gently massaging the baby's tummy also helps in some cases. When all else fails, some parents find their baby is comforted by a car ride. The condition usually first manifests itself within two to four weeks after birth and mostly occurs in the first 12 weeks of life, but in some cases it can carry on for months. Happily, it often resolves after about three months of age.

Remember, colic might not be the only cause of a baby's discomfort. If a baby cries loudly all the time and cannot be comforted, consult a doctor.

## SYMPTOMS

- Legs moving around, and drawing legs up to stomach
- Clenched fists
- Baby out of sorts, particularly in the evenings
- Flushed or red face
- Baby wants to feed constantly
- Intense crying, sometimes for hours
- Abdomen feels hard
- Discomfort after feeding
- Poor sleep

## TREATMENT GOAL

Treatment aims to relieve symptoms and soothe the baby's distress. Contact your doctor if your baby has other symptoms, such as vomiting or diarrhea.

## CONVENTIONAL MEDICINE

A baby with colic who is fussy but has a fever, is extremely agitated, or has any other physical symptoms should be taken to a doctor for evaluation. Do not assume that it is an episode of colic.

**Diet:** Treatment of colic is primarily dietary. While breastfeeding is preferred, switching to a non-dairy formula such as a soy-based milk, goat's milk, or a whey hydrosylate milk may be useful. Less frequently, a lactase-treated milk (lactose free) and low allergen milk can be tried. If the baby is breastfeeding, the mother should go on a low allergen diet, which involves low gluten, low dairy, and cutting out processed foods. Avoiding foods that create gas in the mother (beans, broccoli, onions, spicy foods) is also essential.

**Physical comforting:** Feeding techniques that involve frequent, gentle burping, are encouraged as is rocking, cradling, and comforting the baby. Avoid overstimulating irritable babies when they are crying by reducing visual and auditory inputs. However, serene music and lullabies may be soothing and quieting. Massaging the baby may also be effective.

**Herbal tea:** Some herbal teas, such as peppermint tea, or tea with extract of chamomile, vervain, licorice, fennel, and balm mint have been shown to ease colic. These can be drunk by breastfeeding mothers, or a weak tea can be given directly to infants with a medicine dropper.

**Infant drops:** Simethicone infant drops are worth a try but have had mixed reviews as to their effectiveness. If an infant over six months of age is colicky, dicyclomine is sometimes prescribed, however, it does have side effects such as sedation, blurred vision, dizziness, and dry mouth.

## TRADITIONAL CHINESE MEDICINE

**Herbs:** The following formulas can be used to treat children suffering from colic. The herbs called for in these recipes are available from Chinese pharmacies or online. If the pain is not relieved after taking these remedies, consult a doctor immediately.

• Formula one: Mix 2 g of dried peppermint, or 3 g of fresh peppermint, with 3 g of fresh ginger. Boil these ingredients in 3 cups of water, and simmer for two to three minutes. Strain the tea, add 1–2 tbsp of honey, and stir well. Let your child drink the tea once it has cooled to a warm rather than hot temperature. Give your child 2–4 oz every one to two hours.

• Formula two: Combine 4 g of Jin Yin Hua (honeysuckle flower), 3 g of Shen Gan Cao (raw licorice), and five pieces of Da Zhao (Chinese jujube). Place the ingredients in 3 cups of water and bring to a boil. Simmer for three to five minutes and strain. Give your child 3–5 oz of tea to drink every half an hour to one hour for a total of three to five times.

**Acupressure:** Press the Hegu points, located on the back of the hands between the thumb and first finger, with strong pressure. Press the Nei Guan point, located in the center of the wrist on the palm side about 2 inches below the crease, with medium pressure. Press each point for one to three minutes at a time and repeat to reduce the pain.

---

**TIP:** USE A HOT WATER BOTTLE

Place a warm hot water bottle wrapped in a towel on your lap and lay your baby across, stomach down. This will relax the muscle cramps and calm your baby.

---

## NATUROPATHY

**Diet:** Allergies, particularly an intolerance to milk proteins from a cow's-milk-based formula, may cause colic in some infants. Infants who are sensitive to milk may be given a hypoallergenic formula containing extensively hydrolyzed proteins. If this does not work try a soy-based formula, or even goat's milk. If your child appears allergic to this as well, consult a pediatrician. If a baby is breastfed, certain foods in the mother's diet, such as cows' milk, may provoke an allergic reaction in the baby. Cow milk proteins have been found at higher levels in milk from breastfeeding mothers with colicky infants than in milk from mothers with non-colicky infants.

**Supplements:** Lactobacillus acidophilus and Bifidus provide the bowel with friendly intestinal bacteria (flora), which will ease digestion and may help resolve colic. A breastfeeding mother should take 1 tsp twice a day. Give a bottle-fed baby ⅛ tsp of acidophilus and ⅛ tsp of bifidus powder twice a day dissolved in his or her formula.

**Herbs:** Nursing mothers should drink 1 cup of chamomile tea twice a day. Give a bottle-fed infant 1 tbsp of tea three times a day mixed in formula or water. Fennel has been traditionally used to treat colic. Nursing mothers can drink 1 cup of fennel tea, on its own or mixed with chamomile, up to three times a day, or give a breastfeeding baby 1 tsp of the tea four times a day. Nursing mothers can also drink 1 cup of ginger tea twice a day to relieve colic in their infants.

## HOMEOPATHY

The remedies below can ease the distress and pain of a recent, acute bout of colic. However, regular, severe colic is most effectively dealt with by homeopathic practitioner.

**Nux vomica:** This is a possible remedy for colicky pains in breastfeeding babies whose mothers have been eating spicy food.

**Lycopodium:** If strong colic pain tends to come on in the late afternoon, often lasting until the early evening, try Lycopodium. Symptoms include loud, audible rumbling and gurgling sounds coming from the abdomen. Lycopodium is also an appropriate remedy for colic pain that arises in breastfed babies whose mothers have been eating an excessively high-fiber diet.

**Dioscorea:** This is a possible remedy for easing colicky pains that emerge in breastfed babies whose mothers have been drinking a lot of strong tea. Spasmodic pains centered around the navel are temporarily eased when stretching or arching backwards. Diarrhea, which does not help relieve discomfort, may also be present.

**Mag phos:** To relieve symptoms of colic that develop with teething pains, use mag phos. Excessive amounts of gas are produced that can temporarily give relief to pain and discomfort. Symptoms also include an instinctive pressing of the knees up to the belly in order to try and gain relief. Warmth locally applied and gentle massage feel comforting and ease pain.

**Chamomile:** This is one of the leading remedies for colic. It is appropriate if the baby is extremely fussy, irritable, and inconsolable. Babies may arch their backs when crying, and may seem better after passing gas.

**TIP:** AVOID TRIGGER FOODS
There are certain foods and drinks that have a reputation for aggravating colicky pains, and as a result, they are best avoided by mothers breastfeeding colicky babies. The most common culprits include any of the following: cucumbers, citrus fruit, raw peppers, cabbage, beans, raw onion, Brussels sprouts, alcohol, coffee, and very spicy foods.

## HERBALISM

 Colic is commonly described as excessive, inconsolable crying from an otherwise healthy baby. Some research has suggested that colic is related to excess gas; however, this is not the case with every child. The use of any herbal product orally in children younger than six months should be supervised by a medical herbalist. They should also only be taken in small amounts; a total amount of 3–4 oz a day, depending on the age of the child, should not be exceeded.

**Chamomile:** This plant's sweet, aromatic flowers soothe the stomach, relieve excess gas, and act as a mild sedative. The active constituent, apigenin, calms nerves and relieves anxiety, making chamomile the herb of choice for soothing night terrors and anxiety in children. Infuse 1 tsp of flowers in 1 cup of water. Allow the herb to steep for 10 minutes while covered to prevent the loss of important volatile oils. Give a colicky baby 1–2 oz at a time, up to 3–4 oz per day.

**Fennel seed and root:** Recognized for its antispasmodic action, fennel is well known as a herbal remedy for colic. The essential oils, flavonoids, and plant sterols reduce spasms in the digestive system and decrease the production of gas. Infuse 1 tsp of dried seeds (or fruit) in 1 cup of water. Give babies 1–2 oz at a time, up to 3–4 oz per day.

**Peppermint:** Peppermint essential oils and flavonoids have been found to relieve flatulent colic, digestive spasm, and the pain associated with these conditions. Peppermint tastes good and goes down easily. Infuse 1 tsp (2 g) of herb per cup of water. Give the baby 1 oz no more than three times a day.

**TIP:** LAVENDER MASSAGE
Add a few drops of lavender oil to baby oil and massage a colicky baby's back and chest to release tense muscles and calm the spirit.

# COLITIS

## DIAGNOSIS

Colitis is a type of inflammatory bowel disease where a superficial inflammation of the large intestine results in ulceration and bleeding. It is often mistaken for irritable bowel syndrome as the symptoms are similar. It affects men and women equally, and usually starts to manifest itself between the ages of 15 and 40. The condition goes in cycles, with alternating periods of few or no symptoms, followed by periods of frequent stomach pains and diarrhea mixed with blood. The exact cause of colitis is unknown but there is a hereditary link, which means it does tend to run in families. The different types of colitis include ischemic colitis, ulcerative colitis, antibiotic-induced colitis, and many non-specific forms.

An endoscopy and barium enema X-ray examination is usually performed to determine the extent of the disease in the large intestine and the rectum. Blood tests are also done to help determine the severity of the inflammation, and to check for signs of anemia. Once you have this condition the frequency of flare-ups and the severity of the attacks can be reduced. It is crucial to take preventive treatments, monitor symptoms, and consult your doctor if there is blood in your stools. Medication is usually sufficient to suppress the inflammation. In cases of chronic, ulcerative colitis, if the condition cannot be controlled by medical treatment surgical removal of the large intestine is sometimes required.

**DANGER**: If at any time a high fever, bleeding from the rectum, vomiting, or jaundice develops, get immediate medical help.

## SYMPTOMS

- Bloody diarrhea
- Blood in stools
- Fever
- Stomach pain
- Symptoms can be present most of the time or infrequently

## TREATMENT GOAL

Symptoms can usually be relieved and controlled with medication, but surgery may eventually be necessary.

## CONVENTIONAL MEDICINE

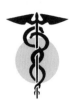

Medical treatment of colitis depends on whether it is an acute (infectious) or chronic (ulcerative) condition.

**To treat infectious colitis:** An episode of acute colitis generally resolves itself in a matter of time. Antibiotics are sometimes prescribed to clear up the infection. Modifying your diet, as described below, is also recommended.

**To treat ulcerative colitis:** Treatment depends on the severity of the disease and the extent of the inflammation in the colon. General methods involve medication, surgery to remove the diseased colon, and modifying your diet to that described below. Stress reduction techniques have been shown to help keep colitis in a state of remission to a certain extent.

**Diet:** Foods that tend to cause inflammation of the colon include gluten (wheat, rye, and barley), dairy products, and soy. Rice is a better choice as a source of carbohydrates. Avoid alcohol and aspirin to decrease the risk of bleeding. Add 1 tbsp of loose psyllium husks to your diet on a daily basis for intestinal health. However, discontinue if you have diarrhea.

**Supplements:** Take a probiotic on a daily basis. Also take a multivitamin, as the body's ability to absorb certain nutrients may be impaired. Take 4 g of fish oil a day to decrease inflammation.

**Medication:** Anti-diarrhea drugs, sulfa drugs (sulfasalazine), medicated enemas, and steroid therapy are sometimes prescribed. In severe cases of chronic disease, immuno-suppressive drugs can be used.

**TIP:** USE A HOT WATER BOTTLE
To relieve cramping, try holding a hot water bottle against the abdominal wall.

## TRADITIONAL CHINESE MEDICINE

**Herbs:** Using any of the herbal combinations listed below, place the herbs in a ceramic pot, add 3 cups of water, bring to the boil, and simmer for 30 minutes. Drink 1 cup twice a day. All the herbs listed are available from Chinese herbalists.

- Formula one: 10 g of Bai Tou Wong (Chinese anemone root), 5 g Huang Lian (coptis root), 10 g of Huang Qin (baical skullcap root), and 12 g of Ma Zhi Xian (purslane).
- Formula two: 12 g of Di Yu (burnet-bloodwort root), 10 g of Huai Hua (pagoda tree flower), and 10 g of Bai Tou Wong (Chinese anemone root).
- Formula three (for severe diarrhea): 10 g of Wu Mei (mume fruit), 15 g of Zhu Ling (polyporus sclerotium), 12 g of Ze Xie (water plantain rhizome), 12 g of Fuling (poria), and 15 g of Qian Shi (euryale seed).

**Acupuncture:** Treatment may be effective for reducing pain and healing the cause of colitis. Consult a practitioner for a treatment plan.

**Acupressure:** Using the tip of your finger or thumb, press the Hegu and Susanli points with strong pressure and the Guan Yuan with median pressure for one to three minutes. Release and repeat. The Hegu points are located on the back of the hands between the thumb and first finger. The Susanli point is on the lower leg, 1 inch outside of and 3 inches below the kneecap. The Guan Yuan point is on the abdomen, about 2 inches below the navel.

**Diet:** Eat foods that are easy to digest such as rice porridge, carrots, zucchini, Daikon radishes, and apple sauce. Avoid eating fatty and raw food.

## NATUROPATHY

**Diet:** Eliminate the most common food allergens from your diet, including dairy, soy, citrus, peanuts, wheat, eggs, and tomatoes, for three weeks. Re-introduce each food one at a time every three days. Watch for any reactions, which may include gastrointestinal upset, mood changes, headaches, flushing, and worsening of symptoms. Carrageenan has been shown in animal studies to cause lesions in the intestinal tract. Carrageenan is used to stabilize proteins and is mostly found in chocolate milk and milk products such as ice cream and cottage cheese. Although this has not been studied in humans, the foods that contain carrageenan should be avoided due to their allergenic properties and potential for intestinal irritation in patients with colitis. A rotation diet in which a different food is eaten every three to four days may be helpful in reducing symptoms. Eat plenty of fiber-rich whole foods such as gluten-free whole grains (for example, spelt or rice) and fresh fruit and vegetables. Vegetables should be eaten steamed not raw as raw vegetables may be difficult for some colitis patients to digest.

**Supplements:** Colitis is associated with low levels of various nutrients due to poor absorption by the body, interactions with medications, or an increase in the body's daily requirements. This can result in a variety of nutritional deficiencies. Take a multivitamin/multimineral, following the directions on the label (a practitioner can recommend a good quality product). Take the following supplements: 200 mg of magnesium, 50 mg of zinc, 3 g of fish oils, 200 IU vitamin E, and 50,000 IU of vitamin A a day—pregnant women should not take more than 10,000 IU of vitamin A a day. Also, taking 1–2 enterocoated peppermint oil capsules after every meal can reduce spasms and bowel irritability. Supplements that are enterocoated can bypass the stomach without disintegrating so that active ingredients are passed on to the intestines.

**Herbs:** The following herbs can be used in tincture form at 30 drops three times a day to treat colitis: marshmallow root, for its soothing effect on the gastrointestinal (GI) tract; wild indigo, to treat GI infections; geranium, to reduce excess secretions in the GI tract; goldenseal, to inhibit the growth of bacteria in the GI tract; poke root, to heal ulcers in the intestines; comfrey, as an anti-inflammatory to promote tissue growth and wound healing; and fennel, to relieve spasm of the GI tract, distention, and flatulence. Do not take comfrey internally as it can damage the liver.

## TIP: USE CASTOR OIL

Apply a castor oil pack directly to the skin of the stomach, covered with a clean cloth and plastic wrap. Place a hot water bottle over the pack for 30–60 minutes to bring relief. Use it as often as needed.

## HOMEOPATHY

Patients who suffer from this condition are likely to find themselves subject to recurrent episodes. As a chronic condition, colitis is best treated and managed by a professional homeopathic practitioner.

## TIP: BE AWARE OF TRIGGERS

Dietary strategies that may be helpful include reducing or eliminating dairy products. Also be aware that certain types of antibiotics can aggravate diarrhea. If you are prescribed antibiotics by your doctor, be sure to inform him or her that you suffer from colitis.

## HERBALISM

There are many types of colitis and some, such as ischemic colitis and ulcerative colitis, are potentially life threatening. The herbs mentioned below are suitable for treating the less severe forms.

**Slippery elm powder:** Demulcents or mucilaginous plants are commonly used to treat skin disorders as they coat and soothe the skin. In the same way, the compounds in these plants can repair the damaged intestinal mucosa of colitis. For example, slippery elm root powder provides a protective layer to the intestinal wall, preventing further damage and healing intestinal mucosa. Add slippery elm root powder to food throughout the day, or add 1 tsp to a cup of liquid to make a thick beverage, sweetened or not, and drink several times a day. This plant is not appreciably absorbed, so there is little worry about internal toxicity with long-term use.

**Aloe vera:** Aloe vera juice can also be taken to help heal the inflamed, injured mucosa of the colon during bouts of colitis. However, care should be taken with the long-term use of aloe vera juice due to the fact that it has stimulant laxative properties; there is the risk of long-term dependency with the use of any stimulant laxatives in order to have normal bowel movements.

**Herbal blend:** One herbal formula for chronic, or ulcerative, colitis recommends combining yarrow, St. John's wort, marshmallow, ginkgo, calendula, frankincense and gentian to bring together herbs with anti-inflammatory, wound-healing, and general gastrointestinal tonic effects. Consult a medical herbalist for a combination that best addresses your individual symptoms.

**Other herbs:** A wide variety of other plants are used for various types of colitis. Dandelion root, barley, lemon balm, and boswellia have all been used to improve symptoms of ulcerative colitis. The antispasmodic, calming effect of lemon balm may ease the inflammation and resulting discomfort. Resin extracts of boswellia, studied in clinical trials, function as anti-inflammatories in ulcerative colitis. To treat ulcerative colitis, a common dose is 350–400 mg of boswellic acid three times daily, standardized to 30% or higher.

# CONSTIPATION

## DIAGNOSIS

Constipation is defined as infrequent or irregular bowel movements. Stools may be hard, small, and dry with a pebble-like consistency. Bowel movements may also cause difficulty or pain. Although most people have a bowel movement at least once a day, there is no standard on what is "normal." A daily bowel movement is by no means essential for good health. It is possible to move your bowels every day and still be constipated if the stools are hard and difficult to pass, and some healthy people regularly do not have a bowel movement for a few days at a time.

Many things can trigger constipation. These include a change in your diet, such as a lack of fiber or too much processed food, an intolerance to certain foods, dehydration, traveling or a change of routine, not getting enough exercise, and emotional stress. The best way to avoid constipation is to eat a balanced diet that is high in fiber, including plenty of fresh fruit and vegetables, and drink at least 8–10 glasses of water a day. Prunes and plum juice can also be beneficial.

## SYMPTOMS

- Going for a long time without having a bowel movement
- Hard stools that are difficult to pass
- Stomach ache, often at mealtimes
- Bloated stomach
- Bad breath
- Abdominal discomfort
- Fever
- Lethargy
- Muscle aches
- Irritability

## TREATMENT GOAL

To relieve the unpleasant symptoms of constipation. Consult your doctor if this in an ongoing problem.

## CONVENTIONAL MEDICINE

**Identify the cause:** Medical treatment of constipation involves multiple therapies, but it is also important to make sure that there are no coexisting diseases causing the constipation. Diseases such as hypothyroidism, diabetes, and depression, some neurological disorders, and connective tissue diseases are linked to constipation. Many medications can also cause constipation, including antihistamines, blood pressure medications, water pills, calcium, iron supplements, and narcotics. Review the medications you are taking.

**Diet and exercise:** General lifestyle measures to relieve constipation include exercising daily (for example, about 20 minutes of rapid walking a day), drinking at least 1.5 liters of water a day, and including plenty of fiber in your diet (ideally about 30 g a day). Take 2 tbsp of psyllium husks a day and eat at least 5 portions of fresh fruit and vegetables a day. If you use stimulant laxatives, decrease the amount you use.

**Laxatives:** Medications for constipation are grouped by category. Bulk laxatives, such as Metamucil®, which is psyllium, Citrucel®, and Fibercon® contain fiber. These are safe to use on a long-term basis. Stool softeners, such as mineral oil and docusate sodium (Colace™), are also less likely to interfere with the body's natural colonic activity. Osmotic laxatives, which include unabsorbed sugars such as sorbitol, polyethylene glycol, and lactose, and salts such as magnesium hydroxide (milk of magnesia), magnesium citrate, and sodium phosphate (fleet enema), are somewhat harsher and should only be used occasionally. Stimulant laxatives, such as aloe vera, senna, castor oil, and bisacodyl (Dulcolax™), are the harshest kind of laxatives. Aloe vera, a natural plant stimulant, can be used for occasional relief while implementing the dietary and lifestyle changes listed above. Rectal enemas and suppositories such as glycerin, tap water enema, and Fleets™ phosphate enema provide direct and immediate relief. A new medication called tegaserod (Zelnorm™) is known as a colonic serotonin receptor binder that speeds up bowel movements and improves consistency of the stool.

## TRADITIONAL CHINESE MEDICINE

**Herbs:** The herbs listed below are available from Chinese herbal stores or online.
• To treat constipation due to excessive heat: Symptoms include one bowel movement every few days, dry stools, yellow urine, possible abdominal pain, feelings of being bloated, and bad breath. The following formula can clean large intestine heat. Combine 10 g Huang Qin (baical skullcap root),

5 g of Di Huang (Chinese foxglove), and 10 g of Huo Ma Ren (hemp seeds) in ceramic pot. Add 3 cups of water and boil for five minutes. Strain the liquid and drink the tea.

• To treat constipation due to yin deficiency: Symptoms may include dry skin, loss of memory, or night sweats. Place 15 g of Zhi Mu (anemarrhena rhizome), 15 g of Xuan Shen (ningpo figwort root), 12 g of Mai Men Dong (ophiopogon tuber), and 12 g of Dang Gui (Chinese angelica root) in a ceramic pot. Add 3 cups of water and boil for five minutes. Drink the tea throughout the day. You can also take the patent Chinese medicine Ma Ren Chang Wan, which has Huo Ma Ren (hemp seeds) as its main ingredient. It helps smooth the intestine and promotes bowel movement.

**Acupuncture:** If the patient's primary complaint is constipation, an experienced acupuncturist will treat the condition by stimulating the large intestine and stomach points. Treatment will be more successful if combined with a herbal remedy. For severe and chronic constipation, a long-term treatment may be required, but the prognosis is usually good. If constipation is a symptom of a more serious illness, it is necessary to treat the primary condition.

**Acupressure:** Press the Guan Yuan point, located on the abdomen, about 3 inches below the navel. You can also press the Zhi Gou point found on the outside of the forearm about 2 inches above the crease of the wrist between the two large bones in the forearm, the radius and ulna. Use the tip of your finger or thumb to press this point for one minute two or three times.

**Diet:** Eat fresh soft vegetables such as spinach and carrots, and fresh fruit such as peach, persimmon, banana, watermelon, and figs. Also recommended are foods that moisten the intestines such as sesame, honey, walnuts, sweet almonds, and pine nuts. Avoid spicy and heat-producing foods heat. Honey soothes the bowel. Take 1 tbsp every morning, or add it to tea. Eating 15 grains of raw rice once or twice a day can help some cases of constipation.

## NATUROPATHY

**Diet:** Drink 10–12 glasses of water a day, sipping throughout the day. Drinking an inadequate amount of fluids is one of the biggest contributors to constipation. A whole food diet consisting of whole grains and fresh fruit and vegetables will provide enough fiber to keep your bowels moving. Other good foods high in fiber are beans, nuts, prunes, and figs. Flaxseeds are highly concentrated in fiber and contain essential fatty acids that are thought to coat your intestines, promoting smooth bowel movements. Do not cook with flaxseeds or subject them to heat; instead, sprinkle 2 tbsp on cereals or salads. Children should take 2 tsp of flaxseeds at a time. Consume fermented products regularly to supply your intestines with healthy flora that can assist in inducing gentle bowel movements. Kefir, unsweetened yogurt, and raw sauerkraut are all excellent choices. Fried foods and simple carbohydrates contribute to constipation. Avoid these foods as much as possible. Caffeine and alcohol are hard on the digestive system and are dehydrating as well. Avoid them as much as possible during episodes of constipation.

**Supplements:** Magnesium helps with acute constipation and improves gut motility. Take 250 mg of magnesium four times a day for four to six weeks, then cut down to twice a day. Take a probiotic product daily that contains at least four billion active organisms to help digestion and elimination. Psyllium husks act as a bulk-forming laxative. Take 1 tsp or 5 g twice daily. Digestive enzymes assist with digestion, which will help with elimination. Take two pills with each meal.

**Herbs:** Cascara sagrada helps with acute constipation. Take 250 mg two to three times a day. Do not use this herb as a long-term solution as it can lead to dependence and gastric irritation. Taking 250 g of dandelion root with each meal stimulates bile flow and improves constipation. Milk thistle improves liver function and bile flow. Take 200–250 mg of a standardized product to 80% silymarin with each meal. Aloe vera juice also improves bowel movements. Drink 1 cup twice daily or as directed on the label.

**TIP:** EXERCISE REGULARLY
Exercise for at least 20 minutes four times a week to help with intestinal contraction. You can do any exercise you enjoy as long as you do it aerobically for 20 minutes without stopping.

## HOMEOPATHY

Constipation can occur as an isolated incident, usually in response to dietary shortcomings or a sudden escalation in stress levels, or it can be a feature of someone's digestive make-up. Either way, the situation must be rectified, since constipation, even in the short term, can lead to headaches, abdominal bloating, and a general sense of fatigue and sluggishness. Most of the homeopathic remedies listed below can help treat a recent episode of constipation. If constipation occurs regularly (whether very little stool is passed from the bowel each day, or nothing at all), it is best to seek a professional homeopathic assessment.

**Bryonia:** Use this remedy to treat constipation that results from dehydration. There is no urge to move your bowels, and when a stool is eventually passed, it is likely to be large, hard, and dry in texture, and therefore difficult to pass. This remedy is helpful for constipation that is associated with a throbbing headache.

**Nux vomica:** If there is a strong, constant urge to move your bowels, but nothing or very little is passed even after a lot of straining, use Nux vomica. The headaches associated with this condition closely resemble a hangover headache and often lodge at the back of the head. Common triggers that call for this remedy include too much stress and tension, and/or a diet that is high in junk foods.

**Lycopodium:** This can be helpful as a remedy for treating an acute episode of constipation that results from traveling. Confirmatory symptoms include bloating and distention in the belly with noticeably loud rumbling and gurgling sounds. Constipation may alternate with diarrhea if there hasn't been a bowel movement for a few days.

**Alumina:** If constipation manifests itself as soft stools that are passed reluctantly and with great difficulty, consider Alumina. Alternatively, stools that have a knotted or hard appearance may require a lot of straining to pass them. When this remedy is indicated there is a noticeable aggravation of the problem when eating a diet high in refined carbohydrates and potatoes.

**Silica:** When this remedy is well indicated here may be what is known as a "bashful stool," where a stool seems ready to pass, but then retreats back into the rectum, leaving an unpleasant sensation of incompleteness.

**TIP:** AVOID THE REGULAR USE OF LAXATIVES
If you have an underlying tendency to constipation, avoid the temptation to rely on laxatives to manage the condition. If they are used as a long-term solution, you may become dependent and it can be progressively more difficult to have a regular bowel movement without them.

## HERBALISM

Herbal medicines relieve constipation in two primary ways: as bulk-forming agents or stimulant laxatives.

**Psyllium seeds:** The husks of psyllium seeds provide a safe source of fiber. Take 2 tsp, which contain about 7 g of fiber, two to three times daily for a total of about 10–30 g. Some people don't need as much as others and the amount of psyllium you should take depends on the severity of the constipation and your tolerance to the herb. Be sure to increase your water intake with any fiber product or it could make symptoms worse. Introduce psyllium slowly, with, for instance, 5 g of seeds twice a day, and increase as necessary.

**Stimulant laxatives:** These increase the motion of the colon and cause changes in the colonic cells that lead to the accumulation of water, thereby improving constipation. The long-term use of stimulant laxatives, however, may cause normal bowel function to decrease and the nerve reflexes to depend on the presence of the stimulant compounds in order to have a regular bowel movement. Stimulant laxatives should only be used in the short term and with care. As the strength of the stimulant laxative goes up, so does the risk of side effects such as cramping, bloating, and diarrhea.

**Aloe vera juice:** This juice is made from the latex from the part of the aloe leaf that contains compounds called anthroquinone glycosides, which act as stimulant laxatives. You should take the minimum amount necessary to produce a soft stool, which is usually 40–170 mg of dehydrated juice in capsule form per day. As with other stimulant laxatives, the use of aloe vera juice for more than seven days in a row can lead to dependency. There are also studies that show that consuming any plant with anthroquinone glycosides regularly for more than a year increases the risk of colon cancer.

**Senna:** This widely used stimulant laxative is usually taken in a cold or hot water tea. Tablets and purified extracts of senna are also available. Take the minimum amount of senna a day necessary to achieve a soft stool. Start with a tea made from 0.5 g (½ tsp) of the ground dried fruit and 1 cup of hot water, and drink once or twice a day. It may be necessary to increase the dosage to 1 g twice daily.

# CYSTITIS

## DIAGNOSIS

Cystitis is a urinary infection that affects the bladder. The E. coli bacteria, which lives in the digestive tract, causes about 80% of all cases of cystitis. Women are particularly prone to this condition, with 40% of women suffering from it at some point. This is thought to be due to the short length of their urethra (the tube that carries urine from the bladder out of the body) and its proximity to the anus. Women should wipe themselves after urinating from front to back, towards the anus, to avoid bringing bacteria from their intestinal tract into their urethra. Many women experience the condition for the first time when they first become sexually active or during periods of increased sexual activity. During intercourse, bacteria are pushed up into the urethra and to the bladder. Urinating before and after intercourse can be preventive, as this flushes out bacteria. Some women are particularly prone to this condition and suffer repeat attacks. Cystitis can also be particularly troublesome during pregnancy when the growing fetus puts pressure on the urinary tract.

## SYMPTOMS

- Painful burning sensation when urinating
- Frequent urge to pass urine
- Cloudy urine that smells unpleasant
- Occasionally, blood in urine
- Pain directly above the pubic bone

## TREATMENT GOAL

To get to the root cause of the cystitis and address it, while providing relief for the painful symptoms of the condition.

## CONVENTIONAL MEDICINE

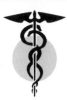

Treatment of cystitis involves identifying the cause and avoiding risk factors wherever possible. Bubble baths, low estrogen, certain spermicides, altered vaginal flora, and toilet hygiene are some factors that contribute to urinary tract infections.

**Drink plenty of fluids:** Drinking enough water is important. Some natural herbs such as cranberry and uva ursa can be taken along with water as preventive measures.

**Antibiotics:** These are used to treat the infection. The antibiotic most frequently used to treat a urinary tract infection is trimethoprim/sulfamethaxazole (Bactrim™), taken twice a day for three days. It is the most cost-effective antibiotic, but does have some side effects such as gastrointestinal problems, depression, and anxiety. Some bacteria have become resistant to Bactrim™, in which case ciprofloxin, taken twice a day for two to five days, is used as an alternative. Nitrofurantoin (Macrobid™) is another common medication used for urinary tract infection. However, again, resistance is occurring and ciproflaxin may be a better choice. A recent study showed that a two- to four-day course of antibiotics is just as effective as longer duration treatments. The medication phenazopyridine (Pyridium™) is used for bladder pain and burning that occurs with a urinary tract infection. It is taken three times a day for two days. This medication causes the urine to turn a red-orange color and should not be used for more than a few days, or at all by children under 12 years old.

## TRADITIONAL CHINESE MEDICINE

**Herbs:** The herbs below are available from Chinese pharmacies.
• Herbal decoction: Combine 10 g of Che Qian Cao (plantago), 10 g of Jin Qian Cao (lysimachia), 10 g of Ze Lan (bugleweed), 12 g of Huang Bai (philodendron), 12 g of Fuling (poria), 12 g of Zhu Ling (polyporus sclerotium), and 8 g of Shen Gan Cao (raw licorice) in a ceramic pot. Add 3 cups of water, bring to the boil, and simmer for 30 minutes before straining the liquid. Drink 1 cup twice a day.
• Herbal decoction to treat yin deficiency and heat: Mix 15 g of Zhi Mu (anemarrhena rhizome), 12 g of Shan Shen (mountain root), 12 g of Huang Bai (philodendron), 12 g of Bai Mao Gen (wooly grass rhizome), 12 g of Cang Zhu (atractylodes rhizome), and 12 g of Jin Qian Cao (lysimachia). Use this mixture to make a decoction as described above.

**Acupuncture:** This method of treatment is effective for both acute and chronic cystitis. The course may vary, but it should reduce the burning sensation and frequency of urination.

**Acupressure:** Use the tip of your finger or thumb to press the San Yin Jiao, Zhong Ji, and Hegu points with medium pressure for one minute several times. The San Yin Jiao point is found on the inside of the leg, about 3 inches above the anklebone. The Hegu points are located on the back of the hands between the thumb and first finger. The Zhong Ji point is on the abdomen, 4 inches below the navel.

**Diet:** Fruits such as watermelon, peach, cantaloupe, mango, and lychee are good for treating cystitis.

## NATUROPATHY

**Diet:** One of the best ways to treat cystitis is to increase the amount of times you urinate. Drink a glass of water every hour throughout the day. Cranberry juice has been used for more than a century to prevent and treat urinary tract infections. Evidence suggests that it is the antioxidant flavonoids called proanthocyanidins that prevent bacteria from adhering to the walls of the urinary tract. Cranberry juice should be unsweetened, especially if it is used by people with suppressed immune systems. Drink three 4 oz glasses throughout the day. Eat watermelons, celery, and parsley, which act as natural diuretics and will help flush out infection from the urinary system.

**Supplements:** Vitamin C enhances immune function, inhibits growth of E. coli (the bacteria most commonly responsible for cystitis), and makes urine more acidic so that bacteria cannot grow as easily. Vitamin A also enhances immune function. Take 25,000–50,000 IU of vitamin C and A daily. Pregnant women should not take more than 10,000 IU a day. Take a probiotic product that contains at least four billion active organisms daily to replace helpful bacteria in your gut. This is especially important if you are taking antibiotics, and the probiotics should be taken at least two hours after taking an antibiotic.

**Herbs:** Take 400–500 mg of cranberry in capsule form twice a day to help prevent bacteria from adhering to the bladder wall. D-mannose, taken at 500 mg four times a day, also prevents bacteria from attaching to the urinary tract and the bladder wall. Uva ursi contains arbutin, a chemical known to have antimicrobial activity against E. coli. Take 250 mg of uva ursi in capsule form or 5 ml of the tincture form four times a day. Horsetail is another herb traditionally used to treat urinary tract infections. Take 500 mg or 2 ml of the tincture four times a day. Juniper berry helps increase urination to rid the bladder of bacteria. You can make juniper tea by adding 1 cup of boiling water to 1 tbsp of juniper berries and allowing the berries to steep for 20 minutes. The usual dosage is to drink 1 cup twice a day. A formula that contains this herb along with the other herbs listed may be more effective.

**Hydrotherapy:** A hot sitz bath is a potent therapy for cystitis. Take it at least once a day and add apple cider vinegar or garlic oil for a stronger effect.

## HOMEOPATHY

The following remedies can help to ease the pain and discomfort, and shorten the duration, of an acute episode of cystitis, provided the symptoms fit the remedy as appropriately as possible. Homeopathy can be used as a first line of defense until a medical evaluation is done, but should not be used as an alternative to conventional care. If cystitis becomes a chronic health problem, consult a professional homeopath who will treat the condition at a deeper level.

**Cantharis:** This is the first choice for treating classic symptoms of cystitis, such as burning sensations before, during, and after urinating. When this remedy is helpful there is a constant, distressing urge to pass water, but only a very small amount of urine is passed at a time. Scalding and burning sensations flare up violently and quickly. Symptoms are characteristically soothed by contact with warmth and massage, while moving around and drinking coffee aggravates symptoms.

**Arsenicum album:** This is a strong candidate if burning pains are associated with a sense of being generally chilly, exhausted, and restless when feeling ill. Symptoms include burning sensations while urinating that are temporarily soothed by taking a warm bath and/or applying warm compresses to the affected area. All symptoms tend to feel more intense at night, including shivering, nausea, and anxiety about being ill.

**Staphysagria:** This can be especially helpful in easing cystitis symptoms that set in after any medical procedures involving catheterization. It can also ease symptoms that are triggered by sexual intercourse. Classic symptoms include an unpleasant sensation of being unable to completely empty the bladder. Urine passed appears dark and concentrated, and stinging, burning sensations occur after urinating.

**Sarsaparilla:** If passing urine is most painful as the bladder becomes more empty, try Sarsaparilla. There may also be a tendency for slight urinary incontinence at night, and symptoms are noticeably worse when premenstrual.

**Apis:** Consider this as an option if stinging pains are made even more distressing by contact with heat and warmth. Cool compresses provide some temporary relief from localized burning sensations. Additional symptoms include a tendency to retain fluid or a violent sense of urgency when needing to urinate.

**Pulsatilla:** If an acute episode of cystitis develops after getting chilly and damp, try Pulsatilla. Symptoms tend to be more intense when resting or lying down. Urinary incontinence occurs if you do not urinate when you feel the urge to, or when coughing, sneezing, and/or exercising. Cystitis may be accompanied by yeast infection symptoms.

**TIP:** DO NOT IGNORE THE NEED TO URINATE

If you develop bladder infections easily, always pass water when you feel the need, however busy you may be. Not doing so can encourage an infection to develop.

## HERBALISM

The following herbs can be taken in combination to treat an infectious condition, or may be used separately for their soothing and healing properties.

**Uva ursi:** An astringent and slightly sweet plant, uva ursi increases urination and renal circulation, while acting as a urinary antiseptic. The key constituent, arbutin, is converted to its active component, hydroquinone, in the alkaline environment that uva ursi creates. This herb may tinge the urine green. Take 2 ml of tincture or boil 1 tsp of dried leaf in a cup of water for 30 minutes and drink four times daily. Do not use if pregnant.

**Buchu:** This herb has a sharp, spicy, and bitter taste. It is a urinary tract anti-inflammatory, diuretic, and antiseptic, and also relieves spasms and soothes pelvic nerves. Buchu may turn urine greenish-brown due to the pigmentation of the leaves. Take 20 drops of tincture or infuse 1 tsp in a cup of water and drink four times daily. Do not use if pregnant.

**Marshmallow root:** This sweet, cooling, nutritious plant has polysaccharides and mucilage properties that soothe and ease pain and inflammation in the urinary tract. Take 30 drops of tincture or boil 1 tbsp per cup of water and drink four times daily. Do not take with other medications, as marshmallow may delay their absorption.

**Usnea:** This cooling lichen has antibacterial and antifungal properties. Usnea also relieves spasm pain in the urinary tract, and reduces fever. Take 30 drops of tincture four times daily.

**Corn silk:** Sweet and cooling, corn silk (the silky threads on a kernel of sweet corn) soothes and coats the urinary tract, while also eliminating microbes and encouraging urination. Corn silk is used to treat inflammation of the bladder and kidneys. Infuse 2 tbsp of dried herb in 1 cup of water or take 30 drops of tincture and drink four times daily.

# DEHYDRATION

## DIAGNOSIS

Water accounts for approximately 55% of your body weight. Dehydration occurs when water and important blood salts like potassium are lost from the body. If you are suffering from dehydration, vital organs such as the kidneys, brain, and heart cannot function as they require a certain amount of water and salt to work effectively. Symptoms of dehydration include thirst, dry lips, and a dry mouth. A more serious form of dehydration is indicated by blue lips, a weak pulse, quick breathing, and confusion. There are various triggers for dehydration. In hot weather, the body regulates its temperature to 98.6°F by sweating, which can result in the loss of body fluid, leading to dehydration and heat stroke. Other causes include persistent vomiting or diarrhea as a result of illness, a high fever, and taking drugs that deplete fluids and electrolytes, such as diuretics. You are more at risk of dehydration if you have had a recent illness with a high fever, and if you have diabetes or chronic kidney disease.

## SYMPTOMS

- Dry mouth and tongue
- Reduction in urination
- Scant amounts of strong, dark urine
- Low blood pressure
- Severe thirst
- Increased heart rate and rapid breathing
- Dizziness
- Confusion
- Rarely, coma

## TREATMENT GOAL

To establish the cause of the dehydration and address the symptoms as quickly as possible to rebalance the body.

## CONVENTIONAL MEDICINE

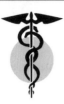

**Prevention:** Dehydration can usually be prevented. Be aware of environments or illnesses that may cause you to become dehydrated, and increase the amount of fluids you take at this time. It is also important to drink plenty of fluids before taking part in a strenuous sporting activity.

**Replace fluids:** Take plenty of liquids and salts to replace the fluids and electrolytes that have been lost. This can be attempted at home unless there is persistent vomiting, diarrhea, dizziness, confusion, or fainting. Medical care must be sought immediately in these cases, and intravenous fluid replacement will be given as well as a diagnosis and treatment of the cause of the dehydration. A Western diet is generally high enough in salt for electrolytes to be obtained by eating and sipping water slowly. This fluid intake should be slow, but constant until symptoms of dehydration, such as dark urine, are resolved. In the early stages of dehydration, sports drinks such as Gatorade™ can be used.

**Oral rehydration solution:** These are available over the counter and should be mixed with water as directed. They can be taken even if diarrhea and vomiting persist. A home oral rehydration solution can be mixed with sugar, salt, and baking soda. This makes a solution very similar to the intravenous fluids administered at a hospital for dehydration. Mix 1 liter of filtered water, 2 tbsp of sugar, ½ tsp of salt, ¼ tsp of potassium chloride, and ½ tsp of baking soda. The solution should be sipped throughout the day until the urine returns to a normal color and urination occurs four to five times a day.

**Intravenous fluids:** If symptoms persist, intravenous fluids containing saltwater (saline solution) at 9% and sometimes other electrolytes and glucose will be given. A doctor will assess the cause of the dehydration, and begin treating any underlying illness as necessary.

## TRADITIONAL CHINESE MEDICINE

For severe dehydration, you should seek emergency medical help.

**Herbs:** To treat acute or severe dehydration, the Chinese medicine formula "Shen Mai Yin" is designed to quickly support body energy and regain the balance. Use the following herbs, available from Chinese pharmacies, to make a tea: 10 g of fresh or 5 g of dried American ginseng, 10 g of Mai Men Dong (ophiopogon tuber), and 3 g of Gan Cao (licorice). Slice the fresh ginseng and put all the herbs in a teapot. Add boiling water and let the mixture steep for 5–10 minutes. Drink the tea as well as liquids that contain electrolytes.

**Acupuncture:** Treatment can support body energy and the flow of body fluids. Dehydration can be caused by various reasons and treating the cause is the key to successfully resolving the condition, no matter which type of therapy you choose.

**Acupressure:** For dehydrated patients who feel weak and dizzy, the Ren Zhong point is helpful. This point is usually used in emergencies to help coma patients regain consciousness. It can be found in the center of the depression between the base of the nose and the upper lip. Press this point with the tip of your finger or thumb with strong pressure for one minute. Repeat two to three times.

**Diet:** Eat fresh fruit such as bananas, watermelon, peach, cantaloupe, apples, mango, and grapefruit. Watermelon and bananas are particularly good.

## NATUROPATHY

Call a doctor if you are concerned about severe dehydration.

**Diet:** Drink a glass of water every hour throughout the day to rebalance the body. You may want to add an electrolyte liquid, sold in most health food stores, to replenish sodium, chloride, and potassium. Drink a fortified drink like Gatorade™ if you are participating in vigorous physical activity, such as a sporting event, or have prolonged fever or diarrhea. Sports drinks can help replenish electrolytes lost by the body in such situations. Avoid caffeine and alcohol, which cause dehydration by inducing urination. Eat five to seven servings of fruit and vegetables every day. Most fruits and vegetables contain at least 70–90% water. They can also provide you with important vitamins and minerals. Excessive consumption of simple carbohydrates and sugars may cause dehydration, so limit your intake of these substances.

## HOMEOPATHY

Because dehydration can constitute a medical emergency (especially in the very young and the elderly), the first priority is to rehydrate the patient as quickly as possible. Once the body's fluid balance is back to normal, the following remedies can help to ease any feelings of trauma that may remain after being so unwell. See Food Poisoning (p. 382), Diarrhea (p.366), and Vomiting (p.489), which can trigger dehydration due to loss of body fluids, for additional remedy suggestions.

**China:** This can be restorative where weakness has followed a case of dehydration, even though rehydration has been completely successful. Along with a profound sense of physical exhaustion there is a distressing, nervous hypersensitivity when exposed to sensory stimulation (such as loud noise and bright lights).

**Aconite:** Consider this remedy to treat the psychological effects of a traumatic illness when, after the event, the patient is left with a sense of extreme panic and a fear of death. Feelings of terror and panic escalate on waking.

## HERBALISM

 Common causes of dehydration include heat exhaustion, diarrhea, vomiting, and chronic conditions such as diabetes and kidney disease. Dehydration is a potentially serious condition and any person at risk should be monitored.

**Fennel seed and peppermint leaf tea:** Rehydration is typically carried out by reintroducing water with electrolytes. The World Health Organization (WHO) recommends the following combination in cases of severe dehydration: Mix 1 liter of filtered water, 2 tbsp of sugar, ½ tsp of salt, ¼ tsp of potassium chloride, and ½ tsp of baking soda. These can be added to a tea of fennel seed and peppermint leaves. The seeds of fennel are full of flavor and are helpful for treating diarrhea. Fennel's carminative action soothes the stomach, allowing the retention of fluids. Peppermint counteracts nausea and vomiting, and soothes irritated and inflamed tissues, especially in the digestive system. Both herbs are very gentle and well-tolerated. Infuse 1 tbsp of each herb in 1 liter of water and sip throughout the day.

**Carob:** This herb is used to treat diarrhea, chronic gastrointestinal conditions such as celiac disease, other nutritional disorders, and vomiting, which can all lead to dehydration. Carob is a very safe and gentle herb that works to replace electrolytes. Studies have found that it is most effective and tolerable when taken as carob bean juice.

**Oats:** Oat is calming and nutritious, and contains small levels of zinc, manganese, calcium, and magnesium, which help to restore electrolyte balance in the body. Infuse 1 tbsp of oat seeds per cup of water or take 2 ml of tincture in water three times daily.

**Marshmallow and chamomile:** Both these herbs have antispasmodic and anti-inflammatory properties that soothe the membranes of the digestive system. Marshmallow contains various sugars, mucilage, starches, and antioxidants, which make it nutritious as well. Boil 1 tbsp of marshmallow root per cup of water, or take 1–2 ml of tincture in water, and infuse 1 tbsp of chamomile flowers per cup of water. Drink three times daily.

# DIABETES

## DIAGNOSIS

Diabetes mellitus is a condition in which the amount of glucose (sugar) in the blood becomes too high because the body cannot process it properly due to insufficient levels of insulin or cellular resistance to insulin. Glucose is produced by the digestion of starchy foods, such as bread, rice, and potatoes, and sugar and other sweet foods, and by the liver. Insulin is a vital hormone produced by the pancreas that helps the body process glucose to be used as fuel. Blood sugar levels that are not regulated, and abnormally high levels of glucose in the blood due to lack of insulin, can lead to a range of problems including impaired circulation.

There are two main types of diabetes. Type 1 develops when the body is unable to produce insulin. This type usually manifests before the age of 40. It is treated by insulin injections, and a diet overhaul and regular exercise are also recommended. With Type 2 the body can still produce some insulin, but not enough, or it produces insulin that cannot exert its effects due to insulin resistance. This type of diabetes is often linked to being overweight and usually appears in people over the age of 40, although it can affect younger people in the South Asian and African-Caribbean communities. Recently, more children are also being diagnosed with the Type 2 condition, some as young as seven. Type 2 diabetes is treated with lifestyle changes such as a healthier diet and weight loss.

## SYMPTOMS

- Frequent urination
- Excessive thirst
- Extreme tiredness
- Weight loss
- Smell of nail polish (acetone) on the breath
- Thrush
- Blurred vision

## TREATMENT GOAL

The main aim of treatment of both types of diabetes is to maintain blood glucose, blood pressure, and cholesterol levels as near to normal as possible. This, together with a healthy lifestyle, will help to improve wellbeing and protect against long-term damage to the body's major organs.

## CONVENTIONAL MEDICINE

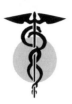

**To treat Type 1 diabetes:** Those with Type 1 diabetes require insulin as none is produced by the pancreas. The amount of insulin needed varies and must be administered several times a day. The insulin pump has been a major advance in improving glucose control in Type 1 or brittle diabetics. The prevention of both low and high blood sugar levels is very important to avoid the complications of diabetes, and blood glucose levels must be checked at least once a day with insulin-dependent diabetes, preferably before each dose of insulin. The dose is adjusted according to exercise levels and food intake, as both of these factors affect the blood sugar. Monitoring the diet for calories, carbohydrates, fat, and protein is also essential. The body's requirements vary according to height, weight, and age, but generally calorie requirements are between 15 and 25 calories per pound of body weight per day. Your diet should be made up of 55% carbohydrates (as whole grains, fruits, and vegetables, not processed food), 25% fat (monounsaturated), and about 20% protein, such as fish, chicken, and vegetable proteins.

**To treat Type 2 diabetes:** This condition initially results when the insulin produced by the body does not work appropriately (known as insulin resistance). It is associated with obesity, and the illness can be prevented by modifying your lifestyle. Studies show that, compared to managing the condition through medication, lifestyle modification more successfully controls sugar levels and the complications of diabetes. Following the diet above, keeping the body mass index under 28, exercising, reducing stress, and keeping alcohol intake to a minimum are usually enough to ensure prevention. At the first signs of insulin resistance, begin a weight loss program, swap carbs for complex, low glycemic index foods (whole grains and fruits and vegetables), and exercise (for example, fast walking) at least 20 minutes a day. The minerals chromium and vanadium are helpful for this condition as are several herbs, fenugreek and cinnamon in particular. Medications used for Type 2 diabetes include several groups of blood-sugar-lowering drugs, such as the sulfonylureas, the biguanides, the glucosidase inhibitors, the thiaxolidinediones, and the meglitinides. Each medication acts in a different way and a doctor will choose the most appropriate one according to the history of illness, other medications being taken, and other diseases suffered. Type 2 diabetes is monitored by family physicians.

**Complications of diabetes:** Each type of diabetes predisposes a person to complications, including cardiac, renal, and neurologic problems, infections, retinal damage in the eyes, and high cholesterol and triglycerides. Those with diabetes should be regularly checked for these complications and referred to a specialist as needed. Most of the associated problems can be prevented by keeping the blood sugar level in a normal range.

# TRADITIONAL CHINESE MEDICINE

Historically, Chinese medicine descriptions of diabetes are much the same as those of Western medicine. Diabetes occurs most commonly in those who have a deficiency of yin. It is often caused by improper diet, emotional disturbance, stress, and exhaustion.

**Herbs:** The herbs listed can be found in Chinese herbal stores. **Caution**: The suggested formulas are best used after consulting with a Chinese medicine doctor. For severe cases of diabetes, and particularly Type 2 diabetes, Chinese medicine treatment can be integrated with Western medicine, but it is not a replacement for conventional medication, and you may also need to use insulin. Consult your doctor before integrating treatments.

• Formula one: This can be used to treat either Type 1 or Type 2 diabetes. Symptoms of dryness in the mouth and on the tongue, thirst, frequent urination, dizziness, and vertigo are usually diagnosed as an insufficiency of kidney yin. Combine 12 g of Bei Mao Gen (wooly grass rhizome), 10 g of Yu Mi Xu (corn silk), 12 g of Xuan Shen (ningpo figwort root), 12 g of Di Huang (Chinese foxglove), 10 g of Shan Zhu Yu (Asiatic cornelian cherry fruit), 12 g of Tian Men Dong (asparagus tuber), and 12 g of Wu Wei Zi (schisandra fruit) with 3–4 cups of water in a ceramic or glass pot. Bring to the boil and simmer for 30 minutes. Strain the liquid and drink 1 cup two to three times a day.

• Formula two: This can be used to treat either Type 1 or Type 2 diabetes. Symptoms include overheating and emotional disturbance, fever, perspiration, anxiety, irritability, anger, constipation, strong thirst, and a yellow, dry tongue. Place 12 g of Zhi Zi (Cape Jasmine fruit), 12 g of Yu Zhu (atractylodes rhizome), 10 g of Huang Qin (baical skullcap root), 12 g of Tian Hua Fen (trichosanthes root), 10 g of Chai Hu (hare's ear root), 12 g of Zhi Mu (anemarrhena rhizome), and 12 g Dan Pi (cortex of tree peony root) in a ceramic pot and add 3–4 cups of water. Bring the mixture to a boil, simmer for 30 minutes, and strain the liquid. Drink this decoction twice a day.

**Acupuncture:** Treatment is beneficial for diabetes in its early or later stages. It is also effective in treating complications. Consult a practitioner regarding the benefits.

**Acupressure:** Using gentle to moderate pressure on the Nei Guan, Shan Yin Jiao, and Tai Xi points is useful for diabetes. The Nei Guan point is located in the center of the wrist on the palm side about 2 inches below the crease. The San Yin Jiao point is on the inside of the leg, about 3 inches above the anklebone. The Tai Xi point is also on the inside of the leg in the depression between the Achilles tendon and the anklebone.

**Diet:** Recommended foods include spinach, turnip, balsam pears, wax gourd, millet, Chinese yam, water chestnuts, duck, goose, rabbit, and cow's milk. Avoid fatty food, alcohol, and spicy food, along with foods high in sugar.

**TIP:** EXERCISE REGULARLY

Exercise regularly to maintain optimal blood sugar levels. Exercise helps reduce weight and lowers blood sugar. It improves insulin sensitivity, the immune system, and circulation. It lowers blood pressure and LDL ("bad") cholesterol, raises HDL ("good") cholesterol, and reduces the risk of heart disease. Find an exercise that you like and try to do at least four sessions a week.

## NATUROPATHY

**Diet:** The most important therapy for diabetes is a healthy diet. Eat plenty of vegetables, beans, nuts, seeds, and whole grains. The high fiber in these foods helps balance blood sugar. Ground flaxseeds should be eaten on a daily basis as well. Sprinkle 2 tbsp on your cereal or salad. Do not expose the flaxseeds to too much heat. Focus on good fats found in foods such as salmon and sardines. Use extra virgin olive oil and flaxseed oil on your salad. Refrain from eating large meals throughout the day. Instead, frequently eat small meals that consist of some good quality protein. Do not go for longer than three hours without eating. Avoid eating simple sugars, including junk foods like sweets, cookies, and carbonated drinks. These foods contribute to blood sugar instability. Avoid cow's milk. Some studies show a link between cow's milk and diabetes in children. Use stevia or xylitol as a sweetener, which are safe for diabetics and are healthier choices.

**Supplements:** Take a high-quality multivitamin as directed to obtain many of the nutrients involved with blood sugar metabolism. Take 200–400 mcg of chromium a day to improve glucose metabolism and balance blood sugar levels. Take 300–600 mg of alpha lipoic acid a day to improve insulin sensitivity and reduce the symptoms of diabetic neuropathy. Vanadyl sulfate improves glucose tolerance; take 100–300 mg a day. Take 3 g of fish oils a day to support the nervous system and assist in proper insulin function. B-complex vitamins are involved in glucose metabolism, and should be taken at 50 mg a day. Biotin, taken at 7,000–15,000 mcg a day, reduces the changes of diabetic neuropathies. This is a B vitamin so consider the amount included in your B-complex vitamin and adjust the dosage accordingly. You can also take 500 mg of magnesium, involved in insulin production and utilization, a day. Reduce the dosage if your stools soften.

**Herbs:** Bitter melon helps balance blood sugar levels. The typical dosage of bitter melon is one small, unripe, raw melon a day, or about 50–100 ml of fresh juice, divided into two or three doses over the course of the day. Bitter melon tastes unpleasant to some, and can be taken in capsule form at 200 mg three times a day. Billberry helps prevent problems with the retinas caused by diabetes. The standard dosage of bilberry is 120–240 mg of an extract standardized to contain 25% anthocyanosides twice a day. Taking 15–30 g of defatted fenugreek three times a day with meals stabilizes blood sugar. Fenugreek seeds are bitter so the herb is best taken in capsule form. Banana leaf has also been shown to lower blood sugar levels. Take 16 mg in capsule form twice a day.

## HOMEOPATHY

Diabetes is a condition for which it is inappropriate to suggest self-help homeopathic prescribing, since both Type 1 and Type 2 diabetes are chronic conditions. As such, any homeopathic treatment that is given will be of a constitutional nature and needs to be provided by an experienced homeopathic practitioner.

## HERBALISM

Herbal medicines used to treat diabetes generally aim to lower blood sugar, protect vascular integrity, and preserve the function of the pancreas. Insulin and other diabetic agents may need to be adjusted if herbal remedies are used in a complementary manner, because of many herbs' hypoglycemic effect. All recommended herbs are safe for both Type 1 and Type 2 diabetics.

**Gymnema:** This woody plant, also called urine honey, was traditionally used to treat diabetes long before its positive results were discovered in clinical trials. Gymnema discourages sugar consumption by inhibiting the taste of sugar placed on the tongue. Studies have also shown that gymnema effectively lowers blood sugar when taken at 400 mg per day. Current research shows that gymnema increases insulin levels or decreases insulin sensitivity, possibly indicating that it regenerates pancreatic beta-cells (insulin-secreting cells). Take 400 mg in capsule form or 5 ml of tincture daily.

**Bitter melon:** The fruit and seeds of bitter melon contain charantin, polypeptide P, and vicine, which are thought to contribute to its hypoglycemic effect. Take 50 mg or 3 ml of tincture daily. Do not use if pregnant.

**Fenugreek:** This herb slows carbohydrate absorption, delays gastric emptying, and increases insulin receptors, all of which have blood sugar lowering effects. In most clinical trials, patients took 50 mg per day to achieve significant effects. Do not use if pregnant.

# DIARRHEA

## DIAGNOSIS

Diarrhea occurs when the mucous membrane lining the intestinal walls becomes irritated and inflamed, causing stool content to pass through too quickly, absorbing a lot of liquid with it. It is usually accompanied by abdominal pains, malaise, nausea, and vomiting. In some cases some blood may also be passed.

Diarrhea is often caused by a virus or bacteria passed from person to person. Simple hygiene measures such as washing your hands with soap and water after using the toilet can help prevent the disease spreading. Diarrhea can be acute (short term, which tends to be caused by anxiety, food poisoning, and medicine such as antibiotics), which generally lasts around 24 hours. It can also be chronic (long term, which is usually a sign of an intestinal disorder such as irritable bowel syndrome, ulcerative colitis, and Crohn's disease), which can last more than two weeks. Those with chronic diarrhea, especially with blood mixed in, should seek medical help immediately. Diarrhea can also be a symptom of an intolerance to food, such as lactose and gluten intolerance. Children can get diarrhea from having too much fruit, fruit juice, or cold foods and drinks.

## SYMPTOMS

- Loose, watery stools/liquid feces
- Frequent bowel movements
- Loss of appetite
- Unpleasant-smelling stools
- Stomach cramps
- Bloating and flatulence
- Nausea and vomiting
- Fever
- Dehydration—symptoms include small amounts of dark urine, drowsiness, and thirst. Dehydration as a result of diarrhea is a particular risk for young children and the elderly

## TREATMENT GOAL

To establish the cause of the diarrhea and take measures to control symptoms and rehydrate the body.

## CONVENTIONAL MEDICINE

To treat diarrhea, conventional medicine focuses on rehydrating the body and getting nutrition levels back to normal. Wash your hands thoroughly and avoid preparing food while ill to prevent the spread of infection.

**Rehydrate the body:** Taking an oral rehydration solution has been shown to be as effective as intravenous therapy in rehydrating the body. To make a solution mix 1 quart of a liter of clean, filtered water with 2 tbsp of sugar and 1/2 tsp each of baking soda and salt. The solution is appropriate for both adults and children and should be sipped continuously throughout the day.

**Diet:** Eat soft complex carbohydrates such as bananas, rice, potatoes, and toast. Drink black tea as it is a natural antidiarrheal. Fruits and vegetables (except those mentioned above) should be excluded from your diet, as should sugary processed foods, dairy products, and fatty foods. Infants may continue to breastfeed, but breast milk should be supplemented with oral rehydration fluid as described above. Probiotics (beneficial bacteria that live in the gut) may be given as a supplement. Some botanical formulas containing mallow licorice and black walnut can be helpful in re-establishing a healthy gut during or immediately after an episode of diarrhea.

**Medication:** Do not give infants or small children over-the-counter or prescription antidiarrheal medications. Loperamide (Lomotil™), Kaopectate™, Imodium™, and bismuth subsalicylate (Pepto Bismol™) may be used in adults and children aged 12 and over as directed, but never for longer than three days.

**Complications:** There is cause for concern if diarrhea is accompanied by light headedness, a high fever, severe abdominal pain, blood and mucus in the stool, or if the diarrhea lasts for more than three days. In any of these cases, an examination of the abdomen and tests of the stool for bacteria, parasites, and blood are carried out. Sometimes liver and kidney testing is also done. Intravenous rehydration is usually given. Extreme care should be taken when diarrhea affects the very young and the very old as these two groups are particularly susceptible to dehydration.

## TRADITIONAL CHINESE MEDICINE

In traditional Chinese medicine, the pathogenic factors of diarrhea include summer heat, dampness, and cold. Improper diet and drinking, deficiency in spleen, stomach, and kidney, and emotional disorders are some other causes of diarrhea.

**Herbs:** The herbal formulas below can help treat diarrhea. Place the herbs in a glass or ceramic pot and add 3–4 cups. Bring to the boil and simmer for 30 minutes. Drink 1 cup twice a day. These herbs should be available from Chinese herbal stores.

• To treat acute diarrhea: Symptoms include clear and diluted stools. Combine 12 g of Ge Geng (kudzu root), 6 g of Chen Pi (tangerine peel), 12 g of Cang Zhu (atractylodes rhizome), 10 g of Hou Po (magnolia bark), 5 g of Gan Cao (licorice), and 5 g of fresh ginger.

• To treat diarrhea due to dampness and heat: Symptoms include yellow-brown stools, abdominal pain, a burning sensation in the anus, thirst, and small amounts of yellow urine. Mix 12 g of Bai Shao (white peony root), 5 g of Huang Lian (coptis root), 10 g of Huang Qin (baical skullcap root), and 10 g of Bai Tou Wong (Chinese anemone root).

• To treat diarrhea due to food poisoning: Symptoms include undigested food mixed with stools, abdominal pain, foul belching, and a dirty, sticky, and coated tongue. Mix 10 g of Shen Qu (massa fermentata), 10 g of Shan Zha (hawthorn fruit), 5 g of Chen Pi (tangerine peel), 10 g of Lai Fu Zi (radish seeds), 12 g of Fuling (poria), and 10 g Lian Qiao (forsythia fruit).

• To treat chronic diarrhea due to spleen deficiency: Symptoms include poor appetite, belching, abdominal distention and pain. Combine 10 g of American ginseng, 12 g of Bai Zhu (white atractylodes rhizome), 12 g of Fuling (poria), 15 g of Shan Yao (Chinese yam), 5 g of Sheng Ma (bugbane rhizome), and 3 g of Gan Cao (licorice).

• To treat diarrhea due to emotional upset: Symptoms include pain in the stomach, sticky stools, anxiety or depression, poor appetite, and belching. Mix 10 g of Chai Hu (hare's ear root), 8 g of Bo He (field mint), 10 g of Mu Xiang (costus root), 12 g of Bai Shao (white peony root), 8 g of Zhi Ke (bitter orange), and 3 g Gan Cao (licorice).

**Acupuncture:** This can be used to treat all types of diarrhea to reduce abdominal pain and the frequency of bowel movements. You can also have acupuncture treatment to address chronic diarrhea. Treatment courses vary depending upon your condition and the stage of the diarrhea.

**Acupressure:** In a sitting position, press the Hegu, Guan Yuan, and Susanli acupressure points for one minute two to three times a day. The Hegu points are located on the back of the hands between the thumb and first finger. The Guan Yuan point is on the abdomen, about 3 inches below the navel. The Susanli point is on the lower leg, 1 inch to the outside of and 3 inches below the kneecap.

**Diet:** Foods those are easy to digest, such as gruel, buckwheat, noodles, and rice are recommended. Avoid foods that are too fibrous or greasy. Avoid raw and cold foods such as celery, Chinese chives, soy, and bean shoots because they are difficult to digest. Also avoid cold drinks and baked foods.

## NATUROPATHY

**Diet:** It is critical to stay hydrated. Drink eight to 12 oz of water throughout the day. In acute cases do not eat solid foods if you do not want to, but stay hydrated with water, soups, vegetable juices, sports drinks with electrolytes, and broths. Try a few tbsp of carob powder in water. This has been shown to reduce the duration of diarrhea.

**Supplements:** Take a probiotic product containing at least 4 billion active organisms of Lactobacillus acidophilus and bifidus a day to help with digestion and fight infection. Saccahromyces has been shown to be effective in treating diarrhea caused by antibiotic use. Take 1,000–3,000 mg of L-glutamine, an amino acid that repairs the gut, three times a day. Lactase enzymes help to digest dairy sugars. Take two with each meal that may contain dairy. Avoid magnesium and vitamin C during active episodes of diarrhea, as they can contribute to the condition.

**Herbs:** Ginger decreases intestinal inflammation. Take 500 mg in capsule form and/or 1–2 cups of ginger tea a day. Goldenseal kills many micro-organisms that may cause diarrhea and helps improve digestion. Marshmallow root is soothing to the digestive tract. Take 500 mg in capsule form three times a day. Drink 3 cups of slippery elm tea each day, or take 500 mg in capsule form every three days, for its soothing effect on the intestines. Red raspberry has traditionally been used to relieve symptoms of diarrhea. To make raspberry leaf tea, pour 1 cup of boiling water over 1–2 tsp of dried leaf. Let the herb steep for 10 minutes, then sweeten to taste. Raspberry leaf generally has a very pleasant taste. In capsule form take 5–10 g daily.

## HOMEOPATHY

The following homeopathic advice can be invaluable in helping to clear up a recent, mild bout of diarrhea that has been triggered by an obvious cause, such as eating something suspect, or feeling tense and anxious. Chronic diarrhea should be treated by a homeopathic practitioner.

**Podophyllum:** If diarrhea is watery and produces little or no pain or cramps, consider Podophyllum. There is a feeling of profound weakness after emptying the bowels, and a very loud gurgling in the gut precedes an episode of diarrhea. Liquid stools are triggered by eating too much fruit or drinking an excessive amount of milk.

**Gelsemium:** To treat painless diarrhea that is brought on by feelings of anxiety and stress, use Gelsemium. Liquid stools are likely to be accompanied by dizzy, faint sensations with an accompanying feeling of exhaustion and heaviness in the limbs. The eyes may take on a heavy, droopy look, while the patient becomes introverted, pre-occupied, and withdrawn thinking about the trigger.

**Carbo veg:** If diarrhea is combined with an unusual amount of trapped wind and gas, with severe, cramping pains accompanying a bowel movement, consider this remedy. Frequent episodes of diarrhea lead to a profound feeling of exhaustion and weakness to the point of being on the verge of collapse. During or after a bout of diarrhea the complexion may become very pale, while the skin may feel cold and clammy to the touch. Contact with fresh air or fanning is reviving, while being in a stuffy, airless room intensifies the sensation of feeling ill.

**Sulphur:** This is a potential candidate if diarrhea is particularly urgent after waking. The diarrhea is especially watery, gushing, and frequent, and leaves the anus feeling sore, raw, and inflamed, and possibly irritated and itchy. As a result, you may put off going to the toilet until the last possible moment, so that involuntary bowel movements sometimes take place. Contact with heat in any form makes discomfort and distress worse.

**Arsenicum album:** If diarrhea is accompanied by a sense of being chilled to the bone and shivery, and if there is a profound sense of restlessness, exhaustion, and anxiety when feeling ill, use Arsenicum album. Burning pains in the digestive tract are temporarily soothed by taking small sips of warm drinks.

**Veratrum album:** If bouts of diarrhea lead to a state of near collapse as a result of cramping pains and straining to clear the bowel, try Veratrum album. The skin takes on a pale appearance and is also likely to feel cold and clammy to the touch. There is also likely to be an unquenchable thirst for long drinks of cold water. Unusually, the appetite is unaffected during a bout of diarrhea.

## HERBALISM

Treatment depends on the cause of the diarrhea. For example, the most effective plants will differ according to whether the diarrhea is caused by a viral infection such as gastroenteritis, irritable bowel syndrome, inflammatory bowel disease, or a food intolerance or allergy. Nonetheless, there are some plants that can be helpful in calming the symptoms of diarrhea until the underlying cause is addressed.

**Astringents:** This class of plants contains compounds called tannins that, when they come into contact with tissue, either skin, or intestinal mucosa, cause drying and healing. In this way, plants with tannins can lessen the loss of water through the intestines. Tannins do not address the underlying cause of the diarrhea, and in cases of food poisoning or infection, when the diarrhea may actually help to rid the body of harmful substances, the overuse of astringents could worsen the problem. One common astringent is carob pod, which can ease the frequency and volume of diarrhea. Add 2 g of a powder to food every two hours to mask the taste and make it easier to take. Raspberry leaf, and the stronger root, both can serve as astringents. Raspberry is best taken as an infusion (leaf) or decoction (root). Bilberry leaf and fruit also serve to calm diarrhea via their tannins. The berries should be dried, powdered, and boiled to make a strong tea, which acts like a laxative. Other astringents occasionally used for diarrhea are agrimony, tormentil, and silverweed.

**Goldenseal:** Use this to treat diarrhea that is presumed to be from an infection in the intestines. The root is most commonly used in tincture form and the antibacterial effects are thought to be primarily due to the alkaloid compound, berberine, that it contains. There are a variety of dosages recommended, including 500–1,000 mg of a capsule three times a day, or 2–4 ml of a 1:10 tincture in 60% ethanol three times a day. Goldenseal is still a threatened plant in its natural habitat due to over harvesting, so any goldenseal product purchased should be from companies that cultivate it or obtain it from growers.

# DIVERTICULITIS

## DIAGNOSIS

Diverticulae are small balloon-like pouches that form in the wall of the large intestine, probably as a result of spasms in the muscle. They rarely occur in those under the age of 40, but become more common as people get older. It is thought that the small pockets may represent natural weak points in the bowel wall that are present from birth, and that develop over time as a result of the natural build-up of pressure that occurs in the intestine, particularly when straining to pass gas or stools. Often they are harmless, do not cause symptoms, and the person with diverticula may not even realize they have them. The problems start if blockages or ruptures develop, leading to inflammation and infection. These can develop into the condition known as diverticulitis. Diagnosis is usually made by endoscopy (looking into the bowel through a camera), barium enema X-ray, or by excluding other causes of the symptoms.

**DANGER**: Occasionally the diverticulae can rupture, allowing fluid to leak into the abdominal cavity, which can cause peritonitis.

## SYMPTOMS

- Sudden intense abdominal pain
- Pain and tenderness in the left lower part of the abdomen (though diverticula can cause symptoms throughout the abdomen, the left lower part is by far the most common area affected)
- Fever and nausea
- Rectal bleeding
- Constipation and diarrhea
- Bouts of pain that last several days

## TREATMENT GOAL

Assessing the extent of the problem and making lifestyle changes to help ease and improve the pain associated with the condition.

## CONVENTIONAL MEDICINE

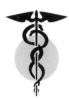

Diverticulosis is an inflammation of the lining of the colon. Diverticulitis occurs when this condition progresses and the area becomes infected. Treatment for diverticulitis involves complete bowel rest, meaning a fluid-only diet until symptoms resolve, as well as antibiotic therapy. Hydration is also essential.

**Antibiotics:** Generally, antibiotic therapy is given intravenously or orally for about 10 days. Ciprofloxacin (Cipro™) is the antibiotic most commonly used, unless peritonitis (an infection of the lining of the abdominal cavity) is suspected, in which case gentamycin or a combination of several antibiotic medications is used.

**Pain relief:** Hyoscyamine, which is prescribed, may be helpful in relieving spasms. Sometimes strong pain relief is also necessary, and this too is determined by a medical examination.

**Blood transfusion:** Occasionally there is severe blood loss and sometimes a blood transfusion is necessary.

**Surgery:** Conservative therapies may be completely effective, and are generally effective in 70% of cases or more. However, complicated or severe conditions may require surgery. For example, if there is a perforation of the bowel, emergency surgery is necessary. This illness is a serious condition and treatment is immediate and aggressive. For cases that do not respond to the medical therapy described above, surgical options are available. Most surgery is laparoscopic (performed with a fiber-optic device). Sometimes a resection of the diseased bowel is performed.

## TRADITIONAL CHINESE MEDICINE

**Herbs:** The herbs listed below are available from Chinese pharmacies and online. To prepare either of the herbal formulas, put the herbs in a ceramic pot, add 3 cups of water, bring to the boil, and simmer for 35 minutes. Drink 1 cup twice a day.

• To treat the heat and dampness type of diverticulitis: Mix 5 g of Huang Lian (coptis root), 10 g of Bai Tou Weng (Chinese anemone root), 10 g of Zi Hua Di Din (Yedeon's violet), and 10 g of Zhi Zi (Cape Jasmine flower).

• To threat Qi and blood stagnation: Mix 12 g of Bai Tou Weng (Chinese anemone root), 12 g of Chi Shao (red peony root), 10 g of Mu Xiang (costus root), and 12 g of Di Yu (burnet-bloodwort root).

• To treat deficiency in spleen and stomach: Take the patent herbal pill Bu Zhong Yi Qi Wan according to the instructions on the label.

**Acupuncture:** Treatment reduces pain and cleans the pathogenic toxin out of the body, as well as helping the body's immune system. You may have treatment twice a week; 10 –12 sessions are recommended as a course and you may need one to three courses.

**Acupressure:** Use gentle to moderate pressure on the Guan Yuan and Nei Guan points for a few minutes at a time. The Guan Yuan point is on the abdomen, about 3 inches below the navel. The Nei Guan is located in the center of the wrist on the palm side, about 2 inches below the crease.

**Diet:** Eat foods that are heat-clearing and cooling such as watermelon, spinach, mung beans, tangerines, string beans, and grapefruit. Avoid foods that are hot and spicy.

## NATUROPATHY

**Diet:** A high-fiber diet, including lots of fruits and vegetables, whole grains, and cereals, is the most important naturopathic treatment for this disease. Avoid eating processed food. Substitute whole grain bread for white, and eat an apple instead of drinking a glass of apple juice. Take psyllium seed bulking agents, following the directions on the packet and taking with plenty of water. Avoid becoming constipated and, if you do, do not use laxatives but instead increase your psyllium and water intake or add bran to your diet. Avoid eating those seeds, nuts, and foods with hard particles that could become lodged in the diverticular sacs, such as strawberries, figs, tomatoes, zucchini, cucumbers, and baked goods that have cracked wheat, poppy, sesame, or caraway seeds. Try prunes and prune juice if you are having difficulty moving your bowels. Drink plenty of fluids every day, including around six to eight glasses of water.

**Herbs:** Flax is a good source of high-quality fiber. Use 1–3 tbsp of crushed flaxseed sprinkled in your food, but do not cook the seeds. Powdery, high-fiber psyllium seeds are the major ingredient in Metamucil™ and a few other bulk-forming commercial laxatives. A few tbsp a day (with plenty of water) provide a healthy amount of diverticulitis-preventing fiber. However, if you develop allergic symptoms after taking psyllium seeds discontinue their use. Glucomannan is a dietary fiber derived from the tubers of Amorphophallus konjac. Take 3–5 g in capsule form a day in divided doses before meals. Glucomannan may cause excess gas, stomach distension, or mild diarrhea. Eat more pineapple and papaya for their potent digestive enzymes that will help reduce inflammation. These symptoms usually abate within a couple of days of treatment, or with a reduction in the dosage. Chamomile is particularly valuable in treating diverticulitis because its anti-inflammatory action soothes the entire digestive system. To make a tea, let 2 tsp of dried chamomile steep in a cup of boiling water for five to 10 minutes. Proteolytic enzymes aid in digestion and reduce inflammation of the colon. Take one or two enzyme pills between meals.

## HOMEOPATHY

Diverticulosis is a condition that is best managed by professional homeopathic treatment, especially if it is administered within the context of an integrated medical approach. This would allow for the exploration of lifestyle factors that can help or hinder the condition, such as your dietary and nutritional status. Conventional medical input will also be a priority if the condition progresses to diverticulitis. This is a more acute phase of underlying diverticular problems, and can give rise to pain and nausea. Any of the remedies for diarrhea may be helpful within the context of complementary help, provided the patient is also receiving conventional medical assessment and treatment (also see Diarrhea, p. 369).

**Podophyllum:** If diarrhea is watery and produces little or no pain or cramps, consider Podophyllum. There is a feeling of profound weakness after emptying the bowels, and a very loud gurgling in the gut precedes an episode of diarrhea.

**Carbo veg:** If diarrhea is combined by an unusual amount of trapped gas, with severe, cramping pains accompanying a bowel movement, consider this remedy. Frequent episodes of diarrhea lead to feeling of exhausted and weak to the point of being on the verge of collapse. During or after a bout of diarrhea the complexion may become very pale, while the skin may feel cold and clammy to the touch. Contact with fresh air or fanning is reviving, while being in a stuffy, airless room intensifies the sensation of feeling ill.

**Arsenicum album:** If diarrhea is accompanied by a sense of being chilled to the bone and shivery, and if there is a profound sense of restlessness, exhaustion, and anxiety when feeling ill, use Arsenicum album. Burning pains in the digestive tract are temporarily soothed by taking small sips of warm drinks.

## HERBALISM

Those with diverticulitis generally require antibiotics. Herbal medicines should primarily be used in conjunction with conventional therapy.

**Slippery elm:** There is evidence that diverticulosis, which is the condition that can lead to diverticulitis, occurs at higher rates in people who have a low-fiber diet. It may be possible to prevent diverticulosis from developing by taking adequate amounts of fiber daily. If you or family members have diverticulosis, it is a good idea to take herbs, except for those that have seeds, to obtain amounts of fiber that are above and beyond the regular nutritional intake. In treating diverticular disease, slippery elm serves two purposes. First, it is a mucilaginous coating agent that soothes the inflamed colonic tissue and helps to promote healing. Also, it provides a gentle, non-seed based fiber supplement to help keep bowel movements regular and decrease the chance of worsening already-present diverticula or the development of new ones.

**Solomon's seal:** Also known as Fo-ti, Chinese cornblind, climbing knootwee, and seal root, Soloman's seal is another gentle laxative useful for treating diverticular disease. This plant is usually ingested as a tea made from 3–5 g of herbs three times daily or in capsule form at 500 mg three times daily. It may also help to improve the connective tissue, defects in which can lead to the formation of diverticula. The use of Solomon's seal is associated with many side effects such as low potassium, dermatitis, and stomach irritation, so use with care and under the guidance of a medical herbalist.

**Other herbs:** Depending on symptoms, other herbs can be helpful. For example, if bleeding is present during an acute attack, then astringent herbs such as witch hazel, bilberry, or cranesbill could be useful. If cramping occurs, use an anti-spasmodic gastrointestinal herb such as chamomile tea or cramp bark. The inflammation of the wall of the colon and surrounding tissues that results from diverticular disease can be addressed by using anti-inflammatory herbs such as yarrow and green tea.

# FLATULENCE

## DIAGNOSIS

Flatulence, often referred to as passing gas or breaking wind, is a common problem that affects everyone from time to time. It occurs when the excess air that builds up in the body naturally throughout the day is expelled through the rectum. Although it can be embarrassing, flatulence is not usually a serious problem. Gas is formed in the large intestine as the result of bacteria acting on undigested food. Flatulence is also triggered by swallowing air while eating, which can often cause discomfort after meals, or by eating non-digestible foods, for example, large amounts of fiber. A food allergy, such as milk intolerance, can also cause problems. Flatulence is also a symptom of a number of diseases, such as irritable bowel syndrome, diverticulosis or diverticulitis, celiac disease, and thyroid dysfunction. It can be a result of the inadequate absorption of nutrients by the body, which is often caused by diarrhea, or due to medications such as antibiotics.

It is difficult to say what is a normal amount of flatulence. It may increase after starting a diet that is high in roughage, but should disappear once the body becomes accustomed to these foods. If symptoms are troubling you and there is no reason to suspect an underlying disease, then try eliminating lactose from your diet. If this is ineffective try cutting out common gas-producing foods such as pulses and beans, broccoli, cabbage, cauliflower, onions, beer, and coffee. Eat more slowly, taking time over meals, and avoid chewing gum and carbonated beverages.

## SYMPTOMS

- Passing gas or wind
- Abdominal pain and bloating
- Rumbling stomach
- Cramps and spasms in stomach

## TREATMENT GOAL

To identify the cause of the flatulence and take avoiding action, and to bring relief of symptoms.

## CONVENTIONAL MEDICINE

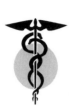

The treatment of flatulence is dependent on the cause of the gas. Celiac disease (the inability to tolerate wheat and gluten), lactose intolerance, constipation and irritable bowel syndrome are all among more serious conditions that may cause gas. More harmless causes include swallowing air, chewing gum, and eating certain vegetables.

**Elimination diet:** Exclude gluten, dairy, soy, and processed foods from your diet for a period of three weeks and then reintroducing these items, one at a time, keeping track of symptoms. This can be helpful to identify foods that cause gas.

**Medication:** Pharmaceuticals that are used to help with the symptoms of gas include simethicone. This can be obtained over the counter and taken as directed on the bottle. Other pharmaceuticals include medications that decrease intestinal motility such as dicyclomine.

## TRADITIONAL CHINESE MEDICINE

**Herbs:** The following formulas can be used to make decoctions. Place the herbs in a glass or ceramic pot, add 3 cups of water, and bring to the boil. Simmer for 30 minutes, strain, and drink 1 cup twice a day.
• To treat flatulence due to stagnation: Symptoms include gas with a strong odor, a bloated abdomen, and constipation. Mix 12 g of Mu Xiang (costus root), 10 g Chai Hu (hare's ear root), 6 g of Sha Ren (cardamon), 12 g of Yu Jin (turmeric tuber), 6 g of Da Huang (rhubarb root and rhizome), and 12 g of Fa Ben Xia (pinellia rhizome).
• To treat flatulence due to digestive system deficiency: Symptoms include a bloated abdomen, passing gas, irregular bowel movements, and/or fatigue. Combine 12 g of Bei Zhu (atractylodes rhizome), 5 g of Chen Pi (tangerine peel), 15 g of Fuling (poria), 15 g of Shan Yao (Chinese yam), 12 g of Tai Zi Shen (pseudostellaria) and 6 g of Sha Ren (cardamon).

**Acupuncture:** Have treatment once or twice a week; you may experience some relief after a couple of treatments. Depending on your condition, the practitioner will decide how many treatments you need. This may be combined with herbal treatment.

**Acupressure:** In a sitting position, press the Susanli and San Yin Jiao points each with the tip of your finger for one minute and repeat. You can repeat this two to three times a day to move stomach and intestinal energy. The Susanli point is on the lower leg, 1 inch to the outside of and 3 inches below the kneecap. The San Yin Jiao point is on the inside of the leg, about 3 inches above the anklebone.

**Diet:** Eat foods that help move stomach and intestinal energy such as bananas, peaches, milk, watermelon, rosemary, sweet basil, and spearmint. Avoid beans and greasy food.

## NATUROPATHY

 **Diet:** Avoid eating foods that are inherently gas-producing, such as beans, cabbage, onions, Brussel sprouts, cauliflower, broccoli, fluffy wheat products such as bread, apples, peaches, pears, prunes, corn, oats, potatoes, milk, ice cream, and soft cheese. Foods that produce minimal gas include rice, bananas, citrus fruits, grapes, hard cheese, meat, eggs, peanut butter, non-carbonated beverages, and yogurt made with live bacteria.

**Supplements:** A probiotics supplement such as Acidophillus, Lactobacillus, and S. boullardii can be taken for a period of 30 days to help improve overall intestinal health. You can also try taking 4 g of glutamine a day, or peppermint and oregano, to relieve symptoms of flatulence.

**Herbs:** The following recipes can be followed to ease flatulence. Pour 1 cup of boiling water over 1 tbsp of chopped dried peppermint leaves. Let this steep for 5–10 minutes, strain, and drink warm three to four times a day. Make fresh fennel tea by pouring 1 cup of boiling water over 1–2 tsp of just-crushed dried seeds. Let the tea steep for 10 minutes, strain, and drink before or after meals. Alternatively, chew ¼ tsp of seeds before or after meals. Chew ½ tsp of dill seeds before or after meals, or prepare dill water by mixing 1 tsp of oil of dill with 4 cups of warm water. Drink 1 cup as needed. Make a mild tea by steeping 1 tsp of ground dill seeds in 1 cup of boiling water for 10–15 minutes. Strain the liquid and drink before or after meals. Mix a few drops of aniseed oil into 1 cup of warm water, or make a tea by grinding 1 tsp of seeds and adding 1 cup of boiling water. Let the tea steep for 5–10 minutes, then strain. Drink either solution before or after meals. Some people may be allergic to anise. The volatile oil components of caraway seeds work as a carminative by promoting gastric secretions and stimulating the appetite. To make a tea, pour 1 cup of boiling water over 1–2 tsp of freshly crushed seeds. Let the tea steep for 10–15 minutes, then strain. Drink 1 cup two to four times a day between meals. Alternatively, chew ½ tsp of seeds after a meal.

**TIP:** USE CHARCOAL TABLETS

Studies have found that activated charcoal tablets are effective in eliminating excessive gas. Check with your doctor if you are taking any medication before using these, as charcoal can soak up medicine as well as gas. Take 1–2 capsules before meals.

## HOMEOPATHY

The advice given below can help to alleviate symptoms of an acute problem, or manage an on-going condition.

**Carbo veg:** This is the classic homeopathic remedy for releasing trapped wind that refuses to move upwards or downwards. This is a common occurrence after surgical procedures or tests such as a laparoscopy or barium enema, or after abdominal surgery. There is likely to be a heavy, full, and nauseous sensation in the stomach with flatulence, plus noticeable swelling and bloating of the belly. The latter is likely to be aggravated by eating, and considerably relieved by belching or passing gas.

**Lycopodium:** If flatulence occurs after eating too much fiber-rich food in one sitting, such as pulses and beans, or bread that is too coarse, use Lycopodium. Alternatively, flatulence and digestive uneasiness may arise in connection with high stress. Signature symptoms include abdominal bloating that is often at its worst in the late afternoon and rumbling and gurgling in the belly, belching, and passing gas.

**Nux vomica:** This is a strong candidate for easing flatulence that is linked to eating too much rich or spicy food, or drinking too much alcohol or coffee. Symptoms include nausea, headache, and constipation. Food lies heavily in the stomach and bitter or sour-tasting burps are ineffective in relieving nausea. The rectum feels full of gas that is reluctant to pass, and there is a sense of uneasiness after passing an incomplete stool.

**TIP:** EAT FREQUENTLY

Eat small, nutritious, and easily digestible meals throughout the day to avoid putting the digestive tract under strain. As a result, it is likely to work far more smoothly and efficiently.

**Bryonia:** This remedy can help to release trapped gas in the stomach that is causing sensations of heaviness, nausea, and tenderness that feel worse for movement of the slightest kind. When this remedy is well indicated, constipation is likely to be present with no urge to empty the bowels. You may be slightly dehydrated, with a dry mouth and thirst for long drinks of cold water.

---

**TIP: EAT SLOWLY**

As you chew, food mixes with saliva, which contains digestive enzymes that begin to break food down. Eating too quickly and not chewing food properly can sometimes result in flatulence.

---

## HERBALISM

**Peppermint:** This hybrid of spearmint and water mint is a carminative, which is commonly used to treat flatulence and the pains associated with gas in the stomach or intestines. Peppermint, particularly as an essential oil, which is primarily composed of menthol, has an anti-spasmodic effect on intestinal muscles. To ease upper intestinal tract gas and spasms, make a tea from peppermint leaf, making sure to cover it as the leaf is steeping to capture as much of the essential oil as possible. Sometimes peppermint tea can worsen heartburn; in these cases, peppermint oil can be taken as an enteric-coated capsule that delivers the oil to the intestines, helping to relieve flatulence without causing heartburn.

**Fennel:** Another common carminative, fennel seeds can simply be eaten after a meal to aid digestion, calm the stomach and intestines, and dispel gas. Alternatively, ½ tsp of the seeds can be powdered and then infused with hot water and consumed throughout the day, or 30–60 drops of a tincture of the seeds can be taken several times daily.

**Anise:** Crush the seeds of this plant and infuse them with hot water to make a tea to be consumed several times daily to relieve flatulence.

**Ginger:** This plant's rhizome can be consumed in a candied form, or a tea of sliced ginger can be made and drunk to warm the stomach, stimulate digestion, and, as a carminative, eliminate gas. It is also possible to purchase capsules of powdered ginger or ginger tincture, both of which can also help with flatulence when taken with meals.

**Sweet flag or calamus:** Used for a variety of stomach ailments, including flatulence associated with colicky pains and abdominal discomfort, a tincture made of the rhizome of sweet flag can be taken at 40–60 drops three times daily.

# FOOD POISONING

**DIAGNOSIS**

Food poisoning is an adverse reaction to a particular substance, usually bacteria in contaminated food or water that attacks the stomach and intestines, resulting in gastrointestinal upset. Salmonella, Campylobacter jejuni, and Staphylococcus, which affect poultry, raw meat, untreated milk, and duck and hen eggs are some of the more common types of food poisoning. E coli, found in undercooked meat, untreated milk, and contaminated water, is a slightly rarer cause. Norwalk virus, found in raw shellfish, salads, and contaminated water, is a common viral cause of food poisoning. In more serious cases, the bacteria may enter the lymph tracts, which carry water and protein to the blood, and the blood itself. Children, pregnant women, the elderly, and people who are already ill or have weakened immunity are particularly vulnerable to food poisoning and may get a serious infection. The symptoms of food poisoning vary quite markedly in intensity, and can range from slight to life-threatening. Most attacks are mild, with symptoms lasting between one and three days.

**DANGER**: Contact your doctor if diarrhea due to food poisoning continues for more than 24 hours, you have severe stomach cramps, there is blood in the feces, there is a fever of 100°F or higher, or there are any signs of dehydration.

**SYMPTOMS**

- Diarrhea
- Headaches
- Stomach cramps
- Nausea and vomiting
- Fever
- Dehydration
- Occasionally, blood in the feces

**TREATMENT GOAL**

To establish the cause of the food poisoning and treat the infection.

## CONVENTIONAL MEDICINE

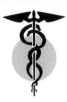

Medical treatment of food poisoning depends on the type of bacteria that caused it, but invariably includes rehydrating the body. Food poisoning causes diarrhea, and sometimes vomiting, both of which can result in dehydration. A diagnosis is made based on the incubation time from ingestion of contaminated food to presentation of symptoms.

**Identify the cause:** A diagnosis is made based on the length of time lapsed between eating the contaminated food and the first sign of symptoms. Determining whether a fever is present also aids in diagnosing the type of bacteria causing the food poisoning and therefore influences the treatment.

**Oral rehydration solution:** A home oral rehydration solution can be mixed with sugar, salt, and baking soda. This makes a solution very similar to the intravenous fluids administered at a hospital for dehydration. Mix 1 liter of filtered water, 2 tbsp of sugar, ½ tsp of salt, and ½ tsp of baking soda. Sip the solution throughout the day until urine is a normal color and urination occurs four to five times a day.

**Antibiotics:** Most infections simply run their course and treatment involves rehydrating the body and avoiding solid foods except for bananas and rice. After rehydrating the body with an oral rehydration solution, a culture of the stool is taken to determine the type of bacteria causing the infection. Antibiotics such as ciprofloxacin (Cipro™) or sulfamethoxazole/trimethoprim (Bactrim™) may be prescribed. Cholera is treated with rehydration and sometimes antibiotics (doxycycline or Vibramycin™ for three days) to shorten the duration of the disease. Salmonella is not treated with antibiotics.

**Complications:** Post-infection problems are associated with some types of food poisoning. See your doctor regarding any new onset of symptoms following an episode of food poisoning. Anyone with a compromised immune system suffering should seek medical treatment at the onset of food poisoning symptoms.

## TRADITIONAL CHINESE MEDICINE

**Herbs:** The herbs listed here are available from Chinese herbal stores.
• To treat diarrhea due to food poisoning: Symptoms include undigested food mixed with stools, abdominal pain, foul belching, and a dirty, sticky, and coated tongue. Mix 10 g of Shen Qu (massa fermentata), 10 g of Shan Zha (hawthorn fruit), 5 g of Chen Pi (tangerine peel), 10 g of Lai Fu Zi (radish seeds), 12 g of Fuling (poria), and 10 g Lian Qiao (forsythia

fruit). Place the herbs in a glass or ceramic pot and add 3–4 cups. Bring to the boil and simmer for 30 minutes. Drink 1 cup twice a day. These herbs should be available from Chinese herbal stores and online.

**Acupuncture:** Treatment will address symptoms such as diarrhea, vomiting, and abdominal pain. It will also help to disperse the toxins and protect the digestive system and other organs. See an experienced practitioner for more advice.

**Acupressure:** Use gentle to moderate pressure on the Nei Guan and Hegu points for a few minutes at a time. The Nei Guan point is located in the center of the wrist on the palm side, about 2 inches below the crease. The Hegu points are located on the back of the hands between the thumb and first finger.

**Diet:** Boil 30 g of fresh ginger and 1 g of ground black pepper in 3 cups of water until the liquid is reduced to one cup. Drink this tea three times a day for vomiting due to upset stomach.

> **TIP:** STORE FOOD PROPERLY
> Separate raw food from cooked food, and store raw food at the bottom of the fridge to avoid juices dripping down and contaminating other food. Make sure that the temperature of your fridge is below 41°F and your freezer below 5°F. Cover all food with lids, tin foil, or plastic wrap. Do not store food in opened tin cans.

## NATUROPATHY

**Diet:** Drink 8–12 glasses of water throughout the day to prevent dehydration. In acute situations do not eat solid foods if you do not feel like them, but stay hydrated with water, soups, vegetable juices, sports drinks with electrolytes, and broths. Miso broth or other clear broths help restore proper fluid and electrolyte balance. Give a child with food poisoning an oral electrolyte formula such as Pedialyte™, available over the counter. Drink barley or rice water, made from 1 cup of raw grain added to 1 quart of boiling water, to soothe an inflamed stomach or intestine. Let the grain steep for 20 minutes, strain the liquid, and drink throughout the day. Charcoal has the ability to absorb substances such as parasites and bacteria, preventing them from being reabsorbed by the body. Charcoal may also be used for relieving indigestion, nausea, vomiting, diarrhea, and intestinal bloating. Take ½ cup of charcoal powder mixed with a glass of water. You can also take 4 charcoal tablets every hour to absorb the toxins from the body.

**Supplements:** Take a probiotic product containing at least four billion active organisms of Lactobacillus acidophilus and bifidus daily to help digestion and fight infection. Alpha-lipoic acid is indicated in some reports as helpful in treating some types of food poisoning. Take 50 mg twice a day or 100 mg once a day. Take 1,000–3,000 mg of L-glutamine, an amino acid that repairs the gut, three times a day. Lactase enzymes help to digest dairy sugars, so take 2 capsules with each meal that may contain dairy. Vitamin A may help the body to rid itself of salmonella, according to some studies, and those people that are vitamin A deficient may actually be more prone to salmonella infection. Take 25,000–50,000 IU a day. Do not take more than 10,000 IU of vitamin A if you are pregnant; children can take 5,000 IU a day.

**Herbs:** Take 500 mg of ginger in capsule form, or 1–2 cups of ginger tea a day, to help ease the effects of food poisoning and decrease intestinal inflammation. Marshmallow root is soothing to the digestive tract. Take 500 mg in capsule form three times a day. Barberry has been traditionally used to treat diarrhea from infectious causes such as E. coli and V. cholera and, therefore, may help ease this symptom in some people with food poisoning. Take 2–3 ml of a tincture three times per day, or standardized extracts containing 5–10% alkaloids.

## HOMEOPATHY

This is a perfect example of an acute condition where homeopathic support can be of immense value in speeding-up recovery. The remedies below will be most successful if used alongside holistic/naturopathic remedies.

**Phosphorus:** If there is marked thirst for cold drinks that initially stay down, but are then vomited up as soon as they are warmed by the stomach, use phosphorus. There is a high level of anxiety when feeling nauseous that is eased by reassurance from a calming, soothing person. Diarrhea is painless but may be severe, especially in the evenings, when there is a real difficulty in controlling bowel movements.

**Ipecac:** For a particularly intense sensation of nausea that leads to episodes of vomiting that do nothing to relieve the awful sensation of sickness, even temporarily, use Ipecac. Nausea is aggravated by movement of any kind, or by stooping and bending forward. Although patients bring up frothy vomit frequently, there is an unusual lack of thirst when this remedy is helpful. The abdomen feels sensitive and distended with spasmodic colicky pains, and there is an unpleasant, constant urge to empty the bowels.

**Arsenicum album:** This and the remedy that follows are specific for situations where diarrhea and vomiting occur simultaneously. Classic symptoms include burning pains in the stomach and abdomen that are temporarily eased by small sips of warm drinks. Contact with warmth in general is very much desired (with the exception of the head and face), since there is a pervading sense of being chilled to the bone. Feelings of anxiety when ill do not respond to the strongest reassurance, and can develop into a feeling of being unable to recover. All symptoms are most intense at night.

**Veratrum album:** This is another strong candidate for treating vomiting and diarrhea that occur together. Symptoms include exhaustion to the point of prostration after vomiting and/or diarrhea. The skin appears exceptionally pale and feels clammy to the touch. There is also a characteristic thirst for cold water, which tends to be vomited up very soon after it has been drunk. Moving around intensifies the distress and intensity of nausea.

---

**TIP: DRINK WATER SLOWLY**

When vomiting and diarrhea occur together, make sure that water is drunk at frequent intervals. If vomiting is a particular problem, avoid the temptation to gulp down a long glass of water quickly, however thirsty you may feel. Instead, take small sips to give yourself the best chance of keeping it down.

---

## HERBALISM

**Antimicrobial botanicals:** Some herbal medicines act to kill the bacteria or viruses responsible for food poisoning. For example, licorice root, purple coneflower root, and osha root may all fight food poisoning stemming from infections. Tinctures of these roots can be taken several times a day during the acute phase of food poisoning.

**Berberine:** This alkaloid has been studied for its ability to combat gastrointestinal infections, and could also be useful for food poisoning. Berberine is found in goldenseal root, but due to the threatened status of goldenseal in its natural habitat, this is not an ideal source for this compound unless the manufacturer is using cultivated goldenseal. A good alternative source of berberine is Oregon grape root, which can be taken in tincture form.

**Antispasmodic herbs:** Chamomile and crampbark can help to ease the acute symptoms of food poisoning, such as diarrhea, abdominal cramping, and nausea. An infusion of dried chamomile flowers can be taken many times a day, but should be avoided by those who are allergic to other plants in the daisy family. You can also infuse 2 tsp of crampbark in water and drink three times daily, or take a dropperful of tincture three times daily to treat symptoms of food poisoning.

**Carob:** Carob powder and any other botanical astringents (see Diarrhea, p.366, and Colitis, p. 341) can also help to control the diarrhea associated with food poisoning. It is important not to completely stop diarrhea, as it is the body's way of ridding the system of toxins that are causing the food poisoning; use the herbs listed above to alleviate some of the symptoms until your body recovers.

# GALLSTONES

## DIAGNOSIS

Gallstones, a consequence of gallbladder disease, are formed in the gallbladder, a small organ positioned near the liver. Bile that is produced in the liver is stored in the gallbladder until it is passed into the intestine to aid in the digestion of fat. If the bile contains an excess amount of cholesterol, it can solidify in the gallbladder to form small solid stones made up of cholesterol, salt, and calcium. These stones can vary in size from a fraction of an inch across to an inch. The condition primarily affects women, but men can get it too, and the possibility of developing gallstones increases with age. Those with a family history of gallstones, who are overweight or have high cholesterol, or who have inflammatory stomach conditions such as Crohn's disease or ulcerative colitis, are more at risk. Women who have had several pregnancies or who are on a birth-control pill are also more susceptible. The symptoms of gallbladder disease vary widely from mild discomfort to a severe pain that usually begins after eating. A poor diet, especially one high in fatty foods, is a contributory factor to the disease. In severe cases the patient can suffer from jaundice, nausea, and fever as the main bile duct can get blocked with migrating gallstones. Around two-thirds of people with gallstones have no symptoms, and around a third of patients experience episodic symptoms. If symptoms are acute, contact your doctor immediately for tests.

## SYMPTOMS

- Pains in the upper right side of the abdomen, or just below the ribs on the right side
- Pain in the right shoulder or between the shoulder blades
- Nausea and vomiting
- Loss of appetite
- Fever
- Frequency and severity of attacks is variable

## TREATMENT GOAL

To identify the cause of the gallstones and make any lifestyle changes necessary to prevent them from developing further. Treatment also aims to relieve symptoms and dissolve or remove any existing gallstones.

## CONVENTIONAL MEDICINE

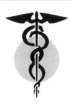

The treatment of gallstones initially depends on an adequate diagnosis. Your doctor may take an ultrasound of the gallbladder to determine whether gallstones are present. If an infection of the gallbladder is suspected, a nuclear imaging study called a HIDA scan is done. The recurrence rate of gallstones is high after treatment unless, of course, the gallbladder is removed. Lifestyle modification, described below, is essential to preventing recurrence.

**Diet:** If you suffer from gallstones, it is necessary to make certain changes to your lifestyle. Substitute polyunsaturated fats in your diet with monounsaturated fats to prevent stones from developing. A slow and steady weight loss (about 2 lb a week is normal) in people who are overweight is appropriate, but rapid weight loss should be avoided as this can precipitate gallstones.

**Surgery:** Gallstones that are symptomatic are treated surgically by a cholecystectomy (removal of the gall bladder). The operation generally requires a short recovery period, particularly when performed through a laparascope. This involves inserting a scope into the abdomen and operating through it rather than cutting through the abdominal wall.

**Dissolving the stones:** Those who are too high risk for surgery, can take a medication that dissolves the gallstones. If there are five or less stones that are made of cholesterol rather than calcium, and that are less than ½ inch in size, ursodiol (Actigall™) is used. The stones can also be dissolved using a solvent called methyl tert-butyl ether (MTBE). The solvent is administered directly into the area of the stone through the skin with a long catheter, through which the solvent is infused before then catheter is drawn out. Finally, the stones can be shocked until they break up into very small pieces in a procedure called extracorporeal shock wave lithotripsy (ESWL).

## TRADITIONAL CHINESE MEDICINE

**Herbs:** The formulas below are designed to dispel gallstones. Using either of the herbal combinations, add 3 cups of water, bring to a boil, and simmer for 30 minutes. Strain the liquid and drink 1 cup two to three times a day. The clinical dosage may be heavier, but is reduced here for you to use safely. It best to see a doctor for a prescription of the Chinese herbal formulas.

• To treat gallstones that have formed as a result of Qi stagnation: Mix 10 g of Chai Hu (hare's ear root), 12 g of Yu Jin (turmeric tuber), 12 g of Xiang Fu (nut-grass rhizome), 18 g of Jin Qian Cao (lysimachia), 10 g of Zhi Ke (bitter orange), and 12 g of Da Huang (rhubarb root and rhizome).

To treat gallstones that have formed as a result of dampness and heat: Mix 10 g of Jin Yin Hua (honeysuckle flower), 10 g of Lian Qiao (forsythia fruit), 12 g of Yu Jin (turmeric tuber), 12 g of Yin Chen (artemisia), 10 g of Mu Xiang (costus root), 10 g of Huang Qin (baical skullcap root), and 10 g of Da Huang (rhubarb root and rhizome).

**Acupuncture:** There are many reports of acupuncture and Chinese herbal medicine successfully treating gallstones. You should consult an experienced practitioner for a treatment plan. Results may vary, but in general you can expect relief from pain and less frequent gallstone attacks. The best results occur when the gallstone is ejected by the treatment naturally.

**Acupressure:** Gently press the Yang Ling Quan, Nei Guan, and Hegu points for one minute. Release and repeat to relieve the pain of a gallstone attack. The Yang Ling Quan point is on the outside of the leg by the knee in the depression just below the top of the fibula bone. The Nei Guan point is located in the center of the wrist on the palm side, about 2 inches below the crease. The Hegu points are located on the back of the hands between the thumb and first finger.

**Diet:** Chicory and corn silk are good for the gall bladder. Make a tea using corn silk (corn style and stigma) by boiling 15–30 g of corn silk for 10 minutes to make a tea. Drink it regularly throughout the day.

## NATUROPATHY

 **Diet:** Studies show that vegetarians have a lower risk of getting gallstones than meat eaters. If you suffer from gallstones, try to reduce the amount of animal products in your diet and increase the amount of vegetables you eat. A fiber-rich diet, including whole grains, fresh fruit and vegetables, and oat bran eaten every day at regular intervals, reduces the likelihood of gallstones. Also eat beets, artichokes, and dandelion greens regularly to improve bile flow. Use good quality extra virgin olive oil in salads to improve bile flow, and limit your consumption of sugar and simple carbohydrates. Note: if you already have gallstones, raw vegetables such as lettuce and broccoli may actually make the symptoms worse.

**Supplements:** Take 1–2 capsules of lipase enzymes with food to improve the digestion of fat. Taking 1,000 mg of lecithin in the form of phophatidylcholine twice a day helps to increase the solubility of gallstones. Take a probiotic product containing at least four billion active organisms of Lactobacillus acidophilus and bifidus daily for help with digestion.

**Herbs:** Dandelion root improves bile flow; take 400 mg of the freeze-dried herb or 1 tsp of liquid extract twice a day. Take 100–175 mg of milk thistle two or three times a day to decrease cholesterol saturation and increase bile flow. Artichoke also improves bile flow. Take 1–2 ml of a tincture or 500 mg in capsule form with each meal. Take 150 mg of turmeric with each meal for its anti-inflammatory effects and its ability to relax the bile duct.

## HOMEOPATHY

The advice given below is intended as a temporary complementary medical strategy for managing the pain and discomfort of gallstones that have begun to move. Once gallstones do begin to move, conventional medical assessment and treatment is needed as complications can develop. After the immediate condition is resolved, consult a homeopathic practitioner regarding preventative long-term treatment, as gallstones tend to recur. In cases that require the surgical removal of the gallbladder, homeopathic treatment can provide pre- and post-operative support.

**Chelidonium:** Consider this remedy if pain is present underneath the right shoulder blade. An intense pain may extend from the back to the chest and stomach, leading to severe nausea and possibly vomiting. Alternatively, pains may seem to flit about in all directions, and feel more severe when bending forwards, backwards, or when coughing. Lying on the belly may give some relief.

**Berberis:** To ease crushing, stitching, and sharp pains around the right shoulder blade use Berberis. Pains are so severe that they render the patient prostrate and exhausted. Pain feels more intense when sitting or lying down, and motion of any kind aggravates it further. The pains are also changeable in nature, and seem to flit about.

**China:** If pains are triggering hyper-excitability and nervous exhaustion, try China. Symptoms include weakness due to the loss of body fluids from profuse, drenching sweating that can accompany intense pain. The pain can also trigger episodes of vomiting and possibly diarrhea. Pain and soreness are likely to settle in the area between the shoulder blades. The slightest movement intensifies pain and leads to palpitations and shortness of breath. There may also be a need to double over in an instinctive desire to apply pressure to the painful area.

**Chamomilla:** If intermittent, colicky pains make the patient verbally abusive and frantic with pain, try Chamomilla. The patient may reach the point of feeling they would rather die than go on suffering pains of such intensity, and, feeling constantly restless with pain, may be driven to pace the floor in search of relief. Cramping pains accompany bilious vomiting and possibly diarrhea.

To avoid recurring gallstones, do not eat foods that are high in saturated fats (including full-fat cheese, red meat, cream, and full-fat milk). Instead opt for foods that are high in unrefined carbohydrates, and eat at least five portions of fresh fruit and vegetables each day. Choose fish as a source of protein rather than meat. If you crave meat from time to time, opt for chicken or turkey, but do not eat the skin, which contains a significant amount of fat. Certain foods, such as artichokes, asparagus, kelp, and barley water, are thought to be beneficial for those who are prone to gallstones and may be worth including in the diet. If you are in any doubt, consult a dietician.

## HERBALISM

The presence of gallstones is potentially life threatening and requires medical evaluation to avoid serious complications such as pancreatitis, cholangitis, and cholecystitis. Conventional medicine should be the first line of treatment, but herbal remedies can be useful as additional therapies, or during the period when definitive treatment is being sought. The two categories of herbs used to treat gallstones are choleretics and cholagogues.

**To prevent gallstones:** Choleretic plants cause the liver cells to make more bile, and cholagogue plants cause this bile to be released. By collectively increasing the flow of bile, these plants may help to clean out the bile duct system or gallbladder. Examples of choleretics are dandelion root and Culver's root. Examples of cholagogues are dandelion root, turmeric, licorice, globe artichoke, and tetterwort or celandine. These plants work best when taken 20–30 minutes before meals, and if you are not constipated. To successfully increase bile flow, treatment must be followed by regular bowel movements so that the bile is eliminated from the body.

**To dissolve gallstones:** Peppermint, milk thistle, and a compound from apple juice called malic acid may help to make cholesterol, a common component of gallstones, more soluble in bile and thereby dissolve stones. Take 200–420 mg of milk thistle a day—a form standardized to 70% silymarin seems to work best. 1,000–2,000 mg of malic acid can be taken under the supervision of a naturopathic physician. Peppermint oil, taken as a tea or in capsule form, can also help gallstones dissolve due to its monoterpene essential oils. Similar oils are present in fennel. Both of these plants also act as antispasmodics and may relieve spasms in the gall bladder that are sometimes associated with gallstones. The internal use of essential oils can have significant toxicity, so should only be carried out for short periods of time and under the care of a medical herbalist.

# GASTRIC FLU

## DIAGNOSIS

Gastric flu is an inflammation of the digestive tract, usually caused by a virus passed on through person-to-person contact. It can also be transmitted by contaminated food or water, by a particular food that produces an allergic reaction in the susceptible person, by a sudden change of diet, for example, if you are on vacation abroad, or by any illness or drug that alters the natural balance of bacteria in the gut. Symptoms vary in severity, but an attack usually resolves itself within 48 hours. In particularly bad cases there is usually repeated vomiting and diarrhea, stomach cramps, fever, and a general feeling of being exhausted and unable to do anything. A mild case may be limited to feelings of sickness and loose stools. Avoid food until the stomach settles down, then stick to a light diet for a few days. In infants and elderly people, gastric flu can be serious as it easily leads to dehydration. The best course of treatment is rest and plenty of fluids, although doctors may prescribe medication to control vomiting and diarrhea if it is serious.

## SYMPTOMS

- Burning pain in abdomen
- Vomiting
- Feeling of being chilly, cold, and clammy
- Symptoms worse at night
- Frothy yellow stools
- Flatulence
- Diarrhea with burning sensation
- Mucus in stools
- A red and itchy anus
- Distended stomach
- General feeling of fatigue and being rundown

## TREATMENT GOAL

To establish the cause of the symptoms and bring relief as quickly as possible, generally with lots of rest and drinking plenty of fluids. It is important to be meticulous about personal hygiene, particularly handwashing after using the toilet, so you do not pass the bug on.

## CONVENTIONAL MEDICINE

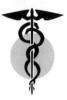

Treatment involves preventing dehydration, and maintaining and normalizing the body's nutritional status. Preventing the infection from spreading is also important. Infected persons should wash their hands regularly and avoid preparing any food.

**Rehydration:** Make an oral rehydration solution by mixing 1 liter of clean filtered water, with 2 tbsp of sugar and a ½ tsp each of baking soda and salt. This solution, suitable for both adults and children, should be sipped continuously. Any signs of dehydration such as dizziness, small amounts of yellow urine, a parched mouth, or dry eyes in young children should be followed up with immediate medical treatment. Intravenous fluids will be administered until hydration is established.

**Diet:** Eat the BRAT diet (bananas, rice, apple sauce, and tea) but focus mainly on fluids as your primary intake.

**Anti-emetics:** This type of medication stops nausea and vomiting. Most commonly chlorpromazine (Phenergan®) is used as a rectal suppository or as an intramuscular shot, as needed. Ginger is a natural anti-nausea remedy and 400–800 mg can be taken at the early onset of symptoms. Larch arabinogalactodes, found in a Thorne product called Arabinex®, is a natural antiviral that seems to speed up recovery. Also, a probiotic product that contains Saccharomyces boullardi, such as Florastore®, taken as directed, can help stop diarrhea and nausea. Over-the-counter anti-diarrhea agents can be utilized as directed, but should not be used by children. Black tea is a good alternative. For children above two years old, add some honey to make it more palatable, or add natural cane sugar for children under two years of age.

**Rest:** Rest is extremely important when recovering from a viral infection. Listen to your body and take as much rest as is needed.

## TRADITIONAL CHINESE MEDICINE

**Herbs:** Using either of the herbal formulas below, make a decoction by combining the raw herbs and adding 3 cups of water. Place in a ceramic pot, bring to the boil, and simmer for 30 minutes. Strain the liquid and drink 1 cup two to three times a day for three to six days. The herbs listed are available from Chinese pharmacies.

• To treat gastric flu with diarrhea and stomachache: Mix 10 g of Huang Qin (baical skullcap root), 6 g of Huang Lian (coptis root), 15 g of Bai Shao (white peony root), 10 g of

Mu Xiang (costus root), 10 g of Bai Tou Wong (Chinese anemone root), 15 g of Bai Zhu (white atractylodes rhizome), and 5 g of Gan Cao (licorice).

• To treat gastric flu with nausea and vomiting: Combine 10 g of Mu Xiang (costus root), 6 g of Sha Ren (cardamon seed), 5 g of Chen Pi (tangerine peel), 15 g of Fuling (poria), 15 g of Bai Zhu (white atratylodes root bark), 12 g of Fa Ban Xia (pinellia rhizome), 5 g of Din Xiang (clove flower bud), 12 g of Zi Shu Ye (perilla leaf), and 6 g of fresh ginger root.

**Acupuncture:** Immediate treatment may reduce symptoms such as nausea, vomiting, and gastric pain, and prevent the condition from getting worse. You may need treatment every other day during the acute and early stages; two to four treatments may be needed.

**Acupressure:** Use the tip of your thumb to press the Hegu point, located on the back of the hand in the depression between the thumb and the first finger, with strong pressure for one to two minutes. Repeat on the opposite hand. Apply median pressure with your fingertips to the Guan Yuan point, found on the abdomen about 3 inches below the navel, for one to two minutes. Repeat three to four times. Follow this treatment two to four times a day to reduce symptoms and assist recovery.

**Diet:** Eat rice, cooked vegetables, and soups. You can eat apples and oranges, but avoid peaches and pears. Avoid raw food, cold food, and cold beverages. You should also avoid eating deep fried, fatty, and greasy food. Eat smaller amounts of food than usual to rest your stomach and digestive system.

## NATUROPATHY

**Diet:** If you do not have an appetite, do not force yourself to eat. Make sure you stay hydrated by drinking herbal teas, water, soups, and broths. Add ginger to broth to warm the body and calm the stomach. When your appetite comes back, eat a nourishing diet composed primarily of whole grains, fresh fruits, and vegetables, and some fish and lean chicken. Avoid saturated fat as studies show it can promote nausea. Also avoid sugar, processed foods, dairy, and junk food as they suppress your immune system. Do not share food or use the same utensils or plates as others, especially children, as gastric flu is contagious.

**Supplements:** Taking a multivitamin/multimineral has been shown to lower the incidence of nausea. Pregnant women should take a specially formulated multivitamin, following the instructions on the label, as some can actually lead to nausea. Talk to your doctor about this possibility. You may need to switch brands, take the product at a different time, or take it with food. Vitamin B6 has been shown to help with nausea in some studies; take 30 mg twice a day. Activated charcoal absorbs toxins in the digestive tract if you have been exposed to micro-organisms from food or water; take 500–1,000 mg throughout the day.

**Herbs:** Ginger alleviates gastric flu symptoms, reduces fever, and has anti-inflammatory effects that can help with aches and pains. You can take ginger as a standardized extract in pill form, 100–200 mg every four hours up to three times a day; as a fresh powder, ½–¾ tsp every four hours up to three times a day; or raw, ¼–½-inch (peeled) slice of ginger every four hours up to three times a day. Ginger tea is available in pre-packaged bags or can be prepared by steeping ½ tsp of grated ginger root in 8 oz of very hot water for 5–10 minutes. A cup of tea, when steeped for this amount of time, can contain about 250 mg of ginger. Drink several cups a day. An 8 oz glass of ginger ale contains approximately 1 g of ginger. Drink several cups a day of a product made with real ginger. You can also take two pieces of crystallized ginger a day; about 500 mg of ginger is present in a 1-inch square, ¼-inch-thick piece. Do not take more than 1 g of ginger a day if you are pregnant. Elderberry is helpful in fighting viral infections. Take 5–10 ml three times a day. Yarrow induces sweat to help break a fever. Take 300 mg in capsule form or 2 ml of fresh tea four times a day. Mix 1–2 drops of peppermint oil into lemonade or other juice to soothe the stomach. You can also make peppermint tea by pouring boiling water through a strainer containing some dried peppermint or spearmint. Let the herb steep for a few minutes, add some sugar or honey if desired, and drink. Do not take peppermint if you are pregnant or have acid reflux. Slippery elm serves as a demulcent and soothes the gastric mucosa. Take 3 ml of tincture or 500 mg in capsule form three times a day. You can also take lozenges of slippery elm.

**Hydrotherapy:** Sit on a chair and place your feet in a bucket of warm water for 15 minutes. Dry them and put on a pair of cotton socks that have been placed in cold water and wrung out. Cover these with a pair of wool socks. Leave the socks on overnight to divert blood flow to the feet and away from the upper body, thus reducing fever and congestion.

## HOMEOPATHY

Although homeopathic remedies can not stop gastric flu it its tracks, they can make you more comfortable and speed up recovery. This is achieved by reducing the frequency and severity of bouts of sickness and/or diarrhea, while also easing a lot of the distress that an illness of this kind can cause. If you find it difficult to get back your natural vitality after a nasty illness of this kind, it is worth considering a consultation with a homeopathic practitioner. Successful homeopathic treatment can give the body the effective kick-start it needs to get the body back on track. Also see the suggestions for remedies of gastroenteritis (p. 403).

**Gelsemium:** If flu symptoms come on gradually and insidiously over a few days, Gelsemium can be an effective remedy. Symptoms include feverishness with an overwhelming feeling of aching, shivering, and exhaustion. There is a lack of thirst, but you may become noticeably thirsty when sweating. Cramping pains in the stomach are more severe and distressing when sitting up. Diarrhea is present, especially if gastric flu symptoms have developed when feeling stressed out and anxious.

**Baptisia:** Consider this remedy if symptoms of complete exhaustion and prostration come on very rapidly with aching, soreness, and restlessness in the muscles. Although you may feel uncomfortable when resting in one position, you are too exhausted to move. Attacks of vomiting and/or diarrhea come on very suddenly and severely with a high temperature.

## HERBALISM

This condition responds well to herbal therapy. The symptoms of gastric flu may include nausea and abdominal pain, or share some of the other symptoms of gastritis; any of the herbs recommended for this condition (see p. 401) may work to relieve symptoms until the infection associated with gastric flu is controlled by the body. Given that gastric flu is usually due to an infection, herbs that help the body eliminate the infection by killing the bacteria or viruses may be useful. Two of the most common herbs with a reputation for this are goldenseal and barberry.

**Goldenseal:** The root of this plant is commonly used in tincture form, and the antibacterial effects are thought to be primarily due to its alkaloid compounds, berberine and hydrastine. Most research has been done on berberine, not on whole goldenseal, so it is not known if goldenseal is the best treatment for infections like gastric flu. There are a variety of dosages recommended, including 500–1,000 mg of a capsule three times a day, or 2–4 ml of a 1:10 tincture of 60% ethanol three times a day. Goldenseal is still a threatened plant in its natural habitat due to over-harvesting, so any goldenseal product purchased should be from companies that cultivate it or obtain it from growers.

**Barberry:** The root bark of barberry contains the alkaloid berberine, which research shows to have antimicrobial effects against some of the common bacteria that may cause gastric flu. Barberry can be ingested as liquid extracts, tinctures, or decoctions of the root to help combat the infection.

**Chamomile tea:** Chamomile is an excellent herb for many gastrointestinal problems, serving as an anti-inflammatory, anti-spasmodic, and a source of fluids, all of which provide relief during a bout of gastric flu.

**Peppermint:** A few drops of the essential oil placed under the tongue, or taken as a tea, can help to control the nausea associated with gastric flu.

# GASTRITIS

## DIAGNOSIS

Gastritis is a broad term for inflammation or irritation of the lining of the stomach. It can come on suddenly, in which case it is known as acute gastritis, or gradually, known as chronic gastritis. Gastritis may be triggered by a viral infection, drinking too much alcohol, an unhealthy diet, smoking, or taking drugs such as aspirin or anti-inflammatory drugs over a long period of time. However, the most common cause of gastritis is the bacteria called H. pylori, the same bug that causes stomach ulcers. If you are showing symptoms of gastritis, avoid solid foods and drink plenty of water and other bland liquids to prevent dehydration. If you have gastritis try to eat a healthy diet, give up smoking, and watch your intake of alcohol and caffeine. You should also avoid foods that are hard to digest, such as hot and spicy meals. You may also want to think about any medication you are on that could be irritating the lining of your stomach.

## SYMPTOMS

- Abdominal discomfort
- Nausea and vomiting
- Diarrhea
- Bad taste in the mouth
- Loss of appetite
- Indigestion

## TREATMENT GOAL

To identify the cause and ease the symptoms. If your gastritis is caused by H. pylori you may need antibiotics to eliminate the bug.

## CONVENTIONAL MEDICINE

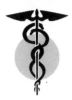

**Prevention:** Avoid any irritating substances, including non-steroidal anti-inflammatory drugs (NSAIDs) such as ibuprofen, alcohol, tobacco, and any foods that cause an increase in irritation of the stomach. Alternatives to non-steroidal drugs include ginger, turmeric, and plant flavonoids, which can be obtained from many natural health products.

**To treat gastritis caused by H. pylori:** A endoscopy and biopsy may be performed to identify the cause of the gastritis. If the H. pylori bacteria is found, a combination of proton pump inhibitor drugs (such as omeprazole) and the antibiotic clarithromycin is given for about 10 days. Other variations on the antibiotic combination can be given and will be determined by the doctor.

**To treat gastritis caused by stress:** To prevent the condition from developing, or worsening, a drug called sucralfate suspension, along with antacid medications such as proton pump inhibitors, are used. Gastritis is aggravated by stress, so stress reduction techniques such as meditation should be put into practice.

## TRADITIONAL CHINESE MEDICINE

**Herbs:** The herbs listed in the formulas below are available from Chinese pharmacies or online. For each formula, place the raw herbs in a glass or ceramic pot. Bring the mixture to a boil and simmer for 30 minutes. Strain the liquid and drink 1 cup twice a day.

• To treat acute gastritis: Symptoms include stomachache and indigestion. Combine 12 g of Mu Xiang (costus root), 12 g of Lian Qiao (forsythia fruit), 10 g of Huang Qin (baical skullcap root), 12 g of Bai Shao (white peony), 10 g of Shen Qu (medicated leaven), 5 g of Chen Pi (tangerine peel) and 12 g of Fa Ben Xia (pinella rhizome).

• To treat chronic gastritis: Mix 15 g of Bai Zhu (white atractylodes rhizome), 15 g of Bai Shao (white peony), 15 g of Shan Yao (Chinese yam), 12 g of Yu Zhu (Solomon's seal rhizome), 15 g of Fuling (poria), 10 g of Tai Zi Shen (pseudostellaria), 3 g of Gan Cao (licorice), and 5 g of fresh ginger.

**Acupuncture:** Treatment can relieve the gastro pain, help digestion, and reduce inflammation. For acute conditions, you need treatment twice a week for two to three weeks. For chronic gastritis, the course of treatment can be much longer. Consult a practitioner regarding a treatment plan.

**Acupressure:** Massage the abdomen with your palm, in a counter clockwise circle, with gentle pressure for 20 circles. This can help digestion and reduce stomachache. You can also press the Nei Guan point, located in the center of the wrist on the palm side, about 2 inches above the crease, to treat nausea. Use firm but gentle pressure for one to two minutes on each side once or twice a day.

**Diet:** Eat food that is well cooked and easy to digest. For acute gastritis, eat soft food such as rice porridge and chicken soup. It is important to avoid cold and raw food and fried, greasy and spicy food.

## NATUROPATHY

**Diet:** Most sufferers of this condition experience loss of appetite. Try to eat several small meals throughout the day to avoid irritating the gastric mucosa. Eat plenty of soluble fiber such as oats and oat bran, dried beans and peas, barley, apples, and flaxseeds. Soluble fiber has been shown to repair the gastric mucosa. Drink at least 5 cups of cabbage juice (made by blending cabbage and water) a day to heal the gastric mucosa. You can mix it with water or carrot juice if preferred. Eat cultured products, such as yogurt, kefir, or raw sauerkraut, for probiotic (friendly bacteria) activity and their ability to fight H. pylori. Use garlic to flavor your meals as it has antibacterial activity that may help fight H. pylori. Avoid foods that irritate the gastric mucosa, including spicy foods, sugar, citrus fruits, coffee, black tea, and alcohol. Avoid possible food allergens, including wheat, corn, soy, and dairy. Milk used to be prescribed for those with ulcer-induced gastritis, but the latest research suggests that milk is a potential problem for this condition.

**Supplements:** Probiotics in the lactobacillus family can inhibit the growth of H. pylori. While this effect does not appear to be strong enough for probiotic treatment to eradicate H. pylori on its own, preliminary studies suggest that probiotics may help antibiotics work better, improving the rate of eradication and reducing side effects. Take a product containing at least four billion active organisms twice daily with meals or 30 minutes after eating. Take 30 mg of zinc, with 2 mg of copper, a day to promote tissue healing. Vitamin C can potentially retard H. pylori growth and produce antioxidant activity in the stomach lining. Take 1,000 mg of the non-acidic form three times a day. L-glutamine also promotes healthy intestines. Take 1,000 mg three times a day.

**Herbs:** Take 500 mg of mastic gum three times a day to heal stomach mucosa and for its antibacterial benefits. Drink 3 cups of fresh chamomile tea a day to relaxe the nervous system and help fight ulcers. Slippery elm serves as a demulcent and soothes gastric mucosa. Take 3 ml of tincture or 500 mg of a capsule three times a day. You can also drink aloe vera juice for its antimicrobial activity and its ability to soothe the lining of the stomach.

## HOMEOPATHY

Any of the following remedies can be helpful in easing the discomfort and speeding up recovery from a recent, mild bout of gastritis. If attacks become more frequent and/or severe, consult a homeopathic practitioner who will be able to work in a complementary way with your doctor.

**Arsenicum album:** Use this remedy to treat symptoms of uneasiness, burning, and acidity in the stomach, especially if symptoms are linked to very high anxiety levels. Unusually, burning in the stomach is eased temporarily by sips of warm drinks, and contact with warmth in general feels soothing and restorative. Symptoms may also be triggered by eating frozen foods, iced drinks, or watery fruit that is overripe. When the appetite returns there is a temptation to eat small amounts often, rather than large meals. There may also be a desire for warm, sweetened milk, which soothes digestive discomfort and uneasiness.

**Nux vomica:** To ease gastritis that has been triggered by a combination of high stress levels combined with too much junk food, alcohol, coffee, and cigarettes, use Nux vomica. Once changes to your lifestyle have been made to avoid these triggers, this remedy can be helpful in easing symptoms of spasmodic pain that radiate from the stomach to the back. It can also help relieve queasiness and heaviness in the stomach.

## HERBALISM

As with other gastrointestinal illnesses where there is an element of mucosal irritation and inflammation, gastritis can benefit from herbs that serve as demulcents, or mucilaginous plants, and anti-inflammatories.

**Licorice:** This is a well-known demulcent. For long-term use take two to four 380 mg tablets of de-glycyrrhizinated licorice (DGL) before meals in order to help with gastritis and, at the same time, avoid the side effects of one of licorice's phytochemicals, glycyrrhizin. **Caution:** The prolonged use of decoctions or infusions of dried, unprocessed licorice root can cause high blood pressure, low potassium, and swelling, due to one of its compounds, glycyrrhizin, also called glycyrrhizic acid.

**Slippery elm root bark powder:** Stir 1–2 tbsp of this demulcent powder into a glass of water and drink after meals and before bedtime. Begin with a smaller amount of powder until you become accustomed to it; if too much powder is mixed in the water, the preparation can be very thick and difficult to tolerate. To improve the taste, it can be sweetened slightly with honey or sugar. Slippery elm is safe, though some of the compounds contained in it can bind medications that are taken at the same time and decrease their absorption. Do not take slippery elm within one to two hours of taking any other medication.

**Marshmallow:** This demulcent herb can relieve symptoms. Make a tea with 5–6 g of marshmallow leaf or root and drink throughout the day. As with slippery elm, medicines taken at the same time may not be absorbed as well.

**Other mucilaginous herbs:** Plantain, ribwort, and Irish moss are all useful in treating gastritis. These plants can be consumed as either capsules or cold water infusions; either way, they should be taken before meals to coat and protect the inflamed stomach lining. As with all demulcents, there may be the risk that they will inhibit the body's ability to absorb any other medication taken, so caution is advised. Take medicines either an hour before or several hours after the herb.

**Bitters herbs:** When even small amounts of a bitter herb are ingested, several nerves are activated to increase the flow of saliva and gastric secretions, and improve the motility of the stomach. All these effects can help to repair and protect an irritated stomach lining, which occurs with gastritis. Tinctures of gentian, centaury, yarrow, and wormwood have been used as bitters in cases of gastritis. Take 5–6 drops of the tincture, depending on the plant and the person's condition, on a short-term basis either with meals or just before until the symptoms resolve.

# GASTROENTERITIS

## DIAGNOSIS

Gastroenteritis is an inflammation of the gastro-intestinal tract, usually due to either food poisoning or a viral illness. It is very common and the usual symptoms include loss of appetite, nausea, vomiting, abdominal pain, and diarrhea. The illness usually lasts for around two to three days, after which the sufferer usually recovers without any specific treatment other than the need to replace the fluids and minerals that have been lost. Mild cases can be treated at home with bed rest and plenty of rehydrating fluids. In babies, small children, and the elderly the illness can be more severe and prolonged as there is a risk of dehydration, and it is often necessary to locate the source of the problem. For severe cases, hospital treatment may be necessary and fluids, and occasionally antibiotics, may be given intravenously. Most infectious organisms are transmitted by unwashed hands, and maintaining good standards of hygiene substantially reduces the risk of infection.

## SYMPTOMS

- Abdominal pain and cramps
- Diarrhea
- Nausea and vomiting
- Weight loss
- Sweating and feeling clammy
- Fever and chills
- Muscle pain and stiffness
- Reduced appetite

## TREATMENT GOAL

The most important goal is to prevent dehydration and the spread of the infection. Treatment also aims to relieve symptoms and discomfort.

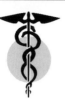

## CONVENTIONAL MEDICINE

In general gastroenteritis, the inflammation and irritation that occur in the stomach and intestines can initially be treated symptomatically, independent of the cause (whether viral, a food allergy, etc.). Diarrhea must be addressed, with the goal being rehydration and maintenance of nutritional status. Please see the section on diarrhea for instructions on how to make an oral rehydration solution and for specific treatment of diarrhea (p. 366). To treat specific causes of gastroenteritis, such as gastric flu and food poisoning, see p. 393 and p. 403 respectively.

**To treat inflammation of the gastrointestinal system:** Rest the bowel for 48 hours if diarrhea is present and follow this with a two- to three-week diet that avoids difficult to digest food types. Specifically, it may be helpful to eliminate dairy, gluten, soy, caffeine, alcohol, and processed artificial foods during this time. Fructo-oligopolysaccharides (which can be found in some health food formulas for intestinal health), glutamine, and probiotics, specifically bifidus and Saccharomyces boullardi, can be helpful. The botanicals slippery elm, althea root, and cranesbill are soothing and healthy for the gastric mucosa.

**Warning:** Great care must be taken to avoid dehydration. If diarrhea is persistent, or if signs of dehydration occur, such as scant urination, dizziness, or confusion, seek urgent medical care for intravenous rehydration.

## TRADITIONAL CHINESE MEDICINE

**Herbs:** To make a decoction, use any of the formulas below. Place the herbs in a ceramic pot and add 4 cups of water. Bring to the boil and simmer for 30 minutes. Strain the liquid and drink 1 cup twice a day. You can purchase these raw herbs from Chinese herbalists or online.

• To treat acute gastroenteritis: Mix 12 g of Fa Ban Xia (pinellia rhizome), 8 g of Huang Qin (baical skullcap root), 5 g of Huang Lian (coptis root), 3 g of dried ginger, and 5 g of Gan Cao (licorice). If gastroenteritis occurs with symptoms of indigestion such as bloating, add 12 g of Shan Zha (hawthorn fruit) and 8 g of Shen Qu (medicated leaven). If you are vomiting mucus, add 12 g of Bai Zhu (white atractylodes rhizome) and 10 g of Tian Ma (gastrodia rhizome). If gastroenteritis occurs due to overheating, such as heatstroke, add 12 g of Zhu Ru (bamboo shavings) and 10 g of Huo Xiang (agastache).

• To treat chronic gastroenteritis: Combine 12 g of Xiang Fu (nut grass rhizome), 10 g of Mu Xiang (costus root), 6 g of Sha Ren (cardamon), 12 g of Fuling (poria), 12 g Bai Zhu (white atractylodes rhizome), and 6 g of Chen Pi (tangerine peel). If accompanied by stress, add 10 g of Chai Hu (hare's ear root), 12 g of Bai Shao (white peony), and 6 g of Bo He (field mint). For chronic stomachache, add 12 g of Ru Xiang (frankincense) and 10 g of Yan Hu (corydalis rhizome).

**Acupuncture:** Treatment can benefit both acute and chronic gastroenteritis. You may have treatment for an acute condition two or three times a week for one or two weeks. For chronic conditions, you may have treatment once a week for three months. You can combine acupuncture treatment with the herbal remedies above.

**Acupressure:** In a sitting position, with both legs up straight, press the Susanli and San Yin Jiao points to strengthen the stomach and digestive system. The Susanli point is found on the lower leg, 1 inch to the outside of and 3 inches below the kneecap. The San Yin Jiao point is located on the inside of the leg, about 3 inches above the anklebone. Press these points with the tip of your finger or thumb for one minute three times. You can press these points three times a day for acute conditions and once a day for chronic conditions. Also in a sitting position, you can press the Qu Chi and Nei Guan points to help with digestion. With the elbow flexed, the Qu Chi point is on the outside of the elbow at the lateral end of the crease. The Nei Guan point is in the center of the wrist on the palm side about 2 inches above the wrist. Press these points with the tip of your finger or thumb for one minute three times, one to three times a day.

**Diet:** Eating rice, particularly sticky and brown rice, sweet potato, Chinese yam, squash, chicken soup, ginger, and dates is recommended. Eat well-cooked food, but avoid deep-fried food as well as anything fatty, since it is harder to digest. Avoid plums (both dried and fresh) and eat less raw food.

## NATUROPATHY

**Diet:** Do not eat if you do not have an appetite, but take lots of fluids, such as water, herbal teas, soups, and broths, to stay hydrated. When you do get an appetite, eat whole grains, fresh fruits, and vegetables, and some fish and lean chicken. Saturated fats can cause nausea and should be avoided, as should sugar, processed foods, dairy, and junk food, which suppress your immune system. Prevent the infection from spreading by not sharing food or serving utensils.

**Supplements:** Taking a multivitamin/multimineral can prevent nausea. Pregnant women should take a specially formulated multivitamin, following the instructions on the label. Some multivitamins can cause nausea, and you may need to switch brands, take it at a different time, or take it with food. Studies have shown that vitamin B6, taken at 30 mg twice a day, can also help with nausea. Take 500–1,000 mg of activated charcoal a day to absorb toxins in the digestive tract. This is helpful if you have been exposed to micro-organisms from food or water.

**Herbs:** Ginger alleviates gastric flu symptoms, reduces fever, and has anti-inflammatory effects that can help with aches and pains. You can take ginger as a standardized extract in pill form, 100–200 mg every four hours up to three times a day; as a fresh powder, ½–¾ tsp every four hours up to three times a day; raw, ¼–½-inch (peeled) slice of ginger every four hours up to three times a day; or crystallized, two pieces a day. Do not take more than 1 g of ginger a day if you are pregnant. Taking 5–10 ml of elderberry tincture three times a day is helpful in fighting viral infections. Take 300 mg of yarrow in capsule form to induce sweating and help break a fever. Mix 1–2 drops of peppermint oil into lemonade or other juices, or drink peppermint tea, to sooth the stomach. Do not take peppermint if you are pregnant or have acid reflux.

## HOMEOPATHY

Any of the following remedies can be helpful in easing the distress of, and speeding up recovery from, gastroenteritis.

**Arsenicum album:** This is a helpful remedy for treating vomiting and diarrhea that occur simultaneously. Symptoms include a burning pain in the stomach and/or gut that is temporarily soothed by taking small sips of warm drinks, and feeling incredibly chilly, restless, and agitated. All symptoms cause particular distress at night and in the early hours of the morning. Feelings of agitation, anxiety, and despair can be so severe that it feels unlikely that symptoms will ever improve.

**Veratrum album:** This remedy is also helpful in situations where vomiting and diarrhea occur together, but is more appropriate if they are accompanied by an unquenchable thirst for long drinks of cold water. The patient will be very sweaty and restless, especially after bouts of vomiting and diarrhea, which are likely to be violent and forcible in nature. Although the patient is incredibly thirsty, vomiting and diarrhea are often much worse after drinking cold water. There is also the unusual symptom of feeling hungry despite episodes of severe nausea and vomiting.

**Phosphorus:** Think of this as a possible choice for treating symptoms of nausea, vomiting, and diarrhea with a marked thirst for drinks of cool water. These give temporary relief to stomach pain and cramps and stay down until they become warmed by the stomach. Once this happens, they are promptly vomited up. Bouts of diarrhea are severe but often painless, and there is an unpleasant sensation of stools being passed involuntarily as though the anus remains open. Severe anxiety accompanies symptoms, but unlike the distress that calls for Arsenicum album, it can be eased by reassurance and attention. All symptoms come on, or may feel more distressing, in the evening.

**Ipecac:** Always consider this for severe nausea that is not relieved in the slightest after vomiting or passing liquid stools. Feelings of queasiness and sickness are made even worse by movement of the slightest kind. You may vomit bile, and diarrhea may look frothy or include traces of mucus.

## HERBALISM

 Gastroenteritis is caused by many different viruses and bacteria, and may have symptoms such as nausea, abdominal pain or cramping, and diarrhea. Any of the recommended herbs for these conditions may work to provide symptomatic relief until the infection is under control. Given that gastroenteritis is usually caused by an infection, herbs that help the body kill bacteria or viruses may be useful. Two of the most popular herbs with a reputation for this are goldenseal and barberry.

**Goldenseal:** This herb has a reputation for killing many of the offending bacteria that cause gastroenteritis, though much of the research was done on one of its isolated alkaloids, berberine. There are a variety of dosages recommended, including 500–1,000 mg of a capsule three times a day, or 2–4 ml of a 1:10 tincture of 60% ethanol three times a day.

**Barberry:** The root bark of barberry contains the alkaloid berberine. Studies show it has antimicrobial effects against some of the common bacteria that may cause gastroenteritis. Barberry can be taken as a liquid extract, tincture (20–40 drops), or decoction (1 cup) of the root to help fight infection.

**Chamomile:** Chamomile tea is an excellent herb for many gastrointestinal problems. It works as an anti-inflammatory and anti-spasmodic, and is a source of fluids, all of which provide relief.

**Peppermint:** Place a few drops of essential peppermint essential oil under the tongue, or drink peppermint tea to help to control the nausea associated with gastroenteritis.

**Marshmallow:** Any of the demulcent herbs used for colitis (see p. 341), such as marshmallow, can help to soothe the inflamed tissue of the intestines and colon, leading to an improvement in symptoms.

**Plantain:** This plant acts similarly to marshmallow, soothing and healing the intestinal mucosa that become inflamed during a bout of gastroenteritis. It is in a class of herbs known as vulneraries, or wound healers, thought to have the ability to heal skin cuts. Some vulneraries, like plantain, heal internal "wounds" too. A tincture of the leaves and roots of plantain can be taken twice a day to help with gastroenteritis.

# HEARTBURN

## DIAGNOSIS

The symptoms of heartburn vary, but it is most commonly described as an uncomfortable burning sensation in the throat or chest just behind the breastbone. It occurs when harsh stomach acid flows up (know as reflux) and comes into contact with and irritates the delicate lining of the esophagus, the tube that connects the mouth to the stomach. This generally occurs when the lower esophageal sphincter (LES), the natural valve that keeps stomach acid in the stomach, does not do its job properly. Various lifestyle and dietary factors, as well as certain medications, can contribute to heartburn. Foods that are problematic for heartburn sufferers include citrus fruits, tomatoes, onions and garlic, vinegar, and anything fatty or spicy. Large meals and eating just before bedtime can also cause irritation, as can caffeinated and carbonated drinks. Episodes of heartburn can also be triggered by body position, certain movements, and/or exertion, such as lying down, bending over, or strenuous exercise. Some prescription and over-the-counter medications can also contribute to heartburn. These commonly include high blood pressure and heart medications. Heartburn commonly occurs during pregnancy as hormones produced during the first trimester can cause problems, and the stomach can be pushed upwards within the abdominal cavity to make room for the growing baby.

## SYMPTOMS

- Burning chest pain moving up towards the throat
- Sensation that food is coming back into the mouth
- Bitter taste at the back of the throat
- Difficulty swallowing
- More painful when lying down or bending over

## TREATMENT GOAL

To relieve any immediate symptoms and put into practice lifestyle changes that will help ease the problem of heartburn.

## CONVENTIONAL MEDICINE

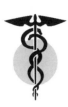

If left unchecked, heartburn can result in more serious conditions, such as damage to the esophagus with bleeding, ulceration, and even cancer. Sometimes the upper airways can become involved, resulting in asthma, chronic cough, and chronic laryngitis. Conventional medical treatment provides relief for the symptoms and discomfort associated with heartburn, while preventing further complications.

**Antacids:** Over-the-counter antacids, which consist of aluminum hydroxide, magnesium carbonate, and magnesium trisilicate preparations, are usually taken five or six times a day between meals. Dissolving 1 tsp of sodium bicarbonate in a glass of water is also effective; however, excessive amounts of sodium bicarbonate can interfere with the acid base balance of the body and add excess sodium to the system, which can contribute to hypertension. Many antacids inhibit the body's ability to absorb minerals, so take vitamin and mineral supplements.

**Lifestyle changes:** Try raising the head of the bed so that acid does not reflux while you are sleeping. Avoid smoking as this irritates acid reflux. Eating a diet of plain, natural organic foods usually leads to an improvement of symptoms. Taking herbs such as althea and mallow root can also be beneficial. Studies show that stress contributes greatly to acid reflux so managing stress levels is important. Weight loss should be considered if you are overweight.

**Medications:** A class of drugs that blocks acid in the stomach, known as H2 receptor antagonists, is used to treat heartburn. It includes medications such as cimetidine, ranitidine, and famotidine. Proton pump inhibitors such as omeprazole and lansoprazole also reduce gastric acid secretion and tend to be more effective than the H2 blockers.

**Surgery:** Surgery to correct acid reflux is rare and is reserved for very severe cases with complications.

## TRADITIONAL CHINESE MEDICINE

Traditional Chinese medicine identifies two types of heartburn: an excessive or deficient condition. Referral to a Western medicine doctor for an examination and diagnosis of the prime causes of symptoms is very helpful, as traditional Chinese medicine can then be used in a complementary manner.

**Herbs:** Combine the ingredients of either of the herbal remedies below in a ceramic pot. Add 3 cups of water, bring to the boil, and simmer for 30 minutes. The herbs listed are available from Chinese herbalists or online.

• To treat excessive heartburn: This is as an acute condition of heartburn and is usually due to improper diet and irregular eating patterns, or a cold or fever. Mix 10 g Zhi Shi (immature fruit of bitter orange), 10 g of Mu Xiang (costus root), 10 g of Zhu Ru (bamboo shavings), 15 g of Fuling (poria), 10 g of Xiang Fu Hua (nut grass), 30 g of Dai Zhe Shi (hematite), 8 g of Shen Qu (medicated leaven), 10 g of Huo Xiang (agastache), 5 g of Sha Ren (cardamon), 5 g of fresh ginger, and 5 g Gan Cao (licorice). Drink 1 cup two to three times a day for three to five days.

• To treat a chronic condition: Symptoms include weakness, fatigue, poor appetite, and indigestion. Combine 12 g of Dan Shen (salvia root), 15 g Bai Zhu (white atractylodes rhizome), 15 g of Fuling (poria), 15 g of Shan Yao (Chinese yam), 10 g of Mu Xiang (costus root), 6 g of Bai Kou Ren (round cardamon fruit), and five pieces of Da Zhao (Chinese jujube). You can use this formula for 7–10 days, or consult a Chinese medicine practitioner regarding long-term use.

**Acupuncture:** You may have acupuncture once or twice a week for one to six months. The length of treatment courses will depend on the individual condition.

**Acupressure:** Use the tip of your thumb to apply medium pressure to the Nei Guan, Hegu, and Tan Zhong points for one minute and repeat. The Nei Guan point is located in the center of the wrist on the palm side about 2 inches above the crease. The Hegu points are located on the back of the hands in the depression between the thumb and the first finger. Tan Zhong point is found on the midpoint between the nipples.

**Diet:** Foods that are good for this condition are corn, rice, tofu, spinach, celery, bamboo shoots, Daikon radishes, carrots, pomegranates, cherries, pears, fish, and water chestnuts. Avoid acidic food, such as tomatoes, oranges, and grapefruit, and hot, spicy food, such as black and white pepper, green and red peppers, chilies, dried ginger, and star anise.

## NATUROPATHY

**Diet:** Eat a whole food diet and eliminate unnatural refined foods. Whole grains, raw vegetables, and raw nuts and seeds are rich in fiber and contain essential nutrients important in relieving gastric symptoms and healing gastric mucosa. Eating bananas seems to be particularly beneficial for relieving heartburn, as they have a natural antacid effect in the body. You may also use ground, dried banana. Drink 8–10 glasses of water a day to maintain good digestive health and neutralize the excess acidity in the stomach. Some foods, including wheat, citrus fruits, and corn, can aggravate the condition. Pay attention to see if symptoms flare up when eating these foods. Avoid foods that contain saturated fats, hydrogenated oils, and partially hydrogenated oils, such as fried and greasy foods, processed foods, heavy sauces, and red meats, as they can lead to acid reflux. Caffeine, alcohol, chocolate, and minty and spicy foods can make symptoms worse and should be avoided. White wine, especially dry young whites from Germany, may cause heartburn as they are very acidic. Avoid overeating and take small meals regularly throughout the day to help soothe the digestive tract. Also avoid eating three hours before bedtime, as sleeping on a full stomach tends to aggravate symptoms.

**Supplements:** Calcium carbonate is a well-known heartburn reliever and the principal active ingredient in antacid tablets such as Tums®. It can provide immediate relief and may be particularly effective for treating sporadic heartburn. Take 250–500 mg of calcium carbonate three times a day with food. Chewable tablets provide the quickest relief. Avoid brands that include peppermint, which has been shown to relax the low esophageal sphincter, the muscle at the base of the esophagus that normally keeps food and digestive acids in the stomach.

**Herbs:** Drinking aloe vera juice between meals is another fast-acting method of soothing an agitated esophagus. Make sure the juice contains 98% aloe vera and no aloin or aloe-emodin. Take 500 mg of mastic gum three times a day to heal stomach mucosa and for its antibacterial benefits. Gamma-oryzanol, also known as rice bran oil, can help repair the entire digestive system. Take 150 mg three times a day for one month.

## HOMEOPATHY

The following remedies can work quickly and effectively to clear up a recent episode of heartburn or acidity that is due to an obvious trigger. Homeopathic remedies may be far more helpful than conventional antacids, which can be associated with acid-rebound when used habitually. If symptoms occur suddenly, with no obvious cause, see a physician. Also seek professional medical attention to treat more established, severe, or recurrent heartburn. Also refer to the remedies suggested in the section on indigestion (p. 428).

**Arsenicum album:** Heartburn and acidity with burning pains in the stomach and severe nausea may be eased by this remedy, especially if symptoms tend to come on at night or in the early hours of the morning. There is a marked anxiety and restlessness when feeling ill, and a tendency to think health issues are grimmer than they are in reality. Distraction and warmth feel desirable and soothing, as well as lying propped up on two or three pillows. Lying too flat aggravates symptoms.

**Lycopodium:** If acid washes up into the gullet from the stomach when anxiety levels are high, or when you eat a lot of high-fiber foods such as wholegrain bread, pulses, and beans or indigestible foods such as onions, use Lycopodium. You may feel ravenous but become full very quickly, or lack an appetite during the day, only to wake up from hunger at night.

## HERBALISM

The herbal approach to dealing with heartburn, as well as with acid reflux, involves using herbs that act in several different ways. Coating, or demulcent, herbs soothe and protect the mucous membranes in the esophagus that may become inflamed with heartburn. Also, anti-inflammatory herbs can improve the symptoms of heartburn and help damaged tissue to heal.

**Licorice:** For long-term use, take two to four 380 mg tablets of de-glycyrrhizinated licorice (DGL), a well-know demulcent, before meals to help with reflux. **Caution:** The prolonged use of decoctions or infusions of dried, unprocessed licorice root can cause high blood pressure, low potassium, and swelling, due to one of its compounds, glycyrrhizin, also called glycyrrhizic acid. Take DGL to avoid this side effect.

**Slippery elm:** Stir 1–2 tbsp of root bark powder into a glass of water and drink after meals and before bedtime. If too much powder is mixed into the water, the liquid can be very thick and difficult to drink, so use small amounts until you get used to making it. You can also sweeten the drink with honey or sugar to improve its taste. Slippery elm is very safe, though some of its compounds can prevent medications from being absorbed by the body.

**Marshmallow:** Make a tea using 5–6 g of marshmallow leaf or root, another demulcent herb, to be drunk throughout the day. As with slippery elm, medicines taken at the same time as marshmallow may not be absorbed well.

**Chamomile:** This anti-inflammatory herb is a popular mild sedative, but it also has anti-spasmodic effects on the intestines. Infuse 1–3 g of chamomile flowers to make a tea and drink three to four times daily. Chamomile is generally well-tolerated, although people who are allergic to other plants in the daisy family may notice that their allergy symptoms worsen; it is best to avoid chamomile if this happens.

# HEMORRHOIDS

## DIAGNOSIS

Hemorrhoids, also know as piles, are small, blood-filled swellings caused by dilated varicose veins in the anal area. They are located just inside the anus, but can sometimes protrude. Constipation and prolonged straining during bowel movements are thought to contribute to the formation of hemorrhoids. If you think you have piles, your doctor will examine the anal canal and lower part of the large intestine using a tube. Some hemorrhoids can get better without medical treatment, particularly those caused by constipation. A doctor may recommend a change of diet that includes more roughage, especially green vegetables, fresh fruit, wholegrain cereals, and bran. Drinking 8–10 glasses of water every day is also advisable. Mild cases can be treated using creams available directly from your local pharmacy. A few days' treatment is usually enough for the irritation to settle. To treat cases of hemorrhoids that protrude from the anus with swelling and pain, resting with a cooling pack applied to the anal area can be helpful. Severe cases need to be treated by a specialist. One possible treatment is rubber band ligation. Sclerotherapy is another option, where a substance is injected that makes the blood in the hemorrhoid clot. The most serious cases require surgical removal, known as a hemorroidectomy.

## SYMPTOMS

- Itchiness in the anal area
- Pain and discomfort
- A lump may be felt in the anus
- Sensation that the bowel has not emptied completely
- Occasionally, anal bleeding after a bowel movement

## TREATMENT GOAL

To ease the pain and discomfort, and resolve the hemorrhoids.

## CONVENTIONAL MEDICINE

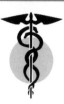

**Stool softeners:** Creating softer stools will ease the pain of bowel movements. Add loose psyllium husks to food to prevent the formation of hard stools, or use the over-the-counter stool softener docusate. Incorporating fiber into your diet and making sure you drink plenty of water also helps in this manner.

**Topical treatment:** Witch hazel can be used topically for its cooling and astringent properties. Over-the-counter topical local anesthetics, which may or may not be mixed with a corticosteroid, can relieve symptoms. These consist of benzocaine 20%, which is applied four times daily as needed for pain and itching, or of lidocaine 5%, which may be applied as required. These are for external use only. Keep in mind that although these are topical agents, they can be absorbed over time. Sitz baths involve sitting in warm water for about 15 minutes three times a day. This can be helpful at the first sign of symptoms.

**Surgery:** Surgical treatments may be needed if the remedies above are unsuccessful or inadequate. An external hemorrhoid excision can be performed to remove any external hemorrhoids. For internal hemorrhoids, rubber band ligation, which involves placing a small rubber band at the base of the hemorrhoid to cut off the blood supply so that it eventually shrinks and falls off, is performed. Infrared coagulation and bipolar electrocoagulation are other possible procedures. These are painless and can be done in a physician's office, but require special equipment that not all doctors have. For advanced hemorrhoids, direct current (DC) therapy is used, where an electric current is applied directly to the hemorrhoid to cut off its blood supply.

## TRADITIONAL CHINESE MEDICINE

**Herbs:** Some external patent herbs may be available from Chinese herbalists, for example, Hua Zhi Gao (a paste that shrinks hemorrhoids). You can also use the formulas below. The herbs listed are available from Chinese pharmacies or online.

• Internal formula for hemorrhoids with constipation: Mix 8 g of Da Huang (rhubarb root and rhizome), 8 g of Chai Hu (hare's ear root), 2 g of Shen Ma (bugbane rhizome), 3 g of Gan Cao (licorice), 8 g of Huang Qin (baical skullcap root), and 10 g of Dang Gui (Chinese angelica root) with 2 ½ cups of water. Bring to the boil, simmer for 30 minutes, and strain the liquid. Drink ½ cup of this decoction three times a day for five to seven days. If you have diarrhea, do not use this formula.

• Internal formula to reduce pain and swelling: Add 15 g of Ku Shen (sophora root) to 3 cups of water. Bring to the boil and simmer for 30 minutes. Remove the herbs and boil two organic eggs, with shells, for five minutes. Remove and peel the eggs and add 30 g of brown sugar to the herbal liquid. Drink the decoction and eat the eggs once a day for five days to complete one course of treatment. You can take two courses of treatment. If you do not see some improvement after one course, see your doctor.

• External herbal formula: Combine 15 g of Ma Zhi Xian (dried purslane), 10 g of Hua Jiao (fruit of Szechuan pepper), 12 g of Wu Bei Zi (gallnut of the Chinese sumac), 15 g of Fang Fen (ledebouriella root), 12 g of Che Bai Ye (biota leaves), 10 g of Zhi Ke (bitter orange), and 15 g of Fuling (poria) in a ceramic pot. Add 6 cups of water, bring to the boil, and simmer for 30 minutes. Strain the herbs, let them cool to a warm temperature, and sit in the herbs. Let the anus soak in the herbs for 10–15 minutes twice a day, in the morning and evening, for five to seven days.

**Acupuncture:** Treatment is effective in helping stop the bleeding and easing the pain. However, it is not common to use acupuncture as the main treatment for this condition.

**Acupressure:** Useful points are the Guan Yuan, Bai Hui, and Qi Hai. Apply gentle pressure with your fingertips to the Guan Yuan point, found on the abdomen about 3 inches below the navel. Use your fingertip to apply pressure to the Bai Hui point, found on the top of the head, on the midpoint of a line running from the top of one ear to the other, for one to three minutes. The Qi Hai point is located on the lower abdomen 1 ½ inches below the navel. Apply downward pressure on this point when you inhale, and repeat for eight breaths. Press these points twice a day.

**Diet:** Oranges, apples, pomegranates, and bananas can ease bowel movements, and do not irritate this condition. If you have hemorrhoids avoid hot, spicy food, such as chilies, black and white pepper, dried ginger, green and red peppers, star anise, and garlic.

## NATUROPATHY

**Diet:** An inadequate amount of fiber in the diet is one of the most common causes of hemorrhoids, and taking fiber has a consistent beneficial effect for relieving symptoms. Base your diet on whole foods like fresh vegetables, fruits, whole grains, beans, nuts, and seeds. Sprinkle ground flaxseeds, which contain high quantities of fiber and essential oils that help with bowel movements, on your cereal, homemade shakes, or salads. If you try to eat too much fiber at one time this may put too much pressure on your intestines, so eat several light meals throughout the day rather than two or three large meals. Avoid trans-fatty acids and hydrogenated oils. They slow down the digestive system and contribute to inflammation. Dehydration worsens hemorrhoids, so drink 8–10 glasses of water throughout the day to keep hydrated and help stools pass more easily.

**TIP:** DO NOT STRAIN YOUR BOWELS

Move your bowels only when you feel the urge and do not spend more than 15 minutes at a time sitting on the toilet. Straining may bring a lot of pressure into the pelvic area, which can lead to hemorrhoids.

**Supplements:** Bioflavonoids are a type of plant compound that stabilizes and strengthens blood vessel walls and decreases inflammation. They have been found to reduce anal discomfort, pain, and discharge during an acute hemorrhoid attack. The major flavonoids found in citrus fruits—diosmin, hesperidin, and oxyrutins—appear to be beneficial. Take a bioflavonoid complex of 1,000 mg three times a day. Also take 500 mg of vitamin C three times a day to strengthen the rectal tissue. Probiotics contain friendly bacteria that help improve constipation. Take a product that contains at least four billion live organisms of lactobacillus and bifidobacterium.

**Herbs:** Witch hazel can be applied topically to the anal area to act as an astringent, decrease the bleeding and relieve the pain, itching, and swelling associated with hemorrhoids. Use a distilled liquid, ointment, or medicated pad as a compress, or apply a cream. You can also add 1 oz to a sitz bath. Butchers broom—also known as knee holly, box holly, and sweet broom—has anti-inflammatory and vein-constricting properties believed to improve the tone and integrity of veins and shrink swollen tissue. Take a standardized extract that provides 200–300 mg of ruscogenins a day. Horse chestnut is often recommended when there is poor circulation in the veins, or chronic venous insufficiency. It relieves symptoms such as swelling and inflammation and also strengthens blood vessel walls. Take 100 mg of standardized aescin daily. Horse chestnut can also be applied externally as a compress. Take a standardized extract of bilberry containing 25% anthocyanosides at 160 mg twice a day to improve circulation and strengthen capillary walls. Stoneroot, taken at 500 mg three times a day, reduces the swelling caused by hemorrhoids.

**Hydrotherapy:** Take two or three sitz baths a day. Sit in a warm bath with your knees raised for 5–15 minutes. To increase circulation, alternate hot and cold sitz baths, sitting for one minute in warm water and 30 seconds in cold.

**TIP:** LIE ON YOUR SIDE IF PREGNANT

If you are pregnant, lying down on your left side and resting for about ½ hour two or three times a day can help prevent hemorrhoids from occurring. It also helps to lie on your left side at night, if you're comfortable in that position, to relieve the pressure of the fetus on the veins serving the lower half of the body.

The selection of homeopathic remedies listed below are the most obvious range of remedies that can be helpful in easing the symptoms of a recently developed, mild to moderate episode of hemorrhoids. If the correct choice is made, taking the homeopathic remedy that most closely matches your individual symptoms should ease pain, discomfort, and/or itching and irritation within a few hours, or a maximum of 48 hours. If you have an established problem with severe hemorrhoids, you will gain greater benefit from seeking treatment from a homeopathic practitioner. This becomes an even greater priority if you experience hemorrhoids in combination with other circulatory problems such as varicose veins. This would suggest that your circulatory system is your vulnerable area, and as a result, needs attention at a constitutional level.

**Nux vomica:** If hemorrhoids are linked to constipation, where although bowel movements occur each day (after lots of straining and urging) the bowel seldom feels cleared, use Nux vomica. Hemorrhoids bleed easily and are distressingly itchy, but are soothed by applying cool compresses.

**Hamamelis:** Use this remedy if hemorrhoids are tender and sore, with lots of prickling stinging pains. Hemorrhoids are likely to bleed quite profusely when very inflamed, and feel especially uncomfortable when touched or when you move suddenly.

**Aloe:** Use this remedy if hemorrhoids burn and itch, especially at night when they make sleeping difficult. There may also be pulsating, throbbing sensations in the rectum, especially after attempting to pass a stool.

**Aesculus:** To relieve acute hemorrhoids that occur due to long-term, underlying constipation and a sluggish bowel, use Aesculus. Pains in the affected area are characteristically sharp and lead to backache, with shooting pains traveling from the rectum up the back. Dryness in the bowel makes passing stools very painful, and there is a persistent feeling of discomfort.

**TIP:** AVOID HEATED SEATS
Heated seats tend to raise the pressure in the veins of the rectum. When traveling by car on long journeys, avoid using heated seats if you are prone to hemorrhoids.

## HERBALISM

The herbal approach to hemorrhoids includes preventing and treating constipation. Please see Constipation for further advice (p. 346).

**Yarrow:** Flowers of yarrow can be used as a poultice or salve to stop bleeding and act, like witch hazel, as an astringent. Both of these actions are important in controlling the swelling and bleeding associated with hemorrhoids. Yarrow's effectiveness is partly due to a compound, called achilleine, which stops bleeding.

**Stone root:** This astringent herb is either taken internally or incorporated into suppositories to treat hemorrhoids. Some herbalists use the whole plant, others use just the root. It contains numerous compounds, such as terpenoids and rosmaric acid, that account for its medicinal effects.

**Multifaceted approach:** There are many other herbs that are useful for treating hemorrhoids. It is important to treat constipation, and use a local, topical herb to help with swelling, bleeding, and pain. Many herbalists also address the health of the vascular system by using plants such as horse chestnut seed to tone the venous system and address any congestion. Open wounds associated with bleeding hemorrhoids can be treated with any of the vulnerary herbs, such as calendula. Also, mucilaginous herbs, such as slippery elm, can soften stools and coat the intestinal wall to make bowel movements more comfortable. Consult a medical herbalist for a comprehensive treatment plan.

# HICCUPS

## DIAGNOSIS

Hiccups are caused when the diaphragm, the muscle under the lungs that helps you breathe in, suddenly contracts. The glottis (located at the top of the windpipe) closes immediately after the diaphragm contracts, which makes the typical "hic" sound. Most people have bouts of hiccups from time to time. It is a reflex action that you cannot stop. However, unlike other reflexes, such as coughing and sneezing, hiccups do not seem to serve any useful purpose. They are harmless, but can be distressing and uncomfortable. In most cases they start for no apparent reason, last a short while, and then stop of their own accord. They are usually due to overeating or eating too fast, drinking carbonated beverages, or swallowing air. Sometimes they can be triggered by very hot or cold food or drinks, taking a cold shower, drinking alcohol, smoking, sudden excitement, or stressful situations. In some rare cases, persistent hiccups are caused by an underlying disease: Over 100 diseases are reported to trigger hiccups, but they usually have other symptoms as well. Some are common, such as acid reflux, while others are much rarer. In some cases of persistent hiccups there is no apparent cause.

## SYMPTOMS

- Producing a "hic" sound that cannot be controlled
- Can cause the abdomen to feel tight and uncomfortable

## TREATMENT GOAL

To bring fast relief if the condition is occasional. To find the underlying cause if the condition is persistent.

## CONVENTIONAL MEDICINE

Conventional medicine operates on the principle that hiccups represent a symptom of another problem, not a disease in itself. As such, although treatment for eradication of hiccups exists, medical therapy involves a search for cause as well.

**Popular remedies:** There is no scientific evidence to support the theory that, for example, drinking a glass of water from the wrong side of a cup can help. However, there are some techniques that have been proven to work. The Valsalva maneuver involves closing your throat and breathing out to press air against it. The oculocardiac reflex involves gently compressing the eyeball with a closed lid for a short period of time. Other techniques that have less supporting evidence are pulling on the tongue, applying bitter substances to the back of the tongue, drinking ice water, and scaring the hiccup sufferer. Also, distracting a sufferer by asking them to hiccup (on demand) often results in that person being unable to do so.

**Medication:** The medication used for hiccups is usually meant for other purposes. These include sedatives (benzodiazepenes), antinausea drugs (Zofran®), analeptics such as Ritalin®, anticonvulsants such as Tegretol®, antipsychotics such as Thorazine®, antidepressants such as Elavil®, calcium channel blockers usually used for blood pressure, lidocaine, antacids, and baclofen. The first choice for treatment is usually 10 mg of Reglan® three times a day for acute hiccups.

**Surgery:** Surgical intervention involves an irreversible destruction of the phrenic nerve, the nerve leading to the diaphragm. This is a very rare and rather new procedure and long-term side effects are not well known.

## TRADITIONAL CHINESE MEDICINE

Traditional Chinese medicine views hiccups as the result of an insufficient or irregular diet, an emotional upset, a deficiency of the digestive system, or a body system failure. Below are some suggested herbal treatments for each type of condition. If hiccups are one symptom of an underlying condition, consult a doctor of Chinese medicine about formulas that can help treat the primary illness.

**Herbs:** For each formula, mix the herbs in a ceramic or glass pot. Add 3 cups of water, bring the mixture to the boil, and let it simmer for 30 minutes. The herbs listed are available from Chinese herbalists or online.

• To treat hiccups due to an irregular diet: If hiccups occur after overeating or wolfing down food, or after eating too much cold or raw food, mix 18 g of Cao Mai Ya (baked wheat), 18 g of Cao Gu Ya (baked rice grain), 12 g of Shan Zha (hawthorn fruit),  8 g of Shen Qu (medicated leaven), and 3 g of Gan Cao (licorice). Drink 1 cup two to three times during the day for three to five days.

• To treat hiccups due to emotional upset: Combine 10 g of Ye Ju Hua (wild chrysanthemum flower), 5 g of Bo He (field mint), 12 g of Chai Hu (hare's ear root), 15 g of Bai Shao (white peony root), 12 g of Yu Jin (turmeric tuber), and 5 g of Gan Cao (licorice). Take 1 cup of the decoction twice a day for 7–10 days.

• To treat hiccups due to digestive system deficiency: Hiccups may be combined with poor appetite, indigestion, diarrhea, and bloating. Mix 15 g of Bai Zhu (white atractylodes rhizome), 15 g of Tai Zi Shen (pseudostellaria), 15 g Fuling (poria), 6 g of Sha Ren (cardamom), 6 g of Chen Pi (tangerine peel), 12 g of Fa Ban Xia (pinellia rhizome), 6 g of Din Xiang (clove flower bud), and 15 g of Shan Yao (Chinese yam). Drink 1 cup three times a day for 10–15 days.

**Acupuncture:** An experienced practitioner will use various acupuncture points to release hiccups; in some cases it can be effective immediately.

**Acupressure:** Apply pressure to the Tian Ding point, located on the lateral side of the neck, just behind the neck muscle (sternocleidomastoid) and about ⅓ inch above the collarbone, for one to three minutes once a day. Press the Nei Guan point on the center of the wrist on the palm side, about 2 inches above the crease, for one to three minutes. In a sitting position, or lying down, have someone press the Ge Shu point on the back, about 1½ inches lateral to the 7th vertebra, with light pressure for one to three minutes. You can press those points one to three times a day.

**Diet:** Eating hawthorn fruit, fresh ginger root and ginger candy, vinegar, honey, lychees, and kiwi are helpful for stopping hiccups. Avoid smoking cigarettes and drinking alcohol.

## NATUROPATHY

**Diet:** Eat slowly and chew each bite of food about 30 times before swallowing. Eating too fast is one of the main causes of hiccups. Mealtimes with friends and family should be a relaxed, enjoyable affair. Sip fluids slowly to avoid hiccups. To prevent infants from getting hiccups, make sure they are burped after every feed. Take care to avoid becoming overweight by practicing good nutrition and maintaining good muscle tone through exercise. Also avoid putting unnecessary strain on abdominal muscles by lifting heavy objects. This may prevent hiccups from occurring.

**Popular remedies:** There are several methods of stopping hiccups. Try putting 1 tsp of sugar under your tongue and drinking 1 cup of water very, very slowly. Some people find that letting 1–2 tsp of sugar dissolve in the mouth works just as well. Blow in and out of a brown paper bag held securely to your lips. Make sure you blow vigorously at least 10 times. You can also try soaking a lemon wedge in angostura bitters and then sucking on it.

## HOMEOPATHY

Choose the most appropriate of the following remedies to deal with an isolated bout of hiccups. If you are prone to hiccups, the tips below can help discourage symptoms from developing.

**Ignatia:** If hiccups develop after an emotional shock and you suddenly feel weepy, try Ignatia. Signature symptoms include a tendency to sigh frequently and involuntarily, and a feeling of being choked with emotion in the throat. When this remedy is suitable, hiccups tend to come on after eating, drinking, or having a cigarette.

**Nux vomica:** Consider this remedy to treat hiccups that develop an hour or so after overindulging in rich food or drink. Common symptoms include hiccups that are combined with lots of empty burping that feels as though it will escalate into retching.

**Arsenicum album:** This is a potentially helpful remedy for treating hiccups that come at frequent intervals, and that are combined with burping and general uneasiness in the stomach. Even the thought of food is disgusting, and symptoms tend to be aggravated by eating or drinking even the smallest amount. Hiccups may be brought on when feeling very anxious and tense, and/or when drinking ice cold drinks.

## HERBALISM

A host of home remedies exist to cure this annoying condition, but there is a lack of specific herbal medicine treatments.

**Wormwood:** It is thought by some that the common bitter herb wormwood may help to relieve hiccups. Wormwood is the major ingredient in Angostura bitters, which has been added to a lemon wedge and used in trials to relieve hiccups. Of course, the effectiveness of this treatment could just as well be due to the lemon itself. Wormwood oil, though occasionally recommended, should be avoided because it is toxic to the liver when taken internally.

# INCONTINENCE

## DIAGNOSIS

Urinary incontinence occurs when the pressure in the bladder is greater than the pressure in the urethra and a person becomes unable to control when urine is released. It is a symptom of another condition rather than a disease in itself and can be caused by a variety of illnesses, including neurological diseases, multiple sclerosis, polio, and degenerative changes associated with ageing. It tends to affect women more than men, as pregnancy and childbirth can weaken the pelvic floor and, after the menopause, estrogen levels are lower, which can mean that muscle pressure around the urethra is weaker. The urethra may be less elastic and unable to close completely so that leaks are more likely to occur. Some medications can also affect the pelvic floor. There are four different types of urinary incontinence. Stress urinary incontinence (SUI) happens while sneezing, coughing, laughing, lifting, or exercising. These activities place extra pressure on the bladder, causing accidental leaks. One in three women experience SUI at some point in their lives. Urge urinary incontinence (UUI) occurs when a person has an urgent need to empty the bladder, but is unable to get to the toilet in time. There is also a need to empty the bladder more frequently than normal, but less urine is passed than usual. Mixed urinary incontinence (MUI) is a combination of SUI and UUI. Overflow urinary incontinence (OUI) usually happens when there's a blockage in the urethra, so that the bladder does not empty completely. When the bladder refills, it puts pressure on the obstruction, which gives way slightly leading to a small leak of urine.

## SYMPTOMS

- Inability to control the release of urine
- A frequent urge to empty the bladder
- Passing less urine than usual

## TREATMENT GOAL

To reduce the pressure on the bladder through lifestyle changes, such as losing weight, taking care about fluid intake, and performing pelvic floor exercises. If these treatments do not work, surgery may be needed.

## CONVENTIONAL MEDICINE

Incontinence is a symptom of an underlying condition, for example, a urinary tract infection, prostate problems, or a side effect of medication. It is necessary to identify and treat the cause.

**Modify your lifestyle:** Lifestyle modification and biofeedback therapies can be helpful. Biofeedback is a treatment technique in which people are trained to improve their health by using signals from their own bodies. For example, make a schedule of consistent times to pass water, or practice Kegel exercises, described below. Eliminating caffeine, alcohol, and other diuretics such as celery, parsley, and dandelion products from your diet can also be beneficial. Avoid eating sugar and processed foods, as well as foods that are diuretic.

**To treat urge urinary incontinence:** Most drugs target UUI. The most commonly used medication is oxybutynin, an anti-spasm drug that affects the bladder muscle. An adult dose is 5 mg three times a day. Transdermal delivery, a patch that gives a controlled dose of the drug through the skin, is another method of taking this medication.

**To treat stress incontinence:** Electrical stimulation, administered by a physical therapist or a nurse, is one option. Medications used for this type of incontinence are pseudoephedrine and imipramine. Sometimes estrogen treatment can be helpful in post-menopausal women with stress incontinence. Natural bioidentical estrogen can be given for this purpose as opposed to the more risky synthetic variety. If these methods fail, surgery, known as cystourethropexy, which raises the neck of the bladder so that urine can not leak out, can be performed.

**To treat overflow incontinence:** One medication used is bethanechol. To treat incontinence in men due to the enlargement of the prostate gland, a condition know as benign prostatic hypertrophy, finasteride is used. For overnight bedwetting, particularly in children, Tofranil® and desmopressin are most commonly used.

**TIP: DO KEGEL EXERCISES**
For incontinence caused during physical stress, such as sneezing, running, or jumping, do Kegel exercises to strengthen the pelvic floor muscles, which surround the bladder and the urethra to help keep urine in. To identify these muscles, try to stop urine midflow while sitting on the toilet. Squeeze these muscles several dozens of times throughout the day. Some practitioners recommend as many as 300 Kegel exercise repetitions over the course of a day. It may take as long as three months to see the full results of this approach.

**Herbs:** Combine the herbs from either formula below in a ceramic pot and add 3 cups of water. Bring the ingredients to the boil and simmer for 30 minutes. Drink 1 cup twice a day. The herbs listed below are available from Chinese pharmacies or online.

• To treat incontinence with symptoms of fatigue, lower backache, and clear urine: Mix 12 g of Huang Qi (milk-vetch root), 10 g of ginseng, 5 g of Sheng Ma (bugbane rhizome), 6 g of Chen Pi (tangerine peel), 10 g of Chai Hu (hare's ear root), 12 g of Wu Mei (mume fruit), 10 g of Jin Yin Zi (cherokee rosehip), 18 g of Mu Li (oyster shell), and 30 g of Qian Shi (euryale seed).

• To treat incontinence due to heat: Mix 10 g of Chai Hu (hare's ear root), 10 g of Long Dan Cao (Chinese gentian root), 8 g of Huang Qin (baical skullcap root), 10 g of Zhi Zi (Cape Jasmine fruit), 10 g of Che Qian Zi (plantago seeds), 12 g of Shen Di Huang (Chinese foxglove root), and 18 g of Mu Li (oyster shell).

**Acupuncture:** Treatment can be effective in some cases. A short-term condition is easier to treat than a long-term one; and patients with stronger constitutions are easier to treat than those who are weaker. An experienced acupuncturist will make a thorough evaluation and advise on the length and frequency of treatment.

**Acupressure:** Use your index fingertip to apply gentle pressure to the Shen Que point on the abdomen in the center of the navel. Press the Guan Yuan point on the abdomen, about 3 inches below the navel. The Bai Hui point is found on the top of the head on the midpoint along the line running from the top of one ear to the other. Use your fingertip to apply pressure to this point for one to three minutes. Also apply downward pressure to the Qi Hai point, located on the lower abdomen 1½ inches below the navel, as you inhale.

**Diet:** Make a porridge using 30 g of walnuts, 50 g of sticky rice, and 4 cups of water. Cook for 45 minutes. Eat this porridge three times a week for as long as necessary. In general, food that nourishes the kidneys, such as black sesame seeds, string beans, sword beans, plums, grapes, tangerines, star anise, chives, duck, egg yolk, and wheat, are good for this condition.

## NATUROPATHY

**Diet:** Drink 8–10 glasses of water daily and eat whole, fresh, unrefined, and unprocessed foods, including fruits, vegetables, whole grains, soy, beans, seeds, nuts, olive oil, and cold-water fish (such as salmon, tuna, sardines, halibut, and mackerel). Avoid sugar, dairy products, refined foods, fried foods, junk foods, and caffeine. In women, lower estrogen levels during the menopause can cause urethral tissue to become thinner, less resilient, and less elastic, leading to urinary incontinence. Adding phyto-estrogens (plant estrogens), compounds found in plants that produce an estrogen-like effect in the body, to the diet can be helpful for women who suffer from incontinence. In most cases, adding phyto-estrogens to the diet is safe and easy. They can be found in roasted soy nuts, soy milk, tempeh, textured soy protein, and tofu.

**Supplements:** Take 3–4 g of fish oils a day; 1 tbsp of flaxseed oil a day; 500 mg of vitamin C two to three times a day; and 400 IU of vitamin E a day for anti-inflammatory support.

**Herbs:** Take 400 mg of bromelain three times a day in between meals. Soy isoflavones, the components of soy with the strongest estrogenic properties, are available in capsule form from health food stores. A typical dose is 50–150 mg daily. Find a herbal formula that contains two or more of the following ingredients: buchu, a soothing diuretic and antiseptic for the urinary system; cleavers, a traditional urinary tonic; corn silk, which has soothing and diuretic properties; horsetail, an astringent and mild diuretic with tissue-healing properties; marshmallow root, which has soothing, demulcent properties; and usnea, which has soothing and antiseptic properties. A herbalist can also make a formula for you. Follow the instructions on the label.

---

**TIP:** USE A PESSARY

A stiff ring called a pessary can be inserted into the vagina to press out against the vaginal walls and urethra to reduce SUI. Ask your doctor for more information.

---

## HOMEOPATHY

This can be an embarrassing problem that can arise for a variety of reasons. The remedies listed below can ease symptoms of mild incontinence that have arisen recently and that have an obvious trigger, such as a cough. However, more often than not, this is a condition that will benefit from professional medical help, particularly an integrated medical approach of conventional and complementary treatment. This is particularly the case if incontinence is brought on by, for example, pregnancy or menopause. Men also may notice symptoms of urinary incontinence as a result of changes in the prostate gland at midlife and beyond. If your child suffers from night-time incontinence, consult a homeopathic practitioner for constitutional treatment.

**Causticum:** If small amounts of urine are released unintentionally, such as during a severe coughing fit, or when laughing, sneezing, and/or blowing the nose, try this remedy. When urinating, the flow may be very slow and hesitant, and men may find they need to sit down to release a reasonable flow of urine. Severe coughing spasms are triggered by a tickling in the throat that may be aggravated by contact with raw, cold air and temporarily eased by taking sips of cold water.

**Pulsatilla:** If urine leaks out when lying down, during sleep, coughing, sneezing, getting very angry, or when passing gas, use Pulsatilla. If urine is held in the bladder for too long, the flow may tend to stop and start rather than pass smoothly. When a cough is present it is likely to be tight, irritating, and tickly at night in bed, and loosen up in the morning. Any mucus producted in yellowish-green in color.

**Sepia:** If urine leaks out as a result of a fright or shock, or when laughing, coughing, and/or sneezing, and is accompanied by a strong bearing-down sensation in the pelvis just above the pubic area, use Sepia. Coughing spasms are characteristically exhausting and draining in nature, and often set off, or are made more intense by, rapid and/or severe changes in temperature.

**TIP:** USE ABSORBENT PADS
Invest in some pads designed for adults with urinary incontinence. These can be a short-term remedy to feelings of frustration and embarrassment until a more permanent solution is found.

## HERBALISM

 Herbs are not the first choice for treating urinary incontinence, but consider a trial of agrimony, and consult a medical herbalist for other treatment ideas.

**Agrimony:** This herb has a traditional use as bitter tonic and for general urinary and gastrointestinal health, but it has also been used for urinary incontinence. It is best to purchase a tincture from a local health food store or herbal pharmacy and take 30 drops three times daily.

# INDIGESTION

## DIAGNOSIS

Indigestion, also known as dyspepsia, is the term used to describe pain or discomfort in the upper abdomen or chest that develops after eating. The stomach produces a strong acid that helps digest food. A layer of mucus that lines the stomach acts as a barrier against this acid, but if this lining becomes damaged the acid irritates the tissues underneath, causing indigestion. The condition tends to occur after eating heavy meals, eating late at night, or eating irregularly, as long gaps between meals allow the acid more time to act. Most people have suffered from indigestion after a large meal at some time or another, but the condition can also be triggered by drinking too much alcohol, smoking, stress and anxiety, drugs such as aspirin and anti-inflammatory medication, pregnancy, and stomach ulcers. Indigestion is sometimes accompanied by heartburn, a burning sensation in the chest (see p. 408).

## SYMPTOMS

- Pain, often in the upper part of the abdomen or chest
- Heartburn, a burning pain caused by reflux of the stomach's contents up the gullet
- Loss of appetite
- Nausea and vomiting
- Flatulence or belching

## TREATMENT GOAL

To introduce lifestyle changes to reduce the long-term occurrence of indigestion, and to relieve any immediate symptoms of burning or discomfort.

## CONVENTIONAL MEDICINE

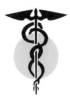

Indigestion is often a symptom of peptic ulcer disease or results from using non-steroidal anti-inflammatory drugs (NSAIDs). Treatment is determined by identifying the cause, which can involve a procedure called an endoscopy, where a tube is inserted through the mouth to view the esophagus and the stomach. This is part of the treatment for patients over 45 years old who have severe and unremitting indigestion. Patients under 45 are often tested for the bacteria associated with ulcers, H. Pylori. If the test is positive, treatment involves eradication therapy, where two antibiotics and a proton pump inhibitor are given simultaneously for a three-week period.

**To treat acute indigestion:** Treatment usually involves using an H2 blocking agent or a proton pump inhibitor. These drugs block the H2 receptor cells in the stomach and the proton pump in the cells to decrease acid production. If these do not work, Reglan® (metoclopramide), which increases stomach motility, is tried. Carafate® may also be used, as well as over-the-counter products such as Maalox®, Mylanta®, and Gaviscon®.

**Modify your lifestyle:** Eliminating wheat and dairy products from your diet may be beneficial. Biofeedback, a treatment that trains your body to listen to its own signals, can also be helpful, as are stress reduction techniques such as breathing and meditation.

## TRADITIONAL CHINESE MEDICINE

**Herbs:** Shan Zha (hawthorn) is a popular fruit in northern China and is widely used for helping digestion. Various formulas that incorporate this herb are detailed below. Hawthorn, as well as the other herbs listed, are available from Chinese herbalists or online.

• To treat indigestion due to overeating and/or acute stomach bloating: Mix 12 g of dried Shan Zha (hawthorn) with 12 g of Bin Long (betel nut), 30 g of Yi Yi Ren (seeds of Job's tears), and 8 g of Shen Qu (medicated leaven). Make a decoction by placing the herbs in a ceramic or glass pot and adding 3½ cups of water. Bring to the boil and simmer for 30 minutes. Strain the liquid and drink 1 cup twice a day.

• To treat indigestion with food retention due to deficiency of spleen and stomach: Combine 12 g of dried Shan Zha (hawthorn) with 12 g of Mu Xiang (costus root), 15 g Fuling (poria), 12 g of Bai Zhu (white atractylodes rhizome), 10 g of Shen Qu (medicated leaven), 12 g of Bai Shao (white peony), and 12 g Fa Ban Xia (pinellia rhizome) in a glass or ceramic pot. Add 3 cups of water, bring to the boil, and simmer for 30 minutes. Strain and drink 1 cup twice a day.

• To treat indigestion with strong abdominal pain: Mix 12 g of Shan Zha (hawthorn), 8 g Qing Pi (immature tangerine peel), 10 g of Zhi Shi (immature fruit of bitter orange), 12 g of Lian Qiao (forsythia fruit), 12 g of Long Dan Cao (Chinese gentian root), 8 g of Huang Qin (baical skullcap root), 10 g of radish seeds, 8 g of Chai Hu (hare's ear root), and 12 g Bai Shao (white peony). Place the herbs in a ceramic or glass pot, add 3½ cups of water, and bring to the boil. Simmer for 30 minutes and strain the liquid. Drink 1 cup twice a day.

**Acupuncture:** You may have treatment once a week, accompanied by the herbal remedies above. Alternatively, see a doctor of traditional Chinese medicine for advice. Usually the doctor will ask you questions about your diet, your eating habits, and your bowel movements. Knowing your mental and emotional condition is also necessary for diagnosis with Chinese medicine. The doctor will determine the frequency of treatment, and the correct combination of acupuncture and/or herbal medicine.

**Acupressure:** To treat indigestion, press the Nei Guan, Hegu, and Tian Shu points. The Hegu point is located on the back of the hand in the depression between the thumb and the first finger. The Nei Guan point is located in the center of the wrist on the palm side about 2 inches above the crease. The Tian Shu point is found on the middle of the abdomen 1 inch to the side of the navel.

**Diet:** Apples, grapefruit, kumquat, mango, barley pineapple, tomato, basil, and sweet rice are all good foods to eat on a daily basis. Avoid eating mango after a big meal, as it will cause the stomach to swell. Avoid foods that may cause gas such as beans, raw and fried onions, and yeast (found in beer). For indigestion due to gastric acid, try eating a few pieces of fresh ginger.

## NATUROPATHY

**Diet:** Eat a whole food diet, eliminating unnatural refined foods. Whole grains, raw vegetables, and nuts and seeds are rich in fiber and the essential nutrients important in relieving symptoms of indigestion and should be staples in your diet. Some natural foods, however, such as wheat, citrus fruits, and corn can aggravate symptoms. Avoid overeating, and eat small meals throughout the day. Drink 8–10 glasses of water a day to maintain good digestive health and neutralize excess acidity in the stomach that can cause indigestion. Saturated fats, hydrogenated oils, and partially hydrogenated oils lead to acid reflux, another potential cause of indigestion. Avoid foods that contain these substances, such as fried and greasy foods, heavy sauces, and red meat. Avoid caffeine, alcohol, chocolate, and minty or spicy foods, as they make symptoms worse. Stop eating three hours before bedtime as sleeping with a full stomach can aggravate symptoms.

**TIP:** TAKE APPLE CIDER VINEGAR
Take 1 tbsp of apple cider vinegar or lemon juice when you are experiencing indigestion. If this eliminates your symptoms you may be deficient in stomach acid.

**Supplements:** If using antacids, avoid brands that include peppermint, as this can relax the low esophageal sphincter. This muscle, at the base of the esophagus, keeps food and digestive acids in the stomach. If relaxed, it can release stomach acid, leading to indigestion. Instead, take 250–500 mg of calcium carbonate three times a day with food. Chewable tablets provide the quickest relief. To restore friendly bacteria to the gut, take a probiotic product in the lactobacillus family that contains at least four billion active organisms twice daily with meals or 30 minutes after meals. Digestive enzymes help you digest food more effectively so that less irritation is caused. The enzymes include lipases that digest fat, proteases that digest proteins, and amylases that digest starch. Take 2 capsules or tablets of a full spectrum enzyme product with each meal. Also take 1–2 betaine hydrochloride capsules to support stomach acid levels.

**Herbs:** De-glycyrrhizinated licorice (DGL), which is safer than other types of licorice, may help to heal damaged mucous lining in the stomach. Take two 380 mg DGL licorice tablets three or four times a day between meals as needed. Slippery elm serves as a demulcent to soothe the digestive lining of the stomach. Take 3 ml of tincture or 500 mg of a capsule three times a day, or lozenges if preferred. Marshmallow is another demulcent that soothes the digestive lining and reduces inflammation in the stomach. Take 300 mg in capsule form or 3 ml of tincture three times a day. Mastic gum has been shown to heal stomach mucosa and has antibacterial benefits. Take 500 mg three times a day. Gamma-oryzanol, also known as rice bran oil, can help repair the entire digestive system. Take 150 mg three times a day for one month.

**TIP:** MANAGE STRESS LEVELS
Unmanaged stress makes indigestion symptoms worse. Exercising regularly is an effective method of reducing stress. Vigorous exercise works for some people while gentler exercises like yoga and T'ai chi work for others.

## HOMEOPATHY

Most people are likely to experience problems with indigestion at some stage, since it's inevitable that eating habits can't always be as healthy as they should be for smooth, comfortable digestive functioning to take place. In addition, lifestyle factors can also impinge on this problem with high stress levels often being a major candidate for triggering the most common features of indigestion. Any of the remedies suggested below should solve the problem of a one-off bout of indigestion that has been caused by an obvious trigger such as those mentioned above. However, indigestion that sets in for no obvious reason, especially if it is beginning to be a regular feature of life, is a symptom that should not be ignored and suppressed temporarily with conventional antacids. Instead, take action by consulting your usual doctor.

**Lycopodium:** If symptoms of indigestion, such as burping, bloating, and/or acid rising into the gullet, occur as a result of eating a lot of high fiber foods, such as sprouts, beans, lentils, and/or very coarse wholemeal bread, try using Lycopodium. Symptoms may also set in when feeling very stressed and anxious. Rumbling, gurgling, and bloating in the belly are so severe that it becomes necessary to loosen the waistband in order to get comfortable. Cold food and drinks aggravate the condition, while warm food and drinks are generally soothing.

**Carbo veg:** To treat trapped gas in the belly accompanied by a heavy, nauseous feeling, and swelling and bloating in the stomach, use Carbo veg. When well indicated, this remedy has a profound capacity for releasing trapped gas, which gives great relief. Signature symptoms include feeling discomfort and distress after eating even the smallest amount when feeling gassy, or while being in stuffy, overheated surroundings. Contact with cool air and being fanned provide temporary relief.

**Pulsatilla:** Use this remedy if indigestion occurs after eating rich and/or fatty foods. Uneasiness and discomfort in the stomach is aggravated by jarring movements, such as walking very quickly. The mouth is dry without thirst, and food eaten tends to "repeat." Lying down makes the uneasiness in the stomach worse, while taking a gentle stroll in the open air gives relief.

**Nux vomica:** If indigestion arises as a result of overindulgence in rich or junk foods, alcohol, strong coffee, or cigarettes, try Nux vomica. If you feel strung out, tense, and highly stressed, this remedy is almost certain to help resolve symptoms. Additional symptoms may include feeling hung over and constipated, which is worse in the morning and slightly improves as the day goes on, especially if it becomes possible to have a bowel movement.

## HERBALISM

The two main classes of herbs used to treat indigestion are carminatives and bitters. Carminative plants stimulate the stomach lining, increase stomach secretions, and promote the flow of bile. Bitter herbs increase the flow of saliva and stomach secretion, and promote the motility of the stomach.

**Peppermint:** This carminative plant is a hybrid of spearmint and water mint. When used in tea form, peppermint leaf may ease upper intestinal tract gas, spasm, and indigestion. It may be more effective if you cover the cup as the leaf is steeping to capture as much of the essential oil (primarily menthol) from the leaf as possible—it can otherwise can be volatile and disperse in the air. Sometimes peppermint tea can worsen heartburn.

**Chamomile:** This carminative has anti-inflammatory, antispasmodic, and soothing effects on gastrointestinal tissue. The beneficial effects of chamomile are probably due to two main classes of compounds, the volatile oils (such as bisabolol) and the flavonoids (such as apigenin). To treat indigestion, steep a heaped tbsp of chamomile flowers in 1 covered cup of hot water for 10 minutes to extract the medicinal flavonoids and some of the volatile oils. This tea can be taken several times a day to help with symptoms.

**Fennel:** Another common carminative, fennel seeds can simply be eaten after a meal to aid digestion, calm the stomach and intestines, and dispel gas. Alternatively, ½ tsp of the seeds can be powdered then infused with hot water and consumed throughout the day, or 30–60 drops of a tincture of the seeds can be taken several times daily.

**Gentian:** Roots and rhizomes of this bitter herb have a long history of use as a gastrointestinal "tonic." Its effects are due to several different medicinal compounds; one of them, amarogentin, a glycoside compound, provides much of the bitter taste. Gentian can be consumed in several different forms. Boil 1 g in ½ cup of water for five minutes to make a liquid decoction that should be taken 30 minutes before meals, up to four times daily. Alternatively, an alcohol-based tincture of gentian can be made and similarly used before meals. Some people may develop a headache after using gentian, or find the bitter taste intolerable.

# IRRITABLE BOWEL SYNDROME

## DIAGNOSIS

Although the exact cause of irritable bowel syndrome (IBS) is uncertain, it is thought to be linked to poor coordination of muscle contraction, and to abnormal bacterial fermentation in the large bowel. When your body digests food, a series of muscular contractions moves the food through the gut, known as peristalsis. IBS occurs when there is a loss of coordination between these muscular contractions. It is the most common condition seen by gastroenterologists and can occur at any age, but usually starts during the teenage years. IBS often results from a combination of physical and psychological factors. For example, there is evidence that patients with irritable bowel syndrome have increased sensitivity to stimuli within the gut. As well as the intestinal symptoms, stress seems to be one of the main triggers. Many people find that the onset of their symptoms is often due to a major life event.

## SYMPTOMS

- Variable and erratic bowel habits, alternating between constipation and diarrhea
- Feeling full after small meals
- Abdominal bloating after meals
- Excessive gurgling noises in the stomach
- Generalized abdominal tenderness with bloating
- Right-sided abdominal pain
- Pain under the left ribs
- Heartburn

## TREATMENT GOAL

Since the cause of IBS is unknown, it is not possible to prevent the condition. There is no single blood test, X-ray, or scan that will diagnose IBS. Changes in diet, exercise, and stress management techniques can all help bring a reduction in distressing symptoms.

## CONVENTIONAL MEDICINE

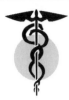

**Diet:** Add 2 tbsp of loose psyllium husk to food a day—it can be sprinkled on cereal or salad. Introduce foods that are high in fiber into your diet. The fiber should be mixed with, or followed by, about 8 oz of water to prevent binding. In the long run this works well, although it may be a little uncomfortable initially. Avoid foods that irritate the gut such as gluten, sugar, and dairy products, although irritants do vary from person to person. Bifidus probiotics and Saccharomyces boullardi introduce and maintain beneficial bacteria in the gut. These are available from health food stores. Black tea is useful for easing episodes of diarrhea.

**Reduce stress:** Stress reduction is very important in IBS. It has been documented that IBS responds best to an integrated mind, body, diet, and medication treatment approach. Meditation, T'ai chi, and yoga are beneficial.

**Medication:** The medication loperamide is used to treat diarrhea. For very severe unresponsive episodes of diarrhea, a medication called alosetron (Lotronex™) can be used. It can cause severe constipation and should be used carefully. Tegaserod (Zelnorm®)is used to treat chronic constipation that does not respond to dietary modification. The antispasmotic dicyclomine (Bentyl®) can be used to treat spasms and bloating pain, although lifestyle and diet modification are usually successful.

## TRADITIONAL CHINESE MEDICINE

**Herbs:** To make either of the decoctions below, mix the necessary herbs in a ceramic or glass pot. Add 3 cups of water, bring to the boil, and simmer for 30 minutes. Drink 1 cup twice a day. The herbs needed for either formula are available from Chinese herbalists or online.

• To treat IBS with digestive function deficiency: Symptoms include irregular bowel movements, diarrhea, and fatigue. Mix 12 g of Zhu Ling (polyporus sclerotium), 12 g of ginseng, 3 g of dried ginger, 8 g of Gui Zhi (cinnamon), 15 g of Fuling (poria), 15 g of Bai Zhu (white atractylodes rhizome), 6 g of Chen Pi (tangerine peel), and 12 g of Fa Ban Xia (pinellia rhizome).

• To treat alternating diarrhea and constipation: Symptoms include bloating after eating, accompanied with anxiety or depression. Combine 12 g of Chai Hu (hare's ear root), 6 g of Chen Pi (tangerine peel), 12 g of Bai Shao (white peony), 10 g of Zhi Shi (immature fruit of bitter orange), 10 g of Xiang Fu (nut grass rhizome), 6 g of Bo He (field mint), and 12 g of Bai Zhu (white atractylodes rhizome).

**Acupuncture:** Treatment can regulate the stomach and intestinal functions. Sessions once or twice a week are usual and you can expect some degree of improvement after about five treatments. However, it will take a few months to one or two years of treatment to achieve maximum results.

**Acupressure:** Self-massage the Susanli and the San Yin Jiao points, once or twice a day. The Susanli point is on the lower leg in a depression 4 inches below and 1 inch to the outside of the knee. The San Yin Jiao point is located in the center of the outside of the leg, about 3 inches above the anklebone. You can also massage the Pi Shu and Wei Shu points while lying on the stomach or in a sitting position. The Pi Shu point is located on the back 1½ inches lateral to the spine at the 11th vertebra. The Wei Shu point is 1½ inches lateral to the spin at the 12th vertebra.

**Diet:** Eat a balanced diet that includes plenty of neutral foods, such as corn, celery, potato, honey, sweet rice, and string beans. Avoid raw food and foods that are hard to digest, like cucumber, onions, and green pepper.

## NATUROPATHY

**Diet:** It is important to follow a high-fiber diet rich in whole grains and fresh vegetables, fruits, and legumes. This will help reduce the irritation of the digestive system and keep your bowels moving. Replenish the healthy flora in your intestines by eating sauerkraut, kefir, and non-sweetened yogurt containing live probiotics. Identify any foods to which you are allergic or intolerant and eliminate them from your diet. Wheat, dairy, corn, soy, and citrus fruits are the most common allergens. Be conscious of how these foods make you feel—for example, lactose produces symptoms of IBS in those who are intolerant to it. Saturated fats, hydrogenated oils, and partially hydrogenated oils lead to acid reflux. Avoid foods that contain these substances, such as fried and greasy foods, heavy sauces, and red meats, as they are hard to digest and may aggravate symptoms. Avoid chilled drinks, as they inhibit digestion and may cause cramping. Also steer clear of the sweetener fructose, as research shows that IBS sufferers are sensitive to it.

**Supplements:** Digestive enzymes help your body digest food more efficiently, reducing irritation. The enzymes include lipases that digest fat, proteases that digest proteins, and amylases that digest starch. Take 2 capsules or tablets of a full spectrum enzyme product with each meal. Betaine hydrochloride supports stomach acid levels and helps with digestion. Take 1–2 capsules with each meal. Probiotics help digestion and prevents overgrowth of candida and other harmful microbes. Take a product containing four billion active organisms daily of lactobacillus acidophilus and bifidus.

**Herbs:** Abdominal pain, the most frequent and disabling symptom of IBS, improves when the intestinal smooth muscles are relaxed. Fennel seed is used to relieve spasms in the gastrointestinal tract, feelings of fullness, and flatulence. Take 1 tsp a day of tincture on an empty stomach. Also take 150 mg of gamma-oryzanol, a natural substance isolated from bran, three times a day for one month. Studies have shown that it protects the mucous lining of the gastrointestinal tract by regulating nervous system control and exerting antioxidant activity, all of which can help with IBS. Gentian root improves overall digestive function by stimulating the secretions of digestive juices; take 300 mg or 10 drops of tincture 15 minutes before meals. Drinking ginger root tea three times a day reduces bloating, gas, and diarrhea. You can also take 500 mg of ginger root in capsule form with each meal.

---

**TIP:** USE A WARM COMPRESS

If you are experiencing abdominal cramping, lie down with a warm compress against your abdomen to relieve pain. Try using a hot water bottle.

---

## HOMEOPATHY

This chronic condition is best treated by a homeopathic practitioner who will be able to help at a level beyond the management of superficial symptoms. The remedies listed below may be helpful, but long-term home prescribing and management of this condition is not encouraged. An experienced homeopath can also give advice on making positive changes to your lifestyle and diet to help you manage your condition more effectively. Homeopathic treatment for IBS can be given on its own or in conjunction with conventional medicine.

**Arg nit:** This remedy may be helpful if symptoms of IBS occur after ingesting too many sugary foods or drinks. Symptoms include passing gas and diarrhea that alternate with bouts of constipation, accompanied by severe bloating and swelling of the belly, which feels as though it's about to burst. High levels of anxiety and nervous tension will also aggravate digestive uneasiness.

**Colocynthis:** This remedy has a reputation for relieving colicky pains that come on in waves after eating and drinking. These are eased temporarily by bending over, which is done instinctively as a way of applying pressure to the abdomen. When this remedy is well-indicated, episodes of watery diarrhea are accompanied by excessive gas. Common triggers of IBS associated with this remedy include anger and/or emotional stress.

**Lycopodium:** If symptoms of IBS are associated with anticipation about an upcoming event, and/or eating too much hard-to-digest, high-fiber foods, such as beans, sprouts, and lentils, try Lycopodium. Common symptoms include alternating bouts of diarrhea and constipation, coupled with a very noisy and distended digestive tract. There is rumbling and gurgling in the abdomen, heartburn, and a tendency for acid to wash up into the throat when belching.

## HERBALISM

 **Peppermint:** Peppermint is the most effective herb in treating IBS and the oil has been shown to decrease intestinal motion by acting on calcium channels in the cells. Menthol is the primary component of peppermint oil and produces many of the clinical effects. For IBS, it is best to use enteric-coated capsules so that the oil passes through to the intestines rather than being absorbed in the stomach, where it may contribute to heartburn. The daily dose is 0.6 ml of peppermint oil in enteric-coated tablets or capsules, often dosed as a 0.2 ml of peppermint oil in a capsule or tablet three times daily before food. Peppermint oil should not be used during pregnancy because it may cause the onset of menstruation, gallbladder disease (due to its activity in stimulating the production of bile), hiatus hernia, or acid reflux disease, because it relaxes the sphincter between the esophagus and stomach.

**Other herbs:** Depending on an individual's symptoms of IBS, there are many other plants that can be helpful. Those that improve digestion, dispel gas, or generally calm the intestines are useful. Examples are teas, tinctures, or capsules of caraway, fennel, and anise. A few pieces of fennel candy, usually offered after a meal in Indian restaurants, may be enough to soothe the symptoms of IBS. Intestinal bitters are calming and healing to the intestines, often because of the astringent tannins present in this class of plants, and are especially useful if diarrhea is the major symptom (see the section on diarrhea, p. 366). A simple, safe, antispasmodic, anti-inflammatory, and general sedative plant, such as chamomile, often relieves IBS. Anxiety may trigger IBS in some people; this can be addressed by using many different plants (see Anxiety, p. 828).

# KIDNEY STONES

## DIAGNOSIS

The cause of most kidney stones is unknown but they do tend to run in families. They generally start off as a minute crystal in the kidneys, usually caused by a high concentration of calcium in the urine. They can also be caused by dehydration, infection, and various kidney disorders. The condition is three times more common in men than women, and tends to be a recurrent problem.

Kidney stones vary greatly in size. Some are as small as a grain of sand whereas others are so big they fill the pelvis and block the flow of urine, which causes the kidneys to swell. If the stone is ¼ inch (5 mm) or smaller, the attack will usually stop after a few hours when the stone is passed in the urine. However, if the stone gets stuck, the process of passing it can take several days. Discharging a kidney stone from the bladder through the urethra is often painless, or at worst will cause a slight pain when urinating. Often people do not even realize they have kidney stones and they are sometimes discovered completely by accident after an X-ray or ultrasound for another medical reason. There are many methods of removing stones. A stone lodged in the ureter can be removed by a cystoscope (via the bladder), but those in the kidneys are accessed via a small cut in the back, using an instrument called a nephroscope, which either pulls out the stone, or breaks it up with shock waves.

## SYMPTOMS

- Sudden, intense pain of an intermittent nature
- Nausea and vomiting
- Blood in the urine
- Reduced urine flow and output
- Frequent urinary infections

## TREATMENT GOAL

To ease the pain of severe attacks and prevent recurrences of kidney stones. This may involve changes to your diet and drinking plenty of fluids.

## CONVENTIONAL MEDICINE

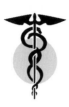

Conventional treatment aims to control pain, identify any complications such as infection or obstruction, and reduce the recurrence of kidney stones. Generally, urgent medical attention is needed if fever and chills are present along with other symptoms of kidney stones. Also, if there is a history of kidney failure, if a sufferer is pregnant, or if the patient has a only single kidney, seek immediate help.

**Pain relief:** Non-steroidal anti-inflammatory drugs (NSAIDs) are used to reduce pain. Effective intravenous NSAIDs such as ketorolac can be given for immediate relief. If this does not work, intravenous narcotic analgesics are given.

**Remove the stone:** It is thought that increasing fluids either orally or intravenously can help to push stones out, but some doctors feel this is dangerous as it may cause an obstruction. Extracorporeal shockwave lithotripsy, or ESWL, (in which sound waves are used to break up stones) is a common method of stone ablation. Percutaneous nephrolithotomy, a procedure done under sedation or anesthesia to remove stone fragments, is performed if stones are too big to be removed by ESWL, or if ESWL fails. The procedure does require a short hospital stay. Ureteroscopy is another procedure that can be performed to remove stones.

**Modify your lifestyle:** Depending on what kind of kidney stone develops (different stones are made up of different minerals), general lifestyle modifications can be taken to prevent recurrence. In general, however, drinking 2 liters of water a day helps to keep the dilution and flow of urine at a level that discourages stone to develop. A high fiber diet is also recommended. Avoid carbonated beverages that contain phosphates as these have been associated with the development of stones. Grapefruit juice should also be avoided as it has been linked to the formation of kidney stones in some studies. Avoiding calcium is generally thought to be unhelpful, and some doctors even advocate calcium supplementation as a preventive measure. Generally, avoiding a high-protein diet, particularly animal protein, is wise. It is recommended that you also avoid too much salt and fat in the diet, alcohol, and foods that are high in oxalate, such as beets, black tea, chocolate, figs, pepper, lamb, parsley, poppy seeds, spinach, soy, and Swiss chard. Oxalate combines with calcium to form a salt that causes kidney stones.

**Supplements:** Taking magnesium (as a salt of aspartate, which does not cause diarrhea) helps inhibit stone formation, as does taking 25–100 mg of vitamin B6 a day. There is some evidence that omega-3 fatty acids found in fish oil (taken at about 4 g a day) reduce oxalate stone formation. Since acidification of the urine is a problem in stone formation, a supplemental greens alkalinizing powder such as Xymogen® BioAlkalizer should be effective, although this has not been the subject of research.

**Medication:** The medications hydrochlorothiazide, chorthalidone, amiloride, cellulose sodium phosphate, allopurinol, potassium citrate, or calcium carbonate, may be recommended for prevention. Again, the medication used depends on what type of stone is identified.

## TRADITIONAL CHINESE MEDICINE

There are some clinical success stories in treating kidney stones with traditional Chinese medicine. A combination of Chinese herbal medicine and acupuncture works best if the stone is smaller then 1 cm in diameter and if the patient has normal kidney function. If the patient has kidney disease or kidney dysfunction, consult a doctor before treatment. If the stone is stuck in the wall of the kidney, or if the patient has a narrow urinary tract, other treatments such as surgery should be considered.

**Herbs:** To make a decoction, mix the herbs of one of the formulas below in a glass or ceramic pot. Add 3 cups of water, bring the ingredients to the boil, and simmer for 30 minutes. Strain the liquid and drink 1 cup twice a day.

• Formula one: Mix 10 g of Jin Qian Cao (lysimachia), 12 g of Xia Ku Cao (common selfheal fruit-spike), 15 g of Hu Tao Ren (walnut), 10 g of Che Qian Zi (plantago seed), 12 g of Shi Wei (pyrrosia leaves), 12 g of Bian Xu (knotwood), and 12 g of Qu Mai (aerial parts and flower of Chinese pink dianthus).

• Formula two: Mix 10 g of Chen Xiang (aloeswood), 10 g of Mu Xiang (costus root), 12 g of Bin Long (betel nut), 12 g of Wang Bu Liu Xing (vaccaria seeds), 10 g of Tao Ren (peach kernel), 15 g of Niu Xi (achyranthes root), 12 g of Zao Jiao Ci (spine of Chinese honeylocust fruit), 12 g of Ru Xiang (frankincense), 12 g of Mo Yao (myrrh), and 12 g of Chuan Lian Zi (sichuan pagoda tree fruit).

• Formula three: Mix 10 g of Dan Shen (salvia root), 12 g of Huang Qi (milk-vetch root), 12 g of Du Hong (safflower), 12 g of Gou Ji Zi (wolfberry), 10 g of Gui Zhi (cinnamon), 12 g of Jin Qian Cao (lysimachia), 12 g of Ze Xie (water plantain rhizome), and 15 g of Hua Shi (talcum).

**Acupuncture:** Treatment may reduce the pain and ease some symptoms. Acupuncture is often combined with Chinese herbal medicine to treat kidney stones. Consult an experienced doctor of traditional Chinese medicine for options.

**Acupressure:** Have someone apply medium pressure to the Shen Shu point, found 1½ inches lateral to the center of the back, just below the top of the hipbone, for one to three minutes. In a sitting position apply medium pressure to the Yang Ling Quan point, on the outside of the leg in the depression about 2 inches from the bottom of the knee, and the Tai Xi point, on the inside of the leg in the depression between the Achilles tendon and the anklebone, for one to three minutes.

**Diet:** Foods that are good for the kidneys are chives, duck, plums, star anise, tangerines, and egg yolk. To help prevent kidney stones forming, drink plenty of water and cranberry juice, and avoid drinking too much black tea. Another helpful recipe is to boil three fresh star fruits in 2 cups of water with 2 tsp of honey. Eat the fruit and drink the liquid once a day.

## NATUROPATHY

**Diet:** Staying hydrated is important in the treatment and prevention of this condition. If you have kidney stones, make sure you drink plenty of water every day. A vegetarian diet may help prevent the formation of kidney stones in the first place, as research shows that vegetarians have a lower rate of developing condition. Follow a diet based on whole grains, fresh vegetables, and legumes. If you do eat meat, opt for lean cuts. Eat foods that are rich in magnesium such as barley, bran, corn, buckwheat, rye, oats, brown rice, potatoes, and bananas. Freshly squeezed lemon juice helps acidify the urine and eases the passage of calcium oxalate stones. Drink an 8 oz glass three times a day. Dilute it with a little water to minimize its tartness. Avoid naturally carbonated and mineral waters, as their calcium content can be high.

**Supplements:** Magnesium prevents the formation of calcium oxalate crystals. The citrate form may be most effective; take 400–500 mg of magnesium daily. Vitamin B6 is deficient in those with kidney stones, and also reduces calcium oxalate levels. Take 50 mg a day. Take 120 mg of IP-6 (inositol hexophosphate) a day as it also reduces calcium oxalate crystals in the urine. Vitamin A deficiency is considered a risk factor for kidney stone formation. Take 5,000 IU daily. Vitamin C supplementation should be kept below 2,000 mg a day. Vitamin C can potentially form oxalates, which make up kidney stones, in high amounts.

**Herbs:** Take 400 mg of a standardized cranberry extract twice a day; it has been shown to reduce urinary calcium in those with a history of kidney stones. Drinking aloe vera juice may also reduce urinary crystals. Uva ursi is traditionally used for urinary tract infections, and relieves pain and cleanses the urinary tract. Take 250–500 mg three times a day, but do not use this herb for more than two weeks. Drink 2–4 cups of juniper berry tea, a strong diuretic kidney cleanser, every day until the stones pass.

Horsetail also has diuretic qualities. You can take 2 g a day of the capsule form or drink 2–3 cups of the tea a day.

**Hydrotherapy:** A hot sitz bath can help relieve pain. Drink lemon juice, tea, or water while sitting in the bath to speed up the elimination of stones.

---

**TIP:** AVOID ANTACIDS
Antacids that contain aluminum are known to contribute to kidney stone formation, especially if taken with milk.

---

## HOMEOPATHY

Since kidney stones tend to be a recurrent problem, they require professional conventional medical and homeopathic support. Treatment from a homeopath will aim to help at both preventive and acute levels (but not simultaneously) to relieve the situation. The long-term aim of homeopathic constitutional treatment (ideally in combination with dietary and nutritional guidance) is to discourage the body from producing kidney stones. Should an acute episode of pain occur, any of the remedies below can be used in a supplementary way to conventional pain relief. If removal of the stone or stones is needed by conventional means, don't forget that your homeopath will also be able to prescribe to support a swift recovery.

**Nux vomica:** To ease spasmodic pain, especially that due to renal colic, which tends to be right-sided, radiating to the genitals and the leg, use Nux vomica. Pain and discomfort are more distressing and intense when lying on the back, and there are severe problems when trying to urinate.

**Berberis:** Use this remedy if there are smarting, burning pains that radiate in all directions and are sharp enough to make the patient hold his or her breath. There is a burning sensation in the urethra, especially between attempts to urinate. Jarring movement and getting up from a sitting position increase the pain.

**Cantharis:** This remedy has a reputation for easing pain and inflammation that affects the kidneys and bladder. When it is well indicated, pains come on quickly and violently, causing unbearable cutting, burning sensations around the kidneys and bladder. Applying pressure to the glans of the penis temporarily eases the pains of renal colic. Trying to urinate increases distress, while massaging and applying warmth to the painful area feel soothing.

**TIP:** USE A COMPRESS

Applying a warm or cool compress can provide some temporary relief, depending on your individual response to either temperature.

## HERBALISM

 The herbal approach to kidney stones is to prevent the formation of stones in the first place, as well as treating symptoms during the passage of a kidney stone. A full examination of the person's digestion and function of the gastrointestinal tract is also necessary, as abnormalities in uric acid and oxalates (common components of kidney stones) should be addressed. Herbal diuretics can help to increase the flow of urine through the kidneys and help to prevent the formation of kidney stones. Some herbal diuretics such as juniper, parsley, and lovage rely on their volatile oils for this effect. However, these cause a loss of water by irritating the kidney tissue, which, over time, can be damaging to the kidney or aggravate pre-existing kidney disease. These herbs should be used carefully, under the guidance of a medical herbalist.

**Goldenrod:** This herbal diuretic may help facilitate the elimination of kidney stones, probably due to its flavonoid and saponin compounds. There are over 100 species of goldenrod that probably have similar diuretic action. Make a decoction by placing 3–5 g of the above-ground parts of the plant in 1 cup of boiling water. Let the herb steep for a few minutes, strain, and drink the liquid several times a day as necessary for acute urinary pain, or once or twice daily as a preventive measure.

**Parsley:** The leaves and roots of this plant can be used in the same manner as goldenrod, as a diuretic. Pregnant women should not use parsley because its volatile oil compounds can also cause uterine stimulation.

**Pain relief:** Several herbs can be useful to control the pain of passing a kidney stone in an acute episode. For example, a tincture of khella seeds can ease the pain by acting as an antispasmodic on the urinary tract muscles. Couch grass rhizome is used in tincture form and is also calming, but it is more of a coating, or demulcent, herb for the urinary system and has a mild diuretic effect. The leaves of bearberry or uva ursi have a long history of use for helping pass kidney stones, either in tincture or powder form as symptoms dictate. Consider adding it to any of the other herbs mentioned here. Finally, an infusion or tincture of *Hydrangea arborescens* root and sandalwood oil calm the urinary system and can help with pain.

# LACTOSE INTOLERANCE

## DIAGNOSIS

Lactose intolerance is a condition where the body is unable to absorb lactose (the sugar found in milk) in the digestive system. An enzyme called lactase that helps the body digest lactose is present in the lining of the small intestine. If the levels of the lactase enzyme are low or absent, bacteria in the stomach causes the lactose to ferment, causing symptoms such as abdominal pain and bloating in the stomach, which can lead to diarrhea. Lactose intolerance is common in babies, in people who have had stomach surgery, and those with celiac disease. There are some simple tests available to establish whether or not you are lactose intolerant. The easiest is a form of self-testing where you eliminate foods that contain lactose for a couple of days then reintroduce them to see if symptoms return. In a lactose tolerance test, your blood sugar levels are measured before and after you drink a liquid containing lactose. Finally there is the breath test, where you are given a lactose solution to drink and the doctor analyzes your breath for hydrogen gas, which is only present if the lactose is fermented.

## SYMPTOMS

- Rumbling stomach
- Abdominal bloating
- Gas
- Diarrhea
- Abdominal pains
- Nausea

## TREATMENT GOAL

Lactose intolerance is a harmless condition. Those with mild symptoms may feel better after reducing the amount of dairy products in their diet. For those with severe symptoms, treatment includes maintaining a lactose-free diet to eliminate the occurrence of symptoms. Ask your physician or consult with a dietician for more information.

## CONVENTIONAL MEDICINE

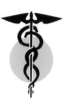

**Diet:** Follow an elimination diet, cutting out foods such as gluten, dairy, and soy. Eventually, gluten and soy may be reintroduced but lactose—found in dairy products—should be omitted from the diet permanently. Eliminating dairy products means eliminating a good source of calcium, so compensate by increasing the quantity of vegetable sources of calcium in your diet, such as broccoli and leafy greens.

**Supplements:** Take acidophilus and S. boullardii, two important intestinal flora components that provide nourishment for the intestines. These are available from health food stores. Include foods with fructo-oligiopolyacharides in your diet, or take a supplement containing this, such as Metagenics Endefen™. Try taking 1,500 mg daily of glutamine to encourage a healthy intestinal lining. It is also advisable to take a vitamin D3 supplement (cholecalciferol in the amounts of 400–1,000 IU daily). Monitor your vitamin D3 levels, and have bone density scans if applicable. A supplement with calcium, vitamin D3, and vitamin K2 (such as Jarrow Formulas Bone Up™) is advised for bone health. Take 1–2 enzyme lactase tablets before each meal that contains lactose.

## TRADITIONAL CHINESE MEDICINE

**Herbs:** Combine 12 g of Bai Zhu (white atractylodes rhizome), 10 g of Mu Xiang (costus root), 12 g of Cao Mai Ya (baked wheat), 8 g of Shen Qu (medicated leaven), and 10 g of Shan Zha (hawthorn fruit) in a glass or ceramic pot. To make a decoction, add 3 cups of water, bring the liquid to the boil, and simmer for 30 minutes. Strain the liquid and drink 1 cup twice a day. These herbs can be purchased from a Chinese herbalist or online.

**Acupuncture:** Treatment may help strengthen body function and regulate digestive energy. Your TCM practitioner may evaluate your whole body condition, to determine how best to achieve balance of the internal system. You may need treatment for one to three months to see some improvement. You may notice that your energy increases, even though acupuncture may or may not cure this condition.

**Acupressure:** The Shan Yin Jiao point is located on the center of inside of the leg, about 3 inches above the anklebone. The Susanli point is located on the lower leg, 1 inch to the outside and 3 inches below the kneecap. Take a seat and apply pressure to either of these points for one minute. Locate the Pi Shu point on the middle of the back along the spine. Lie on your stomach and have someone massage this point.

**Diet:** Avoid dairy products. Also, cut out fatty and greasy foods. Eat food that helps strengthen the spleen and stomach such as beef, rice, potatoes and sweet potatoes, string beans, rosemary, cucumber, carrots, chicken, barley, mung beans, muskmelon, watermelon, squash, and aubergines.

## NATUROPATHY

**Diet:** Eliminate milk and all other dairy products except for yogurt, as it contains organisms that produce lactase, which digests lactose. In some suffers, lactose intolerance is so severe that eating yogurt can cause symptoms. If yogurt makes you bloated and/or gives you diarrhea, exclude it from your diet. If you do eat yogurt, stick to regular yogurt rather than the frozen kind. Frozen yogurt is sometimes re-pasteurized, which kills all the friendly bacteria it otherwise contains. If you must drink milk, try a lactose-free variety. If you must eat cheese, choose hard varieties like Swiss cheese or cheddar as these contain only a trace amount of lactose and are thus less likely to produce digestive upset.

**Supplements:** Take a probiotic (friendly bacteria) product in the Lactobacillus that contains at least four billion active organisms twice a day with meals, or 30 minutes after meals. This restores helpful bacteria in the gut to aid in digestions. Digestive enzymes also help you digest food more effectively so that less irritation is caused. The enzymes found in your gut include lipases, which digest fat; proteases, which digest proteins; and amylases, which digest starch. Take 2 capsules or tablets of a full spectrum enzyme product with each meal.

**Herbs:** De-glycyrrhizinated licorice (DGL), which is safer than other types of licorice, can help heal irritated mucous lining in the stomach. Take 320 mg of DGL in capsule form three or four times a day between meals as needed. Slippery elm serves as a demulcent, soothing the digestive lining of the stomach. Take 3 ml of tincture or 500 mg in capsule form three times a day. You can also take lozenges instead of the fluid or capsule.

## HOMEOPATHY

This tends to be a chronic problem and is best treated by an experienced homeopathic practitioner rather than by self-prescription. However, one of the following acute homeopathic remedies can be helpful as a short-term solution to calm symptoms until you are able to get professional assessment and treatment. If your intolerance to lactose is severe, contact a homeopathic supplier, who can provide you with an acute remedy in liquid form that is free of the lactose used to make homeopathic tablets.

**Carbo veg:** Consider this remedy to treat an acute digestive disturbance that manifests as bloating and trapped gas. Colicky pains are likely to be severe, and there is a real sense of discomfort that is triggered by a tight waistband. Burping does little or nothing to relieve severe nausea. Diarrhea tends to be a symptom, as do cramping pains and gas that feels better for being released.

**Nux vomica:** If belching leaves a sour taste in the mouth and nausea occurs, try Nux vomica. The gut feels bloated with colicky pains and tenderness. Sufferers feel that symptoms would be relieved by passing healthy stools, but bowel movements tend to feel incomplete and there are spasmodic pains in the bowel.

## HERBALISM

 There is no herbal "cure" for lactose intolerance. Sufferers should avoid any food with obvious or hidden lactose. The symptoms of lactose intolerance, however, can be addressed by using herbs. Some possible remedies are listed below, but also refer to the sections on diarrhea (p. 366) and indigestion (p. 428).

**Chamomile:** This carminative has anti-inflammatory, antispasmodic, and soothing effects on gastrointestinal tissue. The beneficial effects of chamomile are probably due to two main classes of compounds, the volatile oils (such as bisabolol) and the flavonoids (such as apigenin). To treat indigestion due to lactose intolerance, steep a heaped tbsp of chamomile flowers in a covered cup of hot water for 10 minutes to extract the medicinal flavonoids and some of the volatile oils. This tea can be taken several times a day to help.

**Gentian:** Gentian can be consumed in several different forms to ease indigestion due to lactose intolerance. Boil 1 g in ½ cup of water for five minutes to make a liquid decoction that should be taken 30 minutes before meals, up to four times daily. Alternatively, an alcohol-based tincture of gentian can be made and similarly used before meals. Some people may develop a headache after using gentian, or find the bitter taste intolerable.

**Carminatives:** Herbs such as peppermint, fennel, anise, or ginger, as explained in the section on flatulence (see p. 377), could also address some of the symptoms of lactose intolerance. If the colon is inflamed and irritated, consider some of the demulcent herbs listed in that section, such as marshmallow and slippery elm. These herbs could be combined to help control symptoms until the lactose is out of the body's system and the gastrointestinal tract has been allowed to heal.

# MOTION SICKNESS

## DIAGNOSIS

Motion sickness occurs when your sense of balance (equilibrium) is temporarily upset. It is triggered when small repetitive movements send the brain mixed messages. When you are traveling in a car, on a ship, or in a plane, the balance mechanism in your inner ear and motion sensors in your body detect changes, and tell your body that it is moving. However, your eyes register that the vehicle you are traveling in is not moving relative to yourself. This discrepancy can trigger the symptoms of motion sickness. Children suffer from motion sickness more often than adults, but fortunately many grow out of it. Smells, such as food or gasoline fumes, can aggravate the condition, as can focusing on a nearby object, such as trying to read a book. Anxiety is another common trigger. Symptoms generally start soon after traveling begins, and tend to get worse over the duration of the journey. If feeling sick when traveling by car, sit in the front seat to get a clear view of the horizon, avoid looking down into your lap, and make sure the car is well ventilated. When traveling by sea, get as much fresh air on deck as possible and focus on the horizon rather than the waves. If you must sit below deck, try to stay in the middle of the ship where the boat moves the least. Similarly, when flying, sit over the wings where the plane is the most stable.

## SYMPTOMS

- A feeling of discomfort in the stomach
- Increased production of saliva
- Feeling hot and clammy, and sometimes hot sweats
- Nausea
- Vomiting
- Occasionally yawning, drowsiness, or depression
- Headache
- Color may drain from the face

## TREATMENT GOAL

To prevent symptoms, or relieve them if they do occur. Try to develop methods for dealing with motion sickness— different techniques work for different people.

## CONVENTIONAL MEDICINE

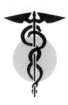

Developing preventive strategies are an important part of treating motion sickness. Several medications, including those discussed below, also exist as preventive aides to motion sickness. Interestingly, biofeedback, a treatment technique in which people are trained to improve their health by using signals from their own bodies, has been shown to be more effective than medication, as it works faster. Acupressure bracelets are also effective.

**Prevention:** Identify situations that bring on the nausea, and avoid them if possible. If they cannot be avoided, take medication prior to long journeys, before symptoms start.

**Medication:** Scopolamine is delivered through the skin via a transdermal patch. It should be used about four hours before commencing your journey. It does cause drowsiness, can cause irregular heartbeat, and can produce withdrawal symptoms if stopped suddenly. It interacts with many medications and should not be used during pregnancy. Dimenhydrinate is an over-the-counter sedating antihistamine that can be used by children. It is good for short trips, but not quite as effective as scopolamine. Promethazine is used infrequently and only for severe nausea. It is a very strong sedative and should not be used by children under two years of age.

**Stay hydrated:** If vomiting causes dehydration, intravenous fluids are administered and a strong, fast-acting drug such as promethazine is given intramuscularly.

## TRADITIONAL CHINESE MEDICINE

**Herbs:** The following patent herbs may be helpful in treating motion sickness. They are available from Chinese herbalists. Some Asian stores may also carry them.
• He Xiang Zhen Qi Wan: This herbal pill is suitable for treating nausea and light headedness, particularly during the summer.
• Bao He Wan: This can help to treat nausea, vomiting, and /or indigestion. Follow the dosage directions on the package.
• Qin Liang You (tiger balm): Using your fingertip, apply a thin layer of tiger balm to your temple at the first sign of travel sickness. This is for external use only.

**Acupuncture:** The acupuncturist will use a few points on your ear that are effective for motion sickness. She/he may either insert or tape a tiny ear staple to those points, or stick some herbal seeds or a magnetic BB to them. These stimulators may help to reduce or stop the sickness. You should see an acupuncturist before you travel.

**Acupressure:** Press the Nei Guan and Tai Yang points with strong pressure for one to two minutes at the first sign of nausea. The Nei Guan point is located in the center of the wrist on the palm side about 2 inches above the crease. The Tai Yang point is situated at the temple in the depression between the lateral end of the eyebrow and eyelid.

**Diet:** Eat a light meal before your journey, making sure it is food that is easy to digest. You can also try chewing 30 g of sugar kumquats slowly, like chewing gum, to combat motion sickness.

## NATUROPATHY

**Diet:** Do not eat heavily processed meals containing saturated fats and oils before traveling. It is also wise to avoid alcohol. Try eating a few whole grain crackers before the trip to settle your stomach.

**Supplements:** Vitamin B6 has been shown to help with nausea. Take 100 mg before the trip and 100 mg two hours later. Also take 300 mg of magnesium, which serves as a nerve tonic, before the trip.

**TIP:** STAY COOL
High temperatures and excess heat can aggravate symptoms.

## HOMEOPATHY

This is one sphere of acute treatment where homeopathy can be of immense help in easing the awful nausea, unsteadiness, and vomiting that can be set off when traveling by boat, train, car, or plane. Homeopathic remedies also have the significant benefit that they can be used safely along with any conventional treatment, or used alone as a first resort. If you know that travel or motion sickness is a problem, bear in mind that an appropriately selected homeopathic remedy can be given a day or so in advance of traveling to prevent the illness from occurring.

**Petroleum:** To ease symptoms of motion sickness that are accompanied by an aversion to contact with open, fresh air, take Petroleum. Motion sickness may have been triggered, or made more intense by, traveling on an empty stomach. When this remedy is indicated, there is likely to be an unpleasant, giddy sensation strongly felt at the back of the head. Unusually, symptoms seem to be eased by contact with warm air.

**Cocculus:** When this remedy is helpful, there is an overwhelming feeling of faintness and prostration when feeling ill or vomiting. Episodes of retching are violent, and an excess amount of saliva is produced when about to vomit. Other symptoms include a severe headache with bouts of vomiting, and a sensitivity to the smell of food that aggravates nausea. Jarring movement makes everything feel worse, while sitting still helps.

**Tabacum:** If symptoms of motion sickness are associated with a sense of disorientation and confusion, consider using Tabacum. When it is indicated, nausea is made worse by even the slightest movement, and is accompanied with unpleasant, drenching sweats. There is also likely to be a sense of pressure around the head with nausea and vomiting.

**Nux vomica:** Consider this remedy when motion sickness triggers distressing episodes of retching, but yet it is difficult to vomit. Once the patient has vomited, he or she feels immediately much better. Sufferers feel trembly and chilly, with a headache that lodges at the back of the neck, or radiates over one eye. Contact with tobacco smoke makes sickness much worse, while having a nap or sipping a warm drink can help.

---

**TIP:** AVOID READING WHEN TRAVELING

Make a point not to read when traveling by car or train, since looking down and focusing can make motion sickness worse. Instead, concentrate on looking ahead at the horizon, since this can actually reduce dizziness, disorientation, and nausea.

---

## HERBALISM

**Ginger:** The underground stem, or rhizome, of ginger is very good for treating motion sickness. Any form of ginger can be useful, from chewing on a piece of candied ginger, or sipping ginger tea. A more pungent method of preparation is to chop ginger root into small pieces until you have about 1–2 tbsp and steep it in water for a few minutes. Strain and drink the liquid before a trip or as soon as you start to experience symptoms. It is also possible to take capsules of powdered ginger, often 500 mg in quantity. Take 2 capsules 30 minutes before traveling, then take 1–2 capsules every four hours as symptoms occur. It seems that ginger acts on the gastrointestinal tract to eliminate the nausea and vomiting that some people experience when traveling, and this effect is probably due to a combination of the volatile oils that give ginger its characteristic aroma, plus nonvolatile components such as shogaols and gingerols. Daily doses up to 2–4 g are thought to be safe, though the taste of ginger can be too strong for some people and may even occasionally aggravate conditions such as heartburn or acid reflux. There is the theoretical concern of increased bleeding with ginger, but it is probably only a concern with doses of 10 g or higher. Do not take more than 1 g of ginger a day if you are pregnant.

**Peppermint:** This is a well-known herb for calming the intestines, so it is no surprise that a tea made of peppermint leaf could be useful to relieve motion sickness. Some herbalists will add it to an infusion or tincture of dried leaves, stems, and flowers of black horehound for its ability to treat nausea, vomiting, and anxiety-related indigestion.

**Meadowsweet:** Travel sickness products may also contain meadowsweet. The above-ground parts of this plant are used to calm the stomach and serve as an antacid, which may stem from the fact that it contains high levels of tannins (strong astringents) and even some salicylic acid (which works in a way similar to aspirin).

**Hyssop:** This plant is a member of the mint family and also contains tannins, which could explain its use for travel sickness.

**Red raspberry leaf:** This can also be useful, serving as an antioxidant and muscle relaxant, perhaps calming the reaction that occurs to cause nausea during a bout of motion sickness.

# NAUSEA

## DIAGNOSIS

Nausea is a term that describes a queasy feeling in the stomach or throat, and feeling as though you might vomit. It is a common symptom of many conditions, including morning sickness, travel sickness, stomach flu caused by a virus, food poisoning, and a hangover. It is also a symptom of more serious medical conditions of the abdomen such as appendicitis, gastritis, pancreatitis, gall bladder disease, and ulcers. Other conditions such as migraines, increased intracranial pressure due to fluid or a tumor, inner ear problems, or even a heart attack may also cause nausea. Occasionally it can occur as a result of a reaction to medication. In some cases, it can be a symptom of cancer and also a reaction to radiotherapy and chemotherapy used to treat the condition. If your symptoms of nausea persist for several days and there is no obvious cause, contact your doctor as they could be an indication of a more serious medical condition.

## SYMPTOMS

- Queasiness in the throat or stomach
- Vomiting
- Diarrhea

## TREATMENT GOAL

To establish the cause of the nausea and take appropriate measures to remedy the situation.

## CONVENTIONAL MEDICINE

It is important to identify and eliminate the cause of the nausea, and to correct any imbalances in body fluid or nutritional deficiencies that may have occurred.

**Diet:** Drink 1–2 liters of clear fluids in small amounts throughout the day. The fluids should include some electrolytes and calories, but sweetened and acidic juices should be avoided. If vomiting occurs with the nausea, eliminate solid foods from your diet. Once liquids are tolerated fully, easily digested foods, such as toast and broth with rice or noodles, can be introduced.

**Medication:** Medication is used to suppress symptoms while the cause of the nausea is being discovered. There are many anti-nausea treatments. Most act on the central nervous system, and can have side effects such as drowsiness and abnormal movements. Compazine, in a class of drugs known as phenothiazines, is one of the most widely used anti-nausea medications. Other common medications include scopolamine patch antihistamine drugs such as Benadryl®, Atarax®, and promethazine (Phenergan®). Metoclopramide (Reglan®) is another anti-nausea medication; Tigan® is in the same category. Most recently, Marinol®, a cannabis-based medication, has been approved as an anti-nausea medication for use in treating chronic nausea cases, for example, as a side effect of chemotherapy.

## TRADITIONAL CHINESE MEDICINE

**Herbs:** To make a decoction, combine the herbs listed in one of the formulas below in a ceramic pot. Add 3 cups of water, bring the liquid to the boil, and simmer for 30 minutes. Strain and drink 1 cup twice a day.

• Formula one: Mix 8 g of Chen Pi (tangerine peel), 12 g of Fa Ban Xia (pinellia rhizome), 15 g of Bai Zhu (white atractylodes rhizome), 8 g of Xiang Fu Hua (nut-grass rhizome), 8 g of Zhi Ke (bitter orange), and 15 g of Fuling (poria).

• Formula two: Mix 12 g of Xiang Fu Hua (nut-grass rhizome), 6 g of Sha Ren (cardamom), 10 g of Chai Hu (hare's ear root), 12 g of Bai Shao (white peony), 6 g of Bo He (field mint), 12 g of Gua Lou (trichosanthes seed), 10 g of Zhu Ru (bamboo shavings), and 10 g of Wu Ze Gu (cuttlefish bone).

**Acupuncture:** Treatment is very affective for nausea, regardless of the cause. Consult a practitioner, and be prepared to disclose your health history as well as your mental and emotional state. This information will be helpful in treating not only the symptoms, but also the underlying cause of the nausea.

**Acupressure:** The Nei Guan point is located in the center of the wrist on the palm side, about 2 inches above the crease. The Hegu points are located on the back of the hands in the depression between the thumb and the first finger. Use the tip of your thumb to press these points with strong pressure for one to two minutes. Exchange sides and repeat. The Shan Yin Jiao point is found on the inside of the leg, about 3 inches above the center of the anklebone. Take a seat and apply pressure to this point for one minute.

**Diet:** Ginger, rice, peppermint, and spearmint are very helpful for dealing with nausea. You can also try eating a small piece of fresh ginger to ease symptoms. Avoid beans, deep fried food, oily food, and raw food.

## NATUROPATHY

**Diet:** Eat a diet low in saturated fat, as studies show this can promote nausea. Eat a nourishing diet composed primarily of whole grains, fresh fruits and vegetables, and some fish and lean chicken.

**Supplements:** Taking a multivitamin/multi-mineral has been shown to lower the incidence of nausea in non-pregnant women. If you are pregnant, make sure you take a prenatal multivitamin, following the instructions on the label. Some prenatal vitamins make some women feel nauseous. If this is the case, you may need to take them at a different time in the day or with food, or switch brands. Take 30 mg of vitamin B6, which has been shown in some studies to help with nausea, twice a day. Activated charcoal, taken at a dose of 500–1,000 mg throughout the day, can absorb toxins in the digestive tract if you have been exposed to bacteria in food or water.

**Herbs:** Ginger can help ease nausea in pregnant and non-pregnant women and children. Do not treat pregnancy-related nausea with ginger for longer than the first two months of pregnancy, and do not take more than 250 mg of ginger four times a day during pregnancy without consulting your obstetrician. Ginger is available in a variety of forms. You can take 100–200 mg of a standardized extract in pill form every four hours up to three times a day; ¼–½-inch of a peeled slice of raw ginger every four hours up to three times a day; or two pieces of crystallized ginger a day (about 500 mg of ginger is in a 1-inch square, ¼-inch thick piece). You can also drink several cups of ginger ale, of a product made with real ginger, a day; an 8 oz glass contains about 1 g of ginger. Ginger tea is also helpful. Use prepackaged teabags or steep ½ tsp of grated ginger root in 8 oz of hot water for 5–10 minutes; a cup of tea can contain about 250 mg of ginger. To treat nausea due to motion sickness, take 100 mg of ginger two hours before departing and then every four hours afterward as needed. Peppermint oil can also soothe a nauseous stomach. Mix 1–2 drops of peppermint oil into juice, or make peppermint tea by pouring boiling water through a strainer containing some dried peppermint or spearmint. Let the tea brew for a few minutes, add some sugar or honey if desired, and drink.

**Essential oils:** These can be helpful in easing symptoms. Massage the abdomen with peppermint oil, which is antispasmodic and helps relieve gas; chamomile oil, which relieves nervous tension in the digestive tract; or lavender oil, which relieves nausea associated with anxiety. You can also try adding these oils to a bowl of hot water and then leaning over it to breathe in the vapors.

## HOMEOPATHY

The remedies below can be effective in easing a recent, acute episode of nausea that has arisen in response to an obvious, isolated trigger. The most common triggers are eating food that is not completely fresh, a stomach bug, feeling stressed out and anxious, traveling, or overindulging in food or alcohol. Symptoms of nausea that arise on a frequent and severe basis for no obvious reason require investigation by your doctor. Depending on the diagnosis, consulting a homeopathic practitioner may be helpful.

**Ipecac:** This remedy is suitable for nausea that feels worse for the slightest movement—even moving the head can trigger a wave of queasiness. Vomiting does nothing to ease symptoms, even temporarily. Feeling queasy may be accompanied by craving something sweet, and is triggered by eating food that is too rich, drinking iced drinks, or overeating.

**Nux vomica:** Consider this remedy to treat nausea that results from overindulgence in food and alcohol. Signature symptoms include sour-tasting burps, and a sense that vomiting, if possible, would relieve nausea. The stomach is also likely to feel knotted, and food tends to lie heavily, refusing to digest. When this remedy is helpful there is also stubborn constipation.

**Arsenicum album:** To ease anxious nausea that is so severe that even the thought of food makes you want to retch, try Arsenicum album. There may be burning sensations in the stomach, possibly with diarrhea, and the digestive tract feels generally tense. Symptoms may be been brought on by a bout of anxiety, and are generally at their most distressing during the night. Although you may be thirsty, drinks of cold water make the nausea worse, and may even trigger vomiting, while small sips of warm drinks have a temporarily soothing effect on the stomach.

**Tabacum:** Consider this as a possible remedy if severe nausea is combined with a tendency for saliva to flood the mouth. Queasiness is made more intense by even the slightest movement, but removing tight clothes from around the abdomen brings relief.

**Sepia:** To treat nausea that is especially severe first thing in the morning, and that is accompanied by a tendency to retch very easily when brushing the teeth and rinsing the mouth, try Sepia. Nausea is made worse by the slightest whiff of a strong odor from perfume or food. Symptoms include exhaustion and feeling mentally drained.

## HERBALISM

 Similar remedies can be used to treat nausea and vomiting. Nausea often progresses to vomiting, so if the nausea can be controlled, vomiting may not set in. The specific herbs used for nausea will depend on the circumstances of the condition, for example, whether it results from pregnancy, traveling, the side effects of medication, anxiety (see p. 828), ulcers (see p. 479), or indigestion (see p. 428).

**Peppermint and spearmint:** The leaves of these plants, when dried, can be steeped in hot water to make a tea that works quickly to alleviate nausea. Many of the medicinal properties from plants in the mint family come from a class of compounds called essential, or volatile, oils, such as menthol, carvone, and limonene. These compounds disappear quickly when heated, so your mint tea may be more effective if it is covered while steeping. It is also possible to buy a small bottle of essential oil of peppermint to carry if you are suffering from nausea from eating certain foods or traveling. One drop of essential oil under the tongue may be enough to calm your digestive tract and stop the nausea. It is important to buy any essential oil from a reputable source, because they can sometimes be adulterated or diluted with other oils that could decrease the effect. Also, do not take any essential oil internally for long periods of time or in high doses because it can have adverse effects on the liver.

**Ginger rhizome:** This is a popular remedy for nausea, whether from morning sickness, gastrointestinal infections, or traveling. Either capsules of dried ginger root, or an infusion of the chopped dried or fresh rhizome can be used to calm the stomach and ease nausea. You can also suck on a slice of fresh root, or chew candied ginger; these methods also deliver the important medicinal compounds to your stomach and may be enough to ease the nausea. The effect of ginger is due to several medicinal compounds, including gingerol, shogaol, and zingerone, which have been extensively studied not only for their nausea-calming effect, but also for their anti-inflammatory properties.

# OBESITY

## DIAGNOSIS

Obesity is the accumulation of excessive amounts of fat in the body's fat storage (adipocyte) cells to such a degree that it rapidly increases the risk of serious related conditions such as heart disease, stroke, and diabetes. The fat may be equally distributed all over the body, or found in problem areas such as the stomach (where it tends to accumulate in men) or the hips and thighs (where it tends to accumulate in women). One way of gauging whether or not you are overweight is by calculating your Body Mass Index (BMI) by dividing your total weight (in kg) by your total height (in meters) squared. Those with a BMI of 25–30 are considered overweight, while people with a BMI of over 30 are classified as obese. Obesity is now a worldwide problem. The occurrence of the condition has increased five fold since the 1940s and experts now believe we are facing an obesity epidemic. The condition can be triggered by many factors. It can be due to heredity, so children of overweight parents are at increased risk; overeating and eating the wrong types of food; comfort eating, where food is used as an emotional buffer; irregular meals and skipping breakfast; a sedentary couch-potato lifestyle and lack of regular exercise. In addition to physical health risks, being overweight can cause several psychological problems, such as poor self-esteem, which can in turn lead to seeking solace from eating yet more food.

## SYMPTOMS

- Presence of excess fat on the body, particularly around the stomach in men and the hips and thighs in women
- Shortness of breath
- Lack of energy
- Sore joints or muscles
- Skin problems

## TREATMENT GOAL

To establish a realistic weight-loss plan to improve your health and lower your risk of serious disease.

## CONVENTIONAL MEDICINE

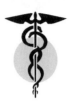

Treating obesity involves incorporating changes in lifestyle that increase energy expenditure and decrease energy intake. Elevated levels of the stress hormone cortisol, as well as some medications, can cause insulin resistance in the body. This can send messages to the body to decrease metabolism and increase the amount of fat cells stored. This, as well as other contributing factors, such as low adrenaline levels, hormonal imbalances, lack of exercise, and overeating, must be assessed and modified. Treatment is also determined by a person's Body Mass Index, or the ratio of height to weight.

**Diet:** It is advisable to have a consultation to establish why you have put on weight, and to develop a customized calorie-reduction program. Most convincing research indicates that focusing on the low glycemic index (how much 1 oz of food makes the blood sugar rise) promotes fat loss. Generally, calorie intake is reduced, the diet is modified to include foods that are low glycemic and non-processed, and a Paleolithic diet (a caveman diet), in which processed foods are eliminated in favor of simple vegetables, fruits, whole grains, and plain meats, is adopted. White foods should be avoided, as should fad diets, such as liquid diets or diet pills, as they do not tend to promote sustainable weight loss.

**Exercise:** Try to find an exercise activity to incorporate into your daily routine that is both physically achievable and enjoyable. It is important to accumulate 30 minutes of aerobic exercise a day. This may be in the form of a rapid walk or a comparable bike ride, swim, or session on the cross trainer. In addition, you should lift weights three times a week to lose fat. Recent studies show that lifting weights at 80% capacity with fewer repetitions is more effective for weight loss than multiple repetition light weight lifting.

**Mindful eating:** Eat at a table and do not watch television during a meal. Focus instead on the food you are eating: the way it looks and smells, where it came from, and who grew it. When placing food in your mouth, give your attention to its texture and taste. Prior to taking the next bite, turn your attention to the stomach and ask yourself: "Am I full?"

**Medication:** Those with a BMI of over 30, or over 27.5 for those with medical problems because of obesity, may take medication to augment weight loss. Orlistat decreases fat absorption and is appropriate for those who have high-fat diets. Sibutramine (Meridia®) is more appropriate when the appetite needs to be suppressed. Fluoxetine (Prozac®) is also used as a weight loss agent.

**Supplements:** 5-hydroxytryptophan (5-HTP) is a tryptophan derivative that increases serotonin and decreases cravings for carbohydrates. Take 50 mg three times a day before meals. Green tea and hydroxycitrate have had some success in suppressing the appetite and carbohydrate metabolism. Drink 600–1,000 mg of tea a day, and take 500 mg of hydroxycitrate three times a day before meals.

**Surgery:** If a person has a BMI of greater than 40, surgery is recommended. Surgical procedures include gastric banding techniques, laparoscopic gastric banding, gastric wrap, intragastric balloon, biliopancreatic diversion, distal gastric bypass, and Roux en Y gastric bypass. These procedures are only performed on those whose obesity is so extreme that it threatens their health. Such surgery can successfully cure some diabetics once weight loss is achieved. Complications, both physical and psychological are quite high for these procedures. Consult your doctor for more information.

## TRADITIONAL CHINESE MEDICINE

**Herbs:** The formulas below can be used to treat symptoms of obesity. Combine the herbs listed in a glass or ceramic pot, add 3 cups of water, bring the liquid to a boil, and simmer for 30 minutes. Strain the liquid and drink 1 cup twice a day. The herbs listed are available from Chinese herbalists or online.

• To treat obesity due to overeating: Symptoms include craving food, stomach bloating, and constipation. Mix 10 g of Zhi Shi (immature fruit of bitter orange), 6 g of Da Huang (rhubarb root and rhizome), 8 g of Shen Qiu (medicated leaven), 12 g of Fuling (poria), 12 g of Ze Xie (water plantain rhizome), 10 g of Huang Qin (baical skullcap root), and 8 g of Huang Lian (coptis root).
• To treat obesity with fatigue: Symptoms include feeling lethargic, headaches, and loose stools. Mix 10 g of Huo Xiang (agastache), 10 g of Zi Su Ye (perilla leaf), 6 g of Chen Pi (tangerine peel), 10 g of Shan Zha (hawthorn fruit), 12 g of Shi Chang Pu (sweetflag rhizome), 12 g of Bai Zhu (white atractylodes rhizome), and 12 g of Fuling (poria).
• To treat dizziness and discomfort of the stomach: There may be phlegm in the throat and weight is usually more concentrated around abdomen. Mix 12 g of Xiang Fu (nut grass rhizome), 6 g of Chen Pi (tangerine peel), 12 g of Fa Ban Xia (pinellia rhizome), 15 g of Fuling (poria), 12 g of Cang Zhu (black atractylodes rhizome), 30 g of Yi Yi Ren (seeds of Job's tears), and 12 g of Da Fu Pi (betel husk).
• To treat obesity with thirst and lower backache: You may still feel dry despite drinking water, and there may be ringing in the ears. Mix 12 g of Shu Di Huang (Chinese foxglove cooked in wine), 12 g of Shan Yu (Asiatic cornelian cherry), 15 g of Shan Yao (Chinese yam), 15 g of Fuling (poria), and 12 g of Ze Xie (water plantain rhizome).

**Acupuncture:** Studies show that acupuncture has some effectiveness in treating obesity as it helps to suppress appetite and boost the metabolism. Acupuncture needles will mainly be placed in your abdomen, arms, and legs. You will need treatment once a week for three to six months.

**Acupressure:** Make a loose fist with your right hand, place it on the abdomen, and use heavy pressure to massage in a clockwise motion for 15 rotations twice a day. You can also try lying on your stomach while your back is massaged, using the palm of the hands. Press along the acupressure points 1½ inches to either side along the spine, repeating 5–10 times until see the skin becomes red. Repeat the treatment every other day.

**Diet:** It is essential to follow a healthy, balanced diet that includes cucumber, squash, pumpkin, Daikon radish, tomatoes, seaweed, celery, ginger, onion, pepper, Chinese chives, mushrooms, pears, purslane, taro root, jellyfish, red beans, mung beans, and corn. Try to avoid fatty, greasy foods, sweets, and alcohol. Eat three meals a day, always eat breakfast, and do not eat heavy meals late at night. Drinking green tea, jasmine tea, or Wu Long tea can help to digest fat.

## NATUROPATHY

**Diet:** Eat a diet that is appropriate for your body type rather than focusing on calorie intake. Some overweight people do well on a high-protein, low-carbohydrate diet and others do well on a low-fat, low-protein, high-complex carbohydrate diet. For more advice consult a dietician. Regardless of the type of diet that is best for you, make sure you eat enough protein every day. Fish, lean organic meats, and whole grains mixed with legumes provide adequate protein. Eat two to three servings of vegetables a day to obtain the nutrients and fiber that most obese people are deficient in. Limit the amount of simple sugars you consume. Foods such as white flour, sugar, sweets, white rice, and baked foods all contribute to blood sugar imbalances and weight gain. Eat small meals throughout the day rather than two or three big meals to keep your metabolism strong. Drink 10–12 glasses of water a day to flush out toxins and keep hydrated.

**Supplements:** A high-quality multivitamin/multi-mineral provides some of the basic vitamins and minerals required for weight loss. Follow the directions on the label for the correct dosage. Take 3–4 g a day of conjugated linoleic acid (CLA), which has been shown to reduce body fat and change body composition in general. Chromium, taken at 500 mcg twice a day, helps to relieve cravings for sweet foods and stabilizes blood sugar. Take 100–300 mg of 5-hydroxytryptophan (5-HTP) three times a day to increase feelings of fullness and decreases carbohydrate cravings. However, do not use this supplement if you are taking antidepressants or medication for anxiety. Pyruvate has shown to help some with weight loss when combined with exercise and a low-fat diet; take 20–40 g daily. Take 100–500 mg of L-carnitine three times a day to help burn fat for energy. Taking 3 g of fish oil, which has DHA (docosahexanoic acid) and EPA (eicosahexanoic acid) can also help to burn fat.

**Herbs:** Take 1,500 mg of green tea extract a day to increase the body's ability to burn energy, which in turn increases metabolism. In addition you can drink green tea two to three times a day. Bladderwrack supports thyroid function to regulate metabolism; take 100 mg in capsule for or 1 ml of tincture twice a day.

**Exercise:** Find the exercise appropriate for you. Exercise is one of the most important parts of any weight loss program. Find an exercise that you enjoy, for example, a 20-minute brisk walk, lifting weights, or yoga. If you are extremely out of shape or have serious health problems, consult a doctor before starting an exercise regime.

**Stress management:** Stress has been shown to contribute to weight gain. Visualization, breathing exercises, physical exercise, T'ai chi, or Qi Gong may all help manage stress levels.

## HOMEOPATHY

Dieting often overlooks the nutritional status of what is eaten in favor of concentrating on reducing calories to lose weight. Although there is no homeopathic slimming formula, homeopathic practitioners, in common with other complementary therapists, will often advise on adopting healthier eating habits to achieve a slow, sustainable weight loss. What follows is some practical advice on making healthy lifestyle changes that can result in maintainable weight loss.

**Avoid "diet" drinks and foods:** These items tend to be a rich source of artificial sweeteners and chemical flavorings. Studies suggest that sweeteners of this kind, although low in calories, increase the body's cravings for more sweet foods and drinks. They also tend to be found in nutritionally deficient foods and drinks, which do nothing to provide your body with essential nutrients.

**Avoid convenient, "low-fat" foods:** These foods often include chemical ingredients, such as trans-fatty acids, that have a negative effect on the body.

**TIP:** KEEP A FOOD DIARY
Keeping a food diary of everything that you eat in a 24-hour period for at least a week can be revealing. Most people considerably underestimate what they consume in the average day and, as a result, can sometimes be unaware as to why they are gaining, or not losing, weight.

**Choose nutritionally sound foods:** Whole grains, unroasted nuts and seeds, pulses, beans, fresh fruit, vegetables, oily fish, and small amounts of poultry and dairy foods are part of a healthy diet. Undesirable foods include cakes, biscuits, pastries, red meat, any fried foods, full-fat milk or white chocolate, alcohol, carbonated drinks, and any foods that are instant and need to be reconstituted by adding water.

**Exercise:** Studies reveal that in order to boost your body's metabolic rate, you must exercise as regularly as possible. In other words, there is very little point in completing a challenging two-hour session at the gym once every two weeks. To stimulate your metabolism, exercise for 40 minutes four or five times each week.

## HERBALISM

Herbs can help people to deal with obesity by supporting the system while on a low-calorie diet, or by actually facilitating weight loss. Despite the claims by many companies, the proof that herbs lead to weight loss is limited and you should be aware that there are some adverse effects.

**Bitter orange:** An extract from the fruit or rind of bitter orange contains a compound called synephrine, which can be found in many weight-loss herbal products. Clinical trials have shown that it has some ability to enhance the metabolism and promote weight loss and the loss of body fat when used in combination with caffeine and other herbs. Some adverse effects have been reported, such as high blood pressure and increased heart rate, with individual case reports of more serious effects such as passing out or strokes. It may work to help obesity, but further research may also show that its side effects are dangerous and unacceptable.

**Green tea:** There are about 40 mg of caffeine in 1 cup of green tea, as well as compounds called catechins or polyphenols, the most well-known of which is epigallocatechin gallate (EGCG). Both caffeine and catechins have been shown to increase the metabolism of fat, which can lead to weight loss. To promote metabolism, consume 3–4 cups of green tea a day, or purchase a green tea extract, labeled as standardized to the catechin or EGCG content. Green tea may increase blood pressure, so people with high blood pressure should be cautious. It also acts as a central nervous system stimulant, which may lead to insomnia or jitteriness in high doses.

**Hoodia:** The sap or the roots and stems of hoodia have traditionally been used as an appetite suppressant, which may be due to a compound called P57AS3. Research into the positive effects of this plant and compound is still in the early stages so it is too soon to tell if this plant will live up to its reputation.

# PINWORMS

## DIAGNOSIS

Pinworms are the most common type of parasitic infection of the intestines. Contrary to popular belief, they are not carried by household pets. The white, thread-like worms are about 0.4 inches (1 cm) long and live in the bowel. They move outside to the anal area and the female worms lay their eggs around the anus, which then becomes irritated and itchy. This causes an infected person to scratch the area, transferring the eggs to the fingers and then possibly into the mouth. Both children and adults can be affected, although it is mostly found in and passed on through children. You can sometimes see pinworms in your child's stools or on his or her bottom. The eggs can spread by direct contact, or by sharing toys and food. Good hygiene, particularly washing hands and scrubbing under nails before eating and after going to the toilet, is essential to stop the infection from spreading. Infected children and adults should keep their nails short as a preventive measure. The eggs can live in clothing and bed linen, so it is also important to wash these items in high temperatures to kill the eggs and prevent re-infection.

## SYMPTOMS

- Itchy feeling around the anus and inside the rectum, usually at night
- Inflammation of the vagina in girls and women, and occasionally painful sensations when urinating
- Restlessness at night and interrupted sleep

## TREATMENT GOAL

Infected children or adults should be treated as soon as possible. Doctors usually recommend that the whole family be treated at the same time. Treatment involves relieving discomfort, eliminating the infection, and preventing the parasites from spreading or re-infecting.

## CONVENTIONAL MEDICINE

As well as treatment, preventing patients from becoming re-infected is important in resolving the condition. Medication is recommended for all household members, and any sexual partners if applicable.

**Mebendazole:** This is a single-dose therapy that is then repeated after three weeks. It does have side effects on the liver and gastrointestinal system, and it has not been approved for children under two years of age. It should also not be used by pregnant women.

**Albendazole:** This drug is very effective at killing parasites, but it has not been proven safe to use by children under six years old, and should not be used by pregnant women. Women should not get pregnant for one month following treatment. It may interact with several medications and, like mebendazole, has some side effects.

**Pyrantel pamoate:** This drug is not proven to be safe in children under two years old. It is probably safer than both mebendazole and albendazole, but can cause similar side effects. Studies on pregnant women have not been performed, but it has not caused problems in animal research.

**Practice good hygiene:** The drugs listed above are effective at killing the parasite but not at killing the eggs. Because of this, clean your house thoroughly, especially the bed linen and toys. Frequent hand washing is important. Change your pajamas and underwear daily and wash all clothes in very hot water. If the eggs are not removed in this manner, re-infection will occur.

## TRADITIONAL CHINESE MEDICINE

**Herbs:**
• Internal formula: Boil 20 g of dried Bai Bu (stemona root), available from Chinese pharmacies, in 2 cups of water for 30 minutes. Children should drink half a cup of this decoction twice a day for three days. For adults, the dose can be doubled. If you have loose stools, do not to use this formula.

• External formula: Boil 18 g of Ku Shen (sophora root), 18 g of Tu Fu Ling (glabrous greenbrier rhizome), 15 g of Bai Bu (stemona root), and 10 g of Jing Jie (schizonepeta stem and bud) in 6 cups of water for 30 minutes. Stain the liquid and pour 3 cups of warm (not hot) liquid into a container. Sit in the decoction to soak the anus area once a day for 15–20 minutes before bed. This liquid will kill the worms and its eggs, as well as stop the itching.

**Acupuncture:** It is not common to treat this condition with acupuncture.

**Acupressure:** It is not common to treat this condition with acupressure.

**Diet:** Eat 10 g of raw or baked pumpkin seeds a day. Pumpkin seeds are widely available in supermarkets and health food stores.

## NATUROPATHY

**Diet:** Cooked rather than raw food is usually recommended. Raw or undercooked beef may contain worms, as can raw fish such as sushi, sashimi, ceviche, and smoked salmon. Cook all meat thoroughly until the juices run clear. Eliminate coffee, refined sugar, white flour, and processed foods from your diet. Carrots, sweet potatoes, and squash are high in beta carotene, a source of vitamin A, which is thought to increase resistance to pinworms. Try eating unsweetened yogurt, miso, and sauerkraut to obtain probiotics, which can help rebuild beneficial intestinal flora. Poor digestion can be a contributing factor. Those with low acid levels in the stomach may not be killing germs in the foods they eat. Pineapple and papaya seeds contain digestive enzymes that can help improve digestion and clear parasites; eat a handful of raw pumpkin seeds and have some papaya juice every day. Turmeric and cloves can also help fight parasites, so add them to food where possible. Have soups made with fresh ginger, garlic, and onions, which have all been shown to have anti-parasitic effects. Drink plenty of fresh water every day.

**Supplements:** Probiotics (friendly bacteria) can inhibit the growth of some microorganisms and raise immunity. Take a product containing at least four billion active organisms twice daily with meals or 30 minutes after eating.

**Herbs:** Take 200 mg or 20 drops of wormwood, a common herbal therapy for intestinal worms and parasites, three times a day. Black walnut has also traditionally been used as a herbal formula to kill parasites. Adults should take 250 mg three times a day or 30 drops three times a day. Oregano oil kills many types of microorganisms, including parasites. Take 500 mg or 5 drops under the tongue three times a day. Goldenseal helps fight infection in the digestive tract. Take 30 drops or 30 mg four times a day. Ginger reduces intestinal cramping and has anti-inflammatory effects. Drink a cup of fresh tea three times a day or take 500 mg three times a day.

## HOMEOPATHY

The following homeopathic remedies can be used in a complementary way together with conventional medicine to treat a recently developing, acute episode of threadworms. If problems are more recurrent, the situation would be outside the realm of home prescribing.

**Teucrium:** If there is a crawling sensation in the rectum after passing a stool, try Teucrium. There may also be frequent and severe itchiness and tingling around the anus, which feel worse during the night when warm in bed. It is difficult to fall and stay asleep due to the amount of tossing and turning caused by the threadworms. When this remedy is well indicated, the nose is noticeably irritated and itchy.

**Cina:** This can be a helpful remedy to treat chubby children who are very hungry, but show signs of weight loss. Irritation from threadworms triggers restlessness, irritability, and petulance. Children may also become very difficult to pacify when feeling discomfort. Tooth grinding and/or night terrors may occur during sleep, and the child may be very twitchy. Although children may not want to be touched, they may feel soothed when being rocked.

## HERBALISM

The herbal approach to threadworms involves improving symptoms at the site of itchiness around the anus, and ridding the body of the offending parasites.

**Anti-parasitic herbs:** There are many herbs that are useful in combating parasitic infections, but most are targeted to more severe infections such as giardiasis, ascariasis, and amebiasis. Protocols have been developed that contain mixtures of herbs, some of which are quite toxic and unsuitable for children, and others that are more amenable for use by children. Determining the right combination of plants to use, and the correct dose to take, to rid the body of any parasite, even threadworms, is best left to a medical herbalist.

**Topical herbs:** Herbs that are useful to treat skin conditions can also be used to address the anal and peri-anal itchiness that occurs with threadworms. For example, a salve that contains calendula would be a good first treatment because of calendula's soothing, anti-inflammatory properties. Any preparation should be used for just a few days because skin around the anal area is very sensitive and becomes irritated easily.

# STOMACHACHE

## DIAGNOSIS

Stomach pains can be caused by a variety of medical conditions. Some of the most obvious ones include heartburn and indigestion, eating something that has disagreed with you, an intolerance to certain foods, food poisoning, and irritable bowel syndrome. Another obvious, but often overlooked, cause is constipation as a result of not including enough fiber in your diet. Stomachache can also be a symptom of more serious conditions such as hernia, gallbladder disease, gastritis, ulcers, diverticulitis, ulcerative colitis, Crohn's disease, appendicitis, and inflammatory bowel disease. Occasionally it can be a symptom of cancer. In women, it can be associated with menstrual problems, endometriosis, ovarian cysts, and fibroids. It can also be triggered by stress and anxiety.

## SYMPTOMS

- Abdominal pain or cramps
- Abdominal bloating
- Feeling constipated
- Possible nausea

## TREATMENT GOAL

To establish the cause of the stomachache and treat it accordingly to bring relief of symptoms.

## CONVENTIONAL MEDICINE

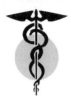

Stomach pain is not a medical condition but a symptom of an underlying illness. As such there is no medical protocol for treating stomachache, however, steps can be taken to relieve symptoms until the cause is determined. If stomach pain is intense, that is greater than a seven on a scale of 10, medical care should be sought as it could be a sign of a more serious condition.

**Diet:** The diet should be modified to clear liquids during times of stomach pain.

**Medication:** Aspirin and non-steroidal anti-inflammatory drugs should be strictly avoided. Sometimes over-the-counter remedies such as bismuth (Pepto Bismol®), aluminum hydroxide (Mylanta®), and simethicone (Gas X™) are worth a try.

**Stress management:** Often, especially in children whose family relationships are under stress, anxiety contributes to stomach pain. Stress reduction techniques such as breathing and, in children, the expression of feelings, should be encouraged, and are helpful regardless of the cause of the pain.

## TRADITIONAL CHINESE MEDICINE

**Herbs:** Using either of the formulas below, make a decoction by placing the herbs in a glass or ceramic pot, adding 3½ cups of water, and bringing the mixture to a boil. Simmer for 30 minutes, strain the liquid, and drink 1 cup twice a day. These herbs are available from Chinese herbalists or online.

• Formula one: If a stomachache is accompanied by chills, feeling full, a poor appetite, or if a large quantity of clear mucus is coming from the stomach, traditional Chinese medicine considers this to be the result of pathogenic cold in the stomach. To warm the stomach use 3 g of dried ginger, 10 g of Zhi Shu (perilla leaf), 6 g of Chen Pi (tangerine peel), 12 g of Xiang Fu (nut grass rhizome), and 12 g of Bai Zhu (white atractylodes rhizome).

• Formula two: If a stomachache is stress related, and there is a sour taste in the mouth, use 12 g of Xiang Fu Hua (nut-grass rhizome), 10 g of Chai Hu (hare's ear root), 12 g of Chuan Xiong (Szechuan lovage root), 8 g of Zhi Ke (bitter orange), 12 g of Bai Shao (white peony), and 6 g of Sha Ren (cardamom).

• Formula three: If a stomachache is combined with phlegm, use 12 g of Fa Ban Xia (pinellia rhizome), 3 g of fresh ginger, 15 g of Fuling (poria), and 10 g of Zhi Shi (immature fruit of bitter orange).

• Formula four: If stomachache results from food stagnation and there is a history of overeating, use 10 g of Mu Xiang (costus root), 12 g of Bin Long (betel nut), 6 g of Chen Pi (tangerine peel), 6 g of Din Xiang (clove flower bud), 10 g of Shen Qu (medicated leaven), 12 g of Lian Qiao (forsythia fruit), and 12 g of Fa Ban Xia (pinellia rhizome).

**Acupuncture:** Treatment can be very effective in both relieving the stomach pain and healing the cause of the pain. Consider having acupuncture treatment for both acute stomachache and chronic conditions. A reduction in pain may be felt immediately. Depending on your condition, sessions once or twice a week may be appropriate.

**Acupressure:** Press the Zhong Wan point, found on the upper abdomen, about 3 inches above the center of the navel. The Nei Guan point is located in the center of the wrist on the palm side, about 2 inches above the crease. The Susanli point is on the lower leg, about 1 inch to the outside of and 3 inches below the kneecap. In a sitting position, use the tip of your thumb to apply medium pressure to these points for one minute. Repeat five to eight times, twice a day.

**Diet:** Try adding honey, fennel seed, and caraway seed to your diet to comfort the stomach and reduce aching. There are also several teas you can drink to relieve symptoms. For example, add 4 g of cinnamon to 1 cup of warm water. Cover for 15 minutes and drink the tea. Place 10 kumquats into 6 cups of water and boil until there are 3 cups of liquid left. Drink 1 cup three times a day. Crush 30 g of dried lychee seeds and boil them in water with 6 g of fresh ginger or dried orange peel. Drink this tea once a day.

## NATUROPATHY

**Diet:** Avoid foods to which you know you are intolerant, such as dairy, wheat, corn, citrus fruits, or soy. Avoid solid foods, and drink chicken and vegetable broths instead. You can add ginger to the broth for faster relief. Drink freshly squeezed juices and tea throughout the day. Avoid alcohol and coffee, which can cause irritation.

**Herbs:** Take 1,000 mg of licorice root between meals two to three times a day. If you have a heart condition or suffer from high blood pressure take de-glycyrrhizinated licorice. This herb helps with the regeneration of the gastric tissue and has antibacterial and anti-inflammatory activity. Drink 3 cups of fresh chamomile tea a day to relax the nervous system and for its anti-ulcer activity. Slippery elm serves as a demulcent and soothes the gastric mucosa. Take 3 ml of tincture or 500 mg of a capsule three times a day. Aloe vera juice has anti-microbial activity and also soothes the lining of the stomach. Take ½–¾ cup three times a day. Activated charcoal can also bring relief of stomachache; mix 2–3 tbsp of activated charcoal powder (available in most health food stores and some pharmacies) with a little water in the bottom of a tall glass. Stir gently, adding water a little at a time until the glass is full, and then drink it through a straw.

**TIP:** USE A HOT WATER BOTTLE

When experiencing stomachache lie down with a heat compress against your abdomen for pain relief. A covered hot water bottle or heating pad is ideal.

## HOMEOPATHY

Any of the following strategies can be useful in clearing up a problem with stomachache that has developed in response to an obvious trigger. Recurrent problems of this kind would render the condition chronic in nature, and as a result, it would be best to seek professional assessment and treatment.

**Nux vomica:** If a stomachache occurs after a meal of an ill-advised mixture of food and drink, take Nux vomica. It is equally suitable for children who may have overeaten at a birthday party, or adults who have had too much food, alcohol, coffee, or cigarettes. The most common symptoms are a headache and colicky, spasmodic pains that feel as though they would be relieved after vomiting or passing a stool. Touch or pressure to the tender area makes things worse, while warmth, rest, and sound sleep are restorative.

**Pulsatilla:** This remedy is specifically for stomachaches that result from eating too much rich, fatty food, such as meat (especially pork), full-fat cheeses, and creamy sauces, in one sitting. Cool drinks temporarily soothe the stomach, while warm drinks make things worse. You are also likely to burp, and trigger foods will "repeat," possibly for hours after you have eaten. Jarring movements upset the stomach, but gentle exercise in the fresh, open air can feel welcome, as can gently massaging the tender area.

**Carbo veg:** If a stomachache is caused by a feeling of trapped gas, try Carbo veg. Along with pain in the stomach, there are also likely to be feelings of exhaustion and queasiness. There may also be a nasty taste in the mouth when bringing up gas, and pressure from clothes around the waist will feel very uncomfortable. Although you may feel chilly, you tend to feel much better when being fanned, or when sitting near an open window.

**TIP:** DRINK PEPPERMINT TEA

Taking sips of peppermint tea can be very soothing to the stomach.

# HERBALISM

The pain and discomfort of a stomachache could have many different causes. A general approach to stomachache may include herbs called carminatives and bitters to improve digestion. As well as the remedies listed below, refer to the sections on indigestion (p. 428), heartburn (p. 408), and gastroenteritis (p. 403).

**Fennel:** This common carminative can be used to improve digestion, thereby easing symptoms of stomachache. Fennel seeds can simply be eaten after a meal, or you can add ½ tsp of powdered seeds to hot water to consume throughout the day. You can also take 30–60 drops of a tincture of the seeds several times daily.

**Gentian:** Roots and rhizomes of this bitter herb have a long history of use as a gastrointestinal "tonic." Its effects are due to several different medicinal compounds; one of them, amarogentin, a glycoside compound, provides much of the bitter taste. Gentian can be consumed in several different forms. Boil 1 g in ½ cup of water for five minutes to make a liquid decoction, which you can take up to four times daily. Alternatively, an alcohol-based tincture of gentian can be taken. Some people may develop a headache after using gentian, or find the bitter taste intolerable.

**Chamomile:** This is a safe and effective gastrointestinal herb, and the tea form is suitable for both adults and children suffering from stomachache. The tea can be sweetened with a little sugar to make it more palatable for children, and can be taken several times a day. Given that chamomile is also a mild sedative, it would partly address any anxiety or stress component that is contributing to the stomachache. For those with allergies to plants in the daisy family, such as ragweed and goldenrod, there is the slight chance that chamomile could worsen rhinitis, asthma, or atopic dermatitis; should this happen, stop using it.

# STRESSED STOMACH

## DIAGNOSIS

Stomach pain can often be a physical manifestation of stress, particularly if it is accompanied by a headache, a racing heart, and sweaty palms. People often refer to this condition as having a knot in the stomach, or say they suffer from a nervous stomach. Stress triggers a hormonal reaction known as the "fight or flight" response. Our muscles become tense, the heart rate increases, and breathing becomes quicker. As a result, tension can accumulate in the abdomen, resulting in a stressed stomach. This can lead to loss of appetite, feelings of nausea, and an upset stomach, often culminating in frequent urination and sometimes diarrhea. It is important to try relaxation techniques if you know you are facing a stressful situation that may leave you feeling worked up and anxious. See your doctor if you suffer from this condition frequently.

## SYMPTOMS

- Stomach pain
- Indigestion
- Nausea
- Racing heart
- Loss of appetite
- Diarrhea
- Frequent urination
- Feeling on edge and restless

## TREATMENT GOAL

To learn to relax and deal with the situation to bring about a reduction in symptoms.

## CONVENTIONAL MEDICINE

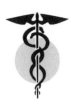

When stressed, the body releases a hormone called cortisol, which in turn releases epinephrine and norepinephrine. This process causes the acid levels in the stomach to rise, and the stomach and intestinal linings to become vulnerable. The treatment of the stressed stomach involves treating the symptoms caused by the stress, as well as modifying the body's response to stress in the long term.

**Diet:** Eliminate dairy, gluten, fructose, sugar, and processed foods from your diet as much as possible. Eating small meals frequently instead of large meals infrequently also helps.

**Reduce stress:** Stress reduction techniques include daily exercise, such as a 20-minute walk, and 20 minutes of meditation or a comparable relaxation program. The goal is to modify the body's response to stress.

**Medication:** To reduce acid, try over-the-counter pharmaceuticals such as aluminum hydroxide (Mylanta®), which neutralizes acid, or Prilosec™, which reduces production of acid. Bismuth (Pepto Bismol®) can help reduce the effect of too much acid on the lining of the stomach, and can be soothing. The over-the-counter remedy simethicone can be used to reduce bloating.

## TRADITIONAL CHINESE MEDICINE

**Herbs:** Combine 3 g of Xu Chang Qing (swallow wort root), 3 g of Mai Men Dong (ophiopogon tuber), 3 g of Dan Shen (salvia root), 4.5 g of Huang Qi (milk-vetch root), 1.5 g of Wu Mei (mume fruit), 1.5 g of Gan Cao (licorice root), and 1.5 g of of green tea. Pestle the herbs into a coarse powder and soak them in 3 cups of boiling water. Drink 1 cup three times every day for three months. All these herbs can be obtained from Chinese herbalists or online.

**Acupuncture:** Treatment can help a stressed stomach by increasing the energy flow, and regulating the circulation in the stomach muscles. You may have acupuncture treatment once a week, for 6–10 weeks. Your acupuncturist will be able to assess how many treatments you may need.

**Acupressure:** To treat a stressed stomach, use the tip of your thumb and apply strong pressure to the Hegu or Nei Guan acupressure points for one to two minutes. The Hegu points are on the back of the hands in the depression between the thumb and index finger.

The Nei Guan point is located in the center of the wrist on the palm side about 2 inches above the crease.

**Diet:** Eat foods that are easy to digest such as rice, cooked vegetables, chicken or vegetable soups, and fresh fruit. Avoid red meat, raw food, watermelon, ice cream, and alcohol as well as fatty meat, and oily and deep fried foods. Eat small meals and avoid drinking large quantities of liquids at a time.

## NATUROPATHY

**Diet:** Unbalanced blood levels can lead to or aggravate a stressed stomach, so eat small meals frequently throughout the day to keep blood sugar levels balanced. Eat whole grains such as oats, quinoa, or brown rice with every meal. These foods contain high levels of B vitamins and fiber, and increase your body's ability to make serotonin, a neurotransmitter that has a calming effect on the body and eases anxiety. B vitamins are also are calming to the nervous system and fiber keeps your bowels moving. Calcium and magnesium, found in sea vegetables, green leafy vegetables, nuts, and yogurt, also have a calming effect. Avoid caffeine, refined sugars, and alcohol, which can make symptoms worse by causing blood sugar imbalances.

**Supplements:** Take 50–100 mg of 5-hydroxytryptophan (5-HTP) two to three times a day to increase serotonin levels, which have a calming effect. Do not take this supplement if you are on antidepressants. Take 200 mcg of chromium twice a day to balance blood sugar levels. Digestive enzymes, such as lipases, proteases, and amylases, help you digest food more effectively so that less irritation is caused in the stomach. Take 2 capsules or tablets of a full spectrum enzyme product with each meal. Also take 1–2 betaine hydrochloride tablets with each meal to support stomach acid levels and help with digestion. Probiotics, friendly bacteria found in the gut, can prevent the overgrowth of candida and other harmful microbes. Take a product containing 4 billion active organisms daily of lactobacillus acidophilus and bifidus.

**Herbs:** Ginger, available in many forms, helps soothe the stomach and increase digestion. You can take 100–200 mg of a standardized extract in pill form; ½–¾ tsp of powdered ginger; or a ¼–½ inch slice of peeled ginger root every four hours or up to three times a day. You can also drink ginger tea or ginger ale (this should be a product made with real ginger), or eat two pieces of crystallized ginger (500 mg) a day. Peppermint oil can reduce abdominal pain, possibly by blocking the influx of calcium into muscle cells and inhibiting excess contraction of intestinal muscles. Take 1–2 enteric coated peppermint oil capsules twice daily between meals. Take 1 tsp of fennel seed tincture a day on an empty stomach to relieve spasm of the gastrointestinal tract, feelings of fullness, and flatulence. Gentian root, taken at a dose of 300 mg in capsule form or 10 drops of tincture 15 minutes before meals, can improve overall digestive function by stimulating the secretions of digestive juices. Aloe vera juice can also be soothing. Take ½–¾ cup of aloe vera juice three times a day between meals. Make sure it contains 98% aloe vera and no aloin or aloe-emodin. Slippery elm serves as a demulcent to soothe the digestive lining of the stomach. Take 3 ml of tincture or 500 mg of a capsule three times a day.

## HOMEOPATHY

Any of the following homeopathic remedies can be useful in relieving discomfort and distress in the stomach that are due to feeling tense and anxious. As always, the choices listed here are most appropriate for easing recently developing symptoms of a disordered stomach. More established problems that have emerged as a repeating pattern will be far more successfully treated by professional homeopathic support.

**Arsenicum album:** This is the remedy to consider for stomach pains that have been triggered by anxiety. Common symptoms include acidity and burning in the stomach, coupled with diarrhea or loose, frequent stools. There will also be a sense of nausea, which may cause vomiting if anxiety levels escalate. Symptoms tend to be most distressing during the night, often waking the patient from sleep in the early hours of the morning. A sense of chilliness, restlessness, and exhaustion are also key symptoms.

**Lycopodium:** This can also soothe a tense, anxious stomach. Symptoms that respond especially well to this remedy are a bloated, gassy belly with alternating diarrhea and constipation. There will be lots of churning and acidity in the stomach, and a burning liquid may reflux into the gullet when burping. There may also be flatulence when feeling stressed and anxious about an upcoming event.

**Nux vomica:** If living in the fast lane leads to a general tension in the digestive tract, try Nux vomica. The complaint manifests as spasmodic pain, intense nausea, and biliousness. There may be a curious symptom of queasiness with hunger, but also a strong aversion to food. Spicy food, alcohol, coffee, and cigarettes all aggravate the symptoms.

**TIP:** TAKE A "DIGESTIVE VACATION"
Avoid foods and drinks that irritate the stomach lining, such as red meat, full-fat dairy items, sugary or rich pastries, fatty foods, deep-fried foods, very spicy dishes, alcohol, and strong tea and coffee. Instead opt for items that are soothing to the stomach and easily digestible, such as lightly cooked vegetables, soups made from fresh vegetables, natural bio-yogurt, organic brown rice, small amounts of fish, and lots of still water. If you crave some seasoning, choose fresh herbs rather than relying on heavy seasoning from salt, pepper, or vinegar.

## HERBALISM

Any number of stressed stomach symptoms are amenable to herbal treatment. In addition to the remedies below, refer to Indigestion (p. 428), Gastritis (p. 398), Acid Reflux (p. 322), Heartburn (p. 408), and Anxiety (p. 828).

**Chamomile:** This general gastrointestinal herb contains compounds that serve as anti-inflammatories as well as overall mild sedatives, which are perfect for someone suffering from stressed stomach. Fill a coffee cup half full of dried chamomile flowers and pour in almost boiling water to fill the cup. Cover the cup and let the flowers steep for 5–10 minutes. Strain the liquid and drink the tea several times a day. It is also possible to buy chamomile teabags.

**Anti-anxiety herbs:** Stress and anxiety can cause physiological changes, which can in turn lead to gastrointestinal symptoms. To help your stomach relax before sleeping, take valerian capsules or a tincture of hops before bed, both of which are mild sedatives. Kava kava is another well-known anti-anxiety herb, but some preparations have dangerous side effects such as liver damage; consult a medical herbalist before adding this herb to your treatment. It is also important to make changes to your lifestyle to reduce stress.

# ULCER

## DIAGNOSIS

An ulcer occurs when an open sore or lesion develops on the inner lining (the mucosa) of the stomach or the upper part of the intestine (duodenum). When the ulcer occurs in the stomach it is called a gastric ulcer, and when it develops in the duodenum it is called a duodenal ulcer. Duodenal ulcers appear in middle age and are more common in men, while gastric ulcers occur later in life and tend to affect women. The most common cause of ulcers is infection, and the H. pylori bacteria is responsible for up to 90% of all cases. The second most common cause is the long-term use of aspirin or non-steroidal anti-inflammatory drugs (NSAIDs) used to treat arthritis, rheumatism, backache, headaches, and period pain. Ulcers can also occur in people weakened by severe conditions such as chronic respiratory disease. Occasionally, a stomach ulcer is caused by cancer; and, rarely, a specific illness, such as Crohn's disease or the excess production of hydrochloric acid in the stomach, is found to be responsible.

## SYMPTOMS

- Pain or a burning sensation in the upper abdomen, often a couple of hours after eating or late at night
- Difficulty swallowing
- Belching or regurgitation
- Bloated stomach
- Persistent nausea and vomiting
- Vomiting blood
- Black, tarry stools
- Unexplained weight loss
- Anemia
- Fatigue
- Sudden, severe attacks of abdominal pain
- Occasionally there are no symptoms

## TREATMENT GOAL

To establish the cause of the ulcer and, with guidance, take the appropriate steps to deal with the symptoms. An ulcer is a serious condition that requires immediate medical attention. If you are suffering from any combination of symptoms, make an appointment to see your doctor.

## CONVENTIONAL MEDICINE

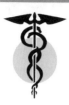

Conventional treatment aims to prevent flare-ups and reduce pain by eliminating the use of any non-steroidal anti-inflammatory drugs (NSAIDs) and eradicating the bacteria H. pylori, which is associated with ulcers. **Caution:** With peptic ulcers, any bleeding in vomit or stools is dangerous and the opinion of a gastroenterologist should be sought.

**Modify your lifestyle:** Lifestyle changes should be carried out. These include giving up smoking and drinking alcohol, and avoiding aspirin and NSAIDs. Stress reduction therapy should also be introduced. Meditation, deep breathing, and exercise are all good stress reducers.

**To treat ulcers caused by H. pylori or NSAIDs:** The presence of H. pylori bacteria is determined by a blood test and is treated first with antibiotics and a proton pump inhibitor such as omeprazole (Prilosec®) and bismuth. The antibiotic combination is usually amoxicillin, or Biaxin® and Flagyl®. If the patient is using NSAIDs, co-therapy with misoprostol (Cytotec®), a drug that decreases acid secretion and protects the gastric mucosa, is recommended to prevent ulcers.

**H2 blockers:** For ulcers not associated with H. pylori or NSAID use, H2 blocker drugs cimetidine (Tagamet®) and ranitidine Zantac® are used. These over-the-counter drugs and have been shown to be effective in ulcers not associated with the above conditions.

**Surgery:** For duodenal ulcers, a surgical procedure called a vagotomy is available. Complicated gastric ulcers that have not responded to aggressive medical treatment are sometimes treated with a surgical procedure called a sub-total gastrectomy.

## TRADITIONAL CHINESE MEDICINE

**Herbs:** The raw herbs listed below are available from Chinese herbalists or online. For each formula, add 3 cups of water to the herbs and bring the mixture to a boil. Simmer for 30 minutes and strain the liquid. Drink 1 cup of the decoction twice a day.

• To treat stomach ulcers: Mix 12 g of Bai Ji Li (caltrop fruit), 8 g of Mu Xiang (costus root), 6 g of Chen Pi (tangerine peel), and 12 g of Bai He (lily bulb).

• To treat an ulcer with symptoms of fatigue, cold hands and feet, clear mucus coming from your stomach, or vomiting watery or sour phlegm: Combine 12 g of Huang Qi (milk-vetch root), 12 g of Bai Shao (white peony), 10 g of Gui Zhi (cinnamon), 5 g of Gan Cao (licorice), 8 g of fresh ginger, and 6 pieces of Da Zhao (Chinese jujube).

• To treat an ulcer if there is also blood in stools, stools are black or dark, and you are vomiting blood: Take this formula along with medication prescribed by your doctor. Mix 6 g of Da Huang (rhubarb root and rhizome), 6 g of Huang Lian (coptis root), 8 g of Huang Qin (baical skullcap root), 8 g of ginseng, 12 g of Bai Ji Li (caltrop fruit), and 10 g of Dan Pi (cortex of tree peony root).

• To treat an ulcer caused by stress or if an ulcer is accompanied with depression: Mix 10 g of Chai Hu (hare's ear root), 12 g of Bai Shao (white peony), 12 g of Dan Pi (cortex of tree peony root), 10 g of Zhi Zi (Cape Jasmine fruit), 10 g of Chuan Lian Zi (sichuan pagoda tree fruit), 6 g of Bo He (field mint), 12 g of Shi Hu (dendrobium), and 10 g of Chen Xiang (aloeswood).

**Acupuncture:** Treatment is beneficial for digestive ulcers. It helps reduce pain and relieve stress, and aids digestion. Treatment may be more effective if combined with herbal remedies. Consult a TCM practitioner for advice.

**Acupressure:** In a sitting position, press the Susanli and Xie Hai points. The Susanli point is found on the lower leg 1 inch to the outside of, and 3 inches below, the kneecap. The Xie Hai point is on the inside of the leg in the depression just above the knee.

**Diet:** Soy bean oil and eggs are good for ulcers. Avoid cinnamon, plums, and lemons. To treat gastric and duodenal ulcers, squeeze the juice out of one Chinese cabbage and drink 1 cup of warm juice twice a day for 10 days.

## NATUROPATHY

**Diet:** You may not feel like eating, but good nutrition is essential for healing ulcers. Eat small meals throughout the day and include cultured products, such as unsweetened yogurt, kefir, miso, and raw sauerkraut, frequently. Eat whole grains and pumpkin seeds for their high zinc content, which is healing to the gastrointestinal tract. Add garlic to your meals for its ability to kill H. pylori bacteria. Avoid sugar, spicy food, citrus foods, coffee, alcohol, and black tea as they contribute to irritation and high levels of gastric acid. Drink 1 glass of fresh cabbage juice twice a day for its remarkable healing qualities. Milk used to be commonly prescribed to treat ulcers, but it is now known that milk and dairy in general can contribute to ulcers and should be avoided whenever possible.

**Supplements:** Probiotics are friendly bacteria in the Lactobacillus family that can inhibit the growth of H. pylori. While this effect does not appear to be strong enough for probiotic treatment to eradicate H. pylori on its own, preliminary studies suggest that probiotics may help standard antibiotic therapy work better, improving the rate of eradication and reducing side effects. Take a product containing at least 4 billion active organisms twice daily with meals or 30 minutes after eating. Also take 30 mg of zinc with 2 mg of copper to promote tissue healing. Vitamin C can potentially retard H. pylori growth and has antioxidant activity in the stomach lining. Take 1,000 mg of the non-acidic form three times a day. Essential fatty acids, such as those found in fish or flaxseed oil, have been shown to help heal gastric and duodenal ulcers. Take 4,000 mcg a day of fish oils or 1 tbsp twice a day of flaxseed oil. Take 400 IU of vitamin E with any essential fatty acid to prevent oxidation. Take 1,000 mg of L-glutamine three times a day to promote healthy intestinal tissue.

**Herbs:** Take 1,000 mg of de-glycyrrhizinated licorice (DGL) between meals two to three times a day. This herb helps with the regeneration of the gastric tissue and has antibacterial and anti-inflammatory activity. Take 500 mg of mastic gum three times a day. It has been shown to heal stomach mucosa and to have anti-bacterial benefits, especially on H. pylori. Drink 3 cups of fresh chamomile tea a day to relax the nervous system and for its anti-ulcer activity. Slippery elm serves as a demulcent and soothes gastric mucosa; take 3 ml of tincture or 500 mg in capsule form three times a day. You can also take lozenges in replacement of the fluid or capsule. Aloe vera juice has anti-microbial activity and soothes the lining of the stomach. Drink ½ cup three times a day.

## HOMEOPATHY

If an ulcer has been diagnosed in the stomach, this is a situation that requires professional homeopathic attention. This is due to the way in which this condition falls into a category of chronic illness, and also to the potential seriousness and severity of the problem. As a result, it is outside the remit of home prescribing for long-term management of the problem. However, the remedies suggested below can be used on a strictly short-term basis (a maximum of 24 hours) for the relief of nausea and vomiting that may be causing distress while a medical opinion is being consulted.

**Ipecac:** To relieve constant, awful nausea that is not eased after vomiting, try Ipecac. Vomiting is made worse by stooping, and it may contain traces of mucus or bile. Nausea may be combined with gripping pains in the belly that are made more intense by movement and eased by keeping as still as possible.

**Phosphorus:** This is a possible remedy for nausea, vomiting, and discomfort that are eased temporarily by drinking cold water. However, once the water becomes warmed by the stomach, it gets vomited up again. There may be a noticeable sore spot in the pit of the stomach that is eased by gentle massage. There is also a burning pain in the stomach that is aggravated by eating.

**Arsenicum album:** Consider this remedy if burning pains are accompanied by a strong desire for ice cold water, which is immediately vomited up after drinking. Sips of warm drinks, however, provide some temporary relief. Nausea is so strong that the thought or smell of food causes immense distress. Symptoms are noticeably worse, or come on, in the early hours of the morning, causing restlessness, distress, and anxiety.

**TIP:** STAY HYDRATED

Since recurrent vomiting can cause dehydration, make sure to replace fluids by taking small sips of water at frequent intervals. Even if you are very thirsty, avoid the temptation to gulp down very cold water, since the stomach is likely to vomit it up again.

## HERBALISM

 A peptic or duodenal ulcer is a serious condition that requires medical supervision and medication to avoid perforation or bleeding of the mucosa. Herbs can be used in a complementary way, aiding the body's ability to heal ulcers. Demulcent or mucilaginous plants (see the section on gastritis, p. 402) can be useful for ulcers. These plants coat the stomach and intestinal lining to prevent further damage from a variety of causes, such as medications or over-production of acid, and allow the ulcers to heal. It is important to be aware of the differences in treating gastric versus duodenal ulcers. For example, bitters (again see the section on gastritis) may help gastric ulcers but worsen duodenal ulcers. Also, weak astringent herbs may be useful for both types, but strong astringents such as cranesbill can help duodenal ulcers but make gastric ulcers worse.

**Licorice:** This well-known demulcent can by used to treat gastric and duodenal ulcers. For long-term use, take two to four 380 mg tablets of de-glycyrrhizinated licorice (DGL) before meals. **Caution:** The prolonged use of decoctions or infusions of dried, unprocessed licorice root can cause high blood pressure, low potassium, and swelling, due to one of its compounds, glycyrrhizin, also called glycyrrhizic acid. DGL is a safer form of licorice as it does not contain glycyrrhizin.

**Herbal blends:** Gentle astringents such as agrimony and meadowsweet, which help heal damaged tissue, anti-inflammatory herbs such as chamomile (see the section on heartburn, p. 408), and wound-healing plants such as calendula and chickweed can also be helpful in treating ulcers. Many herbalists will make a tincture from a combination of all these plants that can be taken three times a day before or with meals to help heal the ulcer.

# URINARY TRACT INFECTION

## DIAGNOSIS

The urinary tract is composed of the kidneys, ureters, the bladder, and the urethra. Most infections affect the bladder and the urethra, which combine to form the lower part of the tract. Cystitis is an infection of the bladder (see p. 352), and urethritis is an infection of the urethra. Pyelonephritis is a more severe infection of the kidneys, triggered by bacteria spreading up from the bladder. A urinary tract infection, also known as a UTI, is defined as the presence of multiplying micro-organisms (bacteria) in the tract through which you pass urine from the kidneys via the bladder. UTI is much more common in women, because of the short length of the female urethra and its proximity to the anus. UTIs are rare in men under 60, but the incidence increases as both men and women get older, until they tend to be equally affected. To establish whether an infection is present, a clean midstream urine sample is taken and sent to the lab for examination. A level of 100,000 bacteria per milliliter of urine is regarded as a significant infection.

## SYMPTOMS

- Burning sensation when passing urine
- Frequent and compelling need to urinate
- Urine can be cloudy
- Urine can have an offensive odor
- Loin pain, with fever and chills (this indicates an upper infection of kidneys or ureters)

## TREATMENT GOAL

Treatment depends on why the infection has occurred. Most patients respond rapidly to antibiotics. A high intake of fluids is essential to help flush out the infection from the system. If UTIs keep occurring, it is essential to identify and treat the underlying cause.

## CONVENTIONAL MEDICINE

**Antibiotics:** Trimethoprim/sulfamethaxazole can be taken twice a day for three days. This antibiotic is generally well tolerated but can affect the skin and central nervous and gastrointestinal systems. If the bacteria causing the UTI is resistant to this antibiotic, ciprofloxacin (Cipro®) or levofloxacin (Levoquin®) can be used, as well as nitrofurantoin (Macrobid®). Symptoms should resolve in one or at the most two days after starting treatment. Phenazopyridine is sometimes prescribed along with an antibiotic to decrease the pain experienced on urination with a urinary tract infection. This medication turns the urine bright orange. It has been associated with infrequent but very severe allergic reactions.

**Lifestyle modifications:** Practice stress reduction techniques, avoid irritating soaps, and take showers rather than baths. Women should wipe front to back after urination.

## TRADITIONAL CHINESE MEDICINE

Traditional Chinese medicine can be an effective treatment for both acute and chronic UTIs.

**Herbs:** To prepare either of the formulas below, mix the herbs in a glass or ceramic pot and add 3 cups of water. Bring the mixture to the boil and simmer for 30 minutes. Strain the liquid and drink 1 cup twice a day. These herbs are available from Chinese herbalists or online.

- To treat acute UTI: Mix 12 g of Pu Gong Ying (dried dandelion), 12 g of Huang Bai (phellodendron), 12 g of Huang Qin (baical skullcap root), 12 g of Che Qian Cao (plantago), 10 g of Zhi Zi (Cape Jasmine fruit), 8 g of Gan Cao (licorice), and 12 g of Bai Mao Gen (wooly grass rhizome). You can take this formula for seven days.
- To treat chronic UTI: Mix 12 g of Sheng Di Huang (Chinese foxglove root), 15 g of Fuling (poria), 15 g of Shan Yao (Chinese yam), 10 g of Huang Bai (phellodendron), 12 g of Zhi Mu (anemarrhena rhizome), 12 g of Han Lian Cao (eclipta), 12 g of Bai Zhu (white atractylodes rhizome), and 12 g of Huang Qin (baical skullcap root). You may take this formula for up to two months. If your stools loosen, stop the treatment.

**Acupuncture:** Acupuncture is usually effective for UTIs. You may have treatment two to three times a week for an acute condition, or once a week for a chronic condition.

**Acupressure:** Use your thumbs to press the Zhong Ji and Guan Yuan points with gentle pressure for one minute. Breathing deeply, release the pressure for one inhalation and exhalation, and then reapply pressure. Repeat this six times once or twice a day. The Zhong

Ji point is on the abdomen, about 4 inches below the navel. The Guan Yuan point is on the abdomen, about 3 inches below the navel.

**Diet:** Eat food that clears heat such as grapefruit, pears, aubergines, mung beans, red beans, watermelon, cucumber, lettuce, and spinach.

## NATUROPATHY

**Diet:** Eat natural diuretics such as watermelon, parsley, and celery, or make a juice out of these foods. Ginger and garlic, which can be added to vegetable broths, have powerful antimicrobial effects. Restrict your sugar intake while battling an infection, as it can feed bacteria. Spicy foods, caffeine, and alcohol can aggravate symptoms and should be avoided. Drink plenty of water, 2–3 liters a day, to increase your urinary output. Also drink two to three glasses of unsweetened cranberry juice a day to flush out the infection. If you are taking antibiotics, eat 1 cup of unsweetened yogurt two to three times a day to replenish some of the friendly bacteria in the gut that antibiotics can cause you to lose.

**Supplements:** Take 1,000 mg of vitamin C four times a day to help enhance immune function, inhibit E.coli bacteria, and acidify the urine to decrease bacterial growth. Probiotics prevent the overgrowth of harmful bacteria and replace healthy flora if you are taking antibiotics. Take a product that contains at least four billion organisms a day (two hours before or after taking antibiotics) for two months.

**Herbs:** Cranberry has been used for more than a century to prevent UTIs. Evidence suggests that it is the antioxidant flavonoids found in cranberry, called proanthocyanins, that prevent bacteria from sticking to the walls of the urinary tract. Take 400 mg of a standardized extract twice daily. Uva Ursi is an antimicrobial that fights E. coli. Take a standardized capsule that contains 250 mg of arbutin four times daily, make a tea by steeping 2 tsp of herb in 1 cup of hot water, or take 1–2 tsp of tincture in warm water. Uva ursi may turn urine green. Goldenseal has a long and well-documented history as a powerful antimicrobial agent. It can be taken as a tea made from 1 tsp of dried herb per cup of hot water, in capsule form at 1,000 mg, or as 1–2 tsp of tincture in warm water. Horsetail is an excellent diuretic and has a long history of use for urinary tract infections. Take 500 mg of the capsule or 2 ml of the tincture four times a day. Take 500 mg of D-mannose a day to prevent bacteria from sticking to the bladder wall. You can also try drinking an herbal tea consisting of buchu, horsetail, thyme leaf, and pipisissewa. To make a tea, steep 2 oz of the herbal mixture in 2 cups of boiling water in a glass or ceramic jar or teapot. Drink 2–5 cups a day for 7–10 days after all the symptoms have cleared. Pregnant women should omit yarrow from the mixture. Marshmallow root has soothing demulcent properties. Soak the herb in cold water for several hours, strain, and drink.

**TIP:** USE A CASTOR OIL PACK

Castor oil packs can be used to treat UTIs with associated bladder cramping or pelvic discomfort. Apply castor oil directly to the skin and cover with a soft piece of flannel and apply heat (such as a hot water bottle) for 30–60 minutes. The anti-inflammatory action of castor oil acts as pain relief.

## HOMEOPATHY

 Any of the following homeopathic remedies can be helpful in easing a recent, mild to moderate bladder infection. The homeopathic approach can be used as a first choice of treatment or as a complementary therapy to conventional medicine. For homeopathic treatment to be most effective, it should be combined with naturopathic measures such as increasing your fluid intake. If problems with UTIs are chronic, seek professional homeopathic support. Over time, symptoms should show signs of being less severe and shorter-lived, and the gaps in between infections should get progressively longer.

**Cantharis:** As soon as the first twinges of a UTI are felt, take Cantharis. When this remedy is helpful, severe burning pains when urinating develop rapidly. Symptoms feel more distressing when you are moving around, but you generally feel better when resting at night.

**Arsenicum album:** This remedy also treats burning pains, but is more suitable for pain that is more distressing during the night and early hours of the morning. Burning sensations feel temporarily eased by contact with warmth, for example, when taking a warm bath or holding a warm compress to the sore area. Symptoms also include shivering and feeling chilly.

**Pulsatilla:** If pain, discomfort, and the urge to urinate are more distressing when lying down at night, try Pulsatilla. This remedy is especially helpful if a UTI results from being in chilly, damp surroundings, and if ignoring the urge to urinate for even a short time brings on slight urinary incontinence. Although you may feel chilly, warmth in any form makes discomfort and distress worse. Symptoms also include feeling weepy when ill, with a noticeable need for sympathy and attention.

**Staphysagria:** If symptoms develop after sexual intercourse, or after being catheterized for surgery, Staphysagria can be immensely helpful. There may be an inability to empty the bladder fully, and urine is likely to look concentrated and dark in color. There are also strong stinging sensations after passing water.

**TIP:** WEAR LOOSE CLOTHING

Avoid wearing clothing and underwear that hugs the body too tightly, such as tights, jeans, leggings, and underwear made from synthetic materials such as nylon. They do not allow for good ventilation around the genital area.

## HERBALISM

**Cranberry:** This fruit has been thought for some time to be of great benefit for those with UTIs. Many studies support its use as a *preventive* measure for people with frequent UTIs. However, data concerning its use to *treat* UTIs is either lacking or indeterminate. Cranberry's capacity to defend against UTIs is said to be from its ability to prevent bacteria from adhering to the bladder and urethra. To prevent, and possibly treat, UTIs it is best to drink 100% pure cranberry juice, which you can find at your local health food store. Most of the cranberry juice you find at the supermarket is highly diluted and contains a lot of added sugar. There is no certain recommended dosage for cranberry juice, though 3 oz has been shown to be beneficial for the prevention of UTIs while as much as 12–32 oz has been used to treat UTIs. The juice can be diluted in water as the pure form is often unpalatable. Cranberry juice has few side effects. Mild stomach upset has been noted, along with the slim possibility of precipitating an attack of kidney stones in people who are already susceptible, but this only occurs in those taking excessive amounts of juice (greater than 32 oz per day).

**Dandelion:** This weed is often referred to as a "restoring" or "purifying" herb for the liver, gallbladder, intestines, and kidneys. Traditionally one of dandelion's purported benefits has been in the treatment of UTIs. There is some evidence that dandelion acts as a diuretic, increasing the flow of urine, which may explain its beneficial effects in the treatment of UTIs. Dandelion can be found in most health food stores in dried or tincture form. If using the dried herb, take 3–4 g as a tea two to three times a day. If using a tincture, take 5–10 ml diluted in water or juice two to three times daily. Dandelion is a member of the daisy/ragweed family, so should be used cautiously by those with allergies to plants in this family. Besides allergic reaction, other reported adverse effects are dermatitis and gallbladder irritation and obstruction. Do not use dandelion if there is a history of gallbladder problems.

**Stinging nettle:** Recent evidence shows promise that this plant can be used effectively to treat enlarged prostate and disorders of the kidneys, bladder, and urinary tract, as well as allergies. For UTIs, the suggested dosage is 1–2 g of the root as a tea two to three times daily. Many health food stores now sell stinging nettles as freeze-dried capsules, which can be a more convenient mode of delivery.

# VOMITING

## DIAGNOSIS

Vomiting is your body's way of ridding itself of an infection or toxins that are causing problems. In most cases, it is caused by a viral gastrointestinal infection. When you vomit, the contents of the stomach are forced up through the esophagus and out of the mouth. It is carried out by a series of complex, coordinated reflexes orchestrated by the brain responding to signals coming from the mouth, stomach, intestines, bloodstream (which may contain medicines or infections), balancing systems in the ear (which trigger motion sickness), and the brain itself (including unsettling sights, smells, or thoughts). Sometimes, just seeing someone else vomit can cause you to be sick as well. Other common triggers include overeating, eating rich foods, food poisoning, stomach bugs, motion sickness, a weak stomach, food allergies, and pregnancy (morning sickness). It is a common condition and affects children, some more than others, and adults. Most cases of vomiting can be safely treated at home. However, if there is blood in the vomit, accompanying severe stomach pain, indications of dehydration, or the vomiting is prolonged, consult a doctor.

**DANGER:** If the vomiting is severe and accompanied by a high fever, headache, and a stiff neck, this could indicate meningitis. Get medical help immediately. If there is a serious pain anywhere in the abdomen or groin, always seek immediate medical advice.

## SYMPTOMS

- Vomiting
- Dry and parched lips and mouth
- Stomachache
- Diarrhea
- Fever and sweating
- Headaches

## TREATMENT GOAL

It is important to stay hydrated and replace any fluids lost by the body. Sip water continuously until the cause of the vomiting is identified and resolved. Treatment aims to relieve symptoms until the cause can be eradicated.

## CONVENTIONAL MEDICINE

**Stay hydrated:** Rehydration should be attempted with a solution containing salts, some sugar, and electrolytes, such as Gatorade®. If fluids cannot be kept down, and signs of dehydration are present, such as dizziness, reduced urination, dry mouth and eyes, and dry skin, then this is a medical emergency that requires intravenous fluid rehydration. Consult your doctor.

**Diet:** Avoid solid foods and instead drink small amounts of cool liquid, but not acidic citric or sweetened juices. Progress to easily digested foods such as toast, crackers, rice, and broth soups. If these are tolerated, plain soft foods such as pasta can be eaten. Fatty foods and dairy products should be avoided.

**Medication:** If dietary changes do not help stop the vomiting, anti-sickness drugs may be needed. Most of them act on the central nervous system and so have sedating side effects. Compazine® and Phenergan® medications can be used rectally, intravenously, or orally. Reglan® (metoclopramide) is another common anti-vomiting drug. These drugs are not normally given to children or pregnant women. Morning sickness can be treated with vitamin B6 (pyridoxine).

## TRADITIONAL CHINESE MEDICINE

**Herbs:** The herbs listed below are available from Chinese pharmacies. For each formula, place the herbs in a glass or ceramic pot and add 3 cups of water. Bring the mixture to the boil and simmer for 30 minutes. Strain the liquid and drink 1 cup twice a day.

• To treat vomiting due to a stomach bug or cold: Combine 10 g of Huang Qin (baical skullcap root), 10 g of Jin Yin Hua (honeysuckle flower), 12 g of Zi Su Gen (perilla), 6 g of Bo He (field mint), 8 g of fresh ginger, and 4 g of dried ginger. For a summer cold, add 10 g of Huo Xiang (agastache), 10 g of Zhu Ru (bamboo shavings), and 10 g of Xiang Ru (aromatic madder). If it is a winter cold, add 10 g of Bai Zhi (angelica root), and 10 g of Zi Su Ye (perilla leaf). Drink one hour before or after meals.

• To treat vomiting due to food poisoning: Mix 10 g of Huang Qin (baical skullcap root), 6 g of Huang Lian (coptis root), 6 g of Chen Pi (tangerine peel), 10 g of Mu Xiang (costus root) 10 g of Lian Qiao (forsythia root), 6 g of Sha Ren (cardamom), 15 g of Bian Dou (hyacinth bean), 8 g of Shen Qu (medicated leaven), and 8 g of Hou Pu (magnolia bark).

• To treat vomiting due to chronic digestive deficiency: Mix 15 g of Fuling (poria), 12 g of Wu Wei Zi (schisandra fruit), 12 g of Tai Zi Shen (pseudostellaria), 12 g of Fa Ban Xia (pinellia rhizome), 6 g of Chen Pi (tangerine peel), 8 g of Sha Ren (cardamom), 10 g of Wu

Zhu Yu (evodia fruit), 15 g of Bai Zhu (white atractylodes rhizome), and 15 g of Shan Yao (Chinese yam).

**Acupressure:** Use the tip of your thumb to apply strong pressure to the Nei Guan point, located in the center of the wrist on the palm side about 2 inches above the crease, for one to two minutes. Also press the Susanli point, on the lower leg, 1 inch to the outside of and 3 inches below the kneecap.

**Diet:** There are several recipes that can help to relieve vomiting.
• Put one piece of Pomello, cut into two, into a pot with 1½ cups of water and boil for 10 minutes. Add one raw egg to the boiling water and 15 g of white sugar. Mix and drink.
• Combine 10 g of loquat leaf with 10 g of reed rhizome and add 3 cups of water. Cook the mixture over a low heat for 20–30 minutes and drink.

## NATUROPATHY

**Diet:** Eat a nourishing diet composed primarily of whole grains, fresh fruits and vegetables, and some fish and lean chicken. Stay hydrated, as dehydration can cause serious problems. Drink herbal tea, broths, soups and water.

**Supplements:** A good multivitamin/multimineral has been shown to lower the incidence of vomiting in non-pregnant women. If pregnant, make sure you take a prenatal multi-vitamin. Follow the instructions on the label. Some prenatal vitamins can lead to feelings of nausea. Talk to your doctor about this. You may need to take them at a different time or with food, or switch brands. In studies, Vitamin B6 has shown to help with nausea. Take 30 mg twice a day. Activated charcoal absorbs toxins in the digestive tract if you have been exposed to micro-organisms in food or water. Take 500–1,000 mg throughout the day.

**Herbs:** Ginger is a useful herb for treating vomiting. However, do not treat pregnancy-related vomiting with ginger for longer than the first two months of pregnancy, and do not take more than 250 mg of ginger four times a day during pregnancy without first consulting your doctor. Ginger is available as a standardized extract in pill form (take 100–200 mg), a fresh powder (take ½–¾ tsp), and a fresh root (take a ¼–½ inch peeled slice). These doses can be taken every four hours or up to three times a day. You can also drink several cups of ginger tea or ginger ale a day, but be sure to buy products that include real ginger. Peppermint is another herb that can soothe the stomach. Mix a drop or two of peppermint oil into juice, or make mint tea. Pour boiling water through a strainer containing some dried peppermint or spearmint. Let the fluid sit for a few minutes, add some sugar or honey if desired, and drink. Do not take peppermint if you are pregnant or have acid reflux.

## HOMEOPATHY

Although unpleasant, the vomiting reflex is an important mechanism that helps the body rid itself of toxins in the stomach. The remedies listed below can bring relief to vomiting due to an obvious trigger, such as a stomach bug or overindulging in food and alcohol. Cases of vomiting that do not have any obvious cause should be assessed by a medical professional, as should vomiting accompanied by severe abdominal pain or blood in vomit.

**Veratrum album:** Consider this remedy to treat violent bouts of vomiting. Vomiting is accompanied by drenching sweats and exhaustion to the point of collapse. Symptoms include an unquenchable thirst for long drinks of cold water and gnawing hunger, despite severe nausea.

**Arsenicum album:** Symptoms are similar to those described above, but there is no hunger and a thirst for small sips of fluids rather than long drinks. In addition, patients are likely to feel chilled to the bone, and are restlessness despite feeling prostrated.

**Nux vomica:** If vomiting results from drinking too much alcohol, try Nux vomica. Symptoms that respond well tend to be those of the classic hangover. Nausea and vomiting is combined with a throbbing headache that radiates from the back of the head to the front. There is also likely to be dizziness and the scalp may feel sensitive. Seek conventional medical advice about headaches that are linked to nausea and/or vomiting.

## HERBALISM

**Mint:** There are many different species of mint, including peppermint and spearmint, and all have a long history of calming stomach troubles that lead to vomiting. The leaves are the part of the plant most often used, and, when dried, can be steeped in hot water to make a tea to decrease vomiting. Many of the medicinal properties from plants in the mint family come from a class of compounds called essential oils, such as menthol, carvone, and limonene. These compounds disappear quickly when heated, so keep mint tea covered when steeping.

**Ginger root:** Either capsules of dried ginger root, or an infusion of the chopped dried or fresh root can be used to calm the stomach and decrease vomiting. The effect of ginger is due to several medicinal compounds, including gingerol, shogaol, and zingerone. Ginger is also useful for vomiting that accompanies motion sickness (see p. 453), and in prudent amounts, nausea and vomiting associated with pregnancy.

# WHEAT INTOLERANCE

## DIAGNOSIS

The cause of wheat intolerance is still not fully known, but it is thought to occur in those who have insufficient amounts of the enzymes necessary for the proper digestion of wheat proteins. Bloating and headaches are the two most common symptoms of this condition. While many people who suffer from bloating believe that they are wheat intolerant, it is in fact quite a rare condition. Dieticians believe that many people who experience such symptoms are actually suffering from other food intolerances—to dairy products for example—or from environmental factors such as stress. If you think you may be intolerant to wheat, keep a food diary for a couple of weeks, note everything you eat and drink along with the times, and observe when you become bloated. Review the diary after two weeks to see if a pattern emerges. If wheat seems to be the culprit, try eliminating it from your diet for two weeks. Remember, besides the obvious sources of wheat such as bread and pasta, wheat is also hidden in biscuits, cakes, pastries, breakfast cereals, beer, soups, and many prepared meals.

**NOTE:** Celiac disease—or gluten intolerance (see p. 332)—is a bowel disease suffered by around one in 1,000 people. It is an extreme form of wheat intolerance that occurs when the intestine finds it difficult to absorb gluten found in wheat, barley, oats, and rye.

## SYMPTOMS

- Bloating and discomfort in the stomach
- Fatigue
- Headaches
- Tiredness
- Dry skin and rashes
- Mood swings

## TREATMENT GOAL

Treatment includes maintaining a wheat-free diet to eliminate the occurrence of symptoms. Ask your physician or consult with a dietician for more information.

## CONVENTIONAL MEDICINE

**Diet:** All food substances containing wheat should be avoided. Oats that are pure whole grain, rolled or steel cut can be eaten, but many oats are mass-produced and contaminated with gluten, so these are best avoided.

**Supplements:** Wheat intolerance can cause chronic diarrhea and inflammation of the digestive tract, which wears out the important absorptive lining in the gut. This decreases the body's ability to absorb certain nutrients, particularly iron, folic acid, the B vitamins (especially B12), calcium, and selenium. Often amino acids are improperly absorbed as well. It is important to restore good bacteria (flora) to the gut. Take a good daily probiotic that includes Saccharomyces boullardii and bifidus species. Herbs such as mallow root help improve the intestinal lining. A high-dose B vitamin and a multivitamin with minerals should be taken as well. Flax oil and fish oil can help relieve the chronic inflammation associated with this condition.

**Medication:** To treat severe wheat intolerance, prednisone is prescribed along with a gluten-free diet.

## TRADITIONAL CHINESE MEDICINE

**Herbs:** Mix 12 g of Bai Zhu (white atractylodes rhizome), 15 g of Shan Yao (Chinese yam), 12 g of Bin Long (betel nut), 8 g of Shen Qu (medicated leaven), 8 g of Chen Pi (tangerine peel), and 12 g of Fa Ban Xia (pinellia rhizome) in a ceramic or glass pot. To make a decoction, add 3 cups of water, bring the liquid to the boil, and simmer for 30 minutes. Strain and drink 1 cup twice a day for up to two months. These herbs, available from Chinese herbalists, help to build a stronger digestive system. Do not use these herbs if you are suffering from diarrhea.

**Acupuncture:** Consult an experienced TCM practitioner about your condition, and in the meantime avoid eating wheat. Treatment aims are to improve your general health, by improving your digestive energy. The length of treatment varies, but it usually lasts for a few months.

**Acupressure:** The Pi Shu point is located in the middle of the back, 1½ inches lateral to the spine at the 11th vertebra. The Wei Shu point is 1½ inches lateral to the spine at the 12th vertebra. Lie on your stomach and have someone massage these points. The Shan Yin Jiao point is on the center of the inside of the leg, about 3 inches above the anklebone. The Susanli point is located on the lower leg, about 1 inch to the outside of and 3 inches below the kneecap. In a sitting position, apply pressure to either of these points for one minute.

**Diet:** Avoid wheat, and wheat products as well as sweet, fatty, and greasy food. Eat foods that are easily digested: these include rice, sweet potatoes, sweet basil, peaches, apples, spinach, squash, celery, chicken, peas, and string beans.

## NATUROPATHY

**Diet:** Eliminate all wheat and wheat products from your diet, including bread and other baked goods, pasta, pancake mixtures, and soy sauce. Also avoid whiskey, gin, beer, and any drink that contains grain.

**Supplements:** Take a probiotic product in the Lactobacillus family that contains at least four billion active organisms twice daily with meals, or 30 minutes after meals. This will restore friendly bacteria in the gut to help with digestion. Digestive enzymes also help you digest food more effectively so that less irritation is caused. Enzymes include lipases, which digest fat; proteases, which digest proteins; and amylases, which digest starch. Take 2 capsules or tablets of a full-spectrum enzyme product with each meal.

**Herbs:** Take two 380-mg de-glycyrrhizinated licorice (DGL) tablets three or four times a day between meals to bring relief and heal any damage to the mucus lining of the stomach. DGL is a safer form of licorice than other types. Aloe vera juice can also be soothing. Take ½–¾ cup of aloe vera juice three times a day between meals. Make sure it contains 98% aloe vera and no aloin or aloe-emodin. Slippery elm serves as a demulcent to soothe the digestive lining of the stomach. Take 3 ml of tincture or 500 mg of a capsule three times a day.

## HOMEOPATHY

As wheat intolerance is a chronic problem, it is best treated by an experienced homeopathic practitioner. However, one of the following acute homeopathic remedies can be helpful as a stop-gap option, calming symptoms until you are able to get professional assessment and treatment. Any homeopathic support given will have the best chance of success if it's combined with a nutrition program that maintains the integrity of your daily diet, while minimizing exposure to substances that trigger symptoms.

**Carbo veg:** This is one of the main homeopathic remedies to consider when symptoms of excess gas and bloating are causing problems. Trapped gas gives rise to severe colicky pains and there is a sense of being unwell and exhausted. Cramping pains accompany diarrhea, and tight clothing around the waist triggers discomfort. Symptoms also include a dull headache that lodges at the back of the head, made worse by lying down or by the pressure of a headband or hat, plus cravings for sweet or salty foods and coffee.

**Lycopodium:** If the stomach is bloated, and makes noisy rumbling and gurgling noises, try Lycopodium. Eating even a small amount of food makes the stomach feel overfull and uncomfortable, and acid tends to wash up into the throat when burping. Because of the general uneasiness in the digestive tract, bouts of diarrhea tend to alternate with constipation, and there is an unpleasant burning in the rectum. High-fiber foods make digestive problems noticeably worse.

**Arg nit:** If diarrhea and cramping pains are obviously worse after eating and/or drinking, take Arg nit. Although the patient craves sugar, it makes nausea and diarrhea worse. Nausea, which is severe enough to end in vomiting, is relieved by eating something small, but stomach pain becomes more intense after eating. Ulcers may develop on the edges of the tongue, and headaches, which are temporarily eased by applying pressure, are also present. Key symptoms also include feeling agitated and chatty when unwell.

## HERBALISM

 As with celiac disease, there are no specific herbs to cure this condition; the best treatment is to avoid all forms of gluten, some of which are "hidden" in foods you would not normally expect. The herbalist approach to wheat intolerance is to relieve symptoms until the body has recovered and is doing well on a wheat-free diet. Although wheat intolerance could lead to colitis (see p. 341) and constipation (see p. 346), a more common reaction to wheat intolerance is diarrhea, which may respond well to astringent herbs. This class of plants contains tannins, which, when they contact the inside of the intestines, cause drying and healing. In this way, plants with tannins can lessen the loss of water through the intestines. As well as the astringents listed below, agrimony, tormentil, and silverweed are occasionally used to treat diarrhea.

**Carob pod:** Add 2 g of this common astringent in powder form to food (such as apple sauce) every two hours. Carob taken in this way can ease the frequency and volume of diarrhea.

**Raspberry:** Both the leaf and the root of this plant can serve as astringents. Make an infusion from the leaf or a decoction from the root and drink the liquid several times a day.

# RESPIRATORY SYSTEM AND CIRCULATION

# ANEMIA

## DIAGNOSIS

Anemia is a deficiency of red blood cells and/or hemoglobin that results in a reduced ability to carry and transfer oxygen to the body's tissues. Consequently, sufferers usually experience unusual levels of tiredness, although mild anemia may not produce any symptoms. Anemia can be divided into two types: that triggered by the decreased production of red blood cells and that caused by an increased loss of red blood cells. Red blood cells are manufactured in the bone marrow and have a life expectancy of approximately four months. To produce red blood cells, the body needs, among other things, iron, vitamin B12, and folic acid (one of the B group of vitamins). If one or more of these ingredients is lacking, anemia will develop. Iron deficiency anemia is the most common type of anemia, particularly among women. The lack of iron is often triggered by heavy blood loss such as through menstruation or childbirth, the body's inability to absorb iron from the diet, or a diet that lacks iron-rich foods. Vitamin B12 deficiency anemia is frequently caused either by the inability of the small bowel to absorb vitamin B12, or by a lack of food in the diet containing vitamin B12. It frequently occurs in elderly people, although it may also be present in the young, particularly women. Folic acid deficiency anemia is caused by lack of folic acid. Folic acid is not stored in large amounts in the body and a continuous supply of the vitamin is needed.

## SYMPTOMS

- Unusual tiredness
- Difficulty in breathing/shortness of breath
- Dizziness/light-headedness
- Headaches
- Paleness

## TREATMENT GOAL

Anemia is usually detected through a routine blood test. It is not a disease in itself, but can be a warning of serious disease. It is vital to get accurate diagnosis and treat the condition before complications develop.

## CONVENTIONAL MEDICINE

The treatment of anemia is dependent on the cause and type of condition.

**To treat iron deficiency anemia:** Diagnostic tests are carried out to first determine that there is no hidden blood loss, for example, due to a heavy period, an ulcer, or other occult gastrointestinal bleeding. If blood loss is detected, medication is prescribed to treat the cause and prevent further loss. Iron pills are also prescribed, usually in the form of ferrous sulfate, in the amount of 60 mg of elemental iron three times a day. Copper is used in conjunction with iron to make red blood cells, so a mineral supplement containing copper at 100% of the recommended daily allowance is needed along with the iron. Iron pills can upset the stomach, but taking the iron with meals and starting at a lower dose than recommended and gradually increasing it can alleviate discomfort. Foods that are high in iron, such as leafy green vegetables and red meat, should be included in your diet.

**To treat anemia caused by a B12 or folate deficiency:** B12 and folic acids levels can be obtained by a blood test. A Schilling urine test is also used to determine if the body is unable to absorb vitamin B12 adequately. Treatment involves B12 and folate injections every two to four weeks. Sub-lingual B12 (given under the tongue) can sometimes be effective.

## TRADITIONAL CHINESE MEDICINE

**Herbs:** Hemoglobin levels are expressed as the amount of hemoglobin in grams (g) per deciliter (dl) of whole blood. A Western medicine doctor can determine your hemoglobin count. If your hemoglobin is under normal range (12–16 g/dl for women and 14–18 g/dl for men), but above 8 g/dl, try the following formula. Mix 15 g of Shu Di Huang (Chinese foxglove cooked in wine), 12 g of Dan Shen (salvia root), 15 g of Bai Zhu (white atractylodes rhizome), 15 g of Fuling (poria), 12 g of Huang Qi (milk-vetch root), 12 g of Dang Gui (Chinese angelica root), and 5 pieces of Da Zhao (Chinese jujube) in a ceramic pot. Add 3 cups of water, bring to a boil, and simmer for 30 minutes. Drink 1 cup twice a day. This decoction may cause loose bowel movements. Reduce the dose if this occurs and consult your doctor. If your hemoglobin levels are lower than 8 g/dl, consult your doctor about taking iron pills or other medication along with this formula.

**Acupuncture:** Treatment is effective for some of the primary causes of anemia. However, a diagnosis with a practitioner is essential. An experienced acupuncturist will evaluate your overall health before deciding on a treatment plan. It is usually best to combine herbal medicine with acupuncture.

**Acupressure:** Guan Yuan and Xue Hai, and Shan Yin Jiao are suggested pressure points for anemia. Apply gentle pressure with your fingertips to the Guan Yuan acupressure point, found about 3 inches below the navel. In a sitting position, also apply pressure on the Xue Hai and Shan Yin Jiao points. With the knees flexed, rest your palms on the top of the thighs, with your fingers on your knees. Point your thumbs towards the floor to find the Xue Hai point, located on the inside of the upper thigh. The Shan Yin Jiao point is on the inside of the leg about 3 inches above the center of the anklebone.

## NATUROPATHY

There are different causes of anemia and treatment is dependent on the correct identification of its cause. The following recommendations are given with this in mind.

**Diet:** Plan your meals around foods that contain iron, such as liver, leeks, cashews, cherries, figs, organic grass-fed beef, and green leafy vegetables—except for spinach. Spinach contains oxalic acid, which inhibits iron absorption. For this reason also avoid rhubarb, tomatoes, chocolate, coffee, carbonated drinks, and black tea. Brewer's yeast is a good source of iron as well as other essential nutrients. Add 1 tbsp to cereals, juices, or salads daily.

**Supplements:** Take 50–100 mg of iron a day if you are iron deficient. Choose a product that includes citrate, gluconate, glycinate, or fumarate rather than iron sulfate (ferrous sulfate), which is not absorbed as well and can cause constipation. Take 500 mg of vitamin C with each pill to help your body absorb the iron. Do not take iron supplements if you do not have iron deficiency anemia. Vitamin B12 helps with all types of anemia, but if your doctor diagnoses you with B12 deficiency anemia then you should take 1,000 mcg of B12 a day, which is higher than the recommended daily amount, or have B12 injections. For folic acid deficiency anemia, take 800–1,200 mcg a day, which is higher than the recommended daily amount. Also take 2,000 mg of spirulina a day, which has been shown to stimulate the production of red blood cells from bone marrow.

**Herbs:** Take 300 mg of gentian root, or 20 drops of tincture, before each meal to increase the gastric juices that help with iron absorption. You can also take 20 drops of yellow dock tincture with each meal, as it contains high levels or iron and helps with its absorption. Dandelion root, taken as 3,000–5,000 mg a day, has high levels of iron and detoxifies the liver. Pau d'Arco has blood-building qualities and can be taken at 100 mg three times a day. Take 300 mg of nettle leaves a day for their rich nutrient content.

## HOMEOPATHY

The remedies suggested below can provide complementary support for iron deficiency anemia that has been thoroughly investigated and diagnosed by your doctor, and that is caused by an obvious reason, such as heavy periods. Other forms of anemia that fall into a chronic category will require professional medical assessment and case management.

**Ferrum phos:** This remedy is suitable for iron deficiency anemia with symptoms of a pale complexion and a tendency to blush easily and rapidly. There may also be, in women, palpitations with a rapid pulse rate and a heady feeling during a period.

**Calc phos:** If symptoms of iron deficiency anemia develop after an illness, consider using Calc carb. Symptoms may be especially noticeable in children who have poor muscle tone, weak digestion, and a history of cold hands and feet indicating poor circulation.

> **TIP: TAKE VITAMIN C**
> Vitamin C appears to increase the absorption of iron. Eat foods rich in vitamin C, such as red, orange, and dark green fruit and vegetables, with every meal.

## HERBALISM

Anemia can be caused by a variety of nutritional, genetic, and environmental factors. While some forms of anemia may benefit from herbal therapy, most are not responsive. Below is a short list of herbs that have traditionally been used to treat anemia.

**Ginseng:** One of the symptoms of anemia is fatigue and ginseng has been shown to increase energy. Although ginseng can be used to treat fatigue, it does not cure the underlying anemia.

**Stinging nettle:** The leaf of this plant is beneficial in treating iron-deficiency anemia owing to its high concentration of iron. Drink a tea made from 1–2 g of nettle two to three times daily. Many health food stores now sell stinging nettles in standardized extracts as freeze-dried capsules.

**Herbs containing vitamin C:** Iron deficiency anemia may respond to vitamin C supplementation. You can take 250–500 mg in vitamin C tablets or incorporate any of a number of herbs high in vitamin C in your meals.

# A S T H M A

## DIAGNOSIS

Asthma is an inflammatory condition that affects the airways. When the tubes (the bronchioles) that carry air to the lungs are irritated, they become swollen and obstruct the flow of air, filling up with sticky mucus in the process. This causes wheezing and breathing problems. Asthmatics tend to be sensitive to various types of irritants in the atmosphere that can trigger a contraction in the airways. Common irritants and triggers include pet fur, feathers, hair, dander, saliva, house dust mites, perfumes and other fragranced products, environmental pollutants such as car fumes, cigarette smoke, and cold and foggy atmospheres, plus exercise, stress, and anxiety. The number of cases of asthma is steadily increasing worldwide, especially among children, although around half of the children with asthma eventually grow out of it. Some experts believe that this is linked with the rise in air pollution. There is also a genetic predisposition to the condition.

**DANGER:** A severe asthma attack that makes breathing extremely difficult is a frightening experience. Other symptoms such as rapid heartbeat may also develop. If a severe asthma attack occurs, seek immediate medical help.

## SYMPTOMS

- Wheezing
- A dry, irritating, persistent cough
- Night-time cough
- Breathlessness
- Persistent coughs and colds
- Gasping when breathing in
- Pains and feelings of tightness in the chest
- Morning cough

## TREATMENT GOAL

Although asthma cannot be cured it can usually be treated so that symptoms can be controlled so as not to inhibit a normal lifestyle. Asthma can range from mild to severe cases—in some cases it can be life threatening—and is a condition that needs conventional medication. Complementary therapies can help to ease symptoms as part of an integrated approach.

## CONVENTIONAL MEDICINE

Status asthmaticus is severe unremitting asthma that does not respond to treatment. It is a major medical emergency and immediate help must be sought from a hospital emergency room, where oxygen, breathing treatments, and intravenous medication can be administered.

**Modify your lifestyle:** It is important to identify and avoid any triggers of asthma attacks, and make lifestyle changes when necessary. Excluding dairy from your diet may be helpful. Keep your surroundings as clear of dust as possible and practice stress reduction techniques such as deep breathing and meditation. Stress (in adults with asthma and in the parents of asthmatic children) has been linked to more frequent and severe asthma attacks.

**Medication:** The type of medication used to treat asthma in adults and children above five years old varies according to the severity of the condition. A short-acting inhaler (belonging to a class of drugs called beta agonists) can be used as needed for immediate, short-term relief from a wheezing episode. This is usually sufficient for cases of asthma where attacks are infrequent. For mild but persistent asthma, a low-dose inhaler of corticosteroid is used. Other classes of medication can be used as well such as cromolyn sodium, montelukast, ipratropium, and theophylline. For severe asthma, combinations of these medications are used. A steroid such as prednisolone may need to be taken for a short period of time.

## TRADITIONAL CHINESE MEDICINE

Traditional Chinese medicine can be used to treat both acute and chronic cases of asthma. The advantage of traditional Chinese medicine is that it treats the original cause of the asthma and helps prevent attacks. The treatment plan is based on each individual patient's condition. It usually includes strengthening the lungs and spleen, tonifying the kidneys and lungs, and complementing conventional medication. Herbal decoctions and pills are not a replacement for inhalers and/or other medication, which must be used as recommended by your doctor. However, you can consult a doctor about the possibility of reducing your medication by utilizing herbal remedies. In severe cases, consult a doctor or go to the emergency room of your nearest hospital.

**Herbs:** The herbs listed below are available from Chinese medicine clinics or online. Place the herbs from any of the formulas in a ceramic pot. Add 3 cups of water, bring the mixture to a boil, and simmer for 30 minutes.
• To strengthen the lungs and spleen: Symptoms include fatigue, frequent cough with white or clear phlegm, and/or loose stools and distention in the abdomen. Combine 10 g of

503

ginseng, 12 g of Bai Zhu (white atractylodes rhizome), 15 g of Fuling (poria), 12 g of Huang Qi (milk-vetch root), 12 g of Wu Wei Zi (schisandra fruit), 12 g of San Bai Pi (mulberry root bark), 6 g of Chen Pi (tangerine peel), 12 g of Fa Ban Xia (pinellia rhizome), and 5 g of Gan Cao (licorice). Drink 1 cup twice a day for three to six months.

• To tonify the kidneys and lungs: This formula is suitable for those who have suffered from asthma due to kidney deficiency for many years. Symptoms include shortness of breathing at the slightest movement, such as walking up stairs, and difficulty inhaling. Combine 12 g of Wu Wei Zi (schisandra fruit), 15 g of Shan Yao (Chinese yam), 12 g of Tu Si Zi (Chinese dodder seed), 15 g of Fuling (poria), 12 g of Shu Di Huang (Chinese foxglove cooked in wine), 12 g of Shan Zhu Yu (Asiatic cornelian cherry fruit), and 8 g of Ru Gui Zhi (inner bark of Saigon cinnamon). Drink 1 cup three times a day for three months.

• Patent herbal pills: Ding Chuang Wan or Zhi Shu Ding Chuan Wan can be taken to complement conventional medication. These pills are formulated to reduce coughs and help breathing. Take as directed on the label or consult a TCM practitioner.

**Acupuncture:** Treatment can be effective in reducing symptoms such as difficulty in breathing, coughing, and wheezing. Reports show that acupuncture can relieve the spasms of the bronchial tube, and reduce inflammation in the respiratory system. You may see results after a few sessions or you may need a longer course of treatment.

**Acupressure:** Have someone press the Ding Chuan and Feng Man points on your back with moderate pressure for one to two minutes on each point once or twice a day. The Ding Chuan points are at the center of the base of the neck (at the seventh cervical vertebra), ½ inch on either side of the center point. The Feng Man points are also located on the center of the spine, about 3 inches below the Ding Chuan point, 1½ inches on either side of the spine (at the second thoracic vertebrae).

**Diet:** Foods that promote lung health include carrots, button mushrooms, garlic, leeks, grapes, honey, pears, radishes, tangerines, and pumpkin. Foods that help dispel phlegm and are good for asthma include apricots, fresh ginger, and lychee.

## NATUROPATHY

**Diet:** Eat a simple diet that includes lightly steamed vegetables, fresh fruit, whole grains, lean poultry and fish (fish consumption in children has been shown to decrease the risk of developing asthma). Eliminate dairy products and foods made from white flour from your diet, as they cause mucus to form. Sprinkle ground flaxseeds on salads and cereals to obtain some of the omega-3 fatty acids that help reduce inflammation. Drink water regularly throughout the day to flush out mucus from your body.

**Supplements:** Take 4–8 g of fish oils a day for their anti-inflammatory components. Magnesium has been shown to relax the bronchial tubes and improve lung function. Take 250 mg three times a day, but reduce it if the stools become loose. Take 1,000 mg of Vitamin C two to four times a day for its anti-allergen benefits, but again cut back if stools loosen. Vitamin B12 reduces asthma symptoms in some people and can be taken at 1,500 mcg orally or 400 mcg sub-lingually (under the tongue). N-acetylcysteine (NAC) is been used with some success in those with respiratory conditions, including asthma. Take 500 mg two to three times a day.

**Herbs:** Take 500–1,000 mg of astragalus twice a day to strengthen the lungs and to prevent respiratory infections. Lycopene, taken at 10 mg three times a day, can help with exercise-induced asthma. Also take 1,000 mg of quercetin three times a day for its anti-inflammatory benefits. Other herbs act as antihistamines (histamines are substances released in the body that produce swelling and constrict bronchial passages) to open air passages and relieve wheezing. These herbs include anise, ginger, peppermint, and chamomile. Studies show that chamomile may slow allergic reactions, such as those that trigger asthma attacks, by increasing the production of cortisone in the adrenal glands, which reduces lung inflammation and makes breathing easier. Make a tea using some or all of these herbs to help with asthma.

**TIP:** HERBAL TEA

Make a tea using 1 tsp each of chamomile flowers, echinacea root, mullein leaves, and passionflower leaves, and ½ a teaspoon each of elecampane root and lemon verbena leaves (if available). Pour boiling water over the herbs in a saucepan and let them steep for 10–15 minutes before straining. For a 50 lb child, give ½ cup of tea at least once a day as a preventive measure, or a few times a day if breathing becomes strained or when anxiety may lead to an attack. If you use a tincture of these herbs, use 15 drops of each to replace each ½ cup of tea. Store extra tea in the refrigerator to use as needed.

## HOMEOPATHY

Asthma is chronic condition, and cannot be adequately managed by home prescribing. The homeopathic remedies suggested below can help ease mild, acute asthma symptoms, but should not be used as long-term remedies. Constitutional treatment from a homeopathic practitioner, however, can have an enormously beneficial effect on patients who suffer from asthma. The need for professional homeopathic assessment and treatment is even greater if asthma symptoms are combined with hay fever and/or eczema. Patients that suffer from these atopic conditions are frequently hypersensitive, and the appropriate homeopathic remedy needs to be chosen carefully to avoid any adverse reactions.

**TIP:** STAY RELAXED

If you begin wheezing when lying down, sit up to allow the chest to naturally expand. However difficult, try to relax your chest as much as you can. The muscles in the chest instinctively tense and tighten in response to feelings of anxiety and panic, making it harder to breathe.

**Kali carb:** If asthma symptoms are aggravated by the slightest movement, or by exposure to very cold or hot conditions, try Kali carb. There is likely to be an unpleasant sour taste in the mouth, and a cold sensation in the chest during coughing episodes. Coughing spasms are frequent in an effort to raise mucus that seems determined to stay in the chest. Symptoms tend to come on, or be more severe, around 2–4 a.m.

**Arsenicum album:** If symptoms tend to come on, or get worse, around 12–2 a.m., Arsenicum album may be a suitable remedy. Signature symptoms include anxiety coupled with an overwhelming sense of mental and physical restlessness. Sufferers may feel chilled to the bone, but although warmth is desirable, the head and face feel better for contact with cool, fresh air. Bouts of coughing and wheezing may be triggered by smoky atmospheres, or strong perfume.

**Aconite:** This remedy is helpful if wheezy symptoms are brought on by exposure to very dry, cold winds. Sufferers may go to bed feeling fine, but wake from a short sleep feeling terrified and short of breath. Coughing spasms are likely to sound hoarse and dry, and there may be a hot sensation in the lungs, followed by a tingling sensation once the coughing spasm is over. Symptoms are also often brought on by shock or fright when feeling panicky, terror-stricken, and restless.

**Pulsatilla:** If tightness in the chest and wheezing are triggered, or aggravated, by being in a stuffy, poorly ventilated room, try Pulsatilla. Shortness of breath and coughing may be noticeable at the end of a severe cold due to a congested respiratory tract. If mucus is raised it is thick and yellowish-green in color.

**TIP:** SIP A WARM DRINK

When a mild episode of asthma has been triggered by exposure to cold winds, rest in a comfortably warm room and sip a hot drink to encourage the airways to relax.

**Boswellia:** The breathing difficulties associated with asthma are due to overactive muscles that line our airways, the excessive production of mucus, and long-term inflammation of the airways. Current research shows that boswellia contains certain chemical compounds that protect against inflammation, making this herb very useful in the treatment of chronic asthma. Most studies have used standardized extracts of boswellia in capsule or pill form at 300–400 mg three times a day. It is important to note that these extracts used were of the resin, which is believed to contain the active components; they did not contain raw plant material. Boswellia is generally considered safe, although there have been reports of mild stomach pain and nausea. Since boswellia acts in much the same fashion as certain prescription asthma medication (such as Singulair®), it should not be taken at the same time as these drugs, as it may increase their effects.

**Lobelia:** The flowers, as well as the rest of this plant, can be harvested and used to treat asthma, bronchitis, and other respiratory conditions. However, it is a powerful herb so consultation with a medical herbalist is recommended. Lobelia is thought to act by many different mechanisms, increasing airway diameter and promoting the secretion and expectoration of mucus. It may be used as a tea by steeping ½ tsp of dried plant in a cup of boiling water, or as a dilution using 1–2 ml of tincture in water or juice. Adverse effects associated with lobelia include nausea, dizziness, diarrhea, and tremors. Do not take this herb if you have gastrointestinal problems, heart disorders, or are pregnant.

**Green or black tea:** The effectiveness of tea in the treatment of asthma is most likely due to a family of chemical compounds called methylxanthines, which include caffeine and theophylline and some prescription drugs used in the treatment of asthma. This family of compounds acts by increasing the diameter of the airways in our lungs to allow easier and more efficient gas exchange. Tea, especially green tea, also contains polyphenol compounds, which are strong antioxidants and anti-inflammatories that may also be useful for asthma. The effectiveness of tea may not be immediately apparent, so try drinking 3–4 cups daily for several weeks to see if it is beneficial. You can also take your regular medicines for an asthma attack and try drinking 1 cup of tea a day to see if there is any added benefit.

**Ephedra:** This powerful, natural stimulant is an effective treatment for asthma, but has potentially serious side effects. Ephedra has been banned for sale in the United States by The US Food and Drug Administration due to its potential to cause cardiovascular problems, such as heart attack and stroke. Despite this, many still believe it is safe when administered for right reason and in the right dose. Always consult a health professional about ephedra, and use this powerful natural product only under his or her guidance.

# BRONCHITIS

## DIAGNOSIS

Bronchitis is an obstructive pulmonary disease. It is caused when a chest infection, triggered by a virus or bacteria, leads to the inflammation and swelling of the airways that connect to the lungs. It is a common disease among smokers and residents of polluted cities, and can be aggravated by cold, damp weather conditions, especially fog. Like many disorders, bronchitis can be acute (short term) or chronic (long term, when symptoms persist and recur at regular intervals). Many people have a tendency to recurrent attacks of bronchitis and chest infections. It usually takes a couple of weeks to recover from an attack but they can persist for much longer. Acute bronchitis usually lasts around 10 days. Most often it accompanies or closely follows a cold or flu, and is contagious. Chronic bronchitis is more severe, and recovery is even harder for those with additional severe illnesses, such as lung diseases or heart conditions. Pulmonary hypertension and chronic respiratory failure are possible complications of chronic bronchitis.

**DANGER:** If you start coughing up mucus tinged with blood, see a doctor. It could indicate a more serious condition such as pneumonia, TB, or lung cancer.

## SYMPTOMS

- Flu symptoms in the upper respiratory tract
- A dry, hacking cough
- Pain and discomfort in the chest
- Chesty cough
- Copious phlegm
- Rapid breathing that is often accompanied by wheezing
- Fever
- Loss of appetite
- General lethargy
- Symptoms may be worse at night

## TREATMENT GOAL

To establish the cause of the bronchitis and treat it accordingly.

## CONVENTIONAL MEDICINE

**To treat acute bronchitis:** Treatment is dependent on several factors. In patients who do not smoke or have lung disease, bronchitis will usually resolve without medical therapy. Rest, fluids, and deep-breathing practices will help ease symptoms. High doses of vitamin C may also be helpful. Occasionally, coughing can interfere with sleep. In these cases, a non-sedating cough suppressant such as benzoate is effective. The cough should be allowed if it is tolerable as it helps to eliminate the virus. Inhalers such as albuterol are sometimes prescribed, but not generally in routine and uncomplicated cases.

**To treat chronic bronchitis:** When bronchitis occurs in smokers, or ex smokers with chronic lung disease, treatment involves taking antibiotics and using an inhaler. Ampicillin, cephalosporins, tetracylines, sulfonamides, and azithromycin are the antibiotics commonly used. These are prescribed, along with an inhaler that relaxes the lungs and eases breathing.

**Preventive measures:** To prevent bronchitis from recurring, identify and eliminate allergens from your diet and the immediate environment. Dairy is a food that is commonly associated with respiratory problems. If you are a smoker, attempt to stop.

## TRADITIONAL CHINESE MEDICINE

**Herbs:** The herbs listed in the formulas below are available from Chinese pharmacies or online. For each formula, place the raw herbs in a glass or ceramic pot, add 3 cups of water, and bring the mixture to a boil. Simmer for 30 minutes, strain the liquid, and drink 1 cup twice a day.

• To treat coughs with thick yellow or green mucus: Mix 10 g of Huang Qin (baical skullcap root), 12 g of Xin Ren (apricot kernel), 6 g of Bo He (field mint), 15 g of Jie Jeng (balloon flower root), 6 g of Chen Pi (tangerine peel), 12 g of Lian Qiao (forsythia fruit), and 6 g of Gan Cao (licorice).
• To treat coughs with clear mucus, and chronic bronchitis: Combine 12 g of Shang Bai Pi (mulberry root bark), 10 g of Zi Su Ye (perilla leaf), 12 g of Jie Jeng (balloon flower root), 15 g of Fuling (poria), 12 g of Bai Zhu (white atractylodes root bark), 10 g of ginseng, 10 g of Chai Hu (hare's ear root), and 6 g of Gan Cao (licorice).

**Acupuncture:** Treatment can be helpful for both chronic and acute bronchitis, and you can combine acupuncture with herbal remedies and/or conventional medication. The cough should be alleviated and the duration of the bronchitis shortened. You may need treatment up to three times a week for an acute condition, and once or twice a week for a chronic condition.

**Acupressure:** Press the Feng Chi and Da Zhui points for one minute at a time, using light to medium pressure. The Feng Chi points are at the back of the head at the base of the skull, 2 inches on either side of the center point. The Da Zhui point is on the spine in the depression below the seventh cervical vertebra (at the base of the neck).

**Diet:** Foods that promote lung health include carrots, button mushrooms, garlic, leeks, grapes, honey, pears, radishes, tangerines, and pumpkin. Foods that help dispel phlegm include apricots, fresh ginger, and lychee.

## NATUROPATHY

**Diet:** Eat a simple diet of steamed vegetables, fresh fruit, whole grains, and lean poultry, and fish. Avoid mucus-forming foods such as dairy products. Instead eat chicken and vegetable soup with garlic, onions, and ginger to thin mucus, support the immune system, and for their anti-inflammatory effects. Sprinkle some ground flaxseeds on your food to obtain some of the omega-3 fatty acids that help ease inflammation. If you are taking antibiotics to resolve bronchitis, add kefir and sauerkraut to your diet to replenish the beneficial flora in your gut that may be lost. Drinking water at regular intervals throughout the day will also help to flush mucus from your body.

**Supplements:** N-acetylcysteine (NAC) thins phlegm and makes it easier to cough up mucus. Take 300–500 mg twice daily. Also take 1,000 mg of vitamin C two to four times a day for its anti-allergenic benefits and its ability to enhance the immune system. If loose stools develop, cut back the dose.

**Herbs:** Astragalus has been used to strengthen the lungs and to prevent respiratory infections. Taking 500–1,000 mg twice a day is an excellent treatment for acute and chronic bronchitis. Take an echinacea and goldenseal combination—500 mg in capsule form or 2ml of tincture every day—to enhance immune function and dry up mucus. Mullein, taken at 500 mg in capsule form or 2 ml of tincture four times a day, promotes mucus discharge and soothes the respiratory system. Licorice can help to reduce coughing and also enhances the immune system. Take 500 mg in capsule form or 1 ml of tincture four times a day, but do not use licorice if you suffer from high blood pressure. It may also be helpful to take a formula that includes horehound, pleurisy root, plantain, marshmallow, and cherry bark, all of which have traditionally been used for bronchitis.

**Aromatherapy:** Add eucalyptus, peppermint, tea tree, and thyme essential oils to a bath or a steam inhalation to drain congestion.

## HOMEOPATHY

Any of the following homeopathic remedies can be helpful in easing the symptoms and speeding recovery from an acute attack of bronchitis. It also helps to know that acute homeopathic support can be used in a complementary way, together with any conventional treatment that may be recommended. However, should a pattern emerge of recurrent attacks of bronchitis that appear to be increasing in severity and frequency, this is a situation that will be best dealt with by a homeopathic practitioner. As always, not only will he/she be aiming to prescribe in a way that will discourage episodes of bronchitis from developing by strengthening the respiratory system, but he/she will also be concerned to provide treatment that aims to boost your overall health.

**Ant tart:** If bronchitis symptoms include rattling mucus in the chest, and coughing fits and shortness of breath that are eased when lying on the right side, try Ant tart. There is a need to sit upright to feel comfortable, and overheated rooms make distress and discomfort more intense. Temporary relief is felt once mucus has been raised from the chest.

**Ipecac:** If coughing spasms are linked to an intense sensation of nausea, consider Ipecac. The effort of raising mucus by coughing causes the face to flush a purple-tinged color, and may result in retching and vomiting. Humidity and extreme temperature changes aggravate symptoms, while rest and exposure to cool air feels comforting.

**Bryonia:** This remedy can help to ease dry, irritating, tickly coughing spasms that come from the throat or top of the chest. The effort involved in coughing leads to a lot of pain in the chest muscles. Coughing is triggered or made worse by moving around, and eased by keeping as still as possible. You may instinctively use your hand to apply pressure to the chest during a coughing spasm to avoid undue movement. Eating and drinking can also trigger bouts of coughing.

**TIP:** STAY RESTED

It may be stating the obvious, but resting as much as possible during an acute attack of bronchitis is extremely important to provide the body with energy to fight the infection. Try to keep your body at a comfortable and stable temperature to prevent the body from using up energy by adapting to major fluctuations in the environment.

## HERBALISM

**Primrose:** The gamma-linoleic acid, an omega-6 fatty acid, found in this herb is thought to be responsible for many of its therapeutic effects in calming the symptoms of bronchitis. The suggested dosage is 1–2 ml of oil three times a day. Potential side effects with primrose oil include nausea, headache, and rash.

**Thyme:** Thyme oil can be helpful in treating bronchitis, especially when mixed with primrose oil. The recommended dosage is 1 ml of oil three times a day. It can also be taken as a tea, made from 1–2 g of dried herb and drunk two to three times a day. Thyme has been known to cause some mild gastrointestinal upset, and allergic reactions. Thyme oil has also been associated with allergic reactions and should be used with caution and under the direction of a medical herbalist.

**English ivy:** This herb has only one known medicinal use: for bronchitis and its associated symptoms. It appears to work by promoting the clearance of mucus from the lungs, and improving overall lung function. There is very limited research to support these claims or provide grounds for recommended dosages. However, most people use 300–800 mg of dried leaf per day up to three times daily.

**Icelandic moss:** There is some recent evidence suggesting that Icelandic moss may help treat bronchitis. Take 4–6 g per day in capsule form or as a tea. Do not use this herb if you have a history of ulcers, as it can be irritating to the stomach.

**Chamomile:** This herb contains two compounds, quercetin and apigenin, which may be anti-inflammatory and inhibit histamine release from mast cells, both of which could help to improve the symptoms of bronchitis. It is widely available in tea, tincture, pill, and capsule form. Choose the form that is best for you. Do not use chamomile if you are allergic to plants in the ragweed/daisy family.

**Garlic:** Garlic can be added to salads, soups, and other dishes to boost the immune system. Cooking garlic may destroy some of its medicinal qualities so try to eat it raw (chopped, pressed, or diced) whenever possible. Garlic is also widely available in pill or capsule form, which can be a more tolerable method of ingestion. Take 500 mg of capsule twice daily. When taken internally at high, therapeutic doses, garlic may interfere with certain anti-thrombotic drugs.

# CHOLESTEROL

## DIAGNOSIS

Cholesterol is a fat-like substance in the blood. Cholesterol in itself is not harmful and the body needs a certain amount to function properly. However, as levels rise, cholesterol begins to clog the arteries, a condition known as atherosclerosis, which can lead to heart disease or a heart attack. If the arteries that carry blood to the brain are affected, a stroke can occur. If there is a genetic predisposition to heart disease in your family, you're overweight, you eat too much saturated fat, you smoke, or you do not exercise, you are more at risk of developing high cholesterol. However, you can still have high cholesterol if none of these conditions apply.

A lipid (fat) test can be taken on a blood sample to determine your cholesterol levels. This test measures levels of triglycerides (fat in the blood), high-density lipid protein (HDL, good cholesterol), and low-density lipid protein (LDL, bad cholesterol). Cholesterol levels are measured in milligrams of cholesterol per deciliter of blood (mg/dL) and fall into the following catergories:

• Desirable level: Cholesterol in the blood is less than 200 mg/dL.

• Borderline high level: Cholesterol in the blood is 200–239 mg/dL.

• High level: Cholesterol in the blood is 240 mg/dL or above.

## SYMPTOMS

There are no symptoms to indicate you have a high cholesterol level, and it is impossible to determine your levels without taking a lipid test. A high cholesterol level in conjunction with the adverse lifestyle factors listed above increases the risk of developing atherosclerosis and cardiovascular disease.

## TREATMENT GOAL

Your doctor will assess your condition on an individual basis, taking into account the number of risk factors in your life for heart disease. If your levels are higher than they should be, treatment aims to lower them through lifestyle modification as well as medication.

## CONVENTIONAL MEDICINE

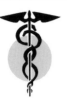

**Diet:** Dietary therapy is a fundamental part of any cholesterol treatment program. Weight loss is a primary goal in patients who are overweight. Losing fat cells is sometimes all that is necessary to lower cholesterol. Studies have shown that a Mediterranean diet lowers LDL (bad cholesterol) and elevates HDL (good cholesterol). This diet consists of monounsaturated fats (olive oil), whole grains, fish, chicken, vegetables and fruit. This diet is effective when combined with about 20 minutes of moderate daily aerobic exercise. Increasing fiber in the diet to 40 g daily or adding 2 tbsp of psyllium husks to your food is also a good idea. In overweight patients, particularly male patients, who also have other risk factors for heart disease, medication as well as diet modification is necessary. Known risk factors are hypertension, smoking, prior cardiac events, diabetes, age, and family history.

**Medication:** Statins, bile acid sequestrants, and intestinal cholesterol absorption inhibitors are the main medications prescribed. The specific medication used depends on the type of high cholesterol, which is measured as different lipoprotein types, that a patient is suffering from. If triglycerides are high, niacin and fish oil are used. Some of the side effects of cholesterol medication, especially from statins, are becoming well known. They include liver enzyme abnormalities due to liver damage and generalized muscle pain. These occur in some individuals but not all.

## TRADITIONAL CHINESE MEDICINE

**Herbs:** The herbs listed below are available from Chinese pharmacies and online.

• Shan Zha (hawthorn): Studies show that this fruit can help the body digest fat and reduce cholesterol. Hawthorn can be used alone, or as part of a formula. Try mixing 12 g of Shan Zha (hawthorn fruit), 12 g of Chi Shao (red peony root), 12 g of Dang Gui (Chinese angelica root), 12 g of Bai Jie Zi (white mustard seed), 6 g of Chen Pi (tangerine peel), 12 g of Fa Ben Xia (pinellia rhizome), and 10 g of San Qi (noto ginseng root). Place these raw herbs in a ceramic pot and add 3 cups of water. Bring the mixture to a boil and simmer for 30 minutes. Strain the liquid and drink 1 cup twice a day.

• San Qi (noto ginseng root): Unlike other types of ginseng, this is beneficial to the blood. It has been proven in China to prevent heart disease and reduce blood cholesterol. It is available as a raw root or in capsule, powder, or pill form. Try adding one or two raw roots (about 5–10 g) to chicken soup, letting it boil for two hours. Eat the soup and root.

**Acupuncture:** Treatment can help with high cholesterol by increasing blood circulation and energy flow. An experienced acupuncturist will choose the point combination that will best address your individual needs. However, in cases of simple high cholesterol, you should try diet modification, herbal remedies, and increased exercise rather than acupuncture treatments.

**Diet:** Celery, shiitake mushroom, seaweed, daikon radishes, sunflower seeds, onions, and dates are all recommended. Avoid fatty, oily foods and egg yolks.

## NATUROPATHY

**Diet:** Eating a high-fiber diet that includes vegetables, fruits, whole grains, nuts, and seeds is one of the best ways to correct high cholesterol. Brown rice, beans, and oats are also high in soluble fiber and bind to cholesterol. You can also sprinkle some ground flaxseeds on oatmeal to enhance its fiber content. Reduce the amount of fat consumed, especially hydrogenated fats. Instead add extra virgin olive oil to your salads, breads, and pastas. Olive oil raises HDL (good cholesterol) and lowers LDL (bad cholesterol). Avoid sugar and alcohol because they stimulate the liver to produce cholesterol.

**Supplements:** Take 3–4 g of fish oil a day to reduce arterial inflammation and lower cholesterol. Niacin, taken at 1,000–2,000 mg a day, reduces cholesterol levels and increases good cholesterol. Take 60–100 mg of coenzyme Q10 (CoQ10) a day, which improves circulation and has been shown to help with heart function. It is even more helpful to take CoQ10 if you are on statins (cholesterol-lowering medications), since they decrease the levels of CoQ10 that may be contributors to liver and muscle abnormalities. Chromium, at 200–400 mcg a day, increases HDL and lowers total cholesterol. Taking 400 IU of vitamin E a day helps with inhibiting cholesterol oxidation.

**Herbs:** Take 1,200 mg of red rice yeast a day with 60 mg of CoQ10. Red rich yeast has been shown to be effective in decreasing cholesterol. Policosanol has also been shown to reduce bad cholesterol (LDL), as well as increase good cholesterol (HDL); take 5–10 mg twice a day. Take 2–3 capsules of garlic a day to lower cholesterol, and perhaps also lower blood pressure. Ginger has also been shown, in some studies, to lower cholesterol by binding to it and inhibiting its absorption. Take 8–10 g of a ginger capsule a day in divided doses and drink ginger tea throughout the day. Do not take more than 1 g of ginger if you are pregnant. Reishi, a mushroom extract that has been shown to lower cholesterol, can be taken at 800 mg twice a day.

## HOMEOPATHY

High cholesterol levels are best treated by an integrated medical approach that can include constitutional homeopathic prescribing. However, for homeopathic treatment to have the greatest chance of success, it needs to be provided by a homeopathic practitioner. The following self-help suggestions can also help in managing cholesterol levels.

**Diet:** Cut down on all forms of saturated fat, including red meat, cream, butter, cheese, and full-fat milk. It will also be helpful to avoid any items that are a source of refined, white sugar, including cakes, pastries, chocolate, and sweet carbonated drinks. Increase the amount of high-fiber foods in your diet, opting for whole grains, pulses, beans, and lentils over red meat and French fries. Oily fish also appears to benefit the heart and circulatory system. Opt for small amounts of cold-pressed virgin olive oil in preference to other cooking oils.

**Garlic:** Add fresh garlic to your food and take a high-potency garlic supplement. Garlic has been shown to have a beneficial effect on the circulatory system, and may help reduce harmful cholesterol.

**Manage stress:** If your stress levels are high, it will be helpful to exercise and practice relaxation therapy regularly. If time is an issue, consider exercise that combines physical fitness with relaxation such as yoga, T'ai chi, or Pilates.

## HERBALISM

The line between potential alternative treatments for high cholesterol and nutritional therapy is often blurred. Many of the remedies listed below are considered to be foods more than herbs, and the dosage recommendations are often to simply increase the amount included in the diet. When it come to high cholesterol, the old adage "let thy food be they medicine" undoubtedly rings true.

**Garlic:** To control high cholesterol, garlic should be considered as a first choice in herbal therapy. Add it to salads, soups, and sandwiches, eating it raw whenever possible. Taking two garlic cloves daily—pressed, chopped, or diced—should be effective, but it may take two to three months before you see a difference. Garlic is also widely available in pill or capsule form, which can be taken at 500 mg twice daily. When taken internally at high, therapeutic doses, garlic may interfere with certain anti-thrombotic drugs.

**Psyllium:** Found in many bulk laxatives and cereals, psyllium has been proven to lower LDL (bad cholesterol), but has no measurable effects on HDL (good cholesterol). Psyllium can be bought in bulk from your local health food store, but recommended dosages vary widely (from 3–45 g daily), so see what works for you. Most people mix psyllium with a glass of water, although this mixture quickly becomes thick and gel-like, which many find unpleasant. Try sprinkling it on cereals or salads instead, but it is extremely important to take psyllium with plenty of water. Side effects are mild and include bloating, gas, and diarrhea. Discontinue use or lower your daily intake if any of these problems arise.

**Soy:** All soy products can potentially lower cholesterol. Soy is similar to psyllium in that it modestly lowers LDL, but has no real measurable effects on HDL. Try incorporating more soy protein into your diet (for example, by introducing tofu in place of red meat) to lower cholesterol.

**Guggul:** This is a relatively unknown herb, but there is increasing evidence that it is a cholesterol-lowering agent. If possible, take a standardized preparation of guggul (often called guggulsterones) two to four times daily; consult your local herbal therapist to determine the dose that is right for you (usually between 25–100 mg). Guggul has been associated with skin reactions, nausea, and headaches.

**Alfalfa:** This common herb can modestly lower cholesterol when taken daily. Steep 5–10 g of dried herbs in a cup of boiling water and drink three times daily. Alfalfa may react with certain drugs such as anticoagulants and diabetic drugs.

**Oats:** Oats have been aggressively marketed as a "heart healthy" food and can reduce cholesterol. Like psyllium, oats have been shown to decrease LDL, but seem to have no effect on HDL. Oats and oatmeal are easily included in a balanced diet.

**Green tea:** This tea contains polyphenol compounds, which are useful in lowering total cholesterol, decreasing the oxidation of LDL cholesterol, and increasing HDL cholesterol. The latter is interesting as there are few other herbs that are useful for increasing HDL cholesterol. Drink 3–4 cups of green tea daily and test your blood cholesterol levels after two to three months. If the caffeine in green tea is intolerable, drink decaffeinated green tea or take capsules of standardized green tea extracts from which the caffeine has been removed.

# CONGESTION

## DIAGNOSIS

Nasal congestion can be a symptom of many conditions. It is most frequently associated with nasal infection from a cold or an allergic reaction. Sinus congestion, or rhinitis, occurs when one or more of the four pairs of sinus passageways in the skull become blocked. This blockage can result from the inflammation and swelling of the nasal tissues, an obstruction by one of the small bones of the nose, or the secretion of mucus. It may be an acute or chronic condition. Acute sinus congestion is most often caused by the common cold. Chronic sinus congestion often results from environmental irritants such as pollen, mold, dust mites, trees, or animal dander. Exposure to various chemicals in the home or workplace may also contribute to nasal congestion, and indoor and outdoor air pollution can be a factor for those who are already susceptible. Smoking and passive smoking have been implicated in chronic nasal congestion and the prevalence of chronic rhinitis among men has been shown to increase with cigarette consumption. Those exposed to chlorine, such as lifeguards and swimmers, may also be at risk of developing this condition.

## SYMPTOMS

- Nasal stuffiness
- Pressure, tenderness, or pain in the area above the eyebrows
- Pressure, tenderness, or pain in the area above the upper molars
- A thick yellow or green discharge
- Postnasal drip
- Bad breath
- Dry, irritating cough

## TREATMENT GOAL

It is important to determine triggers, and careful evaluation by a specialist may help identify contributory factors. Treatment is to alleviate symptoms and prevent the condition from recurring.

## CONVENTIONAL MEDICINE

Treatment for congestion involves investigating the cause and avoiding complications such as infections. If there is an accompanying fever, or breathing is compromised, consult a doctor immediately.

**Diet and supplements:** A healthy diet can markedly improve the symptoms of chronic congestion. Eliminate dairy and gluten from the diet and add anti-inflammatory herbs such as ginger, turmeric, and curcumin to your meals. Taking 4 g of fish oil daily is also beneficial.

**Decongestants:** Medications such as phenylephrine are effective but can have side effects, such as hypertension and elevated heart rate. Other decongestants, such as Afrin®, have fewer side effects but, if used for longer than three days, tend to cause rebound congestion. When this occurs your body adapts to the drug so that congestion persistently recurs unless the drug is used. A saline nasal spray may improve symptoms and has no side effects. If the congestion is severe a steroid nasal spray is sometimes needed. A steam humidifier may also be helpful in relieving congestion.

**Allergy medications:** If the congestion is caused by allergies, an antihistamine such as Claritin® or Allegra® can be used.

## TRADITIONAL CHINESE MEDICINE

**Herbs:** The herbs used in the following formula are available from Chinese pharmacies or online. Combine 12 g of Niu Bang Zi (great burdock fruit), 12 g of Cang Er Zi (cocklebur fruit), 12 g of Fang Fen (ledebouriella root), 10 g of Chuan Xiong (Szechuan lovage root), 10 g of Jing Jie (schizonepeta stem and bud), 10 g of Huang Qin (baical skullcap root), and 5 g of Gan Cao (licorice) in a ceramic pot. Add 3 cups of water, bring to a boil, and simmer for 30 minutes. Strain the liquid and drink 1 cup twice a day.

**Acupuncture:** Treatment, if performed by an experience practitioner, is very effective for sinus congestion. In most cases, the congestion is temporarily reduced immediately after the treatment, and further sessions may enhance the result. If the primary cause of the congestion is an allergy, treatment involves sessions on a regular basis two to four times a month, and the condition may take a few months to improve.

**Acupressure:** Use your fingertip to press the Yin Tang and Ying Xiang points with gentle pressure for one minute and then repeat. The Yin Tang point is located in the depression midway between the eyebrows. The Ying Xiang point is found on the side of and slightly above the lower border of the nostril.

**Diet:** There are several Chinese recipes that can help relieve congestion. To make a chicken broth, slice 50 g (about 2 oz) of chicken livers and boil them until cooked. Eat the soup while it is hot, adding a little salt or other seasoning. You can also try squeezing and drinking the juice from a watermelon. Boil the juice over a high heat, and then lower the temperature until the juice thickens into a syrup. Remove the juice from the heat and let it cool. Add enough sugar to absorb the liquid and let it dry in a warm place. Break the sugared watermelon into small pieces and store it in a jar. Dissolve 15 g (½ oz) in boiling water and drink it three times a day.

## NATUROPATHY

**Diet:** A healthy immune system is the best protection against colds and other causes of congestion, and good nutrition is the key to a healthy immune system. In general, a diet that is rich in vegetables, whole grains, and beans, and low in saturated fat, sugar, mucus-forming foods, and allergenic foods will be beneficial. Sugar depresses the immune system, limiting its ability to clear bacteria and congestion. Foods that promote mucus include dairy, oranges, white sugar, and foods that contain white flour. Potentially allergenic foods include dairy, wheat, soy, fermented foods, and eggs. Try eliminating these from your diet and then reintroduce them one at a time, noting any changes in your symptoms. Eat light meals so that your body's energy is used to eliminate the cause of the congestion rather than digesting heavy foods. Drink plenty of water, herbal tea, diluted vegetable juice, and soup. Avoid fruit juices, dairy, coffee, alcohol, and carbonated drinks as these can make symptoms worse.

**Supplements:** Take 1,000 mg of vitamin C three to five times a day for its antihistamine effects. However, reduce the dosage if diarrhea occurs. Quercetin controls inflammation by reducing the release of histamine and other mediators of congestion from cells. Quercetin also works by stabilizing cell membranes so they are less reactive to allergens. Take 250 mg three times a day. Also take 3 g of fish oil a day for its anti-inflammatory properties, which are beneficial to allergic rhinitis and other causes of congestion. Digestive enzymes, along with Betaine hydrochloride, assist in the digestion of food and reduce the chances of food sensitivities, which can contribute to congestion. Take 1–2 of each with each meal.

**Herbs:** There are several herbs that can help to alleviate congestion. Eyebright reduces congestion and secretions, and can relieve itchy eyes, sneezing, and excess mucus. Gingko contains bioflavonoids and is used as an antioxidant and anti-inflammatory. Milk thistle helps reduce allergic, inflammatory, and histaminic reactions and supports liver function. Red clover helps build the body's resistance to allergies. Stinging nettles can be used as an antihistamine and anti-inflammatory. Yarrow reduces congestion and secretions. You can use one or a combination of these herbs to make a tea. Steep the dried herbs in boiling water and drink 3–4 cups a day. You can also take the herbs in tincture form. Combine several of them and take 1 dropperful three to four times a day.

## HOMEOPATHY

 This is a common problem that can often occur as a lingering side effect of a cold or bout of flu. Any of the remedies included below can be helpful in speeding up dispersal of any mucus in the nose, throat, or chest that has been triggered as a result of a recent cold. However, more recurrent and severe symptoms of congestion in the ears, throat, nose, sinuses, and/or chest will fall into the category of a chronic condition. As a result, they will do best in response to professional homeopathic treatment, rather than attempting to handle the situation through home prescribing measures. This will be even more the case with babies and young children, who can respond exceptionally well to constitutional prescribing at this age.

**Hepar sulph:** If a thick, yellowish mucus that tends to settle in the sinuses and bridge of the nose is causing congestion, use Hepar sulph. The congestion may have followed on from a severe sore throat and swollen, tender glands. Symptoms include a strong aversion to contact with cold drafts of air and a desire for warmth, which feels soothing and comforting. The nose is likely to feel blocked, and there is lots of sneezing and pain in the facial bones.

**Phosphorus:** This remedy can be helpful in relieving swollen and inflamed nasal passages that produce a discharge that alternates between being dry and liquid. If mucus is dislodged, it is likely to be yellowish in color. Nosebleeds occur easily when blowing, and discharges from the nose may be slightly streaked with blood. When the nose is congested there may also be an unusual oversensitivity to smells, while congestion in the sinuses can make the eyes feel drawn, heavy, and tired.

**Pulsatilla:** If a general sense of congestion lingers after a heavy head cold, consider using Pulsatilla. The nose, ears, throat, sinuses, and chest may feel congested and mucus discharges are thick, bland, and yellowish-green in color. The congestion requiring Pulsatilla is made considerably worse by being in warm, stuffy rooms.

**Natrum mur:** This remedy is appropriate if the nose alternates between being completely dry and blocked up and running profusely.

## HERBALISM

**Eucalyptus oil:** This well-known decongestant is found in many over-the-counter medications. Simply place a few drops of eucalyptus oil in a vaporizer and breathe in the steam through the nose. Keep your eyes closed because the volatile oils can cause a stinging sensation. Do not swallow eucalyptus oil. Ingestion can cause severe side effects, including depression of the central nervous system, nausea, and vomiting. Eucalyptus oil is not recommended for use by small children.

**English ivy:** This plant may be useful for congestion. It appears to work by promoting the clearance of mucus from the lungs, and helps improve overall lung function. There is limited research to support these claims or suggest recommended dosages. However, most people use 300–800 mg of dried leaf per day.

**Mullein:** Mullein may be helpful in congestion, especially when combined with coltsfoot and white horehound. Drink a tea make from 1–2 tsp of dried herb, or take 2–6 ml of tincture three times a day. The only reported side effects of mullein are skin irritations.

**White horehound:** This plant has been traditionally used to help clear mucus and congestion and relieve coughs. Adding mullein or coltsfoot to a tea or tincture of white horehound may prove more beneficial. Drink a tea make from 1–2 tsp of dried herb, or take 2–6 ml of tincture three times a day. White horehound may cause diarrhea and has the potential to lower blood sugar.

**Elecampane:** This herb has been used for some time in traditional preparations as a decongestant. Elecampane can be prepared as a tea using a small amount of dried shredded root. You can also take 1–2 ml of tincture two to three times a day. Elecampane is generally considered safe with few reported side effects.

---

**TIP:** USE AN AIR HUMIDIFIER

If nasal congestion is preventing sleep, it can be helpful to humidify the atmosphere. Use a high-energy particulate air (HEPA) filter or place a small bowl of water by a heat source to produce a similar effect.

# COUGH

## DIAGNOSIS

Coughing is a reaction to an irritant, such as a respiratory infection, bacteria, or an allergen, that stimulates the production of mucus in the airways. As such, the coughing reflex is a vital part of the body's defense mechanisms. There are two types of cough: a dry, hard tickly cough and a wet, rattling productive cough that brings up phlegm. Most of the time a cough is nothing to worry about—it is either a simple clearing of the throat or a symptom of a passing cold or respiratory infection. A persistent night-time cough, however, can indicate a more serious problem, such as asthma, and it is important to seek medical advice if this is the case. Triggers and irritants of cough include cold, damp weather conditions, especially fog, air pollution, and cigarette smoke.

**DANGER:** A cough that brings up blood or is accompanied by shortness of breath, or a long-term cough that refuses to resolve, requires medical attention.

## SYMPTOMS

- A dry, irritating cough
- A loose cough that rattles
- Coughing up phlegm that is green, white, or yellow, or foul smelling
- Chest pain
- Shortness of breath or wheezing
- Persistent night-time cough
- Fever and sweating
- Loss of appetite
- General lethargy

## TREATMENT GOAL

Coughing is a symptom rather than a condition in itself. Treatment involves alleviating symptoms while establishing the cause of the cough, and taking appropriate remedial actions to resolve the underlying condition.

## CONVENTIONAL MEDICINE

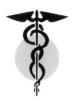

Common causes of chronic cough are acid reflux (see p. 322), postnasal drip, and asthma (see p. 502). A chronic cough can also result as a side effect of a class of anti-hypertensive drugs called ACE inhibitors. A lung, bronchial, or sinus infection are the most common causes of a short-lived cough. Once the cause of the cough is determined, the underlying disease is treated.

**Cough suppressants:** A variety of medications, both narcotic and non-narcotic, exist to treat a cough that is a symptom of an acute upper respiratory tract infection, or to relieve cough symptoms while a diagnosis is being determined. Narcotic cough suppressants may be more effective but do have side effects. They are addictive, can cause constipation, and may interfere with natural sleeping patterns. Another prescription option is benzoanate, which numbs the cough reflex with minimal side effects. Dextromethorphan is a common over-the-counter preparation that can be effective.

**Expectorants:** Expectorants thin secretions so they can be coughed up more easily. They can be used in combination with cough suppressants for added relief.

## TRADITIONAL CHINESE MEDICINE

**Herbs:** The herbs listed in the formulas below are available from Chinese pharmacies. For either formula, place the raw herbs in a glass or ceramic pot and add 3 cups of water. Bring the mixture to a boil and simmer for 35 minutes. Strain the liquid and drink 1 cup twice a day.

• To treat an acute cough: Mix 10 g of Huang Qin (baical skullcap root), 12 g of Xin Ren (apricot kernel), 6 g of Bo He (field mint), 15 g of Jie Jeng (balloon flower root), 6 g of Chen Pi (tangerine peel), 12 g of Lian Qiao (forsythia fruit), and 6 g of Gan Cao (licorice).

• To treat a chronic cough: Combine 12 g of Sang Bai Pi (mulberry root bark), 10 g of Zi Su Ye (perilla leaf), 12 g of Jie Jeng (balloon flower root), 15 g of Fuling (poria), 12 g of Bai Zhu (white atractylodes root bark), 10 g of ginseng, 10 g of Chai Hu (hare's ear root), and 6 g of Gan Cao (licorice).

**Acupuncture:** Treatment may help resolve the underlying illness that is causing the cough, as well as ease the cough. The frequency and length of session may vary from patient to patient. Try acupuncture if your cough does not improve after three days, since sometimes an acute cough can disappear on its own or by a combination of herbal and dietary therapies.

**Acupressure:** While seated or lying on your stomach, have someone apply medium pressure to the Da Zhui and Fei Shu points for one to two minutes. The Da Zhui point is along the spine in the depression below the seventh cervical vertebra (at the base of neck). The Fei Shu points are also on the back, about 3–4 inches below the neck at the third thoracic vertebra, 1½ inches on either side of the spinal cord.

**Diet:** Luo Han Guo (momordica fruit), honey, pomegranates, kumquats, mandarins, tangerines, olives, and thyme are all helpful foods. To treat a prolonged cough, boil 200 g of ginger juice and 200 g of honey in a pan. Dissolve 30 ml of this mixture in boiling water and drink it twice a day. A tea made from 6 g of licorice root, 30 g of honey, and 10 g of vinegar, boiled for 10 minutes, can also be soothing.

## NATUROPATHY

**Diet:** Eat chicken soup made with onions, garlic, and ginger to help raise immunity, decrease inflammation, and dispel toxins. Hot barley soup also helps to reduce phlegm. Eliminate foods that increase mucus production such as dairy, sugar, junk food, and processed, refined foods. Drink a glass of water every hour to thin and dispel mucus.

**Supplements:** Take 500–1,000 mg of vitamin C three times a day to enhance the immune system and for its anti-allergic benefit. N-acetylcysteine (NAC), taken at 300–500 mg twice a day can thin phlegm and make it easier to expectorate.

**Herbs:** Take 500 mg of licorice, or 1 ml in tincture form, to reduce coughing and enhance the immune system. However, do not use licorice if you suffer from high blood pressure. A combination of echinacea and goldenseal enhances immune function and dries up mucus. Take 500 mg in capsule form or 2 ml of tincture of this combination a day. Mullein, taken at 500 mg or 2 ml four times a day, promotes mucus discharge and soothes the respiratory system. Taking 500 mg of wild cherry bark, or 1 ml of tincture, three times a day can help reduce a wet cough. A herbal formula that includes horehound, pleurisy root, plantain, marshmallow, and cherry bark can also be helpful. Follow the instructions on the label.

**Hydrotherapy:** Let the hot water run in your shower for 20 minutes and then sit in the bathroom for 10–20 minutes. This will allow your body to expel toxins and thin mucus secretions. Add eucalyptus, peppermint, tea tree, and thyme oils to a bath or use them in a steam inhalation to ease congestion.

## HOMEOPATHY

Although irritating, a cough is an important mechanism for raising mucus from the chest. However, it can be exhausting when this reflex becomes repetitive and unproductive, and is a more serious issue in those with an underlying chronic chest condition such as asthma (p. 502) and bronchitis (p. 508). The following remedies (especially when combined with positive naturopathic measures) can help speed up recovery from an acute cough. For chronic coughs, it is best to seek the advice of a professional homeopathic practitioner.

**Rumex:** This remedy can be helpful in easing a cough that is set off by touching the throat. Bouts of coughing, choking, and retching are especially disturbing at night and trying to breathe deeply produces a raw, burning sensation in the chest. Any phlegm that is raised from the chest is likely to be thin and frothy.

**Drosera:** To ease bouts of coughing that begin as soon as you go to bed, and that begin with a maddening tickle or irritation, try Drosera. Coughing spasms may be severe enough to trigger a sweat and/or retching. Laughing and talking can aggravate the condition, or bring on a coughing spasm, while exposure to fresh air feels soothing.

**Coccus cacti:** If coughing spasms are triggered by exposure to hot, stuffy rooms, Coccus cacti can help. When this is remedy is appropriate, sufferers swallow constantly in an effort to clear mucus from the throat. The mucus raised by a cough is likely to be stringy, clear, and rather sticky. Coughing spasms tend to be triggered by brushing the teeth and/or rinsing the mouth. Taking a stroll and sipping cool drinks give a temporary sense of relief.

## HERBALISM

A cough can be caused by a variety of underlying factors. Often, it is the body's attempt to clear the airways of an unwanted substance such as mucus that impedes the flow of air. Herbs that relieve congestion may improve a cough at the same time.

**Licorice:** A decoction of licorice root can be taken for a few days to alleviate coughs, especially a dry hacking cough that sometimes produces phlegm and that follows a postnasal drip. Licorice is a classic demulcent or mucilaginous herb, which coats the throat to stop the "tickle" from phlegm that triggers coughing. Boil 2 tbsp of chopped licorice root in 2–3 cups of water for 10 minutes and drink the decoction several times a day. As long as licorice is only consumed for a few days, it is unlikely that the potential adverse effects this herb has on electrolytes and blood pressure will occur.

**Eucalyptus oil:** When this oil is inhaled it has a soothing and calming effect on the respiratory system, which can help alleviate a cough. Add a few drops of the oil to a vaporizer and breathe in, making sure your eyes are closed to protect against the irritating effects of the vapor. Do not swallow eucalyptus oil. Ingestion can cause severe side effects including depression of the central nervous system, nausea, and vomiting. Eucalyptus oil is not recommended for use in small children.

**Lobelia:** The flowers, as well as the rest of this plant, can be used to treat many respiratory conditions from a simple cough to bronchitis. Lobelia is thought to work by increasing airway diameter and promoting the secretion and expectoration of mucus. Make a tea by steeping ½ tsp of dried herb in 1 cup of boiling water, or drink 1–2 ml of tincture diluted in water or juice. Some adverse effects, such as nausea, dizziness, diarrhea, and tremors have been associated with lobelia. Do not take this herb if you have gastrointestinal problems, heart disorders, or are pregnant.

**Thyme:** This herb has been shown to be effective in treating coughs and congestion in recent studies when mixed with English ivy and anise. The recommended dose is 1 ml of tincture three times a day, but it can also be taken as a tea made from 1–2 g of dried herb two to three times a day. Thyme has been known to cause mild gastrointestinal upset and allergic reactions. Do not exceed the recommended dosage.

**English ivy:** This herb works by promoting the clearance of mucus from the lungs and improving overall lung function. There is limited research to support these claims, but the recommended dose is 300–800 mg of dried leaf per day up to three times daily.

**Anise:** To treat a cough, take 3 g of dried anise as a tea three times a day, or a few drops of essential oil mixed in water two to three times a day. As mentioned above anise has been studied in combination with English ivy and thyme for use as a cough suppressant with promising results. General gastrointestinal upset and irritation has been reported.

**Elecampane:** This herb that has been used for some time in traditional preparations as a decongestant. It has antibacterial effects and can serve as an expectorant and mucolytic (to break up mucus). Elecampane can be prepared as a tea, using a small amount of dried shredded root. You can also take 1–2 ml of a tincture two to three times a day. Elecampane is generally considered safe with few reported side effects.

**TIP:** DO NOT TAKE COUGH SUPPRESSANTS IN THE DAY
It is important to allow yourself to cough to expel the phlegm from your chest. This will allow the cough to resolve more quickly. Avoid taking cough suppressants until bedtime, when they can help you sleep undisturbed.

# CROUP

## DIAGNOSIS

Croup is a condition that inflames the airways, resulting in a barking cough and difficulty breathing. It generally affects children under five years old. As a child ages, the chances of developing croup decrease, and symptoms become less severe in those that have the complaint. Some children are prone to the condition, especially those with allergies, and suffer from repeat attacks. It is thought that allergies may trigger recurrent bouts of croup. Croup tends to develop quickly and is usually caused by a viral infection in the upper airways, particularly the larynx and windpipe. In most cases it clears up on its own in a couple of days. However, the coughing and breathing problems that croup causes may last for some time longer. Very rarely, croup is a sign of a much more serious illness, such as diphtheria. The croup virus can be transferred through airborne water droplets by coughing and sneezing, or is passed on by person-to-person physical contact. Children with serious cases of croup may be admitted to the hospital and given oxygen, breathing treatments, and medications.

## SYMPTOMS

- Cold symptoms
- Characteristic deep, barking cough
- Hoarseness and noisy breathing
- Occasionally, voice loss
- Fever and raised temperature
- Symptoms are worse at night and after naps

## TREATMENT GOAL

Croup is a viral infection and cannot be treated with antibiotics. It can generally be treated at home through conventional or alternative therapies to relieve symptoms and prevent recurrence.

## CONVENTIONAL MEDICINE

The medical name for this viral illness is laryngotracheobronchitis. The treatment focuses on protecting the breathing passages.

**Comfort the child:** Most acute cases of croup can be managed at home through rest, hydration, and a light diet.

**Steam inhalation:** Immediate relief may be achieved with hot steam by, for example, standing close to a hot shower, with parental supervision, and inhaling deeply. Releasing cool mist into the room via a humidifier is also suggested.

**When should I see a doctor?** If the condition does not improve within a few days, or if the child is obviously struggling to breath (i.e., you can see the muscles in between the ribs being used, or the muscles around the neck protruding with the tissue in between sinking in), take the child to the emergency room of your nearest hospital where oxygen will be administered. Another danger signal is a breathing sound called stridor (like a wheezing, whistling noise), which is a sign of progressive closure of the airway, likewise needing emergency evaluation. Another treatment is epinephrine released into the airways in a mist every 20 minutes to relax the muscles in the airways. Steroids (usually prednisone) are given intravenously or by mouth.

## TRADITIONAL CHINESE MEDICINE

**Herbs:** The herbs used in the following formula are available from Chinese pharmacies or online. Combine 6 g of Huang Qin (baical skullcap root), 8 g of Lian Qiao (forsythia fruit), 6 g of Jin Yin Hua (honeysuckle flower), 8 g of Zhi Zi (Cape Jasmine fruit), 6 g of Gan Cao (licorice), 8 g of Xin Ren (apricot kernel), 3 g of Ma Huang (ephedra stem), and 5 g of Bo He (field mint) in a glass or ceramic pot. Add 3 cups of water, bring to a boil, and simmer for 30 minutes. Strain the liquid and drink 1 cup twice a day.

**Acupuncture:** Treatment can be useful if the child is cooperative. An experienced acupuncturist will give the patient gentle treatment on certain points to reduce symptoms and larynx infection. Use acupuncture in combination with other methods of treatment, as croup can be a severe condition. Monitor the condition closely, and seek conventional medical treatment if needed.

**Acupressure:** Children may be more cooperative in receiving acupressure than acupuncture. Press the Tian Tu point, found along the central line of the throat at the depression in the collarbone. Also press the Fei Shu points on the back, which is 3–4 inches below the neck at the third thoracic vertebra, 1½ inches to either side of the spinal cord. The Ding Chuan points are on the center of the back at the base of the neck (at the seventh cervical vertebra), ½ inch to either side. Seat the patient and use your fingertip to apply gentle pressure to these points for one to two minutes and repeat three times twice a day. See a doctor to monitor your child's condition.

**Diet:** Eat Daikon radishes and food that is heat cleaning such as watermelon, mung beans, purslane, peppermint, apples, wheat and wheat bran, mandarins, aubergines, spinach, button mushrooms, and cucumber.

## NATUROPATHY

**Diet:** Encourage the child to drink plenty of fluids to thin the mucus and make it easier to cough. To ease coughing spasms, encourage the child to drink either warm soups and drinks or cold beverages, depending on what makes them feel better. Avoid dairy products as these can thicken and increase mucus.

**Herbs:** Prepare a tea using equal parts of marshmallow root (to soothe an irritated throat), mullein (to promote expectoration), osha root (to help clear the lungs) and licorice (for its antiviral and anti-inflammatory properties and to sweeten the tea). Feed your child 3 tbsp three times a day, or mix it with juice.

### TIP: STAY CALM
If your child panics it may aggravate symptoms and make breathing more difficult. Stay calm so that your child feels comforted and secure.

## HOMEOPATHY

Any of the following homeopathic remedies can be used to relieve the symptoms of a mild, acute bout of croup. Should your child experience very severe and recurrent symptoms, this is a situation that will benefit from professional case evaluation and treatment at the hands of an experienced homeopathic practitioner. He/she will be aiming to treat at a level beyond the acute, in order to strengthen your child's system so that the episodes of croup should become less frequent and less severe until they have phased themselves out.

**Aconite:** To treat croup symptoms that develop after your child has been out in dry, cold winds, or has had an upsetting, shocking, or traumatic experience, use Aconite. The child may go to bed seeming fine, but wake abruptly from sleep in a state of panic, anxiety, and distress. There is likely to be a dry, hoarse cough that triggers feelings of fear and tension, making breathing even more difficult.

**Spongia:** If coughs are harsh and rasping, and feel most distressful when talking or inhaling, or when feeling excited, consider using Spongia. When this remedy is indicated, croup symptoms tend to come on just as the child is falling asleep.

**Drosera:** Try this remedy if croup symptoms develop or get more intense after midnight, and when a croupy cough comes on immediately after lying down. The child may be extremely hoarse, and coughing takes so much effort that the child must hold his or her sides and may retch or vomit. Stooping aggravates symptoms, while contact with fresh air may help.

## HERBALISM

Croup is often caused by a virus similar to that which causes influenza. See the section on flu (p. 550) for anti-viral herbal remedies. The section on coughs (p. 523) also provides additional herbal remedies to those listed below.

**Licorice:** A decoction of licorice root can be taken for a few days to alleviate coughs, especially a dry hacking cough. Licorice is a classic demulcent or mucilaginous herb, which coats the throat to alleviate dryness. Boil 2 tbsp of chopped licorice root in 2–3 cups of water for 10 minutes and drink the decoction several times a day. As long as licorice is only consumed for a few days, it is unlikely that the potential adverse effects this herb has on electrolytes and blood pressure will occur.

**Lobelia:** The flowers, as well as the rest of this plant, can be used to treat a cough. Lobelia is thought to work by increasing airway diameter and promoting the secretion and expectoration of mucus. Make a tea by steeping ½ tsp of dried herb in 1 cup of boiling water, or drink 1–2 ml of tincture diluted in water or juice. Some adverse effects, such as nausea, dizziness, diarrhea, and tremors have been associated with lobelia. Do not give this herb to children with gastrointestinal problems or heart disorders.

### TIP: KEEP THE WINDOWS OPEN
Open the windows even during the winter. Cool, moist air can be beneficial in improving and preventing cough attacks.

# DIZZINESS

**DIAGNOSIS**

Dizziness, usually described as a spinning sensation, can be triggered by a range of medical conditions. It is generally associated with feeling lightheaded and unstable on your feet, as though you could topple over at any time, and can ultimately lead to a fainting spell. It may present as vertigo, which is the sensation that you are spinning when you are in fact standing still. It is also a symptom of an anxiety or panic attack, in which case dizziness is accompanied by rapid breathing and a feeling of being overwhelmed. It can also be linked to high blood pressure, low blood sugar levels, and anemia. It is one of the symptoms of ear infections (p. 247) and Meniere's disease (p. 276). Dizziness can also accompany a bad headache or migraine.

**DANGER:** If dizziness follows a head injury, go to the emergency room of your nearest hospital. If dizziness is accompanied by a crushing pain in the chest, or tingling sensations in the arms, you may be having a heart attack. Seek emergency medical help.

## SYMPTOMS

- Lightheadedness
- Loss of balance
- Spinning sensation
- Toppling sensation
- Occasionally, can lead to fainting

## TREATMENT GOAL

To establish the cause of the dizziness and treat the condition accordingly.

## CONVENTIONAL MEDICINE

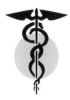

**Identify the cause:** Dizziness has a variety of treatments, all of which depend on the cause of the condition. The first step in conventional medicine is to determine whether or not dizziness is due to a serious illness. Many doctors will make sure that there is not a disease in the brain causing the dizziness by doing an MRI scan of the head. This very uncommon, but serious cause of dizziness, is usually accompanied by other symptoms such as headache.

**To treat dizziness due to ear problems:** Dizziness is sometimes caused by an ear problem, usually the inner ear, which is responsible for balance. This type of problem is thought to result from a viral infection, although this is not always the case. If this is the case, medications such as hydrochlorothiazide, which is a diuretic, may be helpful. A course of steroids such as prednisone can also help, but only as a short-term treatment. Antihistamines such as Benadryl®, Antivert®/Bonine® (meclizine), and hydroxyzine may also help. Occasionally for this type of dizziness, an anti-inflammatory and anti-allergenic diet can be helpful, if the dizziness is caused by fluid in the ear.

**To treat dizziness due to an electrolyte imbalance:** Low or high sodium, potassium, or chloride levels in the body can contribute to dizziness. This type of dizziness is determined by a blood test. Treatment involves replacing electrolytes, and diagnosing and correcting the cause of the deficiency. A multivitamin and mineral supplement may be helpful.

**To treat dizziness due to a neurologic illness:** This type of dizziness is called benign positional vertigo. It manifests as intense dizziness (where the room spins and the patient feels lightheaded) when moving the head. This condition is usually treated with antihistamines, as noted above in the section on ear problems, but may, if it persists, require consultation with a neurologist.

## TRADITIONAL CHINESE MEDICINE

**Herbs:** The herbs listed below are available from Chinese pharmacies or online. For each formula, decoct the herbs by placing them in a ceramic pot with 3 cups of water and bringing the mixture to a boil. Let the herbs simmer for 30 minutes and strain the liquid. Drink 1 cup twice a day.
• To treat dizziness with symptoms of ringing ears, or stress-related conditions: Mix 12 g of Gou Teng (stem and thorns of gambir vine), 10 g of Chai Hu (hare's ear root), 12 g of Niu Xi (achyranthes root), 12 g of Long Dan Cao (Chinese gentian root), 10 g of Zhi Zi (Cape Jasmine fruit), 12 g of Bai Shao (white peony root), 5 g of Bo He (field mint), and 10 g of Ye Ju Hua (wild chrysanthemum flower).

• To treat dizziness accompanied by a poor appetite, and/or mucus in mouth, or indigestion: Combine 12 g of Bai Zhu (white atractylodes rhizome), 15 g of Fuling (poria), 12 g of Shi Chang Pu (sweetflag rhizome), 5 g of Chen Pi (tangerine peel), 12 g of Fa Ben Xia (pinellia rhizome), 12 g of Bai Jie Zi (white mustard seed), and 10 g of Ju Hua (chrysanthemum flower).

**Acupuncture:** Results for treating dizziness vary, as it can be caused by many different illnesses. Long-term treatment may be needed for chronic conditions. For acute conditions, acupuncture may quickly reduce the symptoms. However, preventing the dizziness from recurring can be difficult. Consult a TCM practitioner.

**Acupressure:** The Tai Yang point is situated at the temple in the depression one finger behind the lateral end of the eyebrow and eyelid. The Nei Guan point is located in the center of the wrist on the palm side, about 2 inches below the crease. Apply medium pressure to these points with the tip of your finger, repeating two to three times a day.

**Diet:** Eat 15 g of raw sunflower seeds daily, as well as plenty of fresh vegetables. Drink Ju Hua (chrysanthemum flower) tea and peppermint tea.

## NATUROPATHY

**Diet:** Eat a wholesome diet consisting of fresh vegetables and fruits, beans, and whole grains to guard against nutritional deficiencies, which have been linked to dizziness. Eat several small meals throughout the day to keep your blood sugar levels stable, and avoid foods to which you may be allergic. Also avoid alcohol and reduce your salt intake, as it can potentially upset the inner ear and aggravate other conditions that can cause dizziness.

**Supplements:** A good-quality multivitamin will provide basic nutritional support to protect against various nutritional deficiencies associated with dizziness. Follow the instructions on the label. B-complex vitamins can help fulfill the vitamin B deficiencies often found in those that suffer from dizziness.

## HOMEOPATHY

Any of the following homeopathic remedies may be helpful in easing a mild episode of dizziness in someone who is otherwise in good health. Symptoms of dizziness that arise as a result of an underlying health problem such as Meniere's disease or labyrinthitis will require homeopathic treatment from an experienced practitioner, rather than attempting to manage the situation with self-help alone.

**Aconite:** This is one of the prime remedies to consider in treating dizziness that occurs after hearing traumatic news, or witnessing an accident. Symptoms tend to come on very quickly and abruptly, and can subside just as fast. There is likely to be trembling and a feeling of panic before and after a dizzy spell. Symptoms are generally worse when sufferers are overheated, and eased by moderate temperatures and fresh air.

**Pulsatilla:** If dizziness occurs in women who are premenstrual, pregnant, or menopausal, and comes on in a hot, stuffy, overcrowded room, try Pulsatilla. Being overdressed may aggravate symptoms by raising body temperature, while loosening clothes and walking gently in fresh air can help with recovery. Symptoms include weepiness when feeling dizzy, or after the event, and there is a strong need for sympathy and attention.

## HERBALISM

**Ginkgo biloba:** Most of ginkgo's beneficial effects are derived from the herb's purported ability to increase blood flow. Therefore, conditions are fundamentally caused by a decrease in blood may be amenable to ginkgo's effects. Ginkgo can be obtained easily from your local health food store in pill or capsule form. To treat dizziness try using 60–80 mg in tablets two to three times a day. These should be standardized to the percentage of 24% ginkgolides, which are some of the important compounds in ginkgo. There have been few reported side effects, although there is an increased risk of bleeding, so those who are also taking anticoagulant and anti-thrombotic drugs should be cautious when using gingko.

**Ginger:** It is uncertain exactly how ginger eases symptoms of dizziness, but most feel that it undoubtedly helps with the nausea that is sometimes associated with it, or by decreasing inflammation in the inner ear. Ginger is easily purchased as the raw rhizome or in capsule form. Suggested doses vary, but should not exceed 5 g per day. Do not take more than 1 g of ginger a day if you are pregnant. Ginger can also be taken as a tea or tincture, though these forms may not be as effective. In low doses there are virtually no side effects with ginger.

# EDEMA

## DIAGNOSIS

Edema results when excess fluid builds up in the body tissues and leads to swelling. The skin takes on a puffy, shiny appearance and a spongy feel. Applying pressure can leave an indentation or pitting effect on the surface of the skin. Edema usually occurs in the ankles or legs, as the fluid is pulled down by gravity. It is not a disease in itself but tends to indicate an underlying medical problem. Within the body, fluid in the bloodstream contains not only blood cells, but also oxygen and other vital nutrients. These are carried to different parts of the body through blood vessels and the lymphatic system. Fluid moves through the walls of the blood vessels into body tissues to provide nutrition and water for cells, and then moves back into the blood vessels once the nutrients it contained have been depleted. An abnormal amount of fluid builds up in the tissues when the pressure within the blood vessels increases, or when the amount of protein in the bloodstream decreases, both of which cause fluid to shift out of the vessels and into the surrounding tissues.

Hot weather, periods of immobility (for example, long drives or airplane flights), and pregnancy can lead to changes in hormone levels that affect the rate at which fluid enters and leaves tissues, triggering edema in an otherwise fit and healthy person. These cases usually resolve without recourse to treatment. However, edema can also indicate more serious medical conditions, such as congestive heart failure, kidney disease, or an underactive or overactive thyroid gland.

## SYMPTOMS

- Swollen ankles
- Swollen feet
- Swollen fingers
- Puffy, shiny-looking skin
- Dimpled or puckered skin when pressure is applied

## TREATMENT GOAL

To establish the cause of the swelling and fluid retention, and carry out appropriate treatment.

## CONVENTIONAL MEDICINE

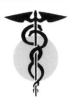

The treatment of edema is dependent on the diagnosis. Edema can be triggered by hormone imbalance, nutritional deficiency, an allergic reaction, injury, poor circulation, varicose veins, and heart, kidney, and liver disease. Each of these conditions requires proper evaluation and treatment of the underlying disease.

**Exercise:** A common and benign condition in which the legs swell after sitting or traveling (known as dependent edema) can be alleviated by improving the circulation of the blood and lymphatic system. Be sure to get up and walk every 15 minutes, or elevate your legs, while sitting for prolonged periods of time. Completing 20 minutes of moderate exercise a day is beneficial.

**Diet:** A diet that is low in protein can trigger edema. The body requires certain levels of amino acids to promote circulation and prevent fluid from leaking out of cells. Amino acids can be added to the diet in the form of lean meats, vegetable proteins such as soy and legumes, or egg whites and low fat dairy products. Men and non-pregnant women should eat about 30 g of protein a day. A protein supplement (20 g) such as whey can be taken daily, otherwise three or more 4 oz servings of protein-rich food a day will provide sufficient amounts of amino acids. High amounts of sodium can also cause edema. Avoiding processed foods, such as canned soups, pre-cooked meals, and take-outs, and stopping adding salt or other condiments to your food will immediately cut down on the amount of salt in your diet. Drink plenty of plain water to help the kidneys remove extra fluid.

**TIP:** WEAR SUPPORT HOSE
Support tights can help in cases where prolonged sitting or standing is necessary. However, they should not be so tight as to cut off circulation.

## TRADITIONAL CHINESE MEDICINE

**Herbs:** The herbs listed in the formulas below are available from Chinese pharmacies or online. To make a decoction, combine the herbs from any of the formulas in a ceramic pot. Add 3 cups of water, bring to a boil, and simmer for 30 minutes. Strain the liquid and drink 1 cup twice a day.

• To treat acute edema due to respiratory infection or an allergic reaction: Mix 15 g of Fuling (poria), 15 g of Bai Zhu (white atractylodes rhizome), 12 g of Xin Ren (almond kernel), 12 g of Fang Fen (ledebouriella root), 12 g of Zhu Ling (polyporus sclertium), 10 g of and Qing Hao (wormwood).

• To treat edema due to kidney failure: Studies show that this formula, when combined with conventional treatment, helps reduce edema. Combine 12 g of Huang Qi (milk-vetch root), 15 g of Bai Zhu (white atractylodes rhizome), 12 g of Dan Shen (salvia root), 12 g of Chi Shao (red peony root), 12 g of Bai Shao (white peony root), 12 g of Shi Hu (dendrobium), 15 g of Zhi Mu (anemarrhena rhizome), 12 g of Huang Bai (phellodendron), and 12 g of Chuan Duan (Japanese teasel root).

• To treat edema due to heart failure: Mix 12 g of Huang Qi (milk-vetch root), 10 g of Gui Zhi (cinnamon), 12 g of Wu Wei Zi (schisandra fruit), 12 g of Wu Jia Pi (acanthopanax root bark), 15 g of Fuling (poria), 15 g of Bai Zhu (white atractylodes rhizome), and 5 g of dried ginger root. **Caution:** Consult a doctor before using this formula.

**Acupuncture:** Treatment can reduce fluid retention by treating the original cause of edema, and by helping circulation and metabolism. Consult an acupuncturist for advice.

**Acupressure:** In a sitting position, use your fingertips to apply pressure to the Yin Ling Qian points, located on the inside of the lower legs, 2 inches below and to the side of the knee. Press for one minute and repeat.

**Diet:** Eat foods that help reduce water retention and that are good for the kidney and spleen. These include black sesame, chives, plums, chestnuts, duck, grapes, string beans, soybeans, apricot kernels, wheat, barley, carrots, squash, and grapefruit. Coconut is thought to be good for edema caused by heart failure.

## NATUROPATHY

**Diet:** A high salt intake can lead to water retention and may worsen edema. Do not add salt to your food and refrain from eating packaged foods, cold cuts, anchovies, and any other foods high in salt. Eat one to two servings of bright-colored foods such as blueberries, cherries, strawberries, and raspberries for their high bioflavonoid vitamin C content. These substances help strengthen the capillaries and improve the immune system. Avoid caffeine, which is found in coffee, carbonated drinks, chocolate, and black tea.

**Supplements:** Take 50 mg of vitamin B complex two to three times a day to reduce water retention. Poor adrenal gland function may contribute to edema. Take 1,000 mg of vitamin C with 250–500 mg of bioflavonoids three times a day to protect against this. Take 400 IU of vitamin E a day to aid circulation. Potassium helps keep body fluids inside the cell walls.

You should obtain most of your potassium from food, but, if not, take 2,000 mg of a supplement a day under the supervision of a doctor. Take 400 mg of flavonoids a day, as they are thought to be beneficial for certain types of edema. Take 2–3 tablets of silica a day as it is a natural diuretic.

**Herbs:** Quercetin, taken at 30–50 mg a day, has been shown to inhibit fluid from leaking out of blood vessels. Bilberry has been used for some types of edema, and 160 mg of a 25% anthocyanoside extract can be taken two to three times a day. Take 1,000 mcg of kelp a day to improve thyroid function, which can have an effect on edema, and supply needed minerals. An inability to digest food can also contribute to edema, so take 500 mg of bromelain three times a day to aid digestion and metabolism. Take 500 mg of horsetail, an excellent diurectic, in capsule form, or 2 ml of tincture, four times a day.

## HOMEOPATHY

The type of edema (fluid retention) that is likely to respond best to the self-help measures below will be of the acute variety that has developed in response to a particular trigger. The best examples of this kind of edema include the puffiness and swelling that often appear in connection with pre-menstrual syndrome, or the transient fluid retention caused by hot weather. More ongoing problems with edema that have been diagnosed as being related to an underlying heart, thyroid, or kidney disorder will require treatment from a homeopathic practitioner. This can be given in a complementary fashion side by side with any conventional treatment that may be necessary.

**Natrum mur:** To ease symptoms of fluid retention that occur before or after a period, try Natrum mur. There is a craving for salty foods and symptoms that tends to be more severe in hot, sunny weather. Massaging the affected areas, rest, and cool bathing bring relief.

**Arsenicum album:** If edema affects the feet and ankles, and is accompanied by symptoms of "restless legs," use Arsenicum album. Symptoms tend to be more noticeable and troublesome at night, and especially in the early hours of the morning. When this remedy is appropriate, exposure to cold is aggravating, while warmth in any form feels welcome.

**TIP: USE FRESH PARSLEY**
Parsley has a gentle fluid-eliminating action. If you suffer from fluid retention before a period, use fresh parsley to season your food.

**Apis:** This remedy can help the body eliminate excess fluid that is worse after resting, and improved by taking gentle exercise. Exposure to warmth aggravates symptoms, while contact with cool air, cool bathing, or applying cool compresses is soothing. If symptoms of fluid retention are accompanied by a noticeable lack of thirst, and if applying pressure to the affected area with your finger leaves an imprint, Apis can be useful.

**TIP: INCREASE YOUR POTASSIUM INTAKE**

Potassium can help to keep sodium levels in the body in an optimum balance. Eat regular portions of dark green leafy vegetables for their potassium content, as well as to obtain antioxidant nutrients such as vitamins A, C, and E.

## HERBALISM

**Horse chestnut seed:** This herb has been attracting attention recently for its effectiveness in treating a host of circulatory problems such as edema, chronic venous insufficiency, and varicose veins. Look for a standardized extract of horse chestnut seed, and take 200–300 mg once to three times per day. See Numbness and Tingling (p. 566) for more info.

**Gotu kola:** This herb has been studied for its use in edema, varicose veins, and other conditions of chronic venous insufficiency, liver problems, and high blood pressure, showing positive results for each. To treat edema try making a tea of gotu kola using 0.5–1 g of dried herb and drink this three times a day. You can also take 30–60 mg in extract form three times a day, or 300–500 mg in capsules three times a day. Gotu kola is a fairly safe herb and has minimal side effects. There are few reports of nausea or cramping. Gotu kola does have the potential to promote drowsiness; therefore you are advised to refrain from using this herb if you are currently taking other drugs that also promote drowsiness, such as sleep aids or cold medications.

**Bilberry:** This plant is packed with vitamin C and other powerful antioxidants. The tiny and delicate fruits of the plant may be helpful in managing edema. The effective dosage is 50–200 mg of bilberry extract three times daily. There have been very few reported side effects of bilberry; diarrhea is the most commonly reported complication.

**Grape seed:** The extract of this seed has been used for some time to treat a wide range of conditions, and may be useful in the management of edema. Look for a standardized extract from local health food stores. The recommended dosage is 100–300 mg, to be taken orally once or twice a day. As with other herbal recommendations in this section do not take grape seed if you are on anti-thrombotic drugs.

# FAINTING

## DIAGNOSIS

Fainting occurs when a person loses consciousness. It is a very common condition and can result from either physical or mental strain. Fainting tends to happen suddenly and unexpectedly, while standing up or when getting up too quickly and causing blood to rush to the head. It is generally not a cause for concern, as it is commonly triggered by a minor incident and only occasionally by a more serious condition. The most common cause of fainting in those under 50 years of age is vasovagal syncope, when, in response to an event, the nervous system dilates the blood vessels and a temporary slowing of the heartbeat triggers a drop in blood pressure. Most people with this condition realize they are going to faint and have time to sit down beforehand or warn people nearby. It is typically preceded by sweating, a loss of color in the face, and a dizzy feeling. Fainting can also be caused by a sudden shock, a stressful situation, excitement, pain, dehydration, or a viral illness. Certain medications, including some blood pressure medications, antidepressants, and tranquillizers, may increase the likelihood of fainting. Sometimes fainting occurs in conjunction with a seizure, where there is a loss of consciousness for a couple of minutes and the body makes jerking movements. After fainting, it rarely takes more than a few minutes to regain consciousness and you may not remember what happened. If someone has fainted, help to position him with head low and legs raised. Once he has regained consciousness, bring him very slowly to a sitting and then standing position.

## SYMPTOMS

- Turning pale
- Sweating profusely
- Feeling nauseous and lightheaded
- Loss of consciousness
- Falling down
- Sensation of weakness or wobbliness in the arms and legs

## TREATMENT GOAL

To establish what is making you faint and treat the cause accordingly. If you tend to faint easily, think about situations that trigger it. If you think you are going to faint, alert people around you.

## CONVENTIONAL MEDICINE

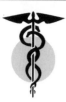

In order to treat fainting it is necessary to first identify the cause. This may be electrolyte imbalance, hypoglycemia, anemia, dehydration, vasovagal response, cardiac problems, or neurological problems. To prevent fainting from occurring it is important to keep the blood, oxygen, and nutrient (especially glucose) supply to the body at healthy levels.

**Stay hydrated:** Make sure that electrolytes are included in the fluids you drink, and drink 2–3 liters of water a day. This amount should be increased to compensate for fluid lost as a result of exercise, a dry environment, a fever, and any situation that involves sweating.

**To treat fainting caused by low blood sugar levels (hypoglycemia):** A medical examination can determine if diabetes or low blood sugar has caused the fainting and a preventive treatment plan can be given. For those with low blood sugar, small, frequent, high-protein meals are a preventive strategy. Avoiding food that is high in sugar is recommended. However, if a fainting episode occurs due to low blood sugar, the immediate treatment is to take a high sugar fluid. If anyone with diabetes faints, seek immediate medical advice.

**To threat chronic fainting:** It is necessary to undergo thorough testing to investigate the heart. Some abnormal heart rhythms can cause fainting and these must be diagnosed and treated. The blood vessels that supply the brain are also investigated, as fainting can sometimes occur when the arteries to the brain are partially blocked.

**Revival:** A person who has fainted can be revived by a strong odor such as ammonia smelling salts, or occasionally amyl nitrate. This should be administered only after trying to arouse the patient vocally, and checking that the patient has a pulse and is breathing. If either is compromised or absent, begin cardiopulmonary resuscitation.

## TRADITIONAL CHINESE MEDICINE

**Herbs:** The herbs used in the following formulas are available from Chinese pharmacies or online. For each of the formulas, place the herbs in a ceramic pot, add 3 cups of water, and bring the mixture to a boil. Simmer for 30 minutes and then drink 1 cup twice a day.

• To treat fainting due to dehydration and low blood sugar: Combine 8 g of ginseng, 12 g of Mai Men Dong (ophiopogon tuber), and 5 g of Gan Cao (licorice).

• To treat fainting due to excessive heat or sunstroke: Mix 8 g of Jin Yin Hua (honeysuckle flower), 8 g of Ye Ju Hua (wild chrysanthemum flower), 5 g if Bo He (field mint), and 5 pieces of Da Zhao (Chinese jujube).

• To treat fainting due to blood deficiency: Combine 12 g of Dan Shen (salvia root), 12 g of Bai Zhu (white atractylodes rhizome), 15 g of Shan Yao (Chinese yam), 12 g of Shu Di Huang (Chinese foxglove cooked in wine), 10 g of Shan Zhu Yu (Asiatic cornelian cherry fruit), 12 g of Dan Shen (salvia root), 12 g of Dang Gui (Chinese angelica root), 12 g of Huang Jing (Siberian Solomon seal rhizome), and 12 g of Fuling (poria).

**Acupuncture:** Treatment can be effective in treating fainting, as well as the underlying cause. Consult a well-trained acupuncturist to determine the most effective points.

**Acupressure:** Use the tip of your finger to apply heavy pressure to the Ru Zhong, Nei Guan, and Bai Hui points. The Ru Zhong point is located in the center of the nipple. The Nei Guan point is located in the center of the wrist on the palm side, about 2 inches above the crease. The Bai Hui point is on top of the head at the midpoint on the line running up and over the head from the top of one ear to the other.

**Diet:** Eat food that tonifies Qi and blood, such as black soy beans, chestnuts, peaches, saffron, sweet basil, buckwheat, mushrooms, and tangerines.

## NATUROPATHY

**Diet:** Low blood sugar sometimes leads to fainting, particularly when it is combined with low blood pressure. Make sure you eat the appropriate amount and type of calories. This is especially important if you are elderly or are prone to fainting. If your body has trouble processing sugar (as in the case with diabetics), you may need to avoid refined foods and sugar, and eat small, frequent meals that are high in protein. It is best to consult a registered dietitian to determine the right nutritional program for your specific needs.

**Supplements:** A good quality multivitamin will provide the basic nutritional support to protect various nutritional deficiencies associated with dizziness and fainting. Follow the instructions on the label. Also take 200–400 mg of chromium a day to help balance blood sugar, as fluctuating levels are a possible cause of fainting.

**Herbs:** Licorice root combined with a high-salt diet can help resolve fainting due to low blood pressure and problems with the nervous system. Take 1–2 g or 2–4 ml of tincture a day. However, you should not use licorice root if you have high blood pressure, low levels of potassium, severe kidney disease, or if you are pregnant. Hawthorn can also be helpful. Take 4–5 ml of tincture or 1 g of the freeze-dried herb a day. Use herbal therapies only under the supervision of an experienced practitioner.

## HOMEOPATHY

The remedies below can support recovery from a fainting episode that has occurred for an obvious reason, such as standing for too long, skipping meals, or receiving a severe shock. An established pattern of fainting needs to be assessed by a medical practitioner, especially related to circulatory problems. Once a diagnosis has been established, consult a homeopath, who may be able to help with the underlying disorder causing the fainting.

**Aconite:** If fainting occurs after sustaining a shock, such as witnessing an accident or being given bad news, use Aconite. When this remedy is appropriate, fainting is accompanied by a profound sense of terror and panic and a genuine fear of dying. This may occur just before or after the fainting episode, and is likely to be accompanied by lots of shaking and trembling.

**Carbo veg:** If a faint is brought on by being in very hot, badly ventilated surroundings, try this remedy. It is also appropriate for fainting episodes that result from physical strain, especially in hot weather. There is a genuine craving for fresh, cool air, and patients feel revived after opening a window or fanning themselves. Additional symptoms include a pale complexion and clammy, sweaty skin that feels cool to the touch.

## HERBALISM

There are no safe, effective herbs that can treat fainting. If fainting occurs simultaneously with dizziness, the following herbs can be used.

**Ginkgo biloba:** Gingko has a reputation for increasing blood flow, which can help protect against dizziness and fainting spells by promoting circulation. Ginkgo is available from health food stores in pill or capsule form. Try taking 60–80 mg in tablets two to three times a day. These should be standardized to the percentage of 25% ginkgolides, which are some of the important compounds in ginkgo. Ginkgo can also be taken as a tea or tincture two to three times daily. There have been few reported side effects, although there is an increased risk of bleeding, so those taking anticoagulant and anti-thrombotic drugs should be cautious when using gingko.

**Ginger:** This herb can ease symptoms of dizziness and nausea, which can lead to fainting episodes. Ginger is available as a raw rhizome or in capsule form. The dosage should not exceed 5 g per day, and not more than 1 g per day if pregnant. Ginger can also be taken as a tea or tincture, though these forms may not be as effective. In low doses there are virtually no side effects with ginger.

# FEVER AND CHILLS

## DIAGNOSIS

A fever occurs when the core body temperature rises above the normal range (an oral reading of 98.6–100°F). A fever generally accompanies infectious ailments, particularly respiratory conditions such as flu, bronchitis, and colds, and acts as the body's mechanism for fighting infection. Occasionally, a fever can develop as a result of other conditions such as gastroenteritis, heatstroke, and dehydration, and more rarely as a result of more serious conditions such as meningitis. As your core temperature rises, your extremities begin to feel cold and send out a signal to the muscles. The muscles begin to shake involuntarily, a condition known as chills. Chills in turn create body heat, which raises a fever. Your body effectively "cooks" the bacteria by generating high temperatures.

**DANGER:** If a fever is accompanied by lethargy, a rash of purple spots, or persists for more than 48 hours, call your doctor as a matter or urgency.

## SYMPTOMS

- Flushed face
- Hot forehead
- Alternating feeling of being burning hot then freezing cold
- Trembling sensation, or involuntary shaking
- General feeling of being unwell

## TREATMENT GOAL

To establish the cause of the fever and treat it accordingly. Treatment also aims to bring down the fever and alleviate any discomfort.

## CONVENTIONAL MEDICINE

The appropriate treatment of a fever is dependent on the causes, the most common of which tend to be dehydration (p. 357), infection, and hyperthyroidism (p. 567). It is important to treat the underlying problem rather than just the fever. In general, a fever of under 103°F in a child and under 102°F in an adult can usually be treated at home unless other symptoms are present. A very high fever can be a sign of a serious problem and requires professional medical help.

**NSAIDs:** To treat a fever associated with a viral infection, treatment usually involves non-steroidal anti-inflammatory drugs (NSAIDs). Ibuprofen is the primary choice for both children and adults. Adults can take up to 800 mg every six hours. Children above two years old can be given 7.5–10 mg per 2.2 lb of body weight every six hours, but no more than three times a day—this should not exceed the adult dosage. NSAIDs should not be taken by anyone with a peptic ulcer, as they may cause gastric irritation or bleeding. Acetaminophen is another treatment option, but do not take this drug if you have liver disease or if you drink alcohol regularly. Aspirin can also lower a fever, but again, the potential for gastric irritation is high in susceptible individuals. Aspirin should not be given to anyone under 16 years of age.

**Keep cool:** Drink cool beverages to relieve any symptoms of dehydration that may occur with a fever. Dehydration may be the cause of the fever, and rehydrating may resolve it. Cool baths are also effective, as are rubbing alcohol and witch hazel massages. Cooling blankets, which are available in First Aid Facilities, can be used if there is no response to the above methods. Intravenous rehydration can also be carried out.

## TRADITIONAL CHINESE MEDICINE

**Herbs:** The following decoction can be used to treat fever and chills that occur simultaneously. The herbs listed are available from Chinese pharmacies or online. Combine 10 g of Gui Zhi (cinnamon), 12 g of Bai Shao (white peony root), 8 g of Huang Qin (baical skullcap root), 10 g of Chai Hu (hare's ear root), 8 g of Jing Jie (schizonepeta stem and bud), 3 pieces of Da Zhao (Chinese jujube), 5 g of Gan Cao (licorice), and 5 g of fresh ginger root. Place the herbs in a ceramic pot and add 3 cups of water. Bring the mixture to the boil and simmer for 30 minutes. Strain the liquid and drink 1 cup two or three times a day. This decoction will help reduce the symptoms and speed up recovery.

**Acupuncture:** If fever and chills are due to an acute cold or flu in its early stages, acupuncture treatment may reduce the symptoms in just one or two sessions. Consult a practitioner.

**Diet:** Make a tea using a 1 oz of ginger chopped into small chips. Place the ginger in a bowl and add boiling water. Cover for 5–10 minutes, then add 1 oz of brown sugar, and stir well. Drink the tea while it is hot. You can also try eating a porridge made from ⅓ cup of rice and 5–6 Chinese jujubes. Place the ingredients in a pot and add 3 cups of water. Bring them to the boil and cook until the rice is soft. Add a chopped green onion. The porridge should have a creamy consistency.

## NATUROPATHY

**Diet:** Eat a diet based on broths, soups, and teas. Avoid solid foods if there is no appetite for them. Add ginger, garlic, and onions to soups and broths to boost your immunity and help the respiratory tract heal. Avoid sugar, processed foods, dairy, and junk foods, which suppress your immune system. Stay hydrated by sipping on water or tea throughout the day. This will also expel toxins and keep the respiratory tract from drying out.

**Supplements:** Take 500 mg of vitamin C several times a day to support the immune system and help healing. If your stools become loose cut back the vitamin C by taking a dose every two hours. Also take 250–500 mg of bioflavonoids a day to stimulate the immune system.

**Herbs:** Take 900 mg of echinacea a day in capsule form, or 2–4 ml of tincture four times a day, to stimulate the immune system. Taking 5–10 ml of elderberry tincture three times a day is helpful in fighting viral infections, which may be causing the fever. Yarrow induces sweat to help break a fever. Take 300 mg in capsule form, 2 ml of tincture, or 1 cup of fresh tea four times a day. Taking 500 mg or 2 ml of ginger can also help to break a fever and reduce inflammation. You can also drink ginger tea throughout the day. Oregano oil, taken at 500 mg three times a day, has antiviral effects. Garlic, at a dosage of 300–500 mg three times a day, combats infection and supports the immune system.

**Hydrotherapy:** Sit on a chair and place your feet in a bucket of warm water for 15 minutes. Dry them and put on a pair of cotton socks that have been soaked in cold water and wrung out. Cover the cotton socks with a pair of wool socks and leave on overnight. This measure diverts blood flow to the feet and away from the upper body, thus reducing fever.

**TIP:** GIVE CHILDREN A HERBAL TEA

Brew a fever-reducing herbal tea using equal parts of lemon balm leaf, chamomile flower, peppermint leaf, licorice root, and elderflower. These herbs promote perspiration, calm and relax the nervous system, and cool fever. Give a child over two years old ½ cup four times a day. A breastfeeding mother can drink 1 cup four times a day.

## HOMEOPATHY

 An appropriately selected homeopathic remedy can do a lot to help support the body in dealing with a fever. For this to be most effective, however, any acute homeopathic home prescribing needs to be done within the context of additional holistic measures that can help bring down a fever. Some of these are mentioned briefly in the next section. **Caution:** Since a very high fever can be a sign of a serious problem, consult the section on conventional medical assessment in order to establish that your situation remains within safe medical boundaries. If it should move beyond these, seek professional medical help.

**Aconite:** Use this remedy to treat a fever that develops after exposure to dry, cold winds. The patient feels fine on going to bed, but wakes from sleep feeling panicky and restless with an accompanying fever. Symptoms emerge dramatically and abruptly, and include a burning, hot head and chilled, shivery body.

**Belladonna:** This remedy is also appropriate for symptoms that develop violently and dramatically. Feeling irritable and having a short temper are key symptoms that call for Belladonna. Additional symptoms include hot, dry, bright-red skin that radiates heat.

**Arsenicum album:** To treat a fever that peaks in the early hours of the morning and causes a significant amount of anxiety and restlessness, try Arsenicum album. Despite having a fever, there is a persistent sense of feeling chilled to the bone. A sufferer feels most comfortable if the body is kept warm, and the head is exposed to fresh air.

**Pulsatilla:** Consider this remedy to treat a fever that has been triggered by exposure to cold and wet conditions. When Pulsatilla is appropriate, warm rooms make feverishness intolerable, while contact with fresh cool air feels soothing.

**TIP:** AVOID EATING

The exertion involved in digesting food can cause the body temperature to rise even further. Therefore, try to avoid eating when a high temperature is present.

Make it a priority to increase your fluid intake when you have a fever. Your thirst reflex does not always provide an accurate guide regarding the amount of liquid that your body requires, so drink a moderate amount of water even if you do not feel thirsty. Drink plain water, and avoid coffee, which has diuretic properties that encourage the body to eliminate rather than conserve fluid.

## HERBALISM

**Willow:** The bark of this tree contains salicylic acid, which is one of the original sources of aspirin. Today, willow bark extract can be used to treat pain and fever in the same way that aspirin is, although different preparations of extract produce different potencies, which makes dosing difficult. Consult a medical herbalist regarding the best source and the most effective dosage. Do not take willow if you have allergies to aspirin that trigger asthma or urticaria, or if you have nasal polyps.

**Yarrow:** This herb is used by some herbalists to treat fever and chills. It is readily available in health food stores as a dried herb or tincture. A suggested dose is 1 oz of dried herb in 1 pint of boiling water; drink a cup of this infusion three times a day. Do not use yarrow if there is a known allergy to plants in the daisy family, as there is a slight risk of an allergic reaction.

**Boneset:** This popular herb is effective in reducing fever. Like yarrow, dosage recommendations are to infuse 1 oz of dried herb in 1 pint of boiling water, and drink 1 cup three times a time. Again, do not take this herb if there is a known allergy to plants in the daisy family. There is a slight chance of nausea and vomiting.

**Meadowsweet:** This plant has components similar to aspirin and is therefore effective at reducing fever. To make meadowsweet tea, steep 5 g of the dried, above-ground parts of the herb in about 150 ml of hot water for 10 mintues. Strain, drink this amount one to three times a day. Do not take meadowsweet if there is a known sensitivity to aspirin or if you have asthma. Potential adverse effects include allergic skin and lung reactions.

# FLU

## DIAGNOSIS

The influenza virus is a highly contagious respiratory infection. It affects everyone at some time or another, and can be a debilitating illness. There are usually several outbreaks of different flu strains every winter. Once you have been infected by a particular strain of flu you become immune to it. Flu shots are designed yearly to fight the flu bug that is prevalent in a particular year, so immunization is necessary on an annual basis. Influenza is spread through sneezing and coughing, when water droplets carrying the virus become airborne and are breathed in by others. It is also passed on through the spread of germs due to poor hand-washing hygiene. Symptoms, which include fever, chills, headache, aches and pains, and exhaustion, begin after an incubation period of one to four days and usually continue for about a week.

**DANGER:** Occasionally, pneumonia can develop from a bad attack of flu. Infants, the elderly, and people with heart or lung disease are more prone to complications.

## SYMPTOMS

- An elevated temperature (above 98.6°F)
- Fever and chills
- Sweating
- A flushed face
- Headache
- Loss of appetite
- Muscular aches and pains
- Weakness
- Feeling lethargic and tired
- Sore throat
- Cough
- Feeling under the weather and rundown

## TREATMENT GOAL

It is usually possible to treat flu at home. Stay in bed and get as much rest as possible. A bad attack of flu can last for up to two weeks. It is not unusual to feel extreme fatigue for a couple of weeks afterwards. Both conventional and complementary therapies aim to relieve symptoms and encourage recovery as quickly as possible.

## CONVENTIONAL MEDICINE

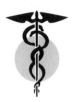

**Flu shot:** It is possible to protect against infection by getting the flu vaccine. However, the vaccine does not protect against every strain of flu. It is recommended for the elderly, debilitated, immune compromised (people who have illnesses that affect their immune systems), asthmatics, and chemotherapy patients. Good hand washing is probably the best preventive measure against spreading flu germs.

**Herbs:** Some herbs with natural viral suppression properties can be taken during the flu season. One that has had some success is larch (found in a Thorne product called Larix®). Elderberry extract can be used in the same way. These herbs can also be used at the onset of flu symptoms.

**Tamiflu®:** Upon exposure to flu, high-risk patients (the elderly, debilitated, immune compromised, asthmatics, and chemotherapy patients) are encouraged to take the drug Tamiflu® within the first 72 hours. It can sometimes lessen the severity and duration of symptoms if taken on the day of exposure.

**Rest and fluids:** Treating an active case of flu involves taking rest, plenty of fluids, and non-steroidal anti-inflammatory drugs for aches and pains are advisable.

**When should I see a doctor?** Complications include dehydration and electrolyte imbalance, pneumonia, and problems related to immobility. If a patient is unable to take oral fluids, is disoriented, has a fever of over 102°F (or 103°F in a child), and does not respond to conventional treatment, seek medical attention.

## TRADITIONAL CHINESE MEDICINE

**Herbs:** The herbs recommended in the following formula are available from Chinese pharmacies or online. Combine 10 g of Jin Yin Hua (honeysuckle flower), 12 g of Lian Qiao (forsythia fruit), 12 g of Ban Lan Gen (isatis root), 10 g of Da Qin Ye (woad leaf), and 3 g of Gan Cao (licorice) in a ceramic or glass pot. Add 3 cups of water, bring the mixture to a boil, and simmer for 30 minutes. Strain the liquid and drink 1 cup two to three times a day for three to five days.

**Acupuncture:** Treatment may help shorten the cause of flu, and may reduce its symptoms.

**Acupressure:** The Feng Chi points are at the back of the head at the base of the skull, about 2 inches on either side of the center point. The Hegu point is located on the back of the hand in the depression between the thumb and the first finger. Press with median pressure for one to two minutes. Repeat five times twice a day.

**Diet:** Eat light food with seasoning such as ginger, garlic, onions, olives, and Daikon radishes. These foods are good for helping recovery.

## NATUROPATHY

**Diet:** Eat light foods such as soups, steamed vegetables, and broths. Add ginger, garlic, and onions to your soup for their antimicrobial and anti-inflammatory effects. If you do not have an appetite, do not eat, but make sure you stay hydrated with water and herbal teas. Try to eat some berries and citrus fruit. These contain bioflavonoids and vitamin C, which help stimulate the immune system. Eliminate foods that weaken your immune system and cause mucus, including refined sugar, dairy products, and any foods to which you are allergic. Caffeine depletes zinc, an important mineral for healing, so avoid black tea, coffee, and chocolate.

**Supplements:** Vitamin C increases white blood cell activity and supports immune function. Vitamin A with beta-carotene has powerful immune-boosting and antioxidant effects. Take 15,000 IU of each vitamin a day. Zinc gluconate lozenges act as immune stimulants. Dissolve 1 lozenge in a glass of water and drink every two hours.

**Herbs:** Elderberry prevents the influenza virus from replicating. Adults should take 1 tbsp four times a day and children should take 1 tbsp twice a day. Lomatium dissectum has strong antiviral activity and is traditionally used by herbalists for flu. Take 500 mg in capsule form or 4 ml four times a day. A combination of echinacea and goldenseal can be taken at 500 mg or 2 ml to enhance immune function and dry up mucus. Take 500 mg of oregano oil four times daily or 300–450 mg of garlic twice a day for their powerful antiviral effects. Andrographis, taken at 400 mg three times a day, can used to prevent flu.

## HOMEOPATHY

Any of the following homeopathic remedies can support the body through a bout of flu, reducing distress and discomfort, and shortening the duration of symptoms. A well-chosen homeopathic remedy may also reduce the possibility of complications setting in, such as congestion in the sinuses.

**Gelsemium:** This remedy can ease classic flu symptoms that develop slowly over two or three days. Symptoms include an overwhelming sense of listlessness, droopiness, and heaviness, accompanied by aching muscles, and shivering. The eyes have a droopy, glassy look, the face is likely to be flushed, and lips may be cracked and dry. Sufferers tend to want to be left alone in peace and quiet to rest.

**Eupatorium perfoliatum:** Use this remedy to treat severe flu symptoms that manifest as aching deep in the bones and a bruised, tender sensation in the muscles. Symptoms include feeling chilly, weak, and restless, with aching in the arms, legs, back, and torso. This remedy can also help treat nausea and lethargy.

**Baptisia:** If a profound sense of exhaustion is combined with a maddening restlessness, try Baptisia. The muscles generally feel very sore and heavy. The throat is also sore and it is very difficult to swallow solids due to pain and inflammation.

**Mercurius:** To ease the later stages of a bout of flu when the initial feverish stage has passed, use Mercurius.

## HERBALISM

**Elderberry:** The fruit of this plant can be used to treat flu. Specific formulations of elderberry juice can be bought at your local health food store—raw elderberry juice can be quite toxic and is not recommended. Although cooking the berry destroys most of these toxins, it is still not considered safe. The recommended preparation of elderberry juice is the specific, store-bought formulations, which eliminate the problem with toxicity. Take the formulated juice orally at the onset of symptoms for three to five days. Diarrhea and vomiting have been reported with use of elderberry juice, although this side effect is greatly decreased with specific formulations.

**Astragalus:** This herb is well known for its immune-stimulating effects. Astragalus root can be used as a tea, or taken in capsule form at 500 mg three times a day. It should not be taken if you are on blood-thinning drugs, immunosuppressive drugs, or have an autoimmune disorder, such as lupus or rheumatoid arthritis.

**Echinacea:** This is another popular and effective immune booster. It has recently been demonstrated that Echinacea may work better if taken as soon as the symptoms of colds and flu develop. There are three main species of Echinacea, but it appears that extracts made from the fresh pressed juice of the above-ground parts of *Echinacea purpurea* are the most effective, but only for adults; most research on the use of echinacea in children has failed to find a benefit.

# HIGH BLOOD PRESSURE

## DIAGNOSIS

High blood pressure (hypertension) is a common condition that tends to run in families and affects around one in six people. There is no cure for high blood pressure and the cause is unknown, although certain lifestyle factors are thought to contribute to the condition.

The heart circulates 5 liters of blood around the body every minute, which carries oxygen and nutrients to the body's major organs, such as the heart, kidneys, liver, and brain. The smaller blood vessels, through which blood passes, produce a resistance to the flow of blood. The heart pumps against this resistance to create the necessary pressure that allows blood to circulate. When the heart contracts, the highest pressure it produces is called the systolic pressure; when it relaxes, the lowest pressure it produces is called the diastolic pressure. Both are important in determining the risk of heart attack and stroke. A normal blood pressure reading might be around 130/80 (often described as 130 over 80)—this is shorthand for a systolic pressure of 130 and a diastolic pressure of 80. Generally blood pressure is thought to be high when it is above 140/90. A permanently raised blood pressure may result in heart attack, stroke, or kidney failure.

## SYMPTOMS

- Most people with high blood pressure do not have symptoms and are unaware that they have the condition
- Those with severe high blood pressure or a rapid rise in pressure may experience headaches or blurred or impaired vision

## TREATMENT GOAL

There is no cure for high blood pressure but treatment exists to lower the pressure and manage the condition. Conventional and complementary therapies aim to find the treatment, or combination of treatments, that suits an individual without causing side effects. Lifestyle factors should also be examined and changes introduced where necessary.

## CONVENTIONAL MEDICINE

**Modify your lifestyle:** Give up smoking and reduce the amount of alcohol you consume a day; men should drink no more that 30 ml a day and women no more than 15 ml. Follow a daily regime of about 20 minutes of moderate aerobic activity, such as a brisk walk. If other cardiac conditions are present, do not begin a vigorous exercise program without first having a medical assessment. Weight loss can also help to lower blood pressure. Cut out fatty foods, reduce the amount of salt you eat, and follow a Mediterranean diet of whole grains, white meat, fruit, vegetables, nuts, and olive oil. Supplements such as fish oil, arginine, hawthorn, and magnesium can be beneficial, and stress reduction is also important.

**Medication:** If an ideal blood pressure reading is not achieved by lifestyle modifications, · or if readings are extremely high, then medication is prescribed. A mild diuretic such as hydrochlorothiazide or a beta blocker such as atenolol is usually the first choice. Sometimes a class of drugs known as "ACE inhibitors" are used, such as enalapril. The third common group is calcium channel blockers, such as diltiazem. The choice of drug really depends on co-existing illnesses and symptoms. Blood pressure medications do have side effects and should be carefully used with close monitoring of blood pressure at the same time each day.

**Severe cases:** Extremely high blood pressure (over 160 systolic and 100 diastolic) should be treated immediately. Symptoms such as headache, impaired vision, and any changes in sensation, cognition, or muscle tone should be immediately evaluated. Pregnant women with high blood pressure should also be treated immediately.

## TRADITIONAL CHINESE MEDICINE

**Herbs:** The herbs listed below are available from Chinese pharmacies or online. For either formula, combine the herbs with 3 cups of water in a ceramic pot. Bring the mixture to the boil and simmer for 30 minutes. Strain the liquid and drink 1 cup twice a day.

• To treat hypertension accompanied by dizziness, or occasional palpitations: Mix 10 g of Tian Ma (gastrodia rhizome), 12 g of Gou Teng (stem and thorns of gambir vine), 12 g of Chuan Niu Xi (Szechuan ox knee), 10 g of Du Zhong (eucommia bark), 12 g of Chuan Xiong (Szechuan lovage root), 12 g of Bai Shao (white peony root), 30 g of Long Gu (fossilized bone), and 30 g of Mu Li (oyster shell).

• To treat hypertension accompanied by the sensation of being overheated, sweating or night sweats, and lower back ache: Combine 12 g of Shu Di Huang (Chinese foxglove cooked in wine), 12 g of Shan Zhu Yu (Asiatic cornelian cherry), 15 g of Shan Yao

(Chinese yam), 15 g of Fuling (poria), 12 g of Dan Pi (cortex of tree peony root), 12 g of Ze Xie (water plantain rhizome), 12 g of Zhi Mu (anemarrhena rhizome), 10 g of Huang Bai (phellodendron), 12 g of Guo Ji Zi (wolfberry), and 10 g of Ye Ju Hua (wild chrysanthemum flower).

• To treat hypertension accompanied by insomnia, stress, and a light headache: Combine 12 g of Dang Gui (Chinese angelica root), 12 g of Bai Shao (white peony root), 12 g of Chuan Xiong (Szechuan lovage root), 12 g of Mu Gua (Chinese quince fruit), 12 g of Shuan Zhao Ren, and 12 g of Mai Men Dong (ophiopogon tuber).

**Acupuncture:** In the early stages of hypertension, a combination of acupuncture treatment and herbal remedies can have good results. For long-term high blood pressure, acupuncture may be used to complement Western medicine treatment. Acupuncture may also be helpful in reducing headache, dizziness, improving the quality of sleep, and reducing stress. Regular treatments once a week for a few months or longer may be recommended by a practitioner.

**Acupressure:** Use your fingertip to apply medium pressure to the Tai Yang point, situated in the depression at the temple, one finger behind the lateral end of the eyebrow and eyelid. The Tai Chong point is located on the sole of the foot in the depression between the first and second toe at the base of the large toe. Press this point for one minute while in a sitting position and repeat two to three times during the day. The Susanli point is found on the lower leg 1 inch to the outside of and 3 inches below the kneecap. Use your fingertip to press this point for one minute while in a sitting position and repeat.

**Diet:** Celery is recommended, and cooked celery with vinegar helps to reduce blood pressure. Other foods to try are peaches, dates, grapefruit, sunflower seeds, Daikon radishes, tomatoes, hawthorn, and corn.

## NATUROPATHY

**Diet:** A whole food diet is key to lowering blood pressure. Your meals should be based on fresh vegetables, beans, nuts, and whole grains. High sodium and low potassium are common in people with hypertension. Eat foods that are high in potassium such as apples, bananas, asparagus, cabbage, tomatoes, kelp, and alfalfa, and restrict your salt intake by cutting out table salt, smoked meats, cheeses, and packaged foods. Add onions, garlic, and parsley to your food; they have been shown to bring down blood pressure. Celery, which can be blended with cucumber to make a juice, has also been shown to lower blood pressure. Avoid saturated fats, hydrogenated, and partially hydrogenated fats, which are found in margarine and refined vegetables oils, as they cause high blood pressure and place a burden on your heart. Dehydration can also contribute to hypertension, so make sure you drink at least eight glasses of water a day. Reduce the amount of caffeine you consume by cutting down on coffee, carbonated beverages, chocolate, and caffeinated tea, as they can contribute to high blood pressure.

**Supplements:** Try to obtain potassium from food, but if you are unable to, take 2,000 mg of a potassium supplement a day under the supervision of a doctor. Also take a combination of calcium (500 mg) and magnesium (250 mg) twice a day, which is commonly prescribed by naturopathic practitioners and other complementary therapists. Take 60–100 mg of coenzyme Q10 twice a day, as it has been shown to lower blood pressure and be supportive for overall heart function. Fish oil also helps lower blood pressure. Take 3–4 g a day, but be aware that you may have to take it for three months before you see any benefits. Taurine, taken at 6 g a day on an empty stomach, is an amino acid that has been shown in research to lower blood pressure.

**Herbs:** Take 250 mg of hawthorn a day; this herb dilates artery walls, decreases blood pressure, and serves as a heart tonic. Garlic has also been shown to lower blood pressure. Take 600 mg of an aged garlic extract twice a day. Passionflower, which can be taken at 250 mg in capsule form or 1 ml in tincture form, helps to decrease blood pressure associated with stress. Dandelion leaf, when taken at 300 mg or 2 ml three times a day, acts as a gentle, natural diuretic to lower blood pressure.

## HOMEOPATHY

Due to its chronic nature, high blood pressure is best treated by a combination of complementary and conventional therapies. If mild symptoms have recently developed, consult a homeopathic practitioner as a first resort to bring blood pressure down to a desirable level. In addition to advising on an appropriate homeopathic remedy, practitioners can assess the condition and provide guidance on making lifestyle changes that can help you manage high blood pressure. Some possible suggestions are listed below.

**Stop smoking:** If heart health and the circulatory system are compromised, give up smoking. If the prospect of giving up seems difficult, consider using complementary therapies, such as homeopathy, acupuncture, herbalism, or hypnotherapy, to support your efforts.

**Manage your stress:** If you know high stress levels are contributing to high blood pressure readings, make a point of taking some time each day to relax. This does not mean slumping in front of the TV, but instead use some tried and tested formal relaxation techniques. Choose from meditation, progressive muscular relaxation, visualization techniques, or a system of movement such as T'ai chi. Alternatively, you may benefit from attending a yoga class that will teach you how to breathe in order to feel relaxed and calm.

**Diet:** Avoid foods that have a reputation for raising blood pressure. These include caffeinated drinks (carbonated drinks as well as tea and coffee), saturated fats such as butter, cheese, cream, and red meat, salty snacks, and convenience "ready meals" and take-out dishes (particularly Chinese food).

## HERBALISM

High cholesterol and high blood pressure often go hand in hand, and many foods that affect one also affect the other. As well as the remedies below, please refer to Cholesterol (p. 513) for suggestions that may help in reducing blood pressure in addition to lowering cholesterol.

**Gotu kola:** To treat high blood pressure try drinking a tea made from 0.5–1 g of dried gotu kola three times a day. You can also take 30–60 mg of extract three times a day, or 300–500 mg in capsule form once or twice a day. Gotu kola is a fairly safe herb with minimal side effects, although there are a few reports of nausea or cramping. Gotu kola can cause drowsiness; therefore, refrain from using this herb if you are currently taking drugs that also promote drowsiness, such as sleeping aids or cold medications.

**Flaxseed oil:** This herb has been shown to be effective in reducing high blood pressure, probably due to the effects of the omega-3 fatty acids it contains. Although not as potent a source of omega-3s as cold-water fish (such as salmon or sardines), it is one of a few plants that contain this highly beneficial oil (walnuts are another option). Flaxseed oil is susceptible to oxidation and can become rancid when exposed to air for a long period of time; it should be refrigerated and used soon after opening. Your best option is to buy fresh flaxseed and store it in the refrigerator. Because the seeds are very durable, and will pass directly through the digestive system, it is best to crush them before use. Use a mortar and pestle or coffee grinder to quickly crush the seeds. Sprinkle them on salads or cereals, or add them to a glass of water.

**Garlic:** Studies show that garlic can lower your blood pressure about five to eight points on average. It can be easily added to salads, soups, sandwiches, and marinades. Cooking garlic at a high temperature destroys some of its medicinal qualities so try to eat it raw whenever possible. Two cloves daily should be sufficient. Garlic is also widely available in pill or capsule form, which do not have the potent odor that raw cloves do. Take 500 mg twice a day. When taken internally at high, therapeutic doses, garlic may interfere with certain anti-thrombotic drugs.

# HYPOGLYCEMIA

## DIAGNOSIS

Hypoglycemia is characterized by lower than normal blood glucose (sugar) levels and often affects diabetics. Glucose levels are measured in units of milligrams per deciliter of blood (mg/dL), and hypoglycemia occurs when levels drop below 70 ml/dL. This causes a "hypo," the name often given to episodes of low blood sugar that trigger a number of symptoms such as dizziness, sweating, and fatigue. Symptoms usually pass 10–15 minutes after eating sugar. Insulin, which is produced in the pancreas, helps the body's cells absorb glucose from the blood. After a meal the glucose level rises to about 140 mg/dL. One to two hours later, glucose levels begin to drop and return to normal: about 70–110 mg/dL. Hypoglycemic episodes can occur in diabetics when the dose of insulin or diabetes tablets taken is too high, or too much is taken by accident. It is also caused by eating less than usual, exercising more than usual, or drinking too much alcohol. If you are prone to hypoglycemic episodes, eat little and often to help maintain blood glucose levels and measure blood glucose levels regularly to avoid severe symptoms.

## SYMPTOMS

- Pale skin
- Shaking and sweating
- A feeling of weakness and fatigue
- Racing heart
- Hunger
- Difficulty concentrating
- Irritability
- Blurred vision

### IN EXTREME CASES

- A temporary loss of consciousness
- Convulsions
- Confusion
- Coma

## TREATMENT GOAL

Normally, hypoglycemia is easily treatable. Conventional and alternative therapies aim to protect against episodes by introducing lifestyle changes that will keep sugar levels stable. However, in serious cases, emergency medical attention may be needed.

## CONVENTIONAL MEDICINE

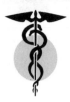

**Modify your lifestyle:** Low blood sugar that occurs in an otherwise healthy person is treated by lifestyle modification. It is important to develop the right balance between what is eaten and when it is eaten relative to activity. Eat high-protein meals and snacks regularly and include low glycemic index (GI), high-fiber carbohydrates in your diet. An item of food's glycemic index is determined by how much it causes the blood sugar to rise relative to a slice of white bread. Low glycemic index foods are those that release sugar into the bloodstream at a slow rate. These foods tend to be high-fiber, whole grain, non-processed foods. Avoid simple sugars, simple carbohydrates, and large, infrequent meals. A simple sugar, such as sweets, causes an immediate elevation but then a big drop in blood sugar.

**Supplements:** There are certain minerals, such as chromium and vanadium, that are important for regulating blood sugar. These can be added to the diet in the form of a multivitamin or separately.

**Exercise:** Exercise within an hour of eating a meal or a snack—the snack should not be high in sugar. Exercising at consistent times relative to meals is helpful, as is stress reduction. Meditation and breathing techniques are good daily practices to adopt.

**Administer glucose:** If someone with diabetes develops hypoglycemia due to excess insulin or other medication, give them glucose immediately. Give the patient fruit juice or, if available, an injection of glucagon, which has a major role in maintaining normal concentrations of glucose in the blood.

## TRADITIONAL CHINESE MEDICINE

**Herbs:** The herbs called for in the following formulas are available from Chinese pharmacies or online. For each formula, place the herbs in a ceramic pot and add 3 cups of water. Bring the mixture to the boil and simmer for 30 minutes. Strain the liquid and drink 1 cup twice a day.

• Formula 1: Mix 12 g of Huang Qi (milk-vetch root), 12 g of Dan Shen (salvia root), 12 g of Bai Zhu (white atractylodes rhizome), 15 g of Shan Yao (Chinese yam), 15 g of Huang Jing (Siberian Solomon seal rhizome), 6 g of Chen Pi (tangerine peel), 3 g of Gan Cao (licorice), and 5 pieces of Da Zhao (Chinese jujube).

• Formula 2: Combine 15 g of Shu Di Huang (Chinese foxglove cooked in wine), 12 g of Sang Shen Zi (mulberry fruit-spike), 12 g of Sang Ji Shen (mulberry mistletoe stem), 15 g of Dan Shen (salvia root), 12 g of Tu Si Zi (Chinese dodder seed), 12 g of Bai Zhu (white atractylodes rhizome), 15 g of Fuling (poria), and 5 g of Gan Cao (licorice).

**Acupuncture:** Treatment can be helpful when combined with Chinese herbal medicine. Acupuncture will boost energy circulation. A weekly session for a few months is a common treatment plan.

**Acupressure:** In a sitting position, use your fingertips to apply pressure to the Susanli point for one minute. The Susanli point is found on the lower leg, 1 inch to the outside and 3 inches below the kneecap.

> **TIP:** EXERCISE
> Regular exercise can help maintain optimal blood sugar levels. Find an activity you like, such as brisk walking, yoga, or tennis, and exercise four times a week.

## NATUROPATHY

**Diet:** Eat smaller meals, but eat frequently with a snack in between meal times. Reduce your intake of simple, processed carbohydrates such as bread, cereals, potatoes, and rice, as the digestive system converts most processed carbohydrates into sugar. Cut out the obvious trigger foods: sugar, honey, cakes, sweets, cookies, ice cream, carbonated drinks, canned fruit, frozen desserts, and any other sweetened foods. Start to read labels carefully. Common sugar additives in food include corn syrup, glucose, molasses, sucrose, lactose, maple syrup, fructose, maltose, and sorghum, all of which should be avoided. Ingredients on labels are listed in descending order of amounts used; a product that counts sugar as its first, second, or third ingredient should be avoided. Just as bad are products that list three different types of sugar. Although they may be near the bottom of the list, indicating a low amount, when the amounts of the different types are added up, you may find that sugar is in fact the main ingredient. Many brands of soup, pasta sauce, ketchup, mayonnaise, and peanut butter also contain sugar. Choose products that do not have sugar as an ingredient. Adding a small amount of protein or fat along with each carbohydrate serving helps most hypoglycemic diets, as it slows the rate of food passing through the stomach, causing blood sugar to increase less rapidly. Olive oil also has the ability to slow digestion in the stomach. Add 1–3 tsp of olive oil to each meal, either spreading it on the food, or eating it directly from the teaspoon. Reduce or eliminate your intake of caffeine and alcohol.

**Supplements:** A high-quality multivitamin will supply your body with many of the nutrients involved with blood sugar metabolism. Follow the instructions on the label. Also take 200 mcg of chromium a day to improve glucose tolerance and balance blood-sugar levels. Fish oils (omega-3s), taken at 3–4 g a day, are useful for proper insulin function and support nerve health. Magnesium is also involved in the production and utilization of insulin. Take 500 mg a day, but reduce the dosage if diarrhea occurs.

## HOMEOPATHY

A chronic, mild condition of this kind, which manifests as low or fluctuating changes in blood sugar levels, is best treated by an experienced homeopathic practitioner. However the practical advice given below may also be helpful in stabilizing the condition.

**Eat frequently:** Do not go for long periods without eating. Skipping meals can bring on hypoglycemic episodes.

**Snack on carbohydrates:** Opt for unrefined carbohydrates, such as organic brown rice cakes with vegetarian pate, hummus, or cottage cheese when snacking, as these release sugar slowly. Additional appropriate snacks include raw vegetables or a small piece of fruit.

**Avoid common triggers:** Some foods have a reputation for giving a short-lived sugar "rush" followed by a sharp slump in energy levels. The most common culprits are refined, white sugar, milk or white chocolate, sweet pastries, sugary carbonated drinks, and coffee. All of these lead to roller-coasting blood sugar levels, and a craving for more sugar once the initial boost has subsided.

## HERBALISM

The following herbs may be helpful in correcting and preventing hypoglycemic episodes.

**Siberian ginseng:** This herb works to bring the body into balance, augmenting some bodily functions while diminishing others. Siberian ginseng may be helpful in providing adrenal support, acting as a tonic to help adjust the hormones produced by the adrenal gland, which helps regulate blood sugar. Siberian ginseng can be used in tincture form, at a dosage of 20 drops two to three times a day, or as a dried extract, at a dosage of 100–200 mg three times a day. Many experts advise against taking Siberian ginseng for more than three consecutive weeks. Side effects are rare and mild, but include drowsiness and paradoxical hypoglycemia. Discontinue use if you notice that hypoglycemia is worsening.

**Licorice root:** Licorice, alone or in combination with Siberian ginseng, may help to strengthen the adrenals. Take 20 drops of tincture two to three times a day, but do not if you have heart disease, high blood pressure, or liver or kidney problems.

# NUMBNESS AND TINGLING

## DIAGNOSIS

Numbness is a loss of sensitivity in the skin, while tingling is a pricking sensation under the surface of the skin often described as "pins and needles." Symptoms of numbness and tingling can be linked with many medical conditions. They commonly occur when sitting in the same position for a long period of time, which causes your leg, arm, or foot, etc., to go numb or "fall asleep." This results from putting too much pressure on a nerve and is easily remedied by shifting your weight, stretching, and changing position regularly. Numbness and tingling can be a symptom of carpal tunnel syndrome (associated with repetitive actions, p. 617), and shingles (if the tingling is in one area of your body and you also have a rash that resembles blisters, p. 956). Sometimes it can indicate a more serious problem, such as stroke (if accompanied by confusion and slurred speech) or spinal cord injuries (if it comes after an accident or injury to the head, neck, or back). If the numbness or tingling is in the feet, it can also be linked with diabetes (p. 361), spinal problems, or other neuropathy.

## SYMPTOMS

- Loss of feeling in the skin
- Affected limb may feel heavy
- Pricking sensation under the skin

## TREATMENT GOAL

To establish the cause of the numbness and tingling and determine whether it is linked to a serious condition. Preventive measures can be introduced if symptoms occur regularly.

## CONVENTIONAL MEDICINE

This condition, usually associated with nerve inflammation, is a symptom of an underlying disease rather than a problem in itself. Conventional medical treatment therefore depends on establishing the cause.

**Reduce inflammation:** Most commonly, numbness and tingling follows a pattern along the body, which can be used to identify the nerve causing the symptoms. Treatment involves reducing the inflammation and compression at the site of the nerve. This can be achieved through physical therapy, non-steroidal anti-inflammatory drugs (NSAIDs), ice, splinting, or surgery.

**Keep moving:** If numbness and tingling occurs as a result of a body part "falling asleep," readjust your body. Exercise, regular movement even when sitting, and wearing loose clothing can guard against this type of numbness and tingling.

**Supplements:** Nutritional deficiencies, particularly of the B vitamins, can sometimes cause numbness and tingling. For example, deficiency of B12 and folate can cause tingling and numbness in the extremities. An overdose of vitamin B6 on a chronic basis can have the same effect. Have the levels of these vitamins in the blood checked and corrected as needed.

**To treat numbness and tingling caused by diabetes:** This complaint can be a complication of diabetes, known as diabetic neuropathy. Treatment predominantly involves prevention by making sure blood sugar levels are within the normal range. Consult a doctor regarding an appropriate therapeutic plan.

## TRADITIONAL CHINESE MEDICINE

**Herbs:** If the symptoms of tingling and numbness are due to poor circulation the following decoction can help. Mix 10 g of Shan Qi Shen (ginseng root), 12 g of Niu Xi (achyranthes root), 12 g of Chuan Xiong (Szechuan lovage root), 12 g of Sang Ji Sheng (mulberry mistletoe stem), 12 g of Dang Gui (Chinese angelica root), and 10 g of Mu Xiang (costus root). Place the herbs in a ceramic pot, add 3 cups of water and bring to the boil. Simmer for 30 minutes, strain the liquid, and drink 1 cup twice a day. These raw herbs are available from Chinese pharmacies or online.

**Acupuncture:** According to traditional Chinese medicine, numbness and tingling are usually caused by blood and Qi (energy) stagnation. Acupuncture is helpful in reducing numbness and tingling by promoting circulation, and releasing the stagnant Qi and blood. It is common to treat this condition once a week, with 10–12 sessions making up one course of treatment. Two to three courses may be recommended.

**Acupressure:** Press the Di Ji points to relieve numbness and tingling in the lower extremities, and the Qu Chi points to treat the upper extremities. With the knee flexed, the Di Ji point is on the inside of lower leg, about 3 inches below the knee and between the fibula and tibia. Apply pressure for one minute once a day while in a sitting position. With the elbow flexed, the Qu Chi point is on the outside of the elbow at the lateral end of the crease. Use the tip of your finger to apply pressure for one to two minutes once a day.

**Diet:** Eat food that is good for blood and Qi circulation, such as tangerines, buckwheat, black soy beans, brown sugar, chestnuts, peaches, saffron, onions, and sweet basil. To treat numbness of skin, fingers, and muscles, boil 3 g of cinnamon sticks in water over low heat, and drink the liquid before bedtime. You can use this tea once or twice a week.

## NATUROPATHY

When watching television, take a few moments during the commercials to uncross your legs, curl your toes, stretch your arms over your head, twirl your wrists, and slowly bend and unbend your fingers. This routine can prevent compressed nerves and lower the risk of numbness and tingling. If you have numbness in a leg, make sure that you do not carry any bulky items, such as a wallet, in your back pockets. Every time you sit down, the lump in the back pocket puts pressure on the sciatic nerve that runs along the buttocks and down the back of the leg. Find another way to carry your cash and credit cards, or move your wallet to your front pocket.

**Supplements:** A variety of vitamin and mineral deficiencies can cause nerve damage. Take a good quality multivitamin/multimineral, following the instructions on the label. Folic acid is helpful for overall nerve function and can be taken at 200–400 mcg a day. Also take 50 mg of zinc two to three times a day to nourish and strengthen the nervous system.

**Herbs:** Ginkgo biloba improves circulation to the whole body. Take 240 mg of the extract (standardized to contain 6% terpene lactones and 24% flavone glycosides) per day, generally divided into two or three doses.

### TIP: STOP SMOKING
Smoking reduces the blood flow to your extremities and increases the likelihood of numbness and tingling in your arms, hands, legs, and feet.

## HOMEOPATHY

Very mild, infrequent symptoms may respond to one of the following remedies. Treatment can help speed up the recovery from an acute episode, but, as always, more established and/or severe problems are best treated by a homeopathic practitioner. Also see Raynaud's disease (p. 582) and carpal tunnel syndrome (p. 619).

**Pulsatilla:** Consider using this remedy if circulation to the fingers and toes is poor. Warmth and resting makes symptoms feel worse, while gentle exercise helps. When this remedy is well indicated, varicose veins tend to become inflamed and painful.

**Arsenicum album:** This is a possible remedy for treating burning, tingling, and itching sensations. Applying heat to the affected area may help to ease any discomfort.

## HERBALISM

**Cayenne:** This herb has been scientifically proven to be effective in treating pain, tingling, and numbness associated with neuralgia and other nerve pains. Cayenne, often referred to as capsicum, contains a compound called capsaicin that is believed to be responsible for its therapeutic effects. Capsicum is now readily available at local health food stores in cream or ointment form. Most preparations contain 0.025–0.075% capsaicin that can be applied to the affected area three to four times daily. Capsicum causes very few side effects, the most prevalent being slight burning and itching around the area on which it is applied. This treatment may make symptoms worse for one to three days until improvement occurs.

**Horse chestnut:** This popular and effective herb is used to treat a host of circulatory problems, including numbness and tingling. Look for a standardized extract of horse chestnut seed. The suggested dosage of horse chestnut seed extract is 200–300 mg one to three times a day. Do not exceed 600 mg in one day. The long-term use of horse chestnut may increase the chances of toxicity to the liver and kidneys. Those who have liver or kidney problems, are pregnant, or have diabetes are advised not to use horse chestnut. It may also interact with certain antithrombotic drugs.

**Ginkgo:** Most of ginkgo's beneficial effects are derived from the herb's purported ability to increase blood flow. Numbness and tingling are two primary manifestations of a decrease in blood flow, so ginkgo could be useful if this occurs. Ginkgo is readily available at local health food stores in pill or capsule form.

# OVERACTIVE THYROID

## DIAGNOSIS

The thyroid gland is located in the neck. It produces thyroid hormones, primarily thyroxine (T4) and triiodothyronine (T3), which regulate the rate of metabolism and are essential to the function of many systems in the body. An overactive thyroid (or hyperthyroidism) is a condition involving the increased activity of the thyroid gland, whereby it produces more of the thyroid hormones than it should. This leads to an increase in the body's metabolic rate, which in turn causes the body's other functions to speed up. The thyroid gland can also become enlarged, which results in the formation of a goiter, where the base of the neck becomes swollen.

The causes of hyperthyroidism are uncertain; however, it is thought that hereditary and environmental factors can contribute to the condition. If your doctor suspects an increase in your metabolic rate, he or she will examine the throat for an enlarged thyroid gland and carry out thyroid function tests.

## SYMPTOMS

- Nervousness, restlessness, and anxiety
- Trembling, shaking hands
- Rapid and pounding heartbeat
- Irritability due to the overstimulation of the nervous system
- Hot, sweaty hands and skin
- Weight loss despite increased appetite
- Severe general tiredness
- Insomnia
- Muscle pains and muscle tiredness
- Frequent bowel movements
- In women, irregular and light periods

## TREATMENT GOAL

To establish the presence of thyroid disease and take appropriate action.

## CONVENTIONAL MEDICINE

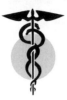

Treatment options for an overactive thyroid vary. Anti-thyroid medications are available, or surgery may be performed to remove all or part of the thyroid. If hyperthyroidism is associated with Grave's disease and bulging eyes, consult an ophthalmologist. As a general rule, eye protection should be worn at all times.

**Modify your lifestyle:** Avoid foods that contain iodine such as kelp, seaweed, spinach, and certain root vegetables. Since this condition increases your metabolism, it is important to also increase your calorie consumption and fluid intake, and avoid extreme physical exertion, particularly when symptoms are present.

**Medication:** Occasionally, Grave's disease (a certain type of hyperthyroidism) heals itself over a period of about six months to two years. Medication can be used to control the disease during this period and is then stopped when the condition resolves. The most common type of medication used is propylthiouracil, which inhibits the synthesis of thyroid in the gland and stops its conversion to an active form that increases metabolism. Another common medication is methimazole. Sometimes beta-blocker drugs are given to slow the heartbeat. This is symptomatic treatment only and does not help the thyroid disease itself.

**Remove the thyroid:** The most popular therapy to treat an overactive thyroid in the US is radioactive iodine ($I^{131}$), which destroys the thyroid. Surgical removal of the thyroid (known as a thyroidectomy) may also be performed. In cases of what is called toxic nodular goiter, where small nodules in the gland produce too many thyroid hormones, removal is the only option.

## TRADITIONAL CHINESE MEDICINE

**Herbs:** The herbs listed in the formulas below are available from Chinese herbalists or online. For either formula, make a decoction by placing the herbs in a ceramic pot, adding 3 cups of water, and bringing the mixture to a boil. Simmer for 30 minutes then strain the liquid. Drink 1 cup twice a day.

• To treat symptoms of constipation, feeling overheated, and sweating profusely: Combine 12 g of Zhi Mu (anemarrhena rhizome), 15 g of Shen Di Huang (Chinese foxglove root), 15 g of Xuan Shen (ningpo figwort root), 12 g of Xia Ku Cao (common selfheal fruit-spike), 12 g of Dan Pi (cortex of tree peony), 12 g of Mai Men Dong (ophiopogon tuber), 10 g of Chai Hu (hare's ear root), and 10 g of Huang Bai (phellodendron).

• To treat symptoms of irritability, phlegm in the chest, and fatigue: Mix 12 g of Chai Hu (hare's ear root), 12 gBai Shao (white atractylodes rhizome), 10 g of Huang Qin (baical skullcap root), 12 g of Tai Zi Shen (pseudostellaria), 15 g of Shan Yao (Chinese yam), 15 g of Fuling (poria), 15 g of Bai Zhu (white atractylodes rhizome), 3 g of Gan Cao (licorice), and 12 g of Gua Lou (trichosanthes).

**Acupuncture:** This treatment method has long been used for treating thyroid problems. Combine acupuncture with herbal remedies to achieve the best results. It is important to inform the practitioner of any conventional therapies being used. You should have regular blood tests to monitor your condition.

**Acupressure:** Use the tip of your thumb to press the Hegu point, located on the back of the hand in the depression between the thumb and the first finger, with strong pressure for one to two minutes. Repeat on the opposite hand. Use the tip of your finger to apply medium pressure to the Nei Guan point, located in the center of the wrist on the palm side about 2 inches above the crease. In a sitting position, press the Tai Chong point, located on the instep of the foot in the depression between the first and second toe, at the base of the big toe for one minute. Repeat two to three times a day.

**Diet:** Eat food that reduces heat and that is calming and cooling. Examples are apples, barley, button mushrooms, lettuce, mangoes, spinach, strawberries, persimmons, licorice, and aubergine.

## NATUROPATHY

**Diet:** Eat Brussel sprouts, cabbage, broccoli, cauliflower, kale, mustard greens, peaches, pears, soybeans, spinach, and turnips several times a day for their ability to suppress thyroid hormone production. Limit the amount of sea vegetables consumed because they contain iodine, which may over stimulate the thyroid gland. Also avoid stimulants such as coffee, carbonated drinks, caffeinated tea, and nicotine, which make symptoms worse. Brewer's yeast has high amounts of vitamin B and other important nutrients. Make a drink from the yeast or sprinkle it on your food.

**Supplements:** Those with an overactive thyroid need vitamin B complex to calm the nervous system. Take 50 mg three times a day. Vitamin C is also important to stabilize stressful conditions. Take 3,000–5,000 mg a day.

**Herbs:** Some studies have suggested that melissa helps to soothe the overactive thyroid gland, particularly if it is associated with Grave's disease. Take 2–4 ml of a tincture twice a day. You can also take 2–4 ml of motherwort tincture twice a day.

## HOMEOPATHY

This is a chronic condition and is best treated by an experienced homeopathic practitioner who will try to rebalance the whole system. The remedies below give a small impression of some of the homeopathic remedies that may be considered to treat an overactive thyroid.

**Phosphorus:** If energy levels are leading to weight loss and veer from being high to low very quickly, Phosphorus may be used. Anxiety and restlessness is very marked, and there is a host of digestive disturbances and discomfort. These may manifest as indigestion, nausea, and burning in the stomach, and may be temporarily eased by cold drinks. Severe diarrhea may also be present. Sleep is likely to be disturbed, and sufferers tend to toss and turn before midnight, and wake feeling sleepy.

**Thyroidinum:** Signature symptoms include weight loss, breathlessness, frequent diarrhea with flatulence and cramping pains, and a marked inclination to be moody and irritable. Symptoms often slightly improve in the evening.

**Calc phos:** If patients tend to tremble, feel breathless, and experience mental and emotional restlessness, Calc phos may be used. Sleep is disturbed and patients may have night sweats and wake feeling totally unrefreshed. Colicky pains accompany diarrhea, as food moves quickly through the gut, and problems with malabsorption are common. Being under stress and pressure can aggravate symptoms, while rest can help.

## HERBALISM

Consult a medical herbalist regarding the recommended dosages of the herbs below. A herbalist will determine the correct dose based on the patient's weight, age, and thyroid parameters.

**Bugleweed:** This unique plant possesses several medicinally active compounds believed to be helpful in treating an overactive thyroid and its associated symptoms. It can be taken as a tea or tincture. Bugleweed is a powerful herb, with largely unknown side effects, so consult a medical herbalist before using it.

**Valerian:** While valerian root does not treat the cause of an overactive thyroid it can be very helpful in mitigating symptoms, providing a calming action on the body. It can be taken as a tea or in capsule form. Avoid driving or operating heavy machinery while taking this herb. Valerian may also interact with other drugs or medications that cause drowsiness, such as alcohol and barbiturates.

# PHLEBITIS

## DIAGNOSIS

Phlebitis is an inflammation of the veins, and usually develops in the legs. It generally occurs in the superficial veins just beneath the skin. The cause of phlebitis is unknown, but it tends to develop in those with poor circulation and who have a predisposition to form blood clots. It can be associated with an infection so antibiotics are sometimes prescribed to resolve the condition, but it is also treated with anti-inflammatory painkillers such as aspirin. It can develop after surgery, and it can affect those with cancer of the breast, ovaries, or pancreas. If left untreated it can spread to deeper veins and can eventually lead to deep vein thrombosis (DVT), where clots form in the large veins of the legs.

## SYMPTOMS

- Skin feels warm to the touch
- Redness and sensitivity in the affected area
- Occasionally, the area can become painful

## TREATMENT GOAL

Treatment aims to bring relief to symptoms, and determine lifestyle changes to prevent the condition from recurring. Phlebitis can lead to serious complications and it is important to be aware of the implications of clotting.

## CONVENTIONAL MEDICINE

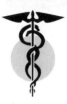

The medical term for phlebitis is superficial thrombophlebitis. It is often treated without resorting to medication.

**Warm compress:** Apply a moist, warm compress to the affected area for 20 minutes every two hours for 48 hours, or as needed.

**Rest:** Usually, you will not need to restrict your physical activity. In extreme cases, however, bed rest and keeping the affected leg elevated helps to improve symptoms.

**Medication:** If the above measures do not bring relief, non-steroidal anti-inflammatory drugs can be taken. If an infected phlebitis is diagnosed, antibiotics are given. In medical evaluation, if it is thought that the phlebitis is progressing into or is initially close to a deep vein, surgical intervention is required. The clot is removed by tying and dividing the vein.

## TRADITIONAL CHINESE MEDICINE

**Herbs:** Prepare a decoction using 12 g of Dang Gui (Chinese angelica root), 15 g of Di Huang (Chinese foxglove), 12 g of Bai Shao (white peony root), 12 g of Chuan Xiong (Szechuan lovage root), 12 g of Sang Ji Shen (mulberry mistletoe stem), 12 g of Bai Hua She She Cao (heydyotis), and 10 g of Si Gua Luo (dried skeleton of vegetable sponge). Combine the herbs with 3 cups of water and place them in a ceramic container. Bring the mixture to a boil and simmer for 30 minutes. Strain the liquid and drink 1 cup twice a day. These herbs can be purchased from Chinese pharmacies or online.

**Acupuncture:** This type of treatment is not recommended for this condition.

**Acupressure:** This type of treatment is not recommended for this condition.

## NATUROPATHY

**Diet:** A high-fiber diet can help by relieving constipation, which can lead to straining and varicosities of the lower body. Base your meals on whole grains, legumes, fruits, and vegetables, adding these foods to your diet wherever possible. Ground flax seeds can also provide plenty of healthy fiber. Take 1–2 tbsp a day sprinkled on your morning cereal or in water.

Consume one to two servings of bright-colored fruit and vegetables, such as berries, cherries, or carrots, every day. These contain powerful antioxidants that will strengthen the walls of the veins and improve their elasticity. Buckwheat naturally contains a flavonoid called rutin, which also strengthens blood vessels, and can be used to make pancakes and bread. Cook with spices such as garlic, onions, ginger, and cayenne pepper for their anti-inflammatory properties and ability to increase circulation. Avoid hydrogenated oils and saturated fats to prevent sluggish circulation and inflammation.

**Supplements:** Take 1,000–5,000 mg of vitamin C and 100–1,000 mg of bioflavonoids in divided daily doses to aid circulation, promote the healing of sores, and strengthen vein walls to prevent dilation. Take 400 IU of a mixed complex vitamin E supplement every day. It promotes blood flow, improves circulation, and sometimes relieves pain. Topical applications of vitamin E oil can be helpful in relieving localized irritation and speeding up the healing of varicose ulcers. You should also take 50 mg of zinc a day to assist with healing and collagen formation.

**Herbs:** Witch hazel has astringent properties that can be effective in treating external varicose veins. It is necessary to apply witch hazel ointment or gel three or more times a day for two or more weeks to see results. It may cause minor skin irritation in some people when applied topically; witch hazel is not recommended for internal use. Horse chestnut can be used both internally and as an external application for venous problems such as weak venous walls and swelling. Take 100 mg of a standardized extract of aescin, horse chestnut's active constituent, a day. You can also apply a horse chestnut ointment, cream, or gel to the affected area two to three times a day. Bilberries support the normal formation of connective tissue and strengthen capillaries and veins in the body. Take a standardized extract containing 25% anthocyanosides at 160 mg twice a day. Also take a standardized extract of butcher's broom—one that gives you 200–300 mg of rucogenins daily—to help reduce inflammation of veins. Take 120 mg of ginkgo twice a day to strengthen blood vessels and improve peripheral circulation. Bromelain can be taken at 500 mg three times a day between meals to reduce inflammation of the veins and help prevent blood clots.

## HOMEOPATHY

The following remedies can help to speed up recovery of the inflammation, pain, and discomfort of an acute episode of phlebitis. However, because of the complications that can develop if this condition is neglected, professional medical assessment is needed to make sure that the condition is resolving.

**Arnica:** This remedy can be helpful in treating phlebitis symptoms that have arisen as a result of an injury. The affected leg is likely to feel sore and achy, and it may be difficult to find a comfortable position in bed at night. This causes sufferers to toss and turn, and jarring movement and touching the affected leg can increase pain and discomfort.

**Hamamelis:** If phlebitis symptoms occur in a leg that is already affected by varicose veins, consider using this remedy. Pain in the affected area is bursting and stinging in nature. Symptoms may have set in after surgery or any investigative procedure that involves inserting needles into a vein.

## HERBALISM

 Although there are no specific herbal remedies to treat phlebitis, or inflammation of the veins, there are herbs that have been used to treat other manifestations of inflammation and maintain blood flow. These may prove helpful in the treatment of phlebitis.

**Gotu kola:** This herb has been used to treat a variety of vascular problems. It can be taken as a tea, made from 0.5–1 g of dried herb, to be drunk three times daily. You can also take 30–60 mg of extract three times a day, or 300–500 mg in capsule form three times a day. Gotu kola is a fairly safe herb with minimal side effects. It does have the potential to promote drowsiness; therefore, it is advisable to refrain from using this herb if you are currently taking other drugs that promote drowsiness, such as sleeping aids or cold medications.

**Boswellia:** This herb contains chemical compounds that protect against inflammation, which may prove useful in the treatment of phlebitis. Most studies use standardized extracts of boswellia in capsule or pill form, which are taken at 300–400 mg three times a day. It is generally considered safe, although there have been some reports of mild stomach pain and nausea.

**Ginger:** This herb acts as an anti-inflammatory agent and also helps to thin the blood. These qualities are both important in the treatment of phlebitis to lessen the inflammation of the veins and prevent clots that may form in these swollen vessels. Ginger is available in many forms and doses. Do not take more than 1 g of ginger a day if you are pregnant. Consult an herbalist for further information.

# PNEUMONIA

## DIAGNOSIS

Pneumonia is an infection or inflammation of the lungs. It has a variety of causes, including infection by viruses, fungi, parasites, and bacteria. The streptococcus bacteria known as pneumococcus is the main cause of the most common type of pneumonia that occurs during the winter months. Although the majority of cases of pneumonia respond well to treatment, the infection can still be a very serious problem. The illness can range from mild to severe, and can even be life threatening in some cases.

The seriousness of the condition is often linked to the health of the patient at the time of infection. The elderly and less mobile have a harder time fighting the infection as it is more difficult for them to shift mucus from the lungs. Small children are equally at risk as their immune systems are still not fully developed. Diabetics and those with heart disease and weakened immune systems are also more prone to severe types of pneumonia. Occasionally, pneumonia develops after an infection of the throat, nose, ears, or sinuses and then spreads into the lungs. Those who are regularly exposed to cigarette smoke are more at risk as smoke injures the airways. For example, those who smoke more than a pack of cigarettes a day are three times more at risk of developing pneumonia than nonsmokers. Toxic fumes, industrial smoke, and other air pollutants may also damage lung function.

## SYMPTOMS

- Shivering fits, chills, fever, pains in the chest, and coughing
- Feeling ill, exhausted, and achy
- Coughing up yellow or brown phlegm, which is sometimes bloodstained
- Fast and shallow breathing
- Breathing and coughing is painful, with sharp pains in the chest
- Confusion (in the elderly)

## TREATMENT GOAL

It is important to determine the type of pneumonia you have in order to treat it in the best possible way. You should get plenty of rest and take plenty of fluids to help flush phlegm out of your system. If you are very unwell you may need to be hospitalized and given intravenous antibiotics.

## CONVENTIONAL MEDICINE

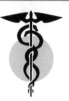

Treatment of pneumonia depends on whether the condition was caused by a virus or bacteria, and how the disease was caught. Generally, an x-ray is taken of the chest and lab tests are carried out to help determine whether pneumonia is present. Patients who are over 60, who smoke, who have cardiovascular conditions, pulmonary disease, immune suppression such as cancer, diabetes, HIV/AIDS, or who have had their spleen removed should receive the pneumococcal vaccine (Pneumovax®).

**To treat bacterial pneumonia:** A two-week course of antibiotics, usually Biaxin®, Levaquin®, or Zithromax®, to be taken orally, is prescribed to otherwise healthy patients. Smokers who suffer from pneumonia should give up cigarettes. Sicker patients are admitted to a hospital and given double the antibiotic treatment. Depending on the oxygen level in the blood, oxygen may also be administered. Hydration is also essential and intravenous hydration is sometimes needed.

**To treat viral pneumonia:** This type of condition requires bed rest and adequate hydration. Viral pneumonia related to flu can be vaccinated against. Amantadine and ribavirin are two medications that can be used to treat certain types of viral pneumonia, but treatment is generally supportive. Maintaining oxygen levels is the primary goal.

## TRADITIONAL CHINESE MEDICINE

**Herbs:** The herbs listed below are available from Chinese pharmacies or online. For each formula, combine the ingredients in a ceramic or glass pot and add 3 cups of water. Bring the mixture to a boil, simmer for 30 minutes, and then strain the liquid. Drink 1 cup twice a day.
- To treat acute pneumonia: Mix 15 g of Yu Xing Cao (houttuynia), 12 g of Pu Gong Ying (dried dandelion), 10 g of Da Qin Ye (woad leaf), 12 g of Bai Jiang Cao (patrinia), and 15 g of Hu Zhang (bushy knotweed root and rhizome).
- To treat pneumonia patients who have lost body fluid from perspiration: In addition to the herbs above, mix 12 g of Zhu Ye (bamboo leaves), 12 g of Tian Hua Fen (trichosanthes root), and 12 g of Sang Bai Pi (mulberry root bark).
- To treat pneumonia patients with excess phlegm: In addition to the herbs used in the first formula, mix 12 g of Gua Lou Ren (trichosanthes seed) and 12 g of Huang Qin (baical skullcap root).

**Acupuncture:** Treatment can be used alongside antibiotics, and with or without herbal medicine. Consult an experienced acupuncturist regarding the frequency of sessions.

**Acupressure:** Use the tip of your thumb to press the Hegu point, located on the back of the hand in the depression between the thumb and the first finger, with strong pressure for one to two minutes. Repeat on the opposite hand. While lying or sitting down, have someone apply medium pressure using the tip of a finger to the Fei Shu points, found 3–4 inches below the back of the neck, 1½ inches on either side of the third thoracic vertebra. Take a seat and apply medium pressure to the Feng Long point, which is approximately halfway between the knee and the foot on the front of the lower leg, for one to two minutes.

**Diet:** Eat Daikon radishes and food that clears heat and phlegm. Examples include peppermint, wild chrysanthemum flowers, purslane, mung beans, red beans, bananas, cucumber, mango, and spinach.

**TIP:** INTEGRATE THERAPIES
Traditional Chinese medicine can be used in combination with conventional medicine to treat pneumonia. Consider integrating therapies to avoid overusing antibiotics.

## NATUROPATHY

**Diet:** Eat small meals that consist of whole grains, fruits, fresh vegetables, and lean proteins frequently. Make sure you are drinking plenty of fluids to prevent dehydration and to thin secretions so that they are easier to cough up. Drink lots of soup, herbal tea, and water. Avoid dairy products, which can increase the production of mucus. Also avoid fats, refined sugars, and caffeine, all of which may depress your immune system.

**Supplements:** Take 15,000 IU of beta-carotene a day to protect the lungs from free radical damage (free radicals are elements that can be harmful to the cells of the body). Take 500 mg of N-acetylcysteine (NAC) two to three times a day; it is being used with some success for respiratory conditions. Vitamin C is an anti-inflammatory and helps stimulate the immune system. It can be beneficial to take 1,000 mg three to four times a day. Emulsified vitamin A, taken at 50,000 IU a day, can help repair immune function. Take 80 mg of zinc gluconate, which is needed for tissue repair and immune function, a day. Take 2–3 proteolytic enzyme capsules a day on an empty stomach to help reduce inflammation. Vitamin B complex, which can be taken at 100 mg three times a day, is important in the formation of red blood cells and antibodies. If your treatment requires an antibiotic, be sure to supplement probiotics such as acidophilus (3–10 billion units/daily) during the treatment and for at least two weeks afterward.

**Herbs:** Take 500 mg of dried ginger powder three times a day to help break up mucus and enhance circulation. Children under six should use one-half of the adult dosage. Licorice helps increase energy, eases coughing, and soothes the lungs. It can be taken at 250–500 mg three times a day, or as a tea made from 14 g of root boiled in 1 pint of water for 15 minutes. Drink 2–3 cups of tea a day. Do not take licorice if you suffer from high blood pressure. Mullein activates the lymph circulation in the neck and chest. To make a tea, pour 1 cup of boiling water over 5–10 g of dried leaves or flowers and let them steep for 10–15 minutes. The tea can be drunk three to four times a day. You can also take 1–4 ml as a tincture three to four times a day, or 3–4 g of a dried product three times a day. Also take 600–900 mg of nettle leaf in capsule or tablet form a day, or 2–4 ml of tincture three times a day.

> **TIP:** USE A HUMIDIFIER
> Using a mist humidifier will help soothe the respiratory tract and thin secretions to facilitate expectoration.

## HOMEOPATHY

The severity of this condition is dependent on the age and vitality of the patient. The suggestions below are appropriate for treating mild symptoms in those who are otherwise in good health. Patients should also seek a conventional medical opinion. Severe cases require prompt conventional medical assessment and treatment, but homeopathy can be helpful after the condition has cleared up. However, treatment is best given by an experienced homeopathic practitioner who will prescribe to strengthen the overall system.

**Aconite:** Consider this remedy if respiratory symptoms come on suddenly in response to exposure to dry, cold air. Coughing spasms sound harsh, and pains in the chest are shooting or burning, and feel much more distressing when not lying on the back. A high fever may also come on suddenly, where the head feels cool while the rest of the body is hot. Sufferers have a strong sense of anxiety and panic.

**Phosphorus:** If coughing bouts are much worse when first lying down, and there is yellow and possibly blood-streaked expectoration from the chest, try Phosphorus. The chest is likely to feel heavy and uncomfortable, with sharp pains in the left lung, or a narrow band of pain behind the breastbone. There is also a tendency to feel hot and bothered with a fever, and most symptoms feel worse in the early evening. Sufferers also tend to feel anxious and have a strong need for emotional reassurance.

**Bryonia:** If pain and distress intensifies with even the slightest movement, try Bryonia. When this remedy is helpful, patients tend to press a hand to the chest when coughing in an effort to keep the area as still as possible. Symptoms that respond well to Bryonia are generally brought on in response to over-exposure to dry, cold winds, but tend to develop slowly and insidiously. When feverish, thirst is marked, and there is a tendency to sweat profusely, especially in the early hours of the morning.

## HERBALISM

If pneumonia is associated with fever, there are several herbs that may be helpful in reducing the fever (see p. 549).

**Astragalus:** This herb is a good choice for the treatment of pneumonia due to its immune-stimulating properties. Astragalus root can be used as a tea, or 500 mg can be taken in capsule form three times a day. Do not take astragalus if you are on blood-thinning drugs, immunosuppressive drugs, or have an autoimmune disorder, such as lupus or rheumatoid arthritis.

**Echinacea:** This herb is another popular and effective immune stimulant. Echinacea works best when it is taken at the first sign of illness. A recommended dose is 250 mg in capsule form two to three times a day, or 20–40 drops of a tincture three times a day. Echinacea should not be taken for more than three weeks. Also, do not take it if there is a known allergy to plants in the daisy family.

**Garlic:** Take garlic capsules as a general immune booster to treat pneumonia. An effective dosage is 1,000 mg three to four times a day. Or, you could simply take two crushed, chopped, or diced cloves of garlic each day for the duration of your illness. Garlic does have the potential to cause stomach irritation, so caution is advised when taking it.

**Lobelia:** This herb can be used to treat a range of respiratory conditions, including pneumonia. Lobelia is thought to act by many different mechanisms, including increasing airway diameter and promoting the secretion and expectoration of mucus. To make a tea, steep ½ tsp of dried herb in 1 cup of boiling water, or you can dilute 1–2 ml of tincture in water or juice. Some adverse effects of lobelia have been reported such as nausea, dizziness, diarrhea, and tremors. Lobelia is a strong herb, so it is best to consult a medical herbalist prior to taking it. Do not take it if you have gastrointestinal problems, heart disorders, or are pregnant.

# RAYNAUD'S DISEASE

## DIAGNOSIS

Raynaud's disease is a condition in which the blood supply to the extremities, usually the fingers and toes but sometimes also the ears and nose, is interrupted. It occurs when the small arteries narrow and cut off the blood supply. During an attack of Raynaud's disease, the affected areas become white, then turn red, and then blue. There is also a painful burning sensation, or numbness or tingling may occur. An attack will often be triggered by exposure to cold air or contact with cold objects. Emotional distress, such as anxiety, can also lead to an attack, as can smoking. The condition can range in severity from minor discomfort to the onset of ulcers or even gangrene. People who work with vibratory tools such as chain saws or pneumatic drills are more prone to Raynaud's disease. The disease often starts in the very young or during the early teens and progresses slowly over time. Primary Raynaud's disease occurs spontaneously, without any underlying condition being present. It can be hereditary, in which case it is usually fairly mild. It affects women nine times more often than it does men. Secondary Raynaud's disease (also known as Raynaud's phenomenon) is less common and is associated with underlying diseases such as lupus and rheumatoid arthritis. This is more serious and early, accurate diagnosis is essential.

## SYMPTOMS

- Fingers or toes turn white, red, then blue
- Numbness in the affected area
- Prickling sensation in the affected area

## TREATMENT GOAL

Prevention of attacks, involving methods such as protecting yourself from the cold with adequate clothing.

## CONVENTIONAL MEDICINE

**Avoid the cold:** Wear gloves, a hat, mittens, and thermal underwear when you go outside during the winter. In the summer months, avoid air-conditioned spaces. When an attack comes on, placing your hands under warm water, or rotating the arms to warm up may help to interrupt it.

**Increase blood flow:** Stress is a contributory factor to Raynaud's disease, so stress reduction techniques are very important. Some techniques actually involve learning to increase the blood flow to the hands. Anything that causes spasm of the blood vessels, such as nicotine, cold medicines, diet pills, and ephedra should be avoided. Certain herbal therapies, especially ginkgo, can also increase blood flow. Avoiding smoking is particularly important if you have Raynaud's disease.

**Medication:** Calcium channel blockers, usually nifedipine, are used to treat Raynaud's disease. Nitroglycerin, which causes the direct dilation of the blood vessels, has also been used topically.

**Surgery:** A surgical intervention called localized digital sympathectomy is available for severe cases in which tissues may be lost. With this procedure, nerve pathways to affected areas are interrupted and the nerves around blood vessels are cut.

## TRADITIONAL CHINESE MEDICINE

**Herbs:** The herbs listed below are available from Chinese pharmacies or online. For either formula, combine the herbs in a ceramic or glass pot and add 3 cups of water. Bring the mixture to a boil, simmer for 30 minutes, and strain the liquid.
• Internal formula: Mix 10 g of Gui Zhi (cinnamon), 12 g of Chi Shao (red peony root), 15 g of Niu Xi (achyranthes root), 15 g of Ji Xue Teng (millettia root), 5 g of Gan Jiang, and 5 pieces of Da Zhao (Chinese jujube). Drink 1 cup twice a day.
• External formula: Mix 15 g of Dan Shen (salvia root), 15 g of Niu Xi (achyranthes root), 10 g of Jing Jie (schizonepeta stem and bud), 12 g of Chuan Xiong (Szechuan lovage root), and 15 g of Chi Shao (red peony root). Wash the affected area with the liquid.

**Acupuncture:** Consult an experienced practitioner for treatment options. You may need 10–20 treatment sessions twice a week. After a few sessions, the fingers and/or toes should become less blue or purple, and you may start feeling warmer. Acupuncture can be combined with herbal treatment, particularly the external herbal treatment mentioned as above.

**Acupressure:** Use Ba Xie, and Ba Feng. The four Ba Xie point are located on the back of the hand at in between the base of each finger and thumb. The Ba Feng points are found on the sole of the foot between the base of each toe. Use your fingers to press each point with gentle pressure for one minute. Repeat this five times twice a day.

**Diet:** Eat food that has warm properties such as dried ginger, cloves, chicken, dates, green onions, grapefruit, coconut, mutton, peaches, sweet basil, shrimp, mustard leaf, and squash.

## NATUROPATHY

**Diet:** Avoid eating too many raw foods as they are cold and contribute to the coldness of your hands and feet. Eat warm foods such as soups and steamed vegetables, adding ginger wherever possible as it has an additional warming effect. Avoid too many cold drinks, as they may aggravate the symptoms. Instead drink warm tea throughout the day. Ginger and cinnamon are warming herbs and can be drunk throughout the day as a tea.

**Supplements:** In one study, fish oil was shown to reduce the severity of blood-vessel spasms in five out of 11 people with Raynaud's disease. Take 4 g of eicosapentaenoic acid (EPA), which is found in fish oil, a day. Niacin (inositol hexaniacinate) has been used with some success to relieve symptoms of Raynaud's disease. Take 3 g per day of inositol hexaniacinate. Take 1 g of L-carnitine three times a day; it has resulted in less constriction in blood-vessels in the fingers of those with Raynaud's disease that develops from cold exposure. Magnesium deficiency can also lead to blood vessel spasm. Take 200–600 mg of magnesium a day. In another study, researchers found low levels of selenium and vitamin C in the blood of women with Raynaud's disease. Take 100–200 mcg of selenium a day, and 1,000 mg of vitamin C three times a day.

## HOMEOPATHY

Very mild, infrequently occurring symptoms may respond to one of the following remedies, speeding up recovery from an acute episode. More established and/or severe occurrences of this condition are best treated by a homeopathic practitioner, especially if Raynaud's disease is combined with additional circulatory problems.

**Lachesis:** If the tips of the fingers have a purple-blue tinge, especially when waking, try Lachesis. Symptoms may be more severe on the left hand, or restricted completely to the left side of the body.

**Pulsatilla:** Consider using this remedy if circulation is generally poor to the fingers and toes, but applying warmth makes symptoms feel worse. Gentle exercise helps, while resting makes symptoms more uncomfortable. When this remedy is well indicated, inflamed and painful varicose veins may also occur.

**Arsenicum album:** If symptoms are accompanied by burning, tingly, and itchy sensations, and if there is a degree of swelling in the fingertips with a blue tinge appearing in the fingernails, try Arsenicum album. Applying heat to the affected area gains some relief and eases burning pains.

**TIP:** EXERCISE
Consider taking up a gentle form of rhythmic exercise, such as walking, to stimulate the circulatory system.

## HERBALISM

**Ginkgo biloba:** Most of ginkgo's beneficial effects are derived from the herb's purported ability to increase blood flow and improve circulation. Take 120–240 mg to three times a day. There have been few reported side effects, but those who are also taking anticoagulant and anti-thrombotic drugs care should take care as there may be an increased risk of bleeding.

**Evening primrose oil:** This oil contains the omega-6 fatty acid gamma-linoleic acid, which is thought to be responsible for many of the oil's therapeutic effects. Take enough evening primrose oil to provide approximately 500 mg of gamma-linoleic acid a day.

**Flaxseed oil:** This oil contains omega-3 fatty acids, which possess a wide array of health benefits and may be helpful in mitigating the effects of Raynaud's disease. It is best to buy small quantities of "cold-pressed" oil. Make sure the oil is refrigerated and stored in dark bottles (to protect the oil from UV light). In addition you can also buy fresh flaxseed. Because the seed itself is very durable and will pass directly through the digestive system, it is best to crush it before use. Use a mortar and pestle or coffee grinder to pulp the seeds. Sprinkle them on salads or cereals, or add them to a glass of water.

# UNDERACTIVE THYROID

## DIAGNOSIS

An underactive thyroid results when the thyroid gland does not produce enough of the thyroid hormones thyroxine (T4) and tri-iodothyronine (T3). Thyroid hormones are extremely important for the regulation of the body's metabolism. If the hormones are not produced in adequate amounts, the body's metabolism slows, leaving you feeling lethargic and run down. Decreased metabolism can affect every organ of the body, including the brain, heart, skin, intestine, and muscles.

The main causes of an underactive thyroid are Hashimoto's thyroiditis (an autoimmune inflammation of the thyroid gland), an inherited problem with the thyroid gland, and complications arising from previous surgery to the thyroid gland. It can also be a side effect of certain medications, or can result from inadvertently taking large amounts of iodine, for example, in food supplements or, at times, shellfish such as shrimp. An underactive thyroid is the most common disorder of the thyroid, and tends to affect women more than men. It is more prevalent among the elderly, but younger people are also susceptible.

## SYMPTOMS

- Increased sensitivity to cold
- Feelings of depression and lethargy
- No desire to exercise
- Weight gain
- Constipation
- Dry, rough, scaly skin
- Thin, dry hair
- Irregular periods
- Voice is deeper and more hoarse
- Loss of memory

## TREATMENT GOAL

A doctor will carry out tests to determine a diagnosis. Permanently decreased metabolism requires lifelong treatment with thyroid medication. Conventional and complementary therapies aim to rebalance hormone levels so that sufferers are able to lead completely normal lives.

## CONVENTIONAL MEDICINE

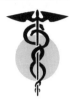

Hypothyroidism usually progresses slowly, but it can reach a dangerous level, especially if the thyroid has been removed. This condition is known as myxedema, and can cause a low temperature, low blood pressure, and a coma. Such cases are emergencies and must be treated at a hospital in Intensive Care.

**Medication:** Conventional medical treatment for an underactive thyroid is levothyroxine (T4), which is a synthetic form of thyroid, or some form of thyroid replacement. This may be given in combination with cytomel (T3). Natural thyroid replacements made by compounding pharmacists, who make up individual prescriptions other than those made by pharmaceutical companies, or Armour® thyroid (pig thyroid) are also available. The dosage varies from person to person, and is adjusted according to levels of thyroid stimulating hormone (TSH) in the blood. It generally takes six to eight weeks for the thyroid values to normalize after an adjustment is made. Because the change is gradual, patients are encouraged to be patient as they await improvement and testing.

**Lifestyle modifications:** A low calorie, high-fiber diet will help combat the effects of an underactive thyroid. Eliminate iodine-blocking foods such as pine nuts, almonds, and dark leafy greens from your diet. Exercise is also important.

## TRADITIONAL CHINESE MEDICINE

**Herbs:** According to traditional Chinese medicine, this condition is caused by a Qi deficiency. The following formula can help to tonify Qi. Combine 12 g of Huang Qi (milk-vetch root), 12 g of Tu Si Zi (Chinese dodder seed), 10 g of Jin Shen (jilin root), 12 g of Bai Zhu (white atractylodes rhizome), 12 g of Shu Di Huang (Chinese foxglove cooked in wine), 12 g of Shan Zhu Yu (Asiatic cornelian cherry fruit), 15 g of Fuling (poria), 15 g of Shan Yao (Chinese yam), and 12 g of Xian Lin Pi (aerial part of epimedium) in a ceramic pot. Add 3 cups of water, bring the liquid to a boil, and simmer for 30 minutes. Strain the liquid and drink 1 cup twice a day.

**Acupuncture:** You may have treatment once a week for a long period of time since this condition responds slowly to the principles of acupuncture. Acupuncture can improve the function of the internal organs and systems and tonify Qi and energy.

**Acupressure:** In a sitting position, use your fingertips to apply pressure to the the Susanli point, found on the lower leg, 1 inch to the outside and 3 inches below the kneecap. Press for one minute on each leg and repeat. Apply medium pressure with your fingertip to the Nei Guan point, located in the center of the wrist on the palm side, about 2 inches above the crease. The Tai Xi point is found in the depression midway between the inside anklebone and the Achilles tendon. With the tip of the finger, apply medium pressure to this point on both legs for one minute.

**Diet:** Eat foods that promote yang energy such as beef, beetroot, chicken livers, Chinese cabbage, carrots, figs, marjoram, peaches, shiitake mushrooms, sunflower seeds, longans, and cinnamon.

## NATUROPATHY

**Diet:** Eat plenty of sea vegetables, such as kelp, nori, dulse, kombu, and wakame. These have high levels of iodine, which nourishes the thyroid gland. Essential fatty acids (EFAs) that are found in walnuts, flaxseeds, and oily fish, are also important for thyroid function. Avoid goitrogens, or foods that suppress thyroid function, such as Brussel sprouts, cabbage, broccoli, cauliflower, kale, mustard greens, peaches, pears, soybeans, spinach, and turnips. Flourine and chloride inhibit the body's absorption of iodine; do not drink fluoride supplemented tap water and use fluoride-free toothpaste.

**Supplements:** Take 500 mg of L-tyrosine, an amino acid used to synthesize thyroid hormone, twice a day. Also take 3,000 g of fish oils a day to obtain the essential fatty acids (EFA) necessary for thyroid function.

**Thyroid glandulars:** Take a tablet of a thyroid glandular, an extract of an animal thyroid gland, three times a day to support thyroid function.

## HOMEOPATHY

This is a chronic condition and is best treated by an experienced homeopathic practitioner who will try to rebalance the whole system. The remedies below give a small impression of some of the homeopathic remedies that may be considered to treat an underactive thyroid.

**Calc carb:** To treat classic symptoms associated with an underactive thyroid, including slow metabolism, easy weight gain, slow digestive processes leading to indigestion and constipation, clammy, sweaty skin, poor circulation, chapped, dry skin, and exhaustion, Calc carb may be used. This remedy can be especially beneficial if an underactive thyroid gland is associated with menopausal symptoms.

**Thyroidinum:** This is a remedy that can be used to treat both under or overactive thyroid glands. Symptoms include unexplained weight gain, sweating of the hands and feet, hair loss, feeling chilly, discomfort after eating, hot flushes, and sharp mood swings. In women, symptoms may improve following a period.

> **TIP:** AVOID TRIGGER FOODS
> Certain foods have a reputation for possibly inhibiting thyroid gland function, and they should be avoided by those who have an underactive thyroid. Common culprits include cabbage, Brussel sprouts, cauliflower, soy, and mustard greens. It may also be beneficial to steer clear of refined foods, white sugar, caffeine, alcohol, and large helpings of dairy products.

## HERBALISM

The primary treatment for an underactive thyroid is thyroid hormone replacement. Herbal remedies can be used to correct any underlying causes of the condition and ease symptoms.

**Bladderwrack:** This type of seaweed treats hypothyroidism and goiter (the enlargement of the thyroid) due to iodine deficiency. It contains high levels of iodine as well as beta-carotene, potassium, zeazanthin, bromine, and mucilages, which heal and soothe the tissues. For the best results, bladderwrack must be taken over a long-term period. Drink a tea made from 1–2 tsp of herb boiled in 1 cup of water or take 30 drops of tincture daily.

**Guggul:** This herb is effective in stimulating the thyroid to produce more thyroid hormone. The active constituent in guggul is a resin, which is secreted by the plant when injured. Because resins are insoluble in water, an alcohol extract must be used. Take 20 drops of tincture three times a day.

**Lemon balm:** If an underactive thyroid is caused by the immune system creating auto-antibodies against the thyroid (e.g., Hashimoto's thyroiditis), lemon balm can be used to decrease the destruction and inflammation of the thyroid. Lemon balm is a slightly warming, sweet-tasting herb that also acts as a mild anti-depressant, a common side-effect of hypothyroidism. Drink an infusion of 1 tbsp in 1 cup of water daily. Drink lemon balm only if you are also taking a thyroid hormone replacement, as it may make symptoms worse.

# WHEEZING

## DIAGNOSIS

Wheezing is a medical condition where breathing becomes labored and noisy. It can range from mild to severe and in some cases—such as when linked to an asthma attack—can be life threatening. The high-pitched whistling sound that characterizes wheezing is produced by air flowing through narrowed airways, especially the smaller airways deep in the lungs. It is common in those who have asthma and chronic obstructive pulmonary disease (COPD). It can be caused by a range of conditions, including bronchiolitis, croup, and allergies. Wheezing can be aggravated by exercise, or exposure to cold air or polluted air, such as a smoky atmosphere. Wheezing is particularly common in young children.

Contact your doctor if an isolated episode of wheezing occurs, or if the skin takes on a blue tone during an attack. Also seek medical attention if wheezing becomes a recurrent, unexplained problem, or if it is caused by an allergic reaction to a bite or medication.

## SYMPTOMS

- Difficulty breathing
- Rapid and shallow breathing
- Shortness of breath
- Noisy breathing, sometimes with a rattling sound

## TREATMENT GOAL

It is important to establish the exact cause of the wheezing. If the patient is diagnosed with a more serious illness such as asthma or COPD, further action to treat and manage the underlying condition is needed.

## CONVENTIONAL MEDICINE

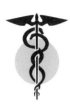

**Diet:** Eliminate processed foods, dairy products, and gluten from your diet if you have asthma. Wheezing is accompanied by the inflammation or swelling of the lining of the airway. Decreasing this inflammation can help to keep the wheezing at bay. Take natural anti-inflammatory nutrients such as fish oil, at about 4 g a day for adults and 2 g for children.

**Avoid allergens:** This condition can occur when the airway reacts to various factors inside and outside the body. When these stimulants are recognized and avoided, the wheezing can generally be prevented. Common allergens that lead to wheezing include dust, pollen, chemicals, smoke, and certain foods.

**Reduce stress:** Stress has been shown to increase wheezing episodes. Stress reduction techniques can be practiced by both children and adults to help decrease attacks.

**Medication:** Albuterol can be inhaled in combination with ipratropium to stop a mild wheezing attack. Corticosteroids can also be inhaled to prevent or treat wheezing, or a class of drugs known as mast cell stabilizers can be used for prevention in place of corticosteroids. Leukotriene receptor antagonists and theophylline are other commonly used preventive drugs. Oxygen is administered in a hospital setting whenever oxygen levels are compromised. **Caution:** Wheezing that does not respond to available medications should be taken seriously. If a patient can not get enough oxygen it is an emergency. Seek immediate medical attention for wheezing that is severe or unresponsive.

## TRADITIONAL CHINESE MEDICINE

**Herbs:** The herbs listed in the formulas below are available from Chinese pharmacies or online. For either formula, combine the herbs with 3 cups of water in a ceramic pot and bring the mixture to the boil. Simmer for 30 minutes and strain the liquid. Drink 1 cup twice a day.

• To treat wheezing that occurs during the winter and is associated with chills and clear or white mucus: Mix 6 g of Ma Huang (ephedra stem), 10 g of Gui Zhi (cinnamon), 12 g of Bai Shao (white peony root), 12 g of Wu Wei Zi (schisandra fruit), 5 g of dried ginger, 12 g of Fa Ben Xia (pinellia rhizome), and 5 g of Gan Cao (licorice).

• To treat wheezing during any season that is associated with a fever, thirst, and yellow mucus: Mix 3 g of Ma Huang (ephedra), 12 g of Xin Ren (almond kernel), 12 g of San Bai Pi (mulberry root bark), 12 g of Huang Qin (baical skullcap root), 10 g of Kwan Dong Hua (coltsfoot flower), 10 g of Zi Su Zi (perilla leaf), 12 g of Bai Guo (ginkgo nut), and 6 g of Gan Cao (licorice).

**Acupuncture:** An acupuncture session can effectively reduce wheezing for a couple of days. In the acute stage, you may have acupuncture up to once a day.

**Acupressure:** Press the Feng Chi, Tan Zhong, and Nei Guan points. The Feng Chi points are located at the back of the head at the base of the skull, 2 inches to either side of the center point. Use the tip of your finger to apply medium pressure to the Nei Guan point, located in the center of the wrist on the palm side, about 2 inches above the crease for one minute. Also apply medium pressure to the Tan Zhong point, found on the chest at the center point in between the nipples for one minute.

**Diet:** Pears, olives, Bi Ba long pepper fruit, and kiwi are all good foods to eat. There are also several recipes that can help with wheezing. Try boiling 30 g of almond kernels and 150 g of sweet rice in 5 cups of water for 45 minutes. Eat this every day for five days.

## NATUROPATHY

 **Diet:** Eat a simple diet by eliminating dairy and food made from white flour that may stimulate mucus production. Instead eat a diet based on steamed vegetables, fresh fruit, whole grains, and lean poultry and fish. Try to eat plenty of fish, since there is a link between fish consumption in children and a decreased risk of developing asthma. Sprinkle some ground flaxseeds on your food to obtain omega-3 fatty acids, which help with inflammation. Be aware of foods that provoke allergy reactions and avoid those foods. Drinking water every waking hour will flush out mucus and phlegm from your body.

**Supplements:** Take 4–8 g of fish oils a day for their anti-inflammatory components. Magnesium has been shown to relax the bronchial tubes and improve overall lung function. Take 250 mg three times a day, but cut back if stools loosen. Take 1,000 mg of vitamin C two to four times a day for its anti-allergic benefits, but again cut back if stools become loose. Take 1,500 mcg of vitamin B12 orally, or 400 mcg sublingually, as it can reduce asthma symptoms in some people.

**Herbs:** Several herbs act as antihistamines to open air passages and relieve wheezing. These herbs include anise, ginger, peppermint, and chamomile. You can make a tea of using some or all of the following herbs. Combine 1 tsp each of chamomile flowers, echinacea root, mullein leaves, and passionflower leaves, and ½ tsp each of elecampane root and lemon verbena leaves (if available). Pour 1 quart of boiling water over the herbs in a saucepan, let them steep for 10–15 minutes, and strain the liquid. Give a 50 lb child ½ cup of tea at least once a day as a preventive measure, or a few times a day if breathing becomes strained or when emotional upset may trigger an attack. If you use a tincture of these herbs, give 15 drops to replace each ½ cup of tea.

## HOMEOPATHY

The following homeopathic remedies can help to ease mild symptoms of wheezing that have arisen following exposure to an obvious trigger, such as inhaling very cold air when exercising, or becoming emotionally stressed or over-excited. Severe episodes of wheezing that are associated with a chronic condition such as asthma require professional assessment and treatment from an experienced homeopathic practitioner.

**Aconite:** If mild wheezing comes on rapidly after an emotionally traumatic experience, or following exposure to harsh, dry cold winds, use Aconite. When this remedy is appropriate, there is likely to be a strong sense of panic in response to feeling wheezy that may be out of proportion to the severity and intensity of symptoms.

**Arsenicum album:** If wheezing comes on at night or in the early hours of the morning, often as a consequence of feeling stressed and anxious, take Arsenicum album. Tightness in the chest is noticeably improved by resting propped up on two or three pillows, and is more intense and distressing when lying flat. Symptoms include a marked sense of restlessness, anxiety, nausea, and chilliness when feeling ill. If a cough is present with mild wheezing it is likely to be dry and tickly, rather than loose and productive.

## HERBALISM

Wheezing can be a sign of a more serious medical state and should always be evaluated by a doctor. Once this is done, there are several herbal medicines that can open the airways and decrease inflammation in the lungs.

**Khella:** This herb contains slightly aromatic, bitter seeds, which open up the bronchioles in the lungs. It acts as a potent antispasmodic, making it ideal for the long-term treatment of asthma. The active constituents of khella also improve blood supply to the heart, and act as an antispasmodic for the bladder. Infuse 1 tsp of crushed seeds per cup of water and drink twice a day or take 20 mg standardized to 12% of the active constituent khellin a day. Khella should not be taken with the medication digoxin.

**Yerba santa:** This herb can be used for any type of lung condition that may cause wheezing and where there is an excessive amount of mucus, such as in asthma, bronchitis, colds, or hay fever. Yerba santa thins the mucus and stimulates expectoration from the lungs. It also opens up the bronchioles, allowing greater airflow through the lungs.

# WHOOPING COUGH

## DIAGNOSIS

Whooping cough is an infection that causes a build-up of mucus and inflamed airways. The ailment is named after the signature coughing and deep breathing that it involves, which produces a sound like a "whoop." It can be serious in babies under the age of one, as their airways are immature, and in the worse cases can cause brain and lung damage. For this reason, babies are vaccinated against whooping cough, and it is now quite a rare condition. It is caused by the bacteria Bordetella pertussis, and is transferred through airborne droplets. It is highly contagious, and if one child in a group contracts it, other children are likely to become infected if they have not already had the disease or been vaccinated against it. Although infants who are breastfed are usually protected against most common childhood infections, they receive no protection against whooping cough. This is why early vaccination is recommended. Anyone who has not been vaccinated is likely to contract the disease simply by spending time in the same room as an infected person. Occasionally those who are vaccinated will still develop a mild case of whooping cough.

Complications of whooping cough include bronchitis, pneumonia, and ear infections, all of which may cause a high temperature. If one or more of these problems occur, they are usually treated with antibiotics. The coughing can continue for up to 10 weeks, a much longer period than for other childhood diseases.

## SYMPTOMS

- A cold
- Coughing bouts
- Distinctive whooping noise when coughing
- Difficulty breathing
- Occasionally, skin around the lips turns blue
- Vomiting (in older children)

## TREATMENT GOAL

Most cases of whooping cough require no specific treatment. Infants and small children with other conditions such as asthma require constant monitoring, which is often done in a hospital.

## CONVENTIONAL MEDICINE

Treatment of whooping cough is directed toward preventing the spread of the infection via vaccination. A routine vaccination is given by the childhood immunization department. All children under one year old who have whooping cough should be evaluated for hospitalization, and children that come into contact with an infected person should be given a prophylactic antibiotic. The local health department should always be notified of any cases.

**Antibiotics:** Although antibiotics have only a minor effect on the disease once the symptoms are present, they are administered as they do shorten the recovery time. They also prevent the spread of the illness. Erythromycin is the antibiotic of choice and a 14-day course is usually required. For people who cannot tolerate this class of drugs, Septra® (trimehoprim-sulfamethoxazole) can be used.

**Treating the cough:** Corticosteroids are sometimes useful in preventing the spasms of coughing in severe cases in infants. Standard cough suppressants do not work and can actually cause coughing spasms.

## TRADITIONAL CHINESE MEDICINE

**Herbs:** The herbs listed in the formulas below are available from Chinese pharmacies or online. For each formula, make a decoction by combining the herbs in a ceramic or glass pot. Add 3 cups of water, bring the mixture to the boil, and simmer for 30 minutes. Strain the liquid and give children 2–3 oz three times a day.

• To treat early whooping cough in the first one to two weeks: Combine 8 g of Jing Jie (schizonepeta stem and bud), 8 g of Yuan Zhi (Chinese senega root), 8 g of Bai Qian (root and rhizome of cynanchum), 8 g of Bai Bu (stemona root), 5 g of Chen Pi (tangerine peel), 12 g of Jie Jeng (balloon flower root), and 3 g of Gan Cao (licorice).

• To treat intermediate whooping cough in the third to sixth week: Mix 8 g of Sang Bai Pi (mulberry root bark), 8 g of Di Gu Pi (cortex of wolfberry root), 6 g of Huang Qin (baical skullcap root), 6 g of Tao Ren (peach kernel), 8 g of Dong Gua Ren (winter melon), 8 g of Yu Xing Cao (houttuynia), and 8 g of Bai Mao Gen (wooly grass rhizome).

• To treat the later stage of whooping cough: Combine 3 g of ginseng, 10 g of Bai Zhu (white atractylodes root), 10 g of Fuling (poria), 12 g of Mai Men Dong (ophiopogon tuber), 10 g of Wu Wei Zi (schisandra fruit), and 3 pieces of Da Zhao (Chinese jujube).

**Acupuncture:** Treatment may help reduce the symptoms, and shorten the course of the disease. However, children may prefer acupressure.

**Acupressure:** In a sitting position, have someone apply gently pressure to the Fei Shu and Din Chuan points with the tip of a finger. The Fei Shu points are located on the back, 1½ inches to either side of the spinal cord and 3–4 inches below the neck at the third thoracic vertebra. The Din Chuan points are also on the back, ½ inch to either side of the base of the neck (at the seventh cervical vertebra). Also use a fingertip to apply medium pressure to the Lie Que point, located on the inside of the forearm about 1½ inches below the crease of the wrist and between the outside muscle and tendon of the thumb.

**Diet:** Yi Yi Ren (seeds of Job's tears), Daikon radishes, almonds, kumquats, mandarin oranges, tangerines, thyme, and ginger are all helpful in easing whooping cough. There are also several recipes that may help with this ailment. Try steaming 5–10 kumquats with 30 g of rock sugar for ½ hour and eat a few twice a day. Make a tea using 6 g of licorice root, 30 g of honey, and 10 g of vinegar. Boil the ingredients in water for 10 minutes and drink. You can also try a tea made from 3 g of licorice and 15–20 g of fresh ginger. Add water and boil for 10 minutes before drinking.

## NATUROPATHY

**Diet:** Children should eat as little as possible. Small meals are best, especially vegetable broths and soups. Add garlic and ginger to these for their immune-boosting effects. Avoid giving your child dairy products as they aggravate symptoms and produce mucus. Instead, encourage your child to drink as much fluid as possible to flush out the mucus.

**Supplements:** Vitamin C helps stimulate the immune system. Give children a product made for them that contains bioflavonoids and follow the instructions on the label. Zinc lozenges for children also stimulate the immune system and promote healing. Give your child one dose twice a day with food.

**Herbs:** Several herbs may be given in a tea or in a tincture form. Licorice has antibacterial properties, soothes the throat and respiratory tract, and tastes sweet. Marshmallow root is soothing to the throat and respiratory tract. Osha root is a mild suppressant and healing to the respiratory tract. Slippery elm bark also soothes the throat and respiratory tract.

## HOMEOPATHY

Any of the following homeopathic remedies can help to ease acute symptoms of a mild bout of whooping cough in an older child. However, more severe symptoms will require professional medical and homeopathic attention, especially in babies under the age of six months.

**Ant tart:** If there is an audible amount of mucus rattling in the chest, try Ant tart. The child may instinctively have to bend slightly backwards during a coughing spasm in order to raise mucus from the chest. Other symptoms include breathlessness before a coughing spasm, and vomiting afterwards. The patient feels generally worse for getting angry (which can trigger coughing bouts), and better after vomiting.

**Carbo veg:** Consider using this remedy if a coughing spasm leads to the child becoming pale, clammy, exhausted, and prostrated. There is a craving for cold air, and a need to be fanned in order to get more comfortable. Stuffy, airless rooms aggravate the discomfort. Speaking triggers coughing bouts, while loosening clothes brings relief.

**Corallium rubrum:** If coughing spasms are preceded by a smothering sensation, and followed by vomiting up stringy mucus, take Corallium rubrum. Coughing bouts tend to occur soon after eating, and one episode follows quickly after another. Body temperature is likely to be very unstable, with a tendency to feel too hot one moment, and too cold the next.

---

**TIP:** EAT LIGHT FOODS

If your child tends to vomit quickly after a bout of coughing, try to give him/her something small and light to eat soon after the bout is over. This will give him a better chance of keeping food down, especially if what you choose is as light and as easily digestible as possible. Such foods include broths made with rice, lightly cooked fresh vegetables, fresh fruit smoothies, scrambled eggs, toast, and small amounts of fresh fish. Foods that generally take longer to digest include any items that are high in fat such as dairy foods (which also increase mucus production) and red meat. Sugary items are also best avoided since they can aggravate a nauseated, sensitive stomach.

---

## HERBALISM

In younger children, especially infants, symptoms of whooping cough must be closely monitored by a doctor and antibiotics may be required. Older children and adults tend to have milder symptoms, although early antibiotic use will decrease the period in which they are contagious. Herbs are used to boost the immune system, relax lung spasms, and soothe the cough reflex. Herbs should be adjusted according to the age of the patient; consult a medical herbalist for specifics. The doses outlined below are appropriate for older children and adults.

**Sundew:** This herb can be used for the treatment of an uncontrollable, excessive spasmodic cough. It has sedative, antispasmodic, demulcent and expectorant properties. Sundew will turn the urine a dark color; do not be alarmed, it is completely safe. Take 30 drops of tincture in water three to four times daily.

**Antimicrobial herbs:** As the mucus produced by whooping cough is often difficult to expectorate, it is best to combine antibacterial herbs with herbs that loosen infected mucus in the lungs. Herbs that strengthen the immune system and fight bacteria directly are echinacea, Oregon grape, garlic, andrographis, and thyme. These herbs should be taken until symptoms have resolved. Combine equal parts of each herb in tincture form and take 60 drops four times daily.

**Antispasmodic and expectorant herbs:** The budding tops of gumweed contain resins that relieve spasms and encourage mucus expectoration from the lungs. Although it is very effective, large doses of gumweed may cause stomach irritation. Elecampane root is another aromatically sweet and pungent herb that promotes expectoration, while decreasing inflammation and boosting the immune system. Add licorice to equal parts of the above in tincture form to create a sweet tincture, and take 60 drops four times daily.

**Demulcents and antitussives:** If the cough is especially harsh, include herbs that soothe the respiratory tract (demulcents) and decrease coughing (antitussives). Antitussive herbs, such as poppy and thyme, act by either performing as a mild analgesic on the lung's tissue or by relieving spasms. Demulcents, such as corn silk, flaxseeds, and oat, often contain mucilages or oils that soothe and heal the lungs.

# ACHES
# AND
# PAINS

# ARTHRITIS

## DIAGNOSIS

Arthritis is a painful condition of the joints. There are several different types of the disease—many are inflammatory while others are more degenerative in nature. It is uncertain what exactly triggers arthritis. It may be partly hereditary and it occurs three times more often in women than in men. People of all ages can develop arthritis—even children can be affected.

Osteoarthritis (also known as degenerative joint disease) is the most common form of arthritis. It is very painful and occurs when the joint cartilage begins to deteriorate and slowly wears away. People become affected by this type of arthritis in middle age. Factors that may contribute to the development of this disease include a genetic predisposition, being overweight, and previous damage to the joints through injury.

Rheumatoid arthritis affects the tissue connecting bones and joints, and is one of the most debilitating forms of arthritis. Pain in the joints almost always begins in the hands, especially in the knuckles, and often occurs in both hands simultaneously. The most obvious areas of damage are to the joints, but it can affect the whole body and in particular the fingers, wrists, elbows, and knees. It can occur at any age but usually starts in early middle age.

## SYMPTOMS

### OSTEOARTHRITIS
- Pain and stiffness in joints, particularly the knees and hips
- Tender joints

### RHEUMATOID ARTHRITIS
- Joints swell and become red, stiff, and sore
- Morning stiffness
- Fatigue and flu-like aches and pains
- Fever
- Loss of appetite

## TREATMENT GOAL

There is no standard treatment for arthritis. Conventional and alternative therapies aim to slow the progressive deterioration as much as possible. Lifestyle changes, such as exercise, can also slow deterioration and relieve pain and stiffness.

## CONVENTIONAL MEDICINE

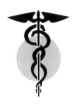

**Exercise:** Lifestyle modifications can be used to augment medication, or even replace it. Daily exercise, particularly aerobic aquatic exercise, is beneficial. Strength building of the muscles also seems to help ease the pain of arthritis, particularly quadriceps work, which is beneficial in the reduction of knee pain. Heat therapy and ultrasound therapy may also be helpful.

**Diet:** Adopt an anti-inflammatory diet. This involves reducing the amount of dairy, gluten, sugar, and processed foods you eat. Using anti-inflammatory herbs such as ginger, curcumin, and turmeric can also be beneficial. Begin a weight loss program if necessary as this can help to ease symptoms.

**Supplements:** Take 4–7 g of fish oil (EPA and DHA in combination) a day. Although recent studies suggest that glucosamine and chondroiten are not as worthwhile as once thought, some case reports indicate otherwise. Some may find that they are beneficial while others do not. Capsaicin cream can be helpful when applied topically, but sometimes causes irritation. Vitamin D3 (cholecalciferol) has surfaced as an important vitamin in osteoarthritis. Doses much higher than the recommended daily allowance are used so consult a doctor regarding an appropriate dose.

**Medication:** Ibuprofen and other non-steroidal anti-inflammatory drugs (NSAIDs) are effective but are generally not recommended for long-term use as gastric bleeding is a side effect. Tylenol® is the medication of choice as it causes the least gastric side effects. Other mediations such as tramadol, propoxyphene, and codeine may be used for pain relief, but have sedating and constipating side effects and can be addictive; however, they do not cause gastric side effects. Cox 2 inhibitors such as celecoxib have less gastric risk but have known risks of increasing cardiovascular problems such as heart attacks. Joint injections with steroids are an effective short-term therapy. If all else fails, surgery, such as joint replacement surgery or osteotomy, which realigns the bones to reduce wear and pain, can be performed.

## TRADITIONAL CHINESE MEDICINE

**Herbs:** Chinese herbal remedies can be combined with acupuncture to treat this condition. The herbs listed in the formulas below are available from Chinese pharmacies or online.
• Internal formula: Combine 10 g of Qing Huo (notopterygium root), 10 g of Du Huo (pubescent angelica root), 12 g of Sang Ji Sheng

(mulberry mistletoe stem), 15 g of Niu Xi (achyranthes root), 15 g of Ji Xue Teng (millettia root), 10 g of Huang Bai (phellodendron), and 12 g of Cang Zhu (black atractylodes rhizome) in a ceramic pot and add 3 cups of water. Bring to a boil and simmer for 30 minutes. Strain and drink 1 cup twice a day.

• External formula: Combine 10 g of Chuan Wu (Szechuan aconite), 10 g of Cao Wu (wild aconite), 12 g of Gui Zhi (cinnamon), 12 g of Tao Ren (peach kernel), 10 g of Hong Hua (safflower flower), and 15 g of Niu Xi (achyranthes root) in a glass or ceramic pot. Add 3 cups of water, bring to a boil, and simmer for 30 minutes. Soak a towel in the warm herbal liquid and apply the towel to the affected joints, or soak the joints in the warm liquid for 20–30 minutes, once a day. Repeat this for five to seven days.

**Acupuncture:** Treatment can help ease the pain and discomfort of arthritis. Acupuncture treatment will more than likely be ongoing since arthritis is a chronic condition. Courses of treatment consist of 12, 30-minute sessions once or twice a week depending on the individual condition. Generally you may expect a reduction in pain and inflammation, and increased mobility.

**Acupressure:** Press the Ba Feng and Ba Xie points, and massage the Yang Lin Qian and Qu Chi points. The Ba Feng point is located on the instep of the foot between the bases of the big and second toes. The four Ba Xie points are located on the back of the hand at the base between each of the fingers. The Yang Ling Quan point is on the outside of the leg in the depression about 2 inches below the knee. The Qu Chi points are about 3 inches to the side of the nostrils in the depression just below the cheekbone.

**Diet:** Traditional Chinese medicine views dampness as one of the major causes of arthritis. Eating green onion, purslane, taro, honey, lychee, squash, and bitter melon are good for reducing dampness and can be combined with herbal remedies and acupuncture to treat arthritis. If arthritis is associated with cold hands and feet or worsens in the wintertime, make a tea by boiling 20 g of cinnamon stick and 30 g of fresh ginger in 2 cups of water. Let the cinnamon and ginger boil until only half the liquid is left, then strain the tea and drink ½ cup twice a day. This formula is not suitable for those who suffer from hot flashes. You can also take 3 oz of hawthorn fruit wine at bedtime to reduce joint pain.

## NATUROPATHY

**Diet:** Dehydration has been linked to arthritis, so drink an 8 oz glass of water every couple of hours to keep your joints lubricated and your body hydrated. Eat foods that are high in essential fatty acids such as salmon, mackerel, and flaxseeds. These have anti-inflammatory properties and the fiber in flaxseeds will help keep your intestines clean. Eat plenty of onions, asparagus, cabbage, and garlic as these foods contain high levels of sulfur, which helps repair cartilage. Avoid non-organic, non-grass-fed meats, fried foods, sugar, dairy, refined carbohydrates, alcohol, and caffeine. Vegetables in the nightshade family, such as tomatoes, eggplant, potatoes, and peppers, contain a substance called solanine that triggers inflammation. Eliminate these foods for three to four weeks and see if you notice any improvement.

**Supplements:** A high-quality multivitamin will provide the proper nourishment to prevent joint damage. Follow the instructions on the container. Glucosamine sulfate, which is usually combined with chondroitin sulfate, reduces joint pain and rebuilds cartilage. Take 1,500 mg daily of glucosamine with 1,200 mg of chondroitin. Take 4,000–8,000 mg of methylsulfonylmethane (MSM) a day; it has natural anti-inflammatory benefits and contains sulfur, an important component of cartilage. Take 4–6 g of fish oil a day to reduce inflammation and lubricate joints, but allow two to three months for the full effects to become noticeable. Niacinamide has been clinically reported to help arthritic patients. It can be taken at 500 mg three times a day, and higher dosages should be supervised by a doctor. Take 250 mg of methionine, a sulfur-containing amino acid (sulfur is important for cartilage structure) that has been shown to have benefits in arthritic patients, four times a day. Take 1–3 g of vitamin C a day; it is beneficial in collagen synthesis repair—a major component of bone. Also take 1–2 capsules of protease enzyme on an empty stomach to reduce inflammation.

**Herbs:** Take 500 mg of bromelain three times a day for its anti-inflammatory effects. Cayenne cream, which depletes the nerves of a neurotransmitter that transmits pain messages to the brain, can be applied to the affected area two to four times a day. White willow relieves pain in the joints. Products should be standardized to contain 240 mg of salicin or 5 ml in tincture form; take this three times a day. Take 1,000 mg of yucca root, which has been traditionally used for arthritic pain, twice a day. Take 1–2 g of ginger, or 2 ml of tincture, three times a day for its anti-inflammatory benefits and pain relief.

**Hydrotherapy:** Soak in a hot bath with epsom salts or mineral salts for at least 20 minutes. The minerals will replenish the body's mineral stores and provide relief.

## HOMEOPATHY

The tips given below may be helpful for relieving the odd, occasional twinge of mild osteoarthritis. Long-term and severe problems that arise as a result of an established case of rheumatoid or osteoarthritis are best treated by an experienced homeopathic practitioner.

**Ledum:** Consider using this remedy to ease pain in the joints that is also relieved by applying cool compresses, or bathing in cool water. Pain tends to move from the feet upwards, and the affected joints may feel cool to the touch and slightly numb with pain.

**Bryonia:** If joints look red and swollen, and get worse as the day goes on but feel less painful while resting, try Bryonia. This is an appropriate remedy if joint pains are related to a low-grade state of toxicity in the system, manifesting itself in the form of constipation and headaches. Jarring movements make the pain more intense, while keeping the affected joint firm and supported relieves the pain and discomfort.

**Apis:** If joints look rosy-pink and puffy, and localized pains are prickling or stinging, try Apis. Acute episodes of pain are likely to flare up quickly and severely, and trigger a restless, fidgety state of mind. Bathing in warm water intensifies the pain, while contact with cool air and cool compresses temporarily soothes and relieves pain.

**TIP: STICK TO AN ANTI-INFLAMMATORY DIET**
Certain foods have a reputation for aggravating inflammation, pain, and stiffness in joints and should be eliminated from the diet, or used in strict moderation. These items include red meat, products made from refined white sugar and flour, citrus fruit, tomatoes, peppers, aubergines, tea, coffee, and alcohol. Also avoid "instant," convenience foods that call for water to be added. These are often a rich source of chemical additives in the form of preservatives and flavorings.

## HERBALISM

 Osteoarthritis treatments that include eliminating food allergies, supplementing deficient vitamins, minerals, and amino acids, stretching and strengthening joints, and herbal approaches tend to be the most successful.

**Counter-irritants:** One interesting approach to decreasing inflammation and pain in a joint is to use a herbal "counter-irritant," which is thought to increase circulation and move toxins from the joint space. Mustard powder, a powerful counter-irritant, is combined with 5–10 parts of corn starch and a small amount of warm water to create a "slurry" or paste that is applied to the affected joint. Smear the mustard paste on a sheet of gauze and cover with a hot pack. Leave the paste on for 15–20 minutes, checking for signs of blistering. Cayenne may also be applied topically for the same effect.

**Devil's claw:** This bitter root is used as medicine to relieve arthritic pain and improve joint mobility. Clinical studies have shown devil's claw to be the most effective when taken in higher doses of 3–6 g of powdered herb or 600–1,200 mg of a 5:1 powdered extract per day. Do not use this herb if you are diagnosed with peptic ulcers or acute gallbladder disease.

**Anti-inflammatory herbs:** Two herbs that are used as gentle, long-term, natural anti-inflammatories are turmeric and Indian frankincense. The powdered rhizome in tumeric inhibits the formation of pro-inflammatory compounds and acts as a strong antioxidant to heal the tissues. Boswellia derives its anti-inflammatory properties from resins, which have been shown clinically to inhibit molecules within the body that promote inflammation and to improve joint circulation. Take 2 ml of a tincture three to four times daily.

# BACK PAIN

## DIAGNOSIS

Back pain or stiffness can be caused by damage to the muscles or nerves. However, it is often difficult to establish the exact cause of the pain, which is why it is often referred to as "non-specific lower back pain." Most back pain is caused by strains or a minor injury rather than something more serious. The pain may start a day or two after an injury occurs, or it may build up gradually over many years, which makes diagnosis even more difficult. The pain often comes on suddenly and is usually triggered by inactivity or a particular movement. Inactivity makes the muscles weak, so that they are not able to support the back properly, making it more vulnerable to damage with certain movements. Usually the problem is due to a strain or tear to the muscles, tendons, or ligaments, which triggers painful muscle tension and spasm. Some of the more common causes of stress and strain on the spine are: poor posture, including slouching in chairs, driving or standing in the wrong position, and hunching over a computer; lifting items incorrectly; sleeping on an old mattress that doesn't give the correct support; being unfit; and generally overdoing it. Even a minor back problem can cause a lot of pain when you stand, bend, or move around. Pain can come on suddenly, or sometimes gradually, but generally lasts just a few days or a week. Persistent back pain can be an indicator of something more major, so you should see a doctor.

## SYMPTOMS

- Pain and stiffness on waking up
- Pain and stiffness at the end of the day
- Pain and stiffness after sitting
- Pain in the buttocks and legs
- Weakness and fatigue

## TREATMENT GOAL

To establish the cause of the back pain and take remedial action. Often the best way to reduce stress and strain on your back is to stay in good physical condition. Exercise can also play a role in treating back pain.

## CONVENTIONAL MEDICINE

Treating back pain involves first diagnosing the cause of the pain. For example, back pain caused by a pulled muscle is treated differently to that caused by a herniated vertebral disc. The goal of treatment is to make sure a serious problem is not present, and to relieve symptoms.

**To treat back pain caused by muscle strain:** This is the most common type of back pain. Treatment may involve ergo-dynamic education (learning how to lift correctly), exercises to strengthen abdominal muscles, and weight loss to decrease strain on back muscles. Massage therapy, heat therapy, and chiropractic adjustments may also be helpful. Muscle relaxation with magnesium aspartate as a nutritional supplement usually helps to relieve muscle spasms, as does valerian root. Medication usually consists of non-steroidal anti-inflammatory drugs (NSAIDs) to help back pain and decrease swelling. Narcotic analgesics can be used in appropriate individuals for 48 hours prior to using NSAIDs. Skeletal muscle relaxants such as cyclobenzaprine (Flexeril®) may be helpful for severe spasm. Local and epidural injections sometimes alleviate chronic back pain.

## TRADITIONAL CHINESE MEDICINE

**Herbs:** In general, you do not have to take herbal medicine for a backache. However, if you have persistent backache and you also experience weakness in your back, along with fatigue, try the following formula: Mix 12 g of Sang Ji Shen (mulberry mistletoe stem), 12 g of Shu Di Huang (Chinese foxglove cooked in wine), 15 g of Niu Xi (achyranthes root), 12 g of Tu Si Zi (Chinese dodder seed), 12 g of Sang Shen Zi (mulberry fruit-spike), 10 g of Shan Zhu Yu (Asiatic cornelian cherry fruit), 12 g of Chuan Xiong (Szechuan lovage root), 12 g of Xu Duan (Japanese teasel root), and 10 g of Du Zhong (eucommia bark). Place the herbs in a ceramic pot, add 3 cups of water, and bring to a boil. Simmer for 30 minutes and then strain the liquid into a container. Drink 1 cup twice a day. These herbs may be purchased from Chinese pharmacies or online.

**Acupuncture:** Treatment can be very effective for back pain. It can help relieve the pain, and also help to treat the cause. A practitioner will first evaluate your back pain and your overall health. Treatment may be given once, twice, or three times a week depending on the severity of the condition. You may feel some initial relief immediately, but it will take a few more sessions to complete treatment for acute back pain. Chronic conditions may need 12–20 sessions to see the maximum results, and to stabilize the condition.

**Acupressure:** Use the base of the palm to press on the back muscles with gentle to medium pressure five times, following the muscle line straight up and down. Also press and massage the Shen Shu, Shang Jiao Shu, and Da Chang Shu points. The Shen Shu points are ½ inch to either side of the back below the second lumbar vertebra (just below the top of the hipbone). The Shang Jiao Shu and Da Chang Shu points are at the same location, just below the first and fourth lumbar vertebrae.

**Dietary therapy:** Eat green onions, purslane, taro, honey, lychees, spearmint, squash, and bittermelon to help with the pain. Cinnamon stick is also good for back pain. Try boiling 20 g of cinnamon stick with 30 g of fresh ginger in 2 cups of water. Boil until only half the liquid is left. Drink 1 cup three times a day. You can also take 30–60 g of hawthorn fruit wine at bedtime for pain management.

**TIP:** USE TUI NA
Tui Na is a Chinese medicine therapy similar to deep-tissue massage and/or chiropractic treatment. It is one of the most effective therapies for back pain. Consult with a well-trained practitioner regarding Tui Na treatment.

## NATUROPATHY

**Diet:** Eat small light meals throughout the day. This will help you keep at a sensible weight and avoid toxic build-up that can aggravate back pain. Eat plenty of fiber to avoid constipation, which may aggravate back pain. Drink at least eight glasses of water a day to keep your body hydrated. This will also help move your bowels more efficiently. Eat plenty of foods high in essential fatty acids for their anti-inflammatory effects. These include walnuts, salmon, mackerel, and ground flaxseeds. Avoid caffeine, alcohol, and refined sugars. They promote inflammation and interfere with weight loss. Green tea or green tea extract though, may help with weight loss.

**Supplements:** A high-quality multivitamin will provide the proper nourishment to prevent joint destruction. Follow the instructions on the container. Take 4,000–8,000 mg of methylsulfonylmethane (MSM) a day for its natural anti-inflammatory properties and ability to reduce pain. Fish oil also reduces inflammation and provides joint lubrication; take 4–6 g a day, but allow two to three months for significant effects to emerge. Take 500 mg of calcium and 250 mg of magnesium a day to alleviate muscle spasm. Also take 1–3 g of vitamin C to strengthen connective tissue, and 1–2 capsules of protease enzyme on an empty stomach to reduce inflammation.

**Herbs:** Take 500 mg of bromelain three times a day for its natural anti-inflammatory effects. Apply cayenne cream to the affected area two to four times a day as it depletes the nerves of a neurotransmitter that transmits pain messages to the brain. Take 1,500–2,500 mg of devil's claw three times a day to help with pain in the joints, but do not take it if you have a history of gallstones, heartburn, or ulcers. Take a white willow product standardized to contain 240 mg of salicin or 5 ml three times a day to relieve pain. Ginger has anti-inflammatory benefits and also relieves pain. Take 1–2 g or 1–2 ml of tincture three times a day.

**Massage:** Find a reputable therapist in your area for a therapeutic massage to help alleviate pain. Try an essential oil mixture that contains arnica oil.

**Hydrotherapy:** Hot water treatments can alleviate pain. Let the hot water hit you in the affected area for 20 minutes. You can also try using a hot water bottle for the same purpose.

## HOMEOPATHY

The following homeopathic remedies may be helpful in easing mild to moderate symptoms of back pain that have developed recently and that are not due to an underlying mechanical cause. The latter type of condition is best treated by other forms of therapy, such as osteopathy, chiropractic therapy, physiotherapy, or surgery, depending on the nature and severity of the problem.

**Gelsemium:** If backache is combined with a heavy, weak sensation in the legs and feelings of unsteadiness, try Gelsemium. Pain and discomfort tends to be most noticeable and distressing at night and moving around after lying still feels very uncomfortable. Damp, cold weather aggravates problems, while gentle, continuous movement may relieve the pain temporarily.

**Hypericum:** This remedy is appropriate for back pain that is more intense when sitting, when pains feel sharp, shooting, and burning. Numbness may follow in the affected area, and the left side may be more affected than the right. Pain may have set in following a fall that has jarred the coccyx at the base of the spine, or at the site of an epidural injection.

**Rhus tox:** If back pain is obviously muscular in nature and pain and stiffness are most intense when resting, use Rhus tox. Pain may be eased by moderate movement, provided it is not overdone. A warm bath or shower also provides temporary relief, while cold, damp conditions aggravate pain and discomfort.

**TIP:** USE THE ALEXANDER TECHNIQUE

If muscle tension and poor postural habits are aggravating or setting off problems with back pain, it may be helpful to have a regular neck, shoulder, and back massage and to consider learning the Alexander Technique. The latter can be an extremely effective way of teaching you good posture and encouraging better postural alignment.

## HERBALISM

Back pain can be very debilitating. Chronic back pain should be evaluated by a doctor to rule out any underlying serious structural abnormalities. See the section on muscle pains for further remedies (p. 671).

**Arnica:** Begin treatment by applying topical arnica to the affected area in gel or lotion form. Arnica is specific for trauma or injury to skin, muscles, tendons, and ligaments, and acts as an anti-inflammatory and circulatory stimulant with mild analgesic properties. Arnica is very safe when used topically; however, using it internally or on an open wound is potentially toxic and must be supervised by a qualified practitioner.

**Essential oils:** These oils are a wonderful way to alleviate muscle spasms and strain, while soothing the senses and relieving pain. Wintergreen and peppermint contain volatile oils that act as analgesics and counter-irritants when placed on the skin. Add 5 drops of each to a ½ tsp of olive or massage oil and apply it to the affected area. Combine these oils with alternating hot and cold towels.

**TIP:** CREATE A PAIN-RELIEVING TINCTURE

Combine herbs that sedate and soothe with herbs that relieve muscle spasms and improve circulation to the area. When the muscles in the back are injured, they tend to swell and begin "guarding" against any further movement, leading to pain and stiffness. Both valerian and passionflower are wonderful examples of herbs that relieve the anxiety and muscle spasm that can accompany back pain. These can be puchased as tinctures (either alcohol or glycerin-based) and combined in equal parts. Take a dropperful of the combination twice or three times daily while the back pain is acute and severe. The passionflower slightly tempers valerian's strong taste. Consult a medical herbalist for other treatment ideas; for example, some people use kava kava to treat cases of back pain, but this should only be taken under strict medical supervision.

# BUNIONS

## DIAGNOSIS

Bunions are one of the most common foot problems. A bunion is a firm bump that appears at the side of the foot by the base of the big toe as a rounded, bony protuberance. This causes the big toe to move towards the smaller toes and, over a period of time, the big toe may even come to rest under the second toe. As the bony protrusion rubs against the shoe, the skin reddens, swells, and becomes painful. The pain may become so severe that it causes the sufferer to limp. Bunions tend to be more common in women than men as women wear high heels, pointy-toed shoes, and other fashionable items of footwear that can manipulate the shape of the foot over time. The complaint also tends to affect more people as they get older, especially if they suffer from arthritis. This condition can lead to a variety of different soft tissue and bone complaints, as well as being distressing and painful to endure on a daily basis. There are various products on the market, such as pads and inserts, to ease discomfort by protecting the bunion. Medication is sometimes needed to help deal with pain and swelling. The patient's foot may become too wide to fit into her normal size shoe, and eventually, bunions may make wearing any shoes difficult. If everything else has failed, a bunionectomy may be necessary, where the bone in the foot is cut and straightened. Walking is difficult for several weeks after surgery.

## SYMPTOMS

- Redness
- Swelling
- Pain and discomfort
- Hammer toe (where the toes curl over like claws) in the second toe
- Corns develop where the skin rubs against shoes

## TREATMENT GOAL

Bunions can be embarrassing, painful, and hard to treat. Conventional and alternative therapies find ways of managing the pain associated with bunions, which includes choosing the most beneficial footwear.

## CONVENTIONAL MEDICINE

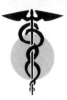

Bunions are often accompanied by Hallux valgus, a deviation of the large toe, and often the other toes bend toward the outside of the foot. They can be treated conservatively, but generally the only way of correcting them is through surgery.

**Apply ice:** Ice can be applied to the affected area to relieve pain. Place ice on the area for 20–25 minutes (or as long as can be tolerated) every couple of hours. After two days, alternate treatment with hot and cold applications. Apply hot towels for three minutes and a cold pack for 30 seconds for three cycles every one to two hours.

**Insoles:** A bunion should be treated as early as possible, since it gets progressively more debilitating as you get older. Initially orthotics (insoles and supports) are recommended, along with footwear that has adequate depth and width.

**Surgery:** A bunionectomy is needed to correct bunions that get progressively worse. It is a relatively well-tolerated surgery in younger people, and it is easily performed under local anesthetic. It is not necessary to use crutches or casts, or be admitted to a hospital as an outpatient.

## TRADITIONAL CHINESE MEDICINE

**Herbs:**
• External formula: Mix 12 g of Chi Shao (red peony root), 12 g of Niu Xi (achyranthes root), 1 g of Xuan Shen (ningpo figwort root), 12 g of Tao Ren (peach kernel), and 10 g of Hong Hua (safflower flower) in a ceramic or glass pot. Add 3 cups of water and bring the mixture to a boil. Simmer for 30 minutes and strain the liquid. Soak your feet for 20–30 minutes once a day for 7–10 consecutive days.
• Zhen Huong Hua: This medicinal oil can be applied to bunions twice a day to help with the pain, and may also reduce swelling.

**Acupuncture:** Treatment may help to reduce the pain and swelling of joints. Consult a practitioner about whether acupuncture will be beneficial for you.

**Acupressure:** Massage the bunion and/or press the Tai Chong and Gong Shun points to increase local circulation. The Tai Chong point is on the instep of the foot in the depression between the first and second toe at the base of the large toe. The Gong Shun point is on the inside of the foot in the depression behind the large toe. In a sitting position, press on each of these points for one minute and repeat two to three times a day.

**Diet:** There is no specific diet to treat bunions, but as a rule of good health eat a well balanced diet with fresh vegetables, fruits, and grains. Also include plenty of liquid in your daily diet.

## NATUROPATHY

 **Diet:** Base your meals on whole grains, fresh vegetables and fruits, and beans to help control inflammation. If you are intolerant or allergic to grains, pain and inflammation may increase, in which case exclude them from your diet. Avoid refined sugars and hydrogenated oils, which increase inflammation.

**Supplements:** A high-quality multivitamin will provide the proper nourishment to encourage tissue healing. Follow the instructions on the bottle. Take 4–6 g of fish oil a day to reduce inflammation and lubricate the joints, but allow two to three months to see the effects. Take 25,000 IU of vitamin A a day for four to six weeks as it has been shown to help soothe bunions.

**Herbs:** Take 500 mg of bromelain three times a day for its natural anti-inflammatory effects. Also take white willow to relieve pain. The product should be standardized to contain 240 mg of salicin or take 5 ml of tincture three times a day. Take 1–2 g of ginger or 1–2 ml of tincture three times a day for its anti-inflammatory benefits and to relieve pain. You can also try soaking the feet in water for ½ hour at night then rub them with St. John's Wort oil. This herb is used to treat pain.

**Prolotherapy injection:** This type of therapy strengthens the weakened ligaments that have caused the bone movement and bone overgrowth. It will not eliminate the toe deformity associated with this condition, but it will eliminate the pain. See a registered practitioner who specializes in giving such injections.

**TIP:** WEAR APPROPRIATE FOOTWEAR
Wear comfortable shoes that do not push your toes together. This is one of the main ways to prevent and treat bunions. You should also rest and elevate the foot as much as possible and refrain from any activity that regularly stresses the foot.

## HOMEOPATHY

Severe bunions tend to need corrective surgery. The following homeopathic remedies can be used pre-and post-operatively to speed up recovery.

**Arnica:** This remedy can be taken internally the day before surgery and for three days following the operation to help ease localized swelling, bruising, and tenderness. Arnica also has an important role in helping the body recover from the physical and psychological trauma that goes along with surgery.

**Hypericum:** As a follow-up treatment to arnica, Hypericum can ease shooting pains and tenderness in the affected area. Pain tends to be much worse when the foot is moved or knocked suddenly.

**Phosphorus:** If there is severe nausea and/or vomiting following surgery in response to an anesthetic, use Phosphorus. Key symptoms include a craving for very cold water, which is usually vomited up once it is warmed by the stomach.

## HERBALISM

Although herbal remedies may help to decrease the swelling of the bunion, surgical correction of the problem is the only cure. Below are some topical treatments that may ease symptoms.

**Essential oils:** Topical anti-inflammatories and analgesics are very helpful at relieving symptoms. Blend together wintergreen, peppermint, camphor, and rue essential oils in combination with arnica gel to create a topical pain reliever. Apply it to the affected area as needed.

**Castor oil:** This oil has been shown to work wonders at decreasing inflammation, healing tissue, and relieving pain. Place 5–10 ml on a washcloth and cover with plastic wrap, such as Saran™ wrap. Cover the wrap with hot towels or a heated clay pack. Replenish the heated towels as necessary to keep the area warm and leave on for 30–45 minutes. Repeat three times daily.

# BURSITIS

## DIAGNOSIS

Bursitis is defined as inflammation of a bursa. Bursas are enclosed, round sacs filled with viscous fluid, located between the bone and the muscle tendons or between skin and tendons. They help cushion the tendon and prevent friction between it and the bone to allow increased range of motion. However, if the tendon is constantly rubbing against the bone in a repetitive motion, the friction can cause the bursa itself to become irritated and inflamed, leading to bursitis. The most commonly affected areas are the elbow, shoulder, hip, knee, ankle, and heel. Symptoms of bursitis are a deep ache at the site of the bursa and local tenderness, warmth, and swelling. Bursitis is commonly associated with rheumatoid arthritis and osteoarthritis, gout, and occupational or sports injuries. For example, a person who repeatedly throws a ball in the same position may begin to develop bursitis in the shoulder or elbow because of the repetitive friction. Bursitis may also develop when the bursa is compressed on a regular basis, for example, when a person sleeps on his or her side, placing a lot of pressure on the shoulder at night. In such cases it only takes a small amount of movement around this already compressed area to cause friction of the bursa.

## SYMPTOMS

- Achy pain and stiffness in the joint
- Burning sensation that surrounds the whole joint around the inflamed bursa
- Localized tenderness
- Pain is usually worse during and after activity
- Bursa and surrounding joint area can become stiffer the following day

## TREATMENT GOAL

Treatment aims to reduce the swelling and pain. It is also important to identify what is causing the condition and avoid any activities or movements that may be triggers.

## CONVENTIONAL MEDICINE

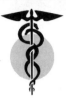

**Diet, supplements, and herbs:** Overweight people who suffer from bursitis should begin a weight-loss program to help relive the pressure and friction on the joints. Supplements such as 4 g of fish oil a day can decrease inflammation, as can anti-inflammatory herbs such as ginger and curcumin.

**Hot and cold compresses:** The initial treatment for bursitis is to apply ice to the affected area for the first two days after the injury, and then to apply heat thereafter. Both ice and heat should be applied for 20 minutes three times a day.

**Physical therapy:** It is important to avoid the activity that triggered the pain. However, do not refrain from all physical activity but instead try to increase your range of motion by performing stretching exercises under the guidance of a physical therapist. Water therapy may also be helpful.

**Medication:** Non-steroidal anti-inflammatory drugs (NSAIDs) are generally used to treat this condition. Lidocaine and methylprednisolone injections into the joint are another treatment method.

**Phonophoresis:** A technique called phonophoresis, which uses ultrasound to enhance the delivery of topically applied drugs and topical corticosteroids may be helpful.

**Surgery:** Surgery is available for severe cases that do not respond to medication. Calcifications in the joint are removed, or the bursa is cleaned out through arthroscopic, or "key-hole," surgery.

## TRADITIONAL CHINESE MEDICINE

**Herbs:** The following formula may help to reduce the inflammation and relieve the pain of bursitis. These herbs needed are available from Chinese pharmacies or online. Combine 12 g of Du Huo (pubescent angelica root), 12 g of Sang Ji Shen (mulberry mistletoe stem), 12 g of Ji Xue Teng (millettia root), 10 g of Huang Bai (phellodendron), 12 g of Chi Shao (red peony root), 10 g of Chuan Xiong (Szechuan lovage root), and 10 g of Gui Zhi (cinnamon) in a ceramic pot. Make a decoction by adding 3 cups of water and bringing the mixture to a boil. Simmer for 30 minutes, strain the liquid, and drink 1 cup twice a day.

**Acupuncture:** You may need acupuncture once or twice a week to treat bursitis. The number of sessions will vary depending on the severity of the condition.

**Acupressure:** Using the tip of the finger or thumb, press the Jian Yu, Jian Qian, and Jian Zhen points, or the three shoulder points, for one minute and then release and repeat. The Jian Yu point is on the shoulder in the depression where the scapula (shoulder) and the humerus (top of the arm) bones meet. The Jian Qian point is on the front of the shoulder, about 1 inch above the armpit. The Jian Zhen point is on the back of the shoulder, about 1 inch above the armpit.

**Diet:** Eat green onions, purslane, taro, honey, lychees, spearmint, squash, and bitter gourds to help ease the pain. You can also drink 30–60 g of hawthorn fruit wine at bedtime for pain management. These should be available from Chinese pharmacies or Asian grocery stores.

## NATUROPATHY

**Diet:** Eat an anti-inflammatory diet, avoiding refined sugars, hydrogenated oils and gluten. Salmon, walnuts, and mackerel have high levels of essential fatty acids, which have anti-inflammatory properties.

**Supplements:** A high-quality multivitamin will provide the proper nourishment to encourage tissue healing. Follow the instructions on the label. Take 4–6 g of fish oil to reduce inflammation and provide joint lubrication. Allow two to three months to see the benefits. Take 1–3 g of vitamin C a day to strengthen connective tissue and build the immune system. Protease enzyme reduces inflammation; take 1–2 capsules on an empty stomach.

**Herbs:** Bromelain has natural anti-inflammatory effects. Take 500 mg three times a day. Take a white willow product that is standardized to contain 240 mg of salicin, or 5 ml of a tincture, three times a day to relieve pain. Ginger has anti-inflammatory benefits and also relieves pain. Take 1–2 g or 1–2 ml of a tincture three times a day.

## HOMEOPATHY

Minor, recently developing problems with bursitis may respond to the most appropriately selected of the following homeopathic remedies. Any of these remedies can be used safely side-by-side with conventional treatment.

**Belladonna:** Use this remedy to treat inflammation in its earliest stages when heat, swelling, and redness are likely to be noticeable. Pain and discomfort is more intense following jarring movements.

**Apis:** If stinging pains and puffy, pink swelling emerge quickly and distressingly, try Apis. Pain becomes more aggravated and distressing following contact with heat in any form, and is temporarily relieved by contact with cool items.

**Rhus tox:** To treat pain that is tearing in nature, and that is more distressing when lying in bed at night, causing lots of restlessness in an effort to get comfortable, try Rhus tox. Applying heat locally feels soothing, as does gentle exercise for short periods of time.

**Bryonia:** Consider this remedy if pain is noticeably worse following the slightest movement and is eased by rest.

## HERBALISM

 **Apply ice:** Ice can be applied to the affected area to relieve pain, especially during the first 24–48 hours. Place ice on the area for 20–25 minutes (or as long as can be tolerated) every couple of hours. After two days, alternate treatment with hot and cold applications. Apply hot towels for three minutes and a cold pack for 30 seconds for three cycles every one to two hours.

**Essential oils:** Topical anti-inflammatories and analgesics are very helpful at relieving symptoms, and promote greater movement of the joint. Blend together wintergreen, peppermint, camphor, and rue essential oils in combination with arnica gel to create a topical pain reliever. Apply it to the affected area as needed.

**Castor oil:** This oil has been shown to work wonders at decreasing inflammation, healing tissue, and relieving pain. Place 5–10 ml on a washcloth and cover with Saran™ wrap. Cover the wrap with hot towels or a heated clay pack. Replenish the heated towels as necessary to keep the area warm and leave on for 30–45 minutes. Repeat three times daily.

**Comfrey:** This herb can be used topically to relieve pain and heal tissue. It is cooling and moisturizing, and acts as a mild analgesic and potent anti-inflammatory. It can be used to heal trauma to the bones, arthritis, bruises, tendonitis, and bursitis. Create a poultice of fresh or moistened roots and leaves by mashing them into a paste (add water if needed). Place the poultice (or paste) on the affected area.

**TIP:** STRETCH
A good stretching motion for stiff shoulder joints is called the cat stretch. Get down on your hands and knees, hands slightly forward of your head. Keep your elbows stiff as you stretch backward and come down on your heels.

# CARPAL TUNNEL SYNDROME

## DIAGNOSIS

Carpal tunnel syndrome (CTS) is triggered when pressure is applied to the median nerve located in the wrist, causing tingling, burning, and aching in the fingers. This nerve transmits impulses that allow feeling in the fingers. Along with nine flexor tendons, the median nerve passes through a narrow channel known as the carpal tunnel and it is in this bottleneck that problems can arise. A rise in pressure in the carpal tunnel, for whatever reason, leads to pressure on the median nerve that interrupts the blood flow, causing the malfunction of the nerve. Compression of the median nerve can also occur in the forearm just below the elbow. This is known as pronator teres syndrome and has symptoms similar but not identical to CTS. CTS can develop as a response to a repetitive manual activity, such as typing at a computer keyboard, or it can accompany conditions such as rheumatoid arthritis. Hypothyroidism and diabetes can also predispose patients to symptoms. The cessation of the trigger activity usually results in the rapid resolution of symptoms.

## SYMPTOMS

- Deep, dull throbbing pain, localized in the wrist and hand
- Occasionally, the pain radiates up along the arm and even to the shoulder
- Numbness and tingling
- Sensory symptoms often develop at night, causing loss of sleep
- Inability to "pinch grip"
- Difficulty manipulating or maneuvering objects, such as picking up a cup

## TREATMENT GOAL

To eliminate the physical cause of the condition, for example by changing the way simple manual tasks are carried out, and to prevent any further deterioration. If a medical cause is suspected, appropriate screening tests are carried out.

## CONVENTIONAL MEDICINE

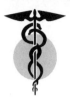

**Rest:** Try to minimize any factors that contribute to the condition, such as repetitive motion. This may require a temporary rest. A wrist splint can also be used to inhibit movement that aggravates the condition. It is also helpful to examine how a trigger activity is carried out, and to try using a different angle of wrist flexion and extension as a preventive measure.

**Diet and supplements:** An anti-inflammatory diet that excludes dairy and gluten may be helpful. Also try to include a high-dose fish oil, ginger, curcumin, and turmeric in your diet. Decreased vitamin B6 levels have been associated with CTS, and vitamin B6 and B12 supplements are recommended.

**Medication:** Non-steroidal anti-inflammatory drugs (NSAIDs) such as ibuprofen, diclofenac, or naproxen can be used to relieve pressure and pain. A local injection of steroids is another therapy that often has successful results.

**Surgery:** Surgical therapy includes decompressing the inflamed nerve by sectioning the flexor tendon. The flexor tendon is separated from the nerve tunnel to make more room and thereby relieve pressure in the area. This is now frequently done by endoscope, which is a less invasive procedure.

## TRADITIONAL CHINESE MEDICINE

**Herbs:** In general, herbs are not taken internally for this condition, but you can try applying some Chinese medicinal ointments topically to the affected area. For example, Wan Hua oil, available from Chinese pharmacies or online, can be applied to the wrist two to three times a day. It helps relieve pain and may reduce inflammation.

**Acupuncture:** Treatment can relieve the pain and discomfort of CTS and help with the healing process. Sessions will last 30 minutes and you may need treatment once or twice a week.

**Acupressure:** Press and knead the Yang Chi and Yang Xi points with the thumb. The Yang Chi point is on the back of the hand at the crease of the wrist in the depression on the ulna (the bone of the outer forearm) side of the tendon. Press and knead in the direction of the ulna. The Yang Xi point is on the edge the wrist below the thumb. When the thumb is tilted upward, it is in the depression between the tendons.

**Diet:** Green onion, purslane, taro, honey, lychee, spearmint, squash, and bitter gourd can help to manage the pain. A healthy diet of fresh fruits, vegetables, and grains is also recommended.

## NATUROPATHY

**Diet:** To combat fluid retention, drink 1 glass of water every couple of hours. Eat foods that are high in vitamin B6, including beans, brewer's yeast, green leafy vegetables, and wheat germ. Eliminate sources of sodium, which contribute to fluid retention and aggravate symptoms.

**Supplements:** A high-quality multivitamin will provide the proper nourishment to encourage tissue healing. Follow the instructions on the pack. Vitamin B6 has been shown in studies to reduce nerve inflammation. Take 100 mg three times a day. A calcium and magnesium combination reduces nerve irritation and muscle tightness. Take 500 mg of calcium and 250 mg of magnesium.

**Herbs:** Take 500 mg of bromelain three times a day for its natural anti-inflammatory effect. Take a white willow product that is standardized to include 240 mg of salicin, or take 5 ml of a tincture, three times a day to relieve pain. Also take 1–2 g of ginger, or 1–2 ml of tincture, three times a day for its anti-inflammatory benefits and ability to relieve pain. Ginkgo biloba, taken at 120 mg twice a day, can help improve circulation. Make sure the product is 24% flavone glycosides.

**Hydrotherapy:** Hot and cold water can be used to improve blood flow and provide pain relief. Submerge the affected hand and wrist in hot water for 3 minutes then in cold for 30 seconds. Repeat this sequence three times.

**TIP:** TAKE BREAKS FROM REPETITIVE ACTIONS
When working on a computer, take breaks every 30–60 minutes. Also use a wrist rest when typing.

## HOMEOPATHY

The following homeopathic remedies, when used appropriately, can be very effective in treating mild or intermittent symptoms of carpal tunnel syndrome. However, if symptoms begin recurring, or become permanent, consult an experienced homeopathic practitioner for advice and treatment.

**Aconite:** Use this remedy to relieve pain, discomfort, and tingling sensations that are especially noticeable at night. Symptoms may be severe enough to wake the sufferer, and trigger distress, restlessness, and anxiety.

**Arnica:** If there is a sense of bruising and pain, as well as localized soreness and/or cramping, consider using Arnica. This remedy is especially helpful for easing recent flare-ups of pain and tenderness that have been triggered by overuse, injury, or trauma.

**Ruta:** If Arnica is initially helpful in easing the symptoms described above, but the benefits are not sustained, use Ruta. Symptoms include a sensation of lameness, stiffness, and pain that is troublesome even when resting the affected area.

**Rhus tox:** If stiffness and pain is aggravated by initial movement, but eased by moderate exercise, try Rhus tox. Symptoms become more intense following contact with damp and cold, and over-exertion. There is also likely to be a strong sensation of weakness in the arms and wrists, and discomfort causes restlessness when trying to sleep at night.

## HERBALISM

 Carpal tunnel syndrome is traditionally treated by splinting the wrist, stretching the hands and wrists, manipulating the carpal bones in the hand, or surgery. Herbal medicines can be used to alleviate swelling and pain.

**Hot and cold compresses:** Hot water promotes circulation, which brings needed healing nutrients to the affected area. Cold water flushes out excess fluid and toxic metabolites created by inflammation. Apply a hot compress to the area for three minutes, followed by a cold compress for 30–45 seconds. Repeat, and always finish with a cold compress. For increased anti-inflammatory action, rub a few drops of menthol, wintergreen, peppermint, and arnica oils onto the area.

**Camphor oil:** This oil is very fragrant and cool to the touch. Camphor acts locally as a counter-irritant and numbs sensation, thereby relieving pain. It is safe when used in the short term in low concentrations of 0.1–11% on unbroken skin.

**Castor oil:** Place 5–10 ml of castor oil onto a washcloth and wrap this around the wrist. Cover the cloth with a thin plastic wrap and place a heated towel over the area for 20–30 minutes. This can help to relieve the pain.

# CHRONIC FATIGUE SYNDROME

## DIAGNOSIS

Chronic fatigue syndrome (CFS) is a condition characterized by profound and severe muscle fatigue. An overwhelming feeling of exhaustion tends to come on suddenly following any form of physical exertion, and is accompanied by problems with memory and concentration. It is an illness that cuts across all classes of society, and it is twice as common in women as men. Children as young as seven years old have been affected. It most commonly develops in those in their early 20s to mid-40s. Many people who feel "tired all the time" consult a doctor regarding CFS, but only a small percentage of these actually have the condition. Illnesses that mimic CFS include anemia, celiac disease, liver disease, lupus, low thyroid function, and multiple sclerosis. Although the basic underlying cause remains uncertain, research suggests that CFS is triggered by a combination of factors, including a genetic susceptibility and repeated infections, particularly of a flu virus.

## SYMPTOMS

- Muscle pain
- Aching joints
- Ongoing flu-like feelings
- Severe headaches
- Waking up still feeling tired
- Sore throat and enlarged glands
- Sensitivity to heat and cold
- Alcohol intolerance
- Low blood pressure
- Sensitivity to bright light and loud noise
- Depression

## TREATMENT GOAL

Although there is no cure at present, a number of drugs are being assessed to treat CFS. The most helpful method of managing this condition involves "pacing," where levels of physical and mental activity are carefully balanced to reflect the stage and severity of the illness. Conventional and alternative therapies look at making lifestyle adjustments, as well as ways of easing symptoms, to reduce the chances of long-term ill health and improve the quality of life.

## CONVENTIONAL MEDICINE

**Medication:** There are several medications that may be used to treat CFS, including antidepressants, non-steroidal anti-inflammatory drugs (NSAIDs) for pain, and triazolopyridine antidepressants such as trazodone for sleep.

**Lifestyle changes:** A low to moderate amount of daily exercise such as graded aerobic exercise is recommended. Performing T'ai chi daily has been shown to be helpful and craniosacral chiropractic techniques (which involve massaging the skull), therapeutic touch, massage, and yoga may also be beneficial. Stress reduction techniques such as meditation are also highly recommended. Support groups and behavioral therapy are often helpful as well.

**Diet and supplements:** Evaluating and optimizing the adrenal and nutritional status of the body should be part of treatment. Eat whole grains, fruits, vegetables, and lean meats, and avoid processed foods to optimize energy. Supplements such as coenzyme Q10 (CoQ10) may be considered, as they also increase energy in the cells. Adequate B vitamins are also essential.

## TRADITIONAL CHINESE MEDICINE

**Herbs:** The herbs needed to make the formulas below are available from Chinese pharmacies or online. For either formula, make a decoction by placing the ingredients in a ceramic or glass pot and adding 4 cups of water. Bring the mixture to a boil and simmer for 30 minutes. Strain the liquid and drink 1 cup two or three times a day.

• To treat fatigue due to Qi deficiency: Symptoms include tiredness, lethargy, poor appetite, and/or loose stools. Combine 12 g of Dan Shen (salvia root), 12 g of Bai Zhu (white atractylodes rhizome), 15 g of Fuling (poria), 15 g of Shan Yao (Chinese yam), 15 g of Huang Jing (Siberian Solomon's seal rhizome), 6 g of Chen Pi (tangerine peel), and 3 g of Gan Cao (licorice).

• To treat fatigue due to blood deficiency: Symptoms include tiredness, a poor memory, lightheadedness, insomnia, or feeling overly sleepy. Combine 12 g of Shu Di Huang (Chinese foxglove cooked in wine), 12 g of Shan Zhu Yu (Asiatic cornelian cherry), 15 g of Shan Yao (Chinese yam), 15 g of Dan Shen (salvia root), 15 g of Niu Xi (achyranthes root), and 12 g of Dang Gui (Chinese angelica root).

**Acupuncture:** Treatment may be administered once or twice a week for a few months or much longer depending on the particular symptoms and causes. The condition should first be evaluated by a practitioner, as determining the underlying causes is at the core of traditional Chinese medicine.

**Acupressure:** The Susanli point is on the lower leg in the depression 4 inches below and 1 inch to the outside of the knee. Press this point using the tip of the finger for about one minute and repeat. The Bai Hui point is on the top of the head at the midpoint of the line running up and over the head from ear to ear. The Guan Yuan point is in the middle of the abdomen, about 2 inches below the navel. Press these points using medium pressure.

**Diet:** Eat food that tonifies blood and Qi and food that nourishes the spleen and lungs. Such foods include black soybean, peach, chestnut, sweet basil, coriander, beef, polished rice, potato, string bean, sweet potato, carrot, grape, and leek.

---

**TIP:** TRY TO EXERCISE

Exercise helps CFS patients get stronger in some cases. However, most fatigue patients do not have the energy to exercise, are not motivated, or feel more tired after exercising. In any case, it is important to know what exercises are adequate and suitable for you. You may try walking or gentle movement like T'ai chi. However, if you feel tired, do not push yourself.

---

## NATUROPATHY

**Diet:** Try following a detoxification and cleansing diet for one to three weeks. This involves avoiding all foods and chemicals that may make symptoms worse, and instead eat a diet of dense nutrients. Eat plenty of sea vegetables and gluten-free grains such as brown rice, millet, and quinoa, and fresh vegetables. Seeds, nuts, and fresh fish are also beneficial. Wheat, dairy, corn, gluten-containing products, sugar, and fermented foods are some of the most common allergens. After three weeks re-introduce the foods into the diet one at a time to identify any triggers. For CFS patients with candidiasis, all types of sugar, including milk products and fruit, should be avoided, as should caffeine, alcohol, and refined carbohydrates such as white flour and white rice. Caffeine depresses the adrenal glands, which secrete the hormones needed for energy. Also avoid refined sugar, which may cause hypoglycemia and induce fatigue.

**Supplements:** Probiotics can greatly improve digestion and reestablish a healthy balance in the intestines. A typical dose is one to two capsules two to three times per day, taken on an empty stomach. Make sure there are at least 4 billion healthy organisms in the formula. Digestive enzymes can supply your body with additional enzymes to digest fats, proteins, and carbohydrates. Products differ greatly—some contain lactase to digest milk, others contain hydrochloric acid to assist the stomach, and still others contain ox bile to help with and still others contain ox bile to help with the emulsification and digestion of fats. A typical dosage is one to two capsules with meals. Vitamin C helps the immune system, is required for healthy adrenal gland function, and helps with liver detoxification; take 3 g throughout the day. Magnesium is involved in more than 300 enzyme reactions in the body and is essential for energy production, muscle function, nerve conduction, and bone health. People with chronic fatigue syndrome often have a deficiency in magnesium and should take 250 mg three times a day. CoQ10 is necessary for energy production and cell function. It also helps with the repair and maintenance of tissues. A typical dose is 60–100 mg daily. Nicotinamide Adenine Dinucleotide (NADH) is a naturally occurring chemical that plays a significant role in cellular energy production. Take 10 mg a day on an empty stomach. Also take 500 mg of L-Carnitine three times a day; it is used by the body to convert fatty acids into energy.

**Herbs:** Those with CFS often have adrenal fatigue or weakness. Licorice can tonify the adrenal glands are as it works to increase levels of cortisol in the body. Take 1,000 mg two to three times daily, and take the de-glycyrrhizinated form if you suffer from high blood pressure. Ginkgo biloba improves circulation and improves memory. Take 60–120 mg twice a day of a standardized product containing flavone glycosides and 6% terpene lactones.

## HOMEOPATHY

This condition demands attention and treatment from an experienced homeopath due to its chronic and complex nature, and its potentially severe symptoms. If the patient's energy levels are severely depleted, choosing the appropriate strength remedy and dosage can be difficult, and is best left in the hands of a trained practitioner. The advice below offers some guidelines on how best to support homeopathic remedies with lifestyle changes.

**Pace yourself:** One of the most important things to bear in mind is not to overdo things on days when you do feel better, as this can trigger a relapse. Instead pace yourself, and stop after achieving about 50% of what you would ideally like to do. As frustrating as this may be, it will give you the best chance of building on your recovery.

**Gentle exercise:** Once your physical strength has shown signs of steadily building and increasing, it can be helpful to engage in some gentle yoga to encourage energy levels to improve, while also having a potentially beneficial effect on the immune system. Consult an experienced practitioner who will be able to tailor his or her advice to your individual situation.

## HERBALISM

Herbal medicines are used to treat CFS to support the adrenals, thereby reducing fatigue, and to modulate the immune system to bring it back into a normal state.

**Licorice:** One theory used to explain fatigue associated with CFS is that adrenal depletion from excessive daily stress leads to lower levels of cortisol, the body's natural anti-inflammatory. A compound in licorice called glycyrrhetinic acid prolongs the life of natural cortisol by inhibiting its breakdown. Licorice is also high in flavonoids, which are potent antioxidants that protect and strengthen tissues, making the body more resistant to infection. Take 2–4 ml of 1:1 tincture of licorice per day. Licorice used in the long-term may cause high blood pressure, so make sure your blood pressure is monitored regularly.

**Bupleurum:** This herb is an antiviral, and a liver and adrenal tonic. It is often used in combination with licorice to treat fatigue. Combine the two herbs to create an adrenal tonic blend.

**Astragalus root:** This herb has been used in Chinese medicine for centuries. It is considered to be a potent herb that tonifies the Qi (life energy) and is nutritive to the life force and body, hence its use in treating fatigue. Current research has shown astragalus to be effective for long-term use in the prevention of infection by supporting the immune system. Active constituents called saponins stimulate immune cells, including NK cells, which are depleted in CFS. Astragalus also demonstrates adaptogenic, diuretic, hypotensive, and antioxidant properties. Boil 10–30 g of dried root in water and drink the decoction daily. Astragalus is safe to use long term, but should not be used during acute infections.

# FACIAL PAIN

## DIAGNOSIS

There are a number of different types of facial pain. Some are severe and persistent, while others are mild and occasional. The pain can be intermittent or continuous, of varying intensity, and can last for years. It may affect a small area of the face, but it can also spread across the whole of the face and mouth. This type of pain is often described as nagging, throbbing, and aching. Facial pain can be triggered by many conditions, but the most common causes are sinusitis, ear infection, dental problems such as an abscess or toothache, headache, herpes (shingles), mumps, and trigeminal neuralgia (severe stabbing pains, often in the lips, gums, or cheeks). Pain in the ear region may be linked to the skin, teeth, tonsils, pharynx, larynx, or neck. Tenderness around the jawbone area may be due to sinusitis, a dental abscess, or a tumor. Facial pain can be precipitated by a specific injury, chewing food, or, on occasion, even the slightest touch to the skin. The condition has also been linked to stress, and it is often associated with pains in other parts of the body, such as irritable bowel syndrome and itchy skin. As a consequence of the pain, many people with this condition are affected by anxiety and depression.

Many types of facial pain can be controlled with medication, but occasionally no cause can be found and the pain does not respond to painkillers. For those affected by conditions such as trigeminal neuralgia, where drug treatment proves ineffective surgery can provide relief. Long-term facial pain should always be investigated by a doctor.

## SYMPTOMS

- Pain, often in the region of the ear
- Tenderness over the jawbone
- Sharp, severe stabbing pain
- Dull, aching pain
- Pain can be intermittent or continuous
- The whole face or part of the face can be affected

## TREATMENT GOAL

Conventional and complementary therapies aim to establish the cause of the pain and treat it accordingly. Pain management is important, as facial pain can be extremely debilitating.

## CONVENTIONAL MEDICINE

**Identify the cause:** Conventional treatment of facial pain is dependent on the cause. Facial pain is a common symptom of a condition called trigeminal neuralgia, which produces excruciating, lightning strikes of facial pain, typically near the nose, lips, eyes, or ears. It is a disorder of the trigeminal nerve, which is the fifth and largest cranial nerve, but may also accompany sinusitis, tooth infection, ear infection, headache, herpes, temporomandibular joint (TMJ) pain and, more rarely, a tumor. It is necessary to carry out tests to exclude tumors and infection. If an infection is causing the pain, this is treated accordingly. If herpes is the source of the pain, this is treated by suppressing the virus.

**Modify your lifestyle:** Make an effort to avoid any potential triggers of the pain, including extremely hot or cold water or environments, or facial stimulation such as shaving.

**To treat trigeminal neuralgia:** Medication prescribed to treat this kind of facial pain includes Tegretol®, Neurontin®, and muscle relaxants such as baclofen. If medication proves unsuccessful, a procedure known as stereotactic radiosurgery may be performed to destroy the trigeminal nerve and thus terminate the pain. Other techniques such as percutaneous radiofrequency, which uses a heated electrode to cause a thermal lesion in the nerve, are also helpful.

## TRADITIONAL CHINESE MEDICINE

**Herbs:** In general, there are no specific herbs that treat facial pain. However, you may see a doctor of traditional Chinese medicine for advice on which herbs may help your specific condition.

**Acupuncture:** Acupuncture can be used to treat both the symptoms and root cause of facial pain. Acupuncture is also commonly used for trigeminal neuralgia, and can relieve sharp pain. Consult with a doctor of traditional Chinese medicine regarding a specific diagnosis and treatment plan. One course of treatment consists of 12 acupuncture sessions, and you will usually need acupuncture once or twice a week.

**Acupressure:** The Xia Guan and Quan Liao points can be used to relieve facial pain. The Xia Guan point is located in front of the ear in the depression above the jaw. The Quan Liao point is about 3 inches away from the nostril in the depression just below the cheekbone. Apply medium pressure to these points with the tip of the finger.

**Dietary therapy:** A healthy, well-balanced diet of fresh fruit, vegetables, and grains is always a good practice, but specifically add green onion, purslane, taro, honey, lychee, spearmint, squash, and bitter gourd to ease the pain.

## NATUROPATHY

 **Diet:** Eat an anti-inflammatory diet, avoiding refined sugars, hydrogenated oils, and glutens. Gluten is a protein found in some grains, especially wheat, that has been shown to be an allergen that causes inflammation. Salmon, mackerel, and walnuts have high levels of essential fatty acids (EFAs), which have anti-inflammatory properties. Flaxseed also has high levels of EFAs and also contains high amounts of fiber. Sprinkle it on your cereal, or in your shakes or juices.

**Supplements:** A high-quality multivitamin will provide the proper nourishment to help heal damaged tissue. Follow the instructions on the label. Take 1,500 mg of glucosamine sulfate a day to reduce joint pain and rebuild cartilage. This is especially helpful if the pain is related to TMJ disease. Methylsulfonylmethane (MSM) is a natural anti-inflammatory and helps with pain; take 4,000–8,000 mg daily. Take 4–6 g of fish oil a day to reduce inflammation and provide joint lubrication. It may take two to three months for significant effects to be seen. Also take one to two capsules of protease enzyme on an empty stomach to reduce inflammation. Taking 50 mg of a B-complex vitamin a day is nourishing to the nervous system and helps with stress. Magnesium, taken at 250 mg two to three times a day, relaxes the nervous system.

**Herbs:** Take 500 mg of bromelain three times a day for its natural anti-inflammatory effects. Cayenne cream can help to inhibit the transmission of pain messages to the brain. Apply the cream directly to the affected area two to four times a day. Devil's claw can ease pain in the joints and is particularly helpful if you have TMJ. Take 1,500–2,500 mg three times a day, but do not take it if you have a history of gallstones, heartburn, or ulcers. Ginger also has anti-inflammatory benefits and relieves pain. Take 1–2 g or 1–2 ml of tincture three times a day.

**TIP:** MANAGE YOUR STRESS
Stress management is important in controlling pain. Learn relaxation techniques that will allow you to deal with stressful events more effectively. A good massage with relaxing oil may also be helpful.

## HOMEOPATHY

If symptoms are consistent with those described below, the following homeopathic remedies can be used to ease mild to moderate facial pain that has recently developed. More recurrent and/or severe symptoms require treatment from a homeopathic practitioner.

**Aconite:** Consider this remedy if facial pain comes on suddenly and without warning after exposure to dry, cold winds. Signature symptoms include intolerance of pain, to the point of being disproportionately restless and panicky.

**Arsenicum album:** If facial pain is burning in nature, try Arsenicum album. Pain is temporarily eased by warmth and aggravated by cold. Symptoms may also be especially troublesome at night and during the early hours of the morning, causing anxiety and restlessness. Pain may also be noticeably more severe on the right side of the face.

## HERBALISM

Herbal medicines can be used to heal trauma, decrease nerve and muscle pain, and relieve pressure in the sinuses.

**Warm compress:** Whether the pain is a result of injury, headache, or sinusitis, a heated clay pack or one or two towels soaked in warm water and placed on the affected area of the face usually brings relief. To soothe the senses, add a few drops of lavender essential oil to the warmed towel and breathe in the vapor. Oil from lavender flowers has been found to relieve headaches due to muscle spasms and calm a nervous disposition. Rosemary essential oil has very similar effects, and is mildly analgesic, especially in rheumatic conditions, and improves circulation. When taken internally, rosemary has been found to improve circulation to the extremities and within the arteries of the heart. For additional pain relief, add a few drops each of wintergreen and peppermint essential oils to the compress above. Be careful not to get the essential oils in your eyes, nose, or mouth.

**St. John's wort:** To treat facial pain due to nerve irritation, which some people describe as "stinging, burning, or shooting" sensations, add a few drops of St. John's wort to ½ tsp of olive oil and apply directly to the affected area on the face or to the warm compress described above. To use internally, take 30 drops of 1:1 tincture or 300 mg in capsule form three times daily. St. John's wort may cause photosensitivity if used in the long term. See the sections on sinusitis (p. 286) and headaches (p. 644) for further treatment options.

# FOOT PAIN

## DIAGNOSIS

Foot pain usually manifests as swelling, bruising, aching, or tenderness. Symptoms are generally caused by a disorder of the bones, joints, or nerves, and may be triggered by a range of common complaints, including arthritis, bunions, corns, calluses, tendonitis, and hammer toe. The most common cause of heel pain is plantar fascitis (also known as heel spur). This condition occurs when the broad band of fibrous tissue that runs along the bottom surface of the foot, from the heel to the toes, becomes inflamed, resulting in a thorn-like protrusion (the heel spur). Symptoms include a dull ache that is felt most of the time and episodes of sharp pain in the heel.

The term neuroma refers to a swelling of a nerve, usually the small nerve that connects the third and fourth toes, resulting in pain in the sole of the foot. This condition begins with numbness or tenderness just behind the third and fourth toes. At a later stage, pain, burning, and tingling sensations can radiate around the foot, and sufferers may experience spontaneous shooting pains. Mechanical problems with the feet include "over pronation," a condition that causes your arches to flatten out when you stand up. This condition is known as being flat-footed and causes your ankles to roll in towards each other, disturbing your normal walking pattern. Flat feet can be painful and may lead to neuroma.

Foot pain that emerges in the heel may be triggered by being overweight, from a sudden increase in weight, and from a sudden increase in the amount of walking or other physical activity you do. Arch pain (often referred to as arch strain) is an inflammation and/or a burning sensation in the arch of the foot.

## SYMPTOMS

- Swelling and redness
- Pain in a particular part of the foot such as the sole or heel
- Numbness in the foot

## TREATMENT GOAL

To establish the cause of the pain, relieve symptoms, and restore the ease of mobility.

## CONVENTIONAL MEDICINE

**Orthotics:** Many foot conditions can be eased by orthotics (products that offer support or cushioning) and by wearing comfortable, supportive shoes.

**Weight loss:** If being overweight is contributing to foot pain, begin a weight reduction program. This should be taken seriously as it greatly relieves many chronic foot pain conditions.

**To treat plantar fasciitis:** Pain on the sole of the foot that is worse first thing in the morning, particularly in long distance walkers or runners, and in people who stand for long periods of time, is usually diagnosed as plantar fasciitis. It is treated by resting, taking non-steroidal anti-inflammatory drugs (NSAIDs), and using night splints and heel cushions.

**To treat a neuroma:** A burning pain and cramping in between the third and fourth toes is usually diagnosed as a neuroma. It is caused by wearing tight fitting, high-heeled shoes and by walking on hard surfaces. Treatment involves wearing wider shoes, using orthotics, and taking NSAIDs. If this treatment fails, local anesthetic steroid injections may be given or a surgical excision may be performed.

**To treat foot pain due to osteoarthritis:** This type of arthritis is another cause of chronic foot pain. It is treated by NSAIDs, physical therapy, and anti-inflammatory nutrients and supplements such as fish oil and ginger.

## TRADITIONAL CHINESE MEDICINE

**Herbs:** The herbs called for in the following formulas are available from Chinese pharmacies or online. For either formula, make a decoction by placing the herbs in ceramic or glass pot and adding 3 cups of water. Bring the mixture to a boil, simmer for 30 minutes, and strain the liquid. Soak the affected foot or feet in the decoction for 20 minutes once a day, or twice a day for severe conditions, to dispel the cold or heat, promote circulation, and reduce the pain.

• To treat pain associated with cold feet and toes: Mix 15 g each of Chuan Xiong (Szechuan lovage root), Ji Shen (jilin root), Xu Duan (Japanese teasel root), Dang Gui Wei (Chinese angelica), Dan Shen (salvia root), Tao Ren (peach kernel), and 10 g of Gui Zhi (cinnamon).

• To treat pain associated with sweaty feet: Combine 15 g each of Huang Bai (phellodendron), Ku Shen (sophora root), Chi Shao (red peony root), Chang Zhu (black atractylodes rhizome), and Niu Xi (achyranthes root).

**Acupuncture:** Treatment can ease the discomfort of foot pain and help with the healing process. Consult an experienced practitioner for treatment. It may be recommended that you have treatment twice a week.

**Acupressure:** To treat foot pain, massage the Tai Xi, Tai Chong, Jie Xi, Jing Gu, and Xuan Zhong points. The Tai Xi point is on the inside of the leg in the depression between the Achille's tendon and the anklebone. The Tai Chong point is found on the instep of the foot in the depression between the first and second toe, at the base of the big toe. The Jie Xi point is in the depression between the instep of the foot and leg. The Jing Gu point is found on the outside edge of the foot, about mid-way back in the depression where the heel begins. The Xuan Zhong point is in the center of the outside of the lower leg, about 3 inches above the ankle.

**Diet:** Include green onions, purslane, taro, honey, lychees, spearmint, squash, and bitter gourds in your diet to help ease the discomfort of foot pain.

## NATUROPATHY

**Diet:** Eat an anti-inflammatory diet, avoiding refined sugars, hydrogenated oils and gluten, which can cause inflammation. Salmon, walnuts, and mackerel have high levels of essential fatty acids (EFAs), which have anti-inflammatory properties. Flaxseeds also have high levels of EFAs and also contain high amounts of fiber. Sprinkle flaxseeds on your cereal, or add them to shakes or juices.

**Supplements:** A high-quality multivitamin will provide the proper nourishment to help heal damaged tissue. Follow the instructions on the label for the correct dosage. Take 4,000–8,000 mg of methylsulfonylmethane (MSM) a day for its natural anti-inflammatory properties and its ability to help with pain. Fish oil reduces inflammation and provides joint lubrication. Take 4–6 g a day, but allow two to three months to see the effects. Also take 1–2 protease enzyme capsules a day on an empty stomach to reduce inflammation. Alpha-lipoic acid has been shown to help with neuropathies of the extremities and in regenerating vitamin C. Take 100–300 mg a day. Vitamin B12 can be taken as methylcobalamin lozenges to help with neuropathies of the extremities that can cause pain. Take 5–40 mg a day.

**Herbs:** Take 500 mg of bromelain three times a day for its natural anti-inflammatory effects. Cayenne cream can help to inhibit the transmission of pain messages to the brain. Apply the cream directly to the affected area two to four times a day. Devil's claw can ease pain in the joints and is particularly helpful if you have temporal mandibular joint (TMJ) dysfunction. Take 1,500–2,500 mg three times a day, but do not take it if you have a history of gallstones, heartburn, or ulcers. Ginger also has anti-inflammatory benefits and relieves pain. Take 1–2 g or 1–2 ml of tincture three times a day.

**Magnet therapy:** A completely different and alternative approach to treat pain in general is to use magnets in what could be called magnetotherapy. Our bodies are made of different electromagnetic fields that interact in complex patterns. Try placing some magnet insoles (available from health food stores or online) in your shoes to relieve symptoms.

**Massage therapy:** Reflexology is an Eastern massage therapy that manipulates the hands and feet. A pleasant exercise using this method can be done while taking a bath. Use the thumb, index, and middle finger to rotate each toe in a circular motion. Make a fist and rotate it slowly around the bottom of the foot. Finally, gently twist each foot as if wringing wet clothes, moving the top and bottom of the foot in opposite directions.

## HOMEOPATHY

If pain and aching has recently developed in the feet for an obvious reason (for instance, after exercising vigorously), the following homeopathic remedies may be helpful. However, more long-term, nagging pains in the feet should be investigated by a podiatrist or your family doctor to determine whether any underlying mechanical problems need to be addressed.

**Arnica:** Use this remedy to ease foot pain that has arisen after over-doing it in the gym, or after a minor accident such as stubbing a toe. Foot pain may be worse when standing or walking for long periods of time.

**Petroleum:** Consider using this remedy if the soles of the feet feel especially painful when walking on a hard surface. Tenderness and aching is especially noticeable in the balls of the feet.

**Rhus tox:** If aching feet are more comfortable when walking, but are more painful when resting at night, use Rhus tox.

## HERBALISM

Foot pain is a common problem, especially in active individuals and the elderly. Many conditions can contribute to foot pain, so the condition must be evaluated carefully. Among the more common conditions that can contribute to foot pain are plantar fasciitis, stress fractures, cysts, arthritis, and sciatica. Plantar fasciitis inflammation of the tissue on the bottom of the foot, is a common complaint. Typically the onset is a result of overuse or increased weight bearing. Luckily, this condition is correctable without resulting to surgery in 90% of cases. Most treatment methods are recommended for prevention as well, such as orthotics, soft foot pad inserts, stretching the lower leg and foot, immobilizing the foot during sleep with a splint, modifying exercises, and losing weight. Other topical and herbal treatment recommendations include icing the foot in combination with topical analgesics, anti-inflammatories and circulation improvement.

**Arnica:** This herb stimulates the healing of swollen and inflamed tissue, whether due to chronic overuse or fracture. After icing the affected area for three to five minutes, place a poultice or oil of arnica onto the foot pad two to three times daily. Create a poultice by infusing 2–3 g of the whole plant or flower heads in 150 ml of hot water for 15 minutes. Place gauze or bandages in the infusion and wrap them around the affected area. You may also create arnica oil by chopping up arnica flowers in five parts of vegetable oil. Arnica should not be placed over open wounds or taken internally.

**Rue:** This is a bitter and cooling herb, and the oil acts as a "rubefacient," improving circulation to the area and healing inflammation of the soft tissues (muscles, tendons, and ligaments), as well as nerve pain due to sciatica. Combine a few drops of rue oil with arnica and apply it topically.

**Anti-inflammatory herbs:** Many people find it helpful to take a blend of anti-inflammatory herbs while pursuing physical therapy treatment for fasciitis, fracture, or sprains to tolerate treatment better and relieve insomnia related to pain. Combine equal parts of tinctures of licorice, which naturally prolongs the life of cortisol, the body's natural steroid; yucca, a cooling and astringent anti-spasmodic and anti-arthritic herb; meadowsweet, which inhibits pro-inflammatory chemicals and contains small amounts of the salicylates found in aspirin; and turmeric, which improves circulation, is high in antioxidants, vitamins, and minerals, and inhibits inflammation. Take 2 ml of the blend three times daily.

# HAND AND WRIST AILMENTS

## DIAGNOSIS

Pain in the hands and wrists can be caused by a range of conditions that affect the bones, joints, and nerves, including rheumatoid arthritis, osteoarthritis, tendonitis, carpal tunnel syndrome, repetitive strain injury, and Raynaud's disease. It can also be triggered by an injury to the bone such as a fracture. Pain in the hands and wrists can be very stressful, as they are vital to a range of everyday functions. The wrist is one of the most common sites of injury, as it is used in a variety of different sports, such as tennis and badminton, and also used extensively when typing. The repetitive motion of certain activities makes some people more susceptible to wrist pain. The majority of falls also result in wrist pain as we naturally stretch out our hands to cushion the fall.

When assessing hand or wrist pain, a doctor should perform a full history and examination of the patient. Particular points to consider are the patient's occupation, any possibility of recent, even minor, trauma, and any features suggestive of referred pain (pain that is felt in an area of the body linked to the site of the injury). The unaffected wrist and hand should also be fully examined, as should all the other joints. It is important to identify the origin of any pain as it may be caused by a more serious condition that can lead to further complications.

## SYMPTOMS

- Swelling and redness
- Stiffness in wrist joints
- Tingling and numbness
- Pain triggered by extreme temperatures

## TREATMENT GOAL

To establish the cause of the pain, relieve painful symptoms, and regain full mobility. Once the cause of pain has been identified it should be treated accordingly. This may include avoiding triggers, or developing different ways of moving to prevent pain from recurring.

## CONVENTIONAL MEDICINE

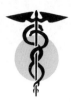

Problems of the hand and wrist may be muscular, joint related, or may be due to nerve problems or a lesion that is causing pressure. Severe pain should be evaluated by a physician. The most common cause for hand and wrist pain is osteoarthritis (see p. 598) or repetitive strain injury (see p. 686). Please refer to the sections on these conditions for further treatment options.

**To treat pain due to musculoskeletal injury:** This type of injury may be treated by resting the hand or wrist, applying ice packs regularly, and taking non-steroidal anti-inflammatory drugs. If the injury does not resolve within two weeks of following this treatment, consult with a physician for a thorough evaluation.

## TRADITIONAL CHINESE MEDICINE

**Herbs:** The following formula can be used to treat severe pain with swollen joints and redness. Mix 15 g of Yan Hu Suo (corydalis rhizome), 10 g of Gui Zhi (cinnamon), 12 g of Ji Shen (jilin root), 15 g of Chi Shao (red peony root), 15 g of Tao Ren (peach kernel), and 15 g of Dan Pi (cortex of wolfberry root) in a ceramic pot. Add 4–5 cups of water, bring the mixture to a boil, and simmer for 30 minutes. Strain the liquid, soak a clean cotton cloth in the warm decoction, and apply it to the affected area.

**Acupuncture:** Since there are a variety of hand and wrist ailments, consult with an experienced practitioner regarding the most appropriate treatment. Acupuncture has proven to be very effective in treating carpal tunnel syndrome and arthritis in the hands and wrists, reducing inflammation and pain. One course of treatment consists of 12 sessions, and each session lasts for 30 minutes.

**Acupressure:** The Hegu points are located on the back of the hands in the depression between the thumbs and index fingers. The Wai Guan point is on the back of the forearm, about 1½ inches above the center point of the wrist crease. The Zhi Gou point is on the outside of the forearm, about 2 inches above the wrist crease and in between the radius and ulna (two bones in the forearm). Use the tip of your thumb to press these points with strong pressure for one to two minutes. Repeat this on the opposite hand and arm.

**Diet:** Eat green onion, purslane, taro, and bitter gourd to help ease the pain. Try drinking a tea made from 20 g of cinnamon stick and 30 g of fresh ginger. Boil the ingredients in 2 cups of water until only 1 cup of liquid remains, and drink the tea. You can also take

30–60 g of hawthorn fruit wine before bed for pain management. This is available from Chinese pharmacies or Asian grocery stores.

## NATUROPATHY

**Diet:** A whole food diet consisting of whole grains, fresh vegetables, and fruits provides the essential nutrients to sustain healthy extremities. Inflammation usually induces pain and discomfort throughout the body, including the extremities, so it is important to follow an anti-inflammatory diet that excludes refined sugars, hydrogenated oils, and glutens. Salmon, mackerel, and walnuts have high levels of essential fatty acids, which have anti-inflammatory properties. Eat vegetables and fruits that are high in vitamin C and bioflavonoids, as these substances strengthen ligaments and tendons, therefore decreasing the occurrences of hand and wrist injuries. Such foods include berries, citrus fruits, green leafy vegetables, and carrots.

**Supplements:** A high-quality multivitamin will provide the proper nourishment to encourage tissue healing. Follow the instructions on the container. Take 4–6 g of fish oil to reduce inflammation and provide joint lubrication. Allow two to three months to see the effects. Also take 1–3 g of vitamin C a day to strengthen connective tissue and build the immune system, and one to two capsules of protease enzyme (to be taken on an empty stomach) to reduce inflammation. Glucosamine sulfate, which is usually combined with chondroitin sulfate, reduces joint pain and rebuilds cartilage. Take 1,500 mg daily of glucosamine with 1,200 mg of chondroitin. Methylsulfonylmethane (MSM) has natural anti-inflammatory benefits and contains the mineral sulfur, which is an important component of cartilage. Take 4,000–8,000 mg daily.

**Herbs:** Take 500 mg of bromelain three times a day for its natural anti-inflammatory effects. Cayenne cream can help to inhibit the transmission of pain messages to the brain. Apply the cream directly to the affected area two to four times a day. Devil's claw can help to ease pain in the joints. Take 1,500–2,500 mg three times a day, but do not take it if you have a history of gallstones, heartburn, or ulcers. White willow can also be taken three times a day to relieve pain in the joints. The product you take should be standardized to contain 240 mg of salicin or 5 ml in tincture form. Yucca root has been traditionally used for arthritic pain. Take 1,000 mg twice a day. Ginger also has anti-inflammatory benefits and relieves pain. Take 1–2 g or 1–2 ml of tincture three times a day.

**Hydrotherapy:** Soak your hands and feet in a hot bath with epsom salt or mineral salts for at least 20 minutes. The minerals will replenish the body's mineral stores and relieve discomfort.

## HOMEOPATHY

Most hand and wrist problems (apart from first-aid type injuries) fall into the category of a chronic condition, and should be treated and managed by consulting a homeopathic practitioner. The following remedies may help with pain related to an injury.

**Arnica:** When an hand or wrist injury has been sustained, this remedy can help the body deal with the systemic shock. It will also help to ease pain and encourage re-absorption of blood from engorged tissues.

**Bryonia:** If Arnica has been initially helpful in reducing pain and swelling, but does not improve the injury any further, try Bryonia. Pain may be aggravated and made more distressing by movement of any kind, and there is an obvious improvement when keeping the affected hand or wrist firmly supported and rested.

**Rhus tox:** If pain and stiffness is made much worse from resting, and obviously improves through gentle movement for a limited period of time, take Rhus tox. This remedy can also follow arnica if the latter has provided initial relief.

**Ruta:** This can follow either Bryonia or Rhus tox to support the final stage of recovery from an established hand or wrist injury. Stiffness and pain tends to lodge in one area, and it feels as though a nail is sticking into the affected joint.

> **TIP: USE ARNICA CREAM**
> Apply arnica cream to the affected area as soon as possible after the injury has been sustained to ease bruising and swelling. However, avoid using this cream if the surface of the skin has been broken, since it may cause inflammation at the edges of the wound.

## HERBALISM

Arthritis and mechanical overuse (for example, carpal tunnel syndrome) are two of the most common triggers of hand and wrist pain. In both cases there is excessive inflammation in the muscles, tendons, ligaments, and joints. To effectively relieve and prevent the recurrence of pain and promote healing, a comprehensive plan of dietary and lifestyle changes must be made. Herbal medicines can be used to alleviate swelling and pain, while promoting muscle and cartilage repair. For other treatment ideas, see Arthritis (p. 598) and Back Pain (p. 604).

**Hot and cold compresses:** Try applying contrasting hot and cold compresses to the affected area. The hot water increases circulation to bring healing nutrients to the area. The cold water flushes out excess fluid and toxic metabolites created by inflammation. Apply a hot compress for three minutes, followed by 30–45 seconds of a cold compress. Repeat, but always finish with the cold. For increased anti-inflammatory action, rub a few drops of menthol, wintergreen, peppermint, and arnica oils onto the area.

**Camphor oil:** This oil is very fragrant and cool to the touch. Camphor acts locally as a counter-irritant and numbs sensation, thereby relieving pain. It is safe when used in the short-term in low concentrations of 0.1–11% on unbroken skin.

**Castor oil:** You can also try applying castor oil to the swollen hand or wrist. Place 5–10 ml of castor oil onto a washcloth and wrap the cloth around the hands and wrists. Cover the cloth with Saran™ wrap and place a heated towel over the area for 20–30 minutes.

# HEADACHE

## DIAGNOSIS

Headaches involve mild to severe pain in one or more parts of the head, and can also cause problems in the neck. A headache can occur for a variety of reasons—and sometimes for no reason at all. They can be triggered by being overtired, feeling stressed, watching too much TV, or sitting in front of a computer for a long period of time. Eating the wrong types of foods can often cause problems, as can missing a meal altogether. Some common medical conditions associated with headaches include colds, flu, sinusitis and catarrh, earache, toothache, dehydration, and sunstroke. While painful, the majority of headaches do not indicate a serious disorder. A tension headache, the most common type of headache, results from the contraction of the head and neck muscles.

**DANGER:** If any of the following symptoms occur, contact your doctor immediately: a sudden, severe headache accompanied by nausea and vomiting; persistent and recurring headaches accompanied by problems with memory; a high fever with neck stiffness; loss of feeling in the arms and legs; and/or convulsion.

## SYMPTOMS

- Head pain can range from a mild ache to a deep throbbing
- Throbbing and pulsating pain may be worse on one side of the head
- Feeling of tightness and constriction in the head
- Pain may be accompanied by other symptoms such as nausea and visual disturbances
- Sensitivity to loud noises and bright lights
- Irritability and tiredness

## TREATMENT GOAL

It may be possible to identify a pattern of when headaches occur and thereby pinpoint a trigger. Treatment aims to relieve acute symptoms, rule out any serious complications, and identify and avoid triggers.

## CONVENTIONAL MEDICINE

In order to treat headaches, it is necessary to identify the type of headache experienced. Headaches can be vascular in nature, such as migraines, tension headaches, or cluster headaches, or due to an infection, trauma medication, high blood pressure, or a tumor. Depression and anxiety can also be associated with headaches. A severe headache that comes on suddenly should be evaluated by a doctor.

**Keep a diary:** A headache diary should be kept so that triggers can be tracked. Once a cause can be isolated, make any necessary modifications to your lifestyle or diet to avoid further episodes.

**Preventive measures:** Magnesium supplements in the form of magnesium aspartate can be helpful in preventing headaches. To treat headaches that occur on a daily basis, tricyclic antidepressants such as amitriptyline can help. Beta-blocker drugs are also used as a preventive measure. Relaxation and stress reduction techniques are also worthwhile and have been shown to help prevent headaches.

**Medication:** The medication usually used to treat tension headaches (the most common type) is acetaminophen or non-steroidal anti-inflammatory drugs. Caffeine is sometimes added to these preparations to enhance the body's ability to absorb the drugs. Biofeedback training (where patients are trained to improve their health by using signals from their own bodies) is another type of therapy that has had good results in treating headaches. Trigger point injections may also provide temporary relief and acupuncture may be beneficial.

## TRADITIONAL CHINESE MEDICINE

**Herbs:** The herbs listed below are available from Chinese pharmacies or online. For each formula, place the herbs in a ceramic or glass pot. Add 3 cups of water, bring to a boil, and simmer for 30 minutes. Strain the liquid and drink 1 cup twice a day. Consult a doctor of Chinese medicine before using the formulas below to get an accurate diagnosis and advice on herbal remedies.

• To treat headaches caused by blood stagnation: Symptoms include nausea, sharp spasms of pain, and irritation from bright lights and sounds. Mix 10 g of Chuan Xiong (Szechuan lovage root), 12 g of Chi Shao (red peony root), 10 g of Dang Gui (Chinese angelica root), 12 g of Yan Hu Suo (corydalis rhizome), and 12 g of Niu Xi (achyranthes root).

• To treat sinus headaches: Symptoms include pain and pressure in the sinuses. Mix 10 g of Bai Zhi (angelica root), 12 g of Fang Fen (ledebouriella root), 10 g of Chai Hu (hare's ear

root), 12 g of Bai Shao (white peony), 3 g of Gan Cao (licorice), and 12 g of Niu Bang Zi.
• To treat headaches due to Qi and blood deficiency: Symptoms include a dull pain in the head, tiredness, and dizziness. Mix 12 g of Huang Jing (Siberian Solomon seal rhizome), 12 g of Huang Qi (milk-vetch root), 12 g of Tai Zi Shen (pseudostellaria), 12 g of Dan Shen (salvia root), and six pieces of Da Zhao (Chinese jujube).

**Acupuncture:** Acupuncture is an effective method of treating headaches. It can reduce the pain, and in some case will address the cause of the headache and achieve long-term results. Consult a Chinese medicine doctor to determine the type of headache you have before receiving acupuncture. A typical session will last for 30 minutes, and the frequency and number of sessions will depend on the individual condition.

**Acupressure:** Press the Tai Yang, Feng Chi, and Shu Gu points. The Feng Chi points are at the back of the head and at the base of the skull, 2 inches from either side of the center point. The Tai Yang point is at the temple in the depression between the lateral end of the eyebrow and eyelid. Press these points and hold for one minute. The Shu Gu point is on the outside edge of the foot. Beginning at the little toe, move your finger along the edge of the foot until you feel a depression. Press this point with the tip of your finger for one minute.

**Diet:** Sweet basil, peppermint, spearmint, rosemary, green onion, radishes, watermelons, bananas, and spinach are recommended to help ease headaches. It is also important to drink an adequate amount of water every day.

## NATUROPATHY

 **Diet:** Eat whole foods that are low in refined sugars and food additives, which can contribute to headaches. Headaches can also be linked to constipation, so eat foods that are high in fiber, such as fresh vegetables and fruits, beans, and whole grains, and drink 8–10 glasses of water a day as a preventive measure. Consuming calcium and magnesium can also prevent against headaches. Good sources are green leafy vegetables, beans, almonds, walnuts, and wheat germ. Salmon and mackerel are high in omega-3 fatty acids, which may also help in preventing headaches. Be mindful of foods that trigger headaches and eliminate them from your diet. The most common food allergens are wheat, dairy, eggs, corn, citrus fruits, soy products, chocolate, alcohol, pork, and yeast. Additives such as monosodium glutamate (MSG) can trigger headaches as well as artificial flavoring and nitrates, which can be found in cold cuts and hot dogs. Avoid sugary foods and junk food at all costs.

**Supplements:** Take 250 mg of magnesium three times a day as it has been shown to alleviate headaches and prevent them. Take 50 mg of vitamin B6 a day. It is partially involved in the synthesis of serotonin, a neurotransmitter found to be deficient in those that suffer from migraines. Take 400 mg of riboflavin (vitamin B2) a day and 100 mg of 5-hytroxytrptophan (5-HTP) three times a day, both of which have been shown to be effective in preventing migraines. Take 5 g of fish oils daily for their anti-inflammatory effect, and 1,000 mg of calcium a day for its ability to relax the nervous system and muscles.

**Herbs:** Feverfew has been shown to reduce the duration and frequency of headaches. Take 250–500 mcg daily of a product standardized to contain parthenolides. You can also try applying peppermint and menthol cream to the temple area to relieve tension headaches. Take 60–120 mg of white willow bark a day as it is an effective pain reliever. Ginger has anti-inflammatory benefits and relieves pain. Take 1–2 g or 1–2 ml of a tincture three times a day.

---

**TIP:** PEPPERMINT OR LAVENDER OIL COMPRESS

Peppermint or lavender oil can help relieve pain in some patients. Add 2 drops of peppermint or lavender oil to 1 cup of water. Soak a cloth in the solution and apply it as a compress to the head.

---

## HOMEOPATHY

The following remedies can help the body deal with symptoms of a recent, mild-to-moderate headache that has set in as a response to an obvious trigger (such as dehydration, high levels of stress, or too much alcohol). To treat recurrent, severe conditions, consult a professional homeopath.

**Nux vomica:** If a headache has symptoms of a hangover, whether too much alcohol has been consumed or not, try Nux vomica. Classic symptoms include pain that may lodge at the back of the head and neck, or radiate over one eye, queasiness and nausea, and a general sense of feeling "toxic." Pain and discomfort is more intense and distressing when getting up and moving around, while some relief is gained from resting in a quiet, peaceful room, or holding the head still.

**Bryonia:** Consider using this remedy if headaches have been set off by low-grade dehydration, which is often accompanied by constipation. Pain tends to lodge at the front of the head, often setting in above the right eye and radiating to the back of the neck. Discomfort is made worse by the slightest movement, and bending forwards. Pain feels eased by cool air and cool compresses, by applying firm pressure, and when resting in one position.

**Pulsatilla:** Recurrent or cluster (several simultaneous) headaches may respond well to this remedy, especially if they are associated with hormonal changes that occur premenstrually. Symptoms, which include dizziness and nausea, are worse when in stuffy, overheated surroundings, while taking gentle exercise in fresh air helps.

---

**TIP: RELAX**

If stress and tension levels are high, try to keep your face and jaw muscles relaxed. Loosen your neck and shoulders to avoid tight back muscles. If trying to consciously let go and relax these areas isn't enough, try taking up yoga, T'ai chi, or Pilates.

---

## HERBALISM

**Pain-relieving tea or tincture:** Sitting for hours at a desk, daily stress, poor diet, and lack of exercise and sleep all result in inflammation and spasm in the muscles of the back, shoulders, neck, and scalp, which can lead to a headache. A combination of several herbs in tea or tincture form can relax the muscles and provide anti-inflammatory relief. The pungent and sharp-tasting root of kava is exceedingly effective at relieving stress-induced anxiety, and acts as an analgesic and anti-inflammatory. Clinical trials show that kava greatly reduces anxiety, muscle tension, and insomnia when 100 mg of an extract standardized to 70% of kava-lactones, the main active constituent, is taken three times a day. Consuming more than 9 g of kava per day has been shown to elevate liver enzymes temporarily; due to concerns about liver toxicity, only use kava under the direction of a medical herbalist. Willow bark, from which aspirin was originally derived, contains mildly anti-inflammatory salicylates. Willow bark is used to relieve pain related to muscle and joint inflammation. Other herbs with pain-relieving properties include meadowsweet, turmeric, and cayenne. Combine equal parts of all herbs, except cayenne, which should make up only 2–5% of the blend. Infuse 1 tbsp per cup of water and drink, or take 3 ml of a combined tincture every three to four hours as needed.

**To treat headaches due to insomnia:** If stress and insomnia are the causes of the headache, create a soothing blend of herbs to stop the mind chatter and allow you to let go of the day's events. Chamomile can be used to treat nervous irritability and mental restlessness. Lavender relieves muscle spasms, which result in headaches, and calms nervous exhaustion. Linden flower is sweet and slightly astringent, and indicated for headaches that are worse with heat and high blood pressure. Skullcap is a bitter, cooling plant from the mint family used to relieve fear, anxiety, and restless sleep. Combine equal parts of these herbs and infuse 1 tbsp per cup of water and drink, or take 3 ml of a combined tincture every three hours as needed.

# HERNIA

## DIAGNOSIS

A hernia is formed when the intestine pushes against a weak spot in the abdominal wall and slips through it to form a lump. It can be caused by being overweight or pregnant, lifting heavy items, coughing, and straining when constipated.

The most common hernias are those found in the groin (also known as inguinal hernias). The inguinal ligament, a band found between the thigh and the stomach, has several weak spots. Inguinal hernias are generally treated by surgery, but in many cases the hernia recurs and the surgery has to be repeated. Occasionally baby boys can be born with an indirect inguinal hernia, which is usually discovered when it descends into the scrotum. Although surgery can be performed immediately after birth to repair the hernia, some surgeons prefer to wait until the child is older. Femoral hernias occur near the groin and affect mostly middle-aged and overweight women. Incisional hernias develop in the abdomen, particularly around the navel. The treatment, again, is surgery.

**DANGER:** A hernia can be dangerous if it becomes trapped in the weak spot in the abdominal wall. This is known as a strangulated hernia. Gangrene and peritonitis, which can be life-threatening, may occur as a result. This is an emergency requiring urgent surgery.

## SYMPTOMS

- A bulge in the abdomen
- Vomiting and nausea (if the hernia becomes strangulated)

## TREATMENT GOAL

A hernia in itself is harmless. Treatment aims to correct the hernia where possible and prevent complications from occurring.

## CONVENTIONAL MEDICINE

Conventional medicine focuses on reducing the hernia to prevent strangulation, which arises when the hernia cannot be pushed back through the defect in the abdominal wall. It also aims to immediately repair the defect if strangulation has already occurred.

**Truss or hernia belt:** These devices can be used to hold the reduced hernia in place. They can help to improve discomfort and are generally used while the patient is waiting for an operation, or is unfit for surgery. A truss, however, is not a cure. It is a temporary measure and does not replace the need for surgical evaluation.

**Surgery:** The only definitive cure of a hernia is surgical repair through a herniorrhaphy. Immediate surgical repair is needed if the hernia cannot be reduced. Surgical techniques include open repair and laparoscopic repair. Sometimes mesh gauze is used during the operation to reinforce the abdominal wall. An antibiotic such as cefoxitin can be prescribed if infection is suspected.

**Modify your lifestyle:** Several lifestyle changes can prevent hernias from occurring and recurring. These primarily include weight loss and exercise to increase abdominal muscles. Consult a doctor before beginning an exercise regime if a hernia is present.

## TRADITIONAL CHINESE MEDICINE

**Herbs:** To treat a hernia, Chinese herbal medicine is usually accompanied by acupuncture. Consult a doctor of traditional Chinese medicine for a Chinese herbal medicine treatment that is appropriate for your condition.

**Acupuncture:** Consult an experienced practitioner to see if acupuncture is suitable to treat your type of condition. It is usual to have treatment for a few months or longer, beginning with one full course of 12 treatments sessions. Treatment may be needed once or twice a week.

**Acupressure:** Use the tip of your finger to press the Bai Hui point for about one minute, and repeat. The Bai Hui point is found on the top of the head, at the midpoint along the line running up and over the head from ear to ear.

**Diet:** To ease the pain of a hernia, crush 60 g of lychee seeds and 15 g of caraway seeds, boil them in water, and drink the liquid once a day. You can also boil 30 g of dried peaches and mango in water. Eat these twice a day to relieve pain.

## NATUROPATHY

**Diet:** Inflammation is one of the main causes of the pain and discomfort of hernias. There are some foods that contribute to inflammation more than others, such as gluten, dairy, and corn. Eliminate these from your diet for three weeks and then reintroduce them one food at a time for one week. Take note of how you feel on a daily basis to identify any triggers. Eat spices such as ginger, tumeric, and garlic. These have anti-inflammatory effects and help strengthen the immune system. Salmon, mackerel, and walnuts have high levels of essential fatty acids, which also have anti-inflammatory properties. Eat these foods two to three times a week. Eat vegetables and fruits that are high in vitamin C and bioflavonoids, including berries, citrus fruits, green leafy vegetables, and carrots, as they strengthen the ligaments and tendons. Also drink 8–10 glasses of water a day and 1–2 freshly squeezed vegetable juices a day to stay hydrated and provide nutrients to nourish the surrounding tissues.

**Supplements:** A high-quality multivitamin will provide the proper nourishment to prevent further deterioration and strengthen surrounding ligaments. Follow the instructions on the container. Take 4,000–8,000 mg of methylsulfonylmethane (MSM) a day for its natural anti-inflammatory benefits. Taking 4–6 g of fish oil a day also reduces inflammation, but allow two to three months to see significant effects. Protease enzymes also reduce inflammation. Take one to two capsules on an empty stomach.

**Herbs:** Take 500 mg of bromelain three times a day for its natural anti-inflammatory effects. Cayenne cream can deplete the nerves of a neurotransmitter that transmits pain messages to the brain. Try applying the cream to the affected area two to four times a day. Take a white willow product standardized to contain 240 mg of salicin to relieve pain, or take 5 ml of a tincture three times a day. Ginger, taken at 2–4 g or 1–2 ml of tincture three times a day, has anti-inflammatory benefits and relieves pain. Do not take more than 1 g of ginger a day if you are pregnant. Dimethyl sulfoxide (DMSO) is a sulfur-containing substance derived from wood pulp. It may relieve pain, stiffness, and inflammation. Talk to your physician about this option.

## HOMEOPATHY

Although surgical intervention is the most common treatment for a hernia, homeopathy can still have a useful role in treatment. Remedies can help prevent the problem from recurring, and can help to prepare the body for surgery and facilitate a quicker recovery. The advice below is given with the latter in mind.

**Arnica:** This remedy can encourage the body to heal quickly and efficiently, and help with the psychological trauma and shock of surgery. It is especially valuable in promoting the re-absorption of blood, healing bruising, tenderness, and swelling around the site of surgery.

**Staphysagria:** Consider this remedy to treat pain and sensitivity that remains around the site of the wound once superficial healing has taken place. When it is appropriate, there will be an excruciating sensitivity to touch or pressure, and some relief is gained by contact with warmth.

**Nux vomica:** This remedy can be used in the short-term to relieve some of the pain and discomfort of a hernia while waiting for surgery. Symptoms include spasmodic, shooting pains and a sensation of heaviness that triggers irritability. Following surgery, Nux vomica can be a helpful remedy in easing nausea, retching, and/or stubborn constipation.

## HERBALISM

 Be advised to avoid any activity that will increase pressure in the intra-abdominal cavity, such as heavy lifting or straining while having a bowel movement. After surgical repair, prevention of additional ruptures includes reducing risk factors such as losing weight, treating constipation and strengthening connective tissue by taking the herbs below.

**Gotu kola:** The tissue that normally holds our abdominal contents in place is weakened after a hernia, therefore it is important to strengthen this tissue. Gotu kola, a spicy, cooling herb from the parsley family, is used to build and strengthen connective tissue. However, this is not its only medicinal ability. Gotu kola also calms the nervous system, supports adrenal fatigue from daily stress and acts as a mild laxative. Whether used topically or internally, gotu kola hastens recovery periods and reduces scar formation. Drink an infusion of 1 tbsp of the whole plant per cup of water, or take 2 ml of a 1:1 tincture or 60 mg in capsule form three times daily.

**Horsetail:** This is a slightly sweet, cooling, and astringent plant, closely related to ferns. The early spring stems are used to make medicine, as the mature plant contains higher levels of potentially irritating silica. Horsetail increases the tone and strength of connective tissue, while also acting as a mild diuretic. Infuse 1 tbsp per cup of fresh stems in cold water for 12 hours, or take 2 ml of a 1:1 tincture in water and drink throughout the day. Be aware that long-term use of horsetail will deplete vitamin B1 (thiamin) and potassium levels in the body due to the diuretic effect. Take 30 mg of vitamin B1 and 40 mg of potassium daily as a preventive measure.

# KNEE PAIN

## DIAGNOSIS

Knee complaints are very common and arise from a variety of causes. Pain, swelling, bruising, or tenderness in or around the knee is usually an indication that you have injured it in some way. The knee joint often takes the full weight of the body, and is therefore vulnerable and susceptible to injury. Problems may occur in the knee bones, joint, or ligaments.

The causes of pain in the knee can be divided into several different categories. Pain can result from diseases such as arthritis and other bone problems; mechanical problems such as tendonitis and bursitis; and/or direct traumas such as sports injuries, accidents, or falls, which can lead to a fracture, dislocation, sprain, strain, or torn ligaments.

## SYMPTOMS

- Swelling
- Redness
- Tenderness
- Soreness
- Pain

## TREATMENT GOAL

To establish the cause of the pain in the knee and treat it accordingly. Conventional and complementary therapies aim to relieve any pain and discomfort and restore full mobility.

## CONVENTIONAL MEDICINE

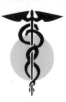

The cause of the knee pain must first be established to determine an appropriate treatment. Some sources of pain require surgical intervention, while others, such as knee fracture, dislocation, ligament tears, or infection, require immediate medical evaluation.

**To treat patellofemoral joint pain:** One of the most common causes of chronic and acute knee pain is patellofemoral joint pain. This occurs when the knee cap tracks improperly on the thigh bone during movement, leading to pain around the knee cap. This is generally treated with rest from strenuous activity, although weight-bearing, physical exercises to strengthen the muscles and ligaments around the knee are encouraged. Exercises focus on hamstring stretching and on strengthening the thigh muscles. Pain can also be relieved by taking non-steroidal anti-inflammatory drugs (NSAIDs). Orthotics (supportive braces and splints) can also be helpful. After the knee has healed and the patient can resume physical activity, a patellar band (which can be purchased at drug stores) can be worn around the knee to prevent further injury.

**To treat a meniscal injury:** A meniscal injury involves the cartilage within the knee. To treat this type of injury rest the knee and take NSAIDs to manage the pain. If there is no resolution, surgical intervention to repair the cartilage and to remove damaged cartilage may be needed.

**To treat bursitis of the knee:** This type of injury is usually treated with rest, NSAIDs, and cortisone injections as well as applying ice packs. Also see Bursitis (p. 613).

## TRADITIONAL CHINESE MEDICINE

**Herbs:** Combine 12 g of Ji Shen (jilin root), 15 g of Niu Xi (achyranthes root), 12 g of Chi Shao (red peony root), 12 g of Yu Jin (turmeric tuber), 10 g of Yan Hu Suo  (corydalis rhizome), 10 g of Ru Xiang (frankincense), 12 g of Du Zhong (eucommia bark), and 18 g of Ji Xue Teng (millettia root). To make a decoction, place the herbs in a ceramic pot and add 3 cups of water. Bring the liquid to a boil and simmer for 30 minutes. Strain the liquid and drink 1 cup twice a week. The herbs listed are available from Chinese pharmacies or online.

**Acupuncture:** Treatment can be effective for knee pain. It may be recommended that you have 30 minute sessions once or twice a week.

**Acupressure:** The Du Bi point is located on the knee, in the depression just to the outside of the kneecap when the knee is flexed. Apply pressure to this point with the tip of your finger.

**Diet:** Take 30–60 g of hawthorn fruit wine before bed to manage the pain. Also add green onion, purslane, taro, honey, lychee, spearmint, squash, and bitter gourd to your diet to help relieve pain.

## NATUROPATHY

**Diet:** Knee pain can be caused by several factors, but inflammation is generally involved. Eat an anti-inflammatory diet, avoiding refined sugars, hydrogenated oils, and glutens. Gluten is a protein found in some grains, especially wheat, that has been shown to be an allergen to some people, causing inflammation. Other common allergens include soy, dairy, egg, and corn. Foods that contain essential fatty acids, such as salmon, mackerel, and walnuts, also have anti-inflammatory properties. Eat vegetables and fruits high in vitamin C and bioflavonoids, such as berries, citrus fruits, green leafy vegetables, and carrots. These substances strengthen ligaments and tendons therefore, decreasing the occurrences of sprains.

**Supplements:** A high-quality multivitamin will provide the proper nourishment to prevent further deterioration and strengthen the ligaments. Follow the instructions on the container. Glucosamine sulfate, which is usually combined with chondroitin sulfate, reduces knee pain and rebuilds cartilage. Take 1,500 mg of glucosamine daily with 1,200 mg of chondroitin. Take 4,000–8,000 mg of methylsulfonylmethane (MSM) a day for its natural anti-inflammatory benefits. Niacinamide has been clinically reported to help arthritis, which can present as knee pain. Take 500 mg three times a day. Higher doses should be supervised by a doctor. Methionine is a sulfur-containing amino acid that is important for cartilage structure, and has also been shown to have benefits in arthritic patients. Take 250 mg four times a day.

**Herbs:** Cayenne cream can deplete the nerves of a neurotransmitter that transmits pain messages to the brain. Try applying the cream to the affected area two to four times a day. Devil's claw, taken at 1,500–2,500 mg three times a day, helps with pain in the knee joints. However, it should not be taken if you have a history of gallstones, heartburn, or ulcers. Ginger, taken at 2–4 g or 1–2 ml of tincture three times a day, has anti-inflammatory benefits and relieves pain. Do not take more than 1 g of ginger a day if you are pregnant. Dimethyl sulfoxide (DMSO) is a sulfur-containing substance derived from wood pulp. It may relieve pain, stiffness, and inflammation. Talk to your physician about this option.

## HOMEOPATHY

The remedies below may help with knee injuries that are caused by sprains or other minor injuries. Also see Arthritis (p. 598).

**Arnica:** When an injury has been sustained, this remedy can help the body deal with the systemic shock. It will also help to ease pain and encourage re-absorption of blood from engorged tissues.

**Bryonia:** If arnica has been initially helpful in reducing pain and swelling, but does not improve the injury any further, try Bryonia. Pain may be aggravated and made more distressing by movement of any kind, and there is an obvious improvement when keeping the knee firmly supported and rested.

**Rhus tox:** If pain and stiffness is made much worse from resting, and obviously improves through gentle movement for a limited period of time, take Rhus tox. This remedy can also follow Arnica if the latter has provided initial relief.

## HERBALISM

It is important to distinguish between acute injuries to the knee and pain due to chronic injuries, as they may be managed differently. Herbal medicines can be used to support the healing of knee tissue and improve circulation in an area that is normally known to have decreased blood flow. Herbs work best when combined with physical therapy and other nutritive support such as glucosamine sulfate.

**Compresses:** You can quickly relieve swelling and pain in acute injuries by applying ice to the knee for three to five minutes, as often as can be tolerated, in the first 24–48 hours.

**Anti-inflammatory tincture:** Alfalfa is very nutritious, and contains high amounts of vitamins, minerals, and protein, all of which are necessary for healing tissue. Alfalfa is also a mild anti-inflammatory and diuretic, relieving excess fluid from around the knee. Due to the vitamin K content, alfalfa should not be taken with blood-thinning medications. Another anti-inflammatory herb used for chronic degeneration of the knee is chaparral. Its bitter resins are drying and cooling, high in antioxidants, and antibacterial. Do not use chaparral if you have liver disease. Combine additional anti-inflammatory herbs, such as licorice, willow bark, bromelain, and curcumin to maximize the effect. Combine equal parts of the above herbs in tincture form and take 30–60 drops three times daily.

# LEG PAIN

## DIAGNOSIS

Leg pain is a common complaint, and problems range from muscle strains linked to sports activities to degenerative joint diseases such as arthritis. Exercise and overexertion when performing routine activities may cause strain in the legs. In addition, many conditions in the trunk of the body may produce symptoms that trigger pain in the legs. Some types of leg pain are caused by obvious injuries from a fall or other trauma, while leg cramps, one of the more common leg pain complaints, can result after exercise or can be due to an imbalance in the body's chemicals. Circulatory problems, such as blocked arteries and blood clots, can also be a cause of leg pain.

One common trigger of leg pain is nerve compression or inflammation that begins in the lower back. Any pain that originates here can be carried down the leg through spinal nerve roots, a condition known as sciatica (see p. 702). Spinal stenosis, which may cause the compression of spinal nerves, can also manifest itself as pain in the legs. For further causes and symptoms, consult the sections on knee pain (p. 649), muscle cramps (p. 663), and varicose veins (p. 164).

## SYMPTOMS

- Aching legs
- Pain
- Swelling

## TREATMENT GOAL

Conventional and complementary treatments aim to relieve pain by treating the cause. Additional management may involve lifestyle modification (to improve circulation), medication, physiotherapy, maintaining a healthy weight, getting regular exercise, and giving up smoking.

## CONVENTIONAL MEDICINE

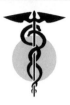

Leg pain can result from compressed nerves, from not getting enough blood supply (claudication), or from muscle or tendon injury, which is usually associated with exercise. Leg pain can also result from bone injury or a tumor. Conventional medical treatment is dependent on first identifying the reason for the leg pain.

**To treat claudication:** If leg pain is brought on by exercise and then stops with rest, claudication is suspected. Certain lifestyle changes, such as stopping smoking and maintaining a healthy diet to lose weight (if appropriate), lower cholesterol, and prevent diabetes are essential. It is also important to exercise on a daily basis. If these conservative measures do not relieve symptoms, a medication called Trental® is prescribed. Failing this, surgical intervention may be necessary.

**To treat pain due to spinal nerve compression:** Leg pain can be due to problems with the back and the compression of spinal nerves as they leave the spinal cord. This should be evaluated by a doctor and treatment will be determined based on how far the disease has progressed. Unremitting leg pain with no obvious cause should also be evaluated by a doctor to rule out serious disease.

## TRADITIONAL CHINESE MEDICINE

**Herbs:** Mix 12 g of Niu Xi (achyranthes root), 12 g of Chi Shao (red peony root), 12 g of Yu Jin (turmeric tuber), 10 g of Yan Hu Suo  (corydalis rhizome), 10 g of Ru Xiang (frankincense), 12 g of Du Zhong (eucommia bark), and 15 g of Ji Xiu Teng (millettia root) in a ceramic pot and add 3 cups of water. Bring the mixture to a boil and simmer for 30 minutes. Strain the liquid and drink 1 cup twice a day. The above herbs are available from Chinese pharmacies or online.

**Acupuncture:** Treatment may be needed once or twice a week depending on the individual condition. Consult an experienced practitioner.

**Acupressure:** Use the tip of your finger to apply medium pressure to the Yang Lin Quan and Cheng Shan points for one minute, and then repeat. The Yang Ling Quan point is on the outside of the leg, about 2 inches from the lower edge of the knee. The Cheng Shan point is on the back of the lower leg in the depression in the center, at the base of the large calf muscle.

**Diet:** As a general recommendation, eat green onion, purslane, taro, honey, lychee, spearmint, squash, and bitter gourd to help with any pain. You can also drink 30–60 g of hawthorn fruit wine before bed to manage pain.

## NATUROPATHY

Leg pain can be caused by many factors, including osteoarthritis, rheumatoid arthritis, gout, sciatica, shin splints, tendonitis, and varicose veins. As with most types of pain, inflammation is a primary contributor. One of the basic natural treatment goals is controlling inflammation.

**Diet:** There are some foods that contribute to inflammation more than others, such as gluten, dairy, and corn. Eliminate these from your diet for three weeks and then reintroduce them one food at a time for one week. Take note of how you feel on a daily basis to identify any triggers. Eat spices such as ginger, tumeric, and garlic. These have anti-inflammatory effects and help strengthen the immune system. Salmon, mackerel, and walnuts have high levels of essential fatty acids, which also have anti-inflammatory properties. Eat these foods two to three times a week. Eat vegetables and fruits that are high in vitamin C and bioflavonoids, including berries, citrus fruits, green leafy vegetables, and carrots, as they strengthen the ligaments and tendons. A whole food diet consisting of whole grains and fresh vegetables and fruits will provide the essential nutrients to support the body's healing process.

**Supplements:** A high-quality multivitamin will provide the proper nourishment to prevent further deterioration and strengthen the ligaments. Follow the instructions on the container. Glucosamine sulfate, which is usually combined with chondroitin sulfate, reduces leg pain and rebuilds cartilage. Take 1,500 mg of glucosamine daily with 1,200 mg of chondroitin. Take 4,000–8,000 mg of methylsulfonylmethane (MSM) a day for its natural anti-inflammatory benefits. Taking 4–6 g of fish oil a day also reduces inflammation, but allow two to three months to see significant effects. Niacinamide has been clinically reported to help arthritis, which can present as leg pain. Take 500 mg three times a day. Higher doses should be supervised by a doctor. Methionine is a sulfur-containing amino acid, which is important for cartilage structure, that has also been shown to have benefits in arthritic patients. Take 250 mg four times a day. Take 1–3 g of vitamin C, with is beneficial in collagen repair. Protease enzymes also reduce inflammation. Take 1–2 capsules on an empty stomach.

**Herbs:** Take 500 mg of bromelain three times a day for its natural anti-inflammatory effects. Cayenne cream can deplete the nerves of a neurotransmitter that transmits pain messages to the brain. Try applying the cream to the affected area two to four times a day. Devil's claw, taken at 1,500–2,500 mg three times a day, helps with pain in the knee joints.

However, it should not be taken if you have a history of gallstones, heartburn, or ulcers. Take a white willow product standardized to contain 240 mg of salicin to relieve pain, or take 5 ml of a tincture three times a day. Ginger, taken at 2–4 g or 1–2 ml of tincture three times a day, has anti-inflammatory benefits and relieves pain. Do not take more than 1 g of ginger a day if you are pregnant. Take 1,000 mg of yucca root, which has been traditionally used for arthritic pain, twice a day. Dimethyl sulfoxide (DMSO) is a sulfur-containing substance derived from wood pulp. It may relieve pain, stiffness, and inflammation. Talk to your physician about this option.

**TIP:** WEAR COMFORTABLE SHOES
Wear comfortable shoes that fit properly. If necessary get insoles that mold to the shape of your foot and help with biomechanical problems. If you are a runner, make sure to change you running shoes every three to six months and purchase shoes that fit appropriately. It is a good idea to buy running shoes in a runner's store where you will get the proper guidance from staff.

## HOMEOPATHY

 The suggestions below may be helpful in easing a recent mild to moderate episode of leg pain. For more established or severe symptoms, homeopathic constitutional prescribing may be helpful, ideally after diagnosis by a conventional medicine doctor.

**Belladonna:** Consider this remedy to treat throbbing, "rheumatic" pains in the legs that develop suddenly. Painful shooting sensations may move around, changing location frequently. This remedy can also relieve muscle cramps.

**Arnica:** This is a classic remedy for aching and soreness in the legs that sets in after an ambitious exercise program, or after taking up sport after years of inactivity. Pains are typically bruised and aching, making it very difficult to rest at night.

**Pulsatilla:** If pains in the leg are associated with varicose veins, try taking Pulsatilla. Legs feel typically heavy during the day, and ache a lot at night. Pain and discomfort is aggravated by heat and rest, and relieved by taking a gentle stroll in the fresh air.

**Guaiacum:** If thigh muscles feel uncomfortable and tight, or pain moves upwards from the ankle to the rest of the leg, use Guaiacum. Touch, movement, and cold, damp weather intensify pain and discomfort, while applying cold compresses and stretching the muscles provide some relief. This remedy may be appropriate for muscle pains that develop in children who are growing very rapidly.

## HERBALISM

Causes of leg pain include muscle spasm, strains, sprains, tendonitis, nerve pain that radiates from the back (sciatica), or insufficient blood supply. More serious conditions, such as clots in the leg or deep skin infections, should be assessed immediately by a doctor. Please refer to Muscle Pains (p. 667), Back Pain (p. 604), and Arthritis (p. 598) for further suggestions.

**Soothing bath:** Immerse the legs in a warm bath filled with 2–3 cups of Epsom salts. This can provide relief to leg pain due to strain or nerve irritation. The salts provide essential minerals that the body absorbs to relieve spasms in the muscles. Add a few drops each of willow bark, rue, wintergreen, and peppermint essential oils to the bath or mix them with ½–1 tsp of olive or massage oil and apply them to the legs topically.

**Witch hazel:** This can be used both internally and topically to ease painful, swollen legs due to venous insufficiency or injury. Witch hazel bark is very astringent, cooling, and drying. Combine it with arnica topically to heal unbroken skin injuries. If you have an open wound, use witch hazel alone as the tannins present within the plant encourage the formation of a protective layer of skin and speed up the process of healing. Witch hazel can be used internally to heal painful varicose veins. Decoct 2 tsp of bark per cup of water, or take 30 drops three times daily. Do not use witch hazel in the long-term as the tannins can be harmful.

**Juniper berries:** Small daily doses of sweet and pungent juniper berries decrease symptoms of pain in the legs, especially when they are due to chronic arthritis or sciatica. This is possibly due to its ability to inhibit pro-inflammatory prostaglandins made by the body. It also acts as a diuretic, improving circulation through the kidneys, leading to improved excretion of toxins. Infuse 1 tsp of berries per cup of water twice daily. Do not use juniper berries if you have a history of kidney disease.

# MIGRAINE

## DIAGNOSIS

A migraine is a headache that is so severe that it prevents you from continuing with your normal everyday activities. It is a common condition, and affects up to 15% of the population. Women appear to be more vulnerable than men, and it is thought that a predisposition to migraines runs in families. Migraines are believed to be caused by the release of the chemical serotonin into the bloodstream, resulting in changes in the neurotransmitters and blood vessels in the brain. Exactly what causes this to happen is still uncertain; however, various factors have been identified that may trigger attacks in susceptible people, including stress, poor diet, environmental issues, fatigue, and hormones such as estrogen. For most people it is not just one trigger, but a combination of several aggravating factors that cause an attack.

## SYMPTOMS

- Intense throbbing pain on one side of the head
- Visual disturbances such as distorted vision and flashing lights
- Nausea, vomiting, and/or diarrhea
- Increased sensitivity to light, smells, and sounds
- Stiff neck
- Lack of concentration

## TREATMENT GOAL

There is no cure for migraines, although it is possible to reduce the severity of attacks. Treatment aims to relieve the often debilitating symptoms of a migraine and identify triggers to prevent future episodes.

## CONVENTIONAL MEDICINE

The goal of conventional treatment is to prevent headaches from occurring or to reduce the frequency of attacks. A severe migraine that does not respond to treatment should be evaluated immediately by a doctor.

**Medication:** Once a migraine has occurred, it is treated by acetaminophen or non-steroidal anti-inflammatory drugs (NSAIDs). Trials show that these medications are more effective than a placebo, but they are not specific for migraine headaches. A more appropriate first-line migraine treatment is a class of drugs called triptans. Sumatriptan and naratriptan are in this category. Ergotamines can also be used to treat severe headaches, unless the patient has a history of coronary artery disease. Sometimes anti-emetic drugs are added to treat the nausea and vomiting that can accompany a migraine. Prophylactic treatment, which protects those prone to migraines, includes beta blockers, tricyclic antidepressants, gabapentin, and verapamil.

**Prevention:** Eliminate foods that trigger migraines (these may include caffeine, alcohol, nitrites, coffee, and cheeses) and reduce your stress levels as much as possible. Magnesium aspartate and B vitamins, especially niacin, along with the herbs butterbur and feverfew have been shown to be effective in treating migraines. Acupuncture and chiropractic treatment may also be worthwhile.

## TRADITIONAL CHINESE MEDICINE

**Herbs:** The herbs listed in the formulas below are available from Chinese pharmacies or online. For each formula, make a decoction by mixing the herbs in a ceramic pot and adding 3 cups of water. Bring the herbs to a boil and simmer for 30 minutes. Strain the liquid and drink 1 cup twice a day.

• Formula one: Mix 12 g of Tian Ma (gastrodia rhizome), 12 g of Guo Teng (stem and thorns of gambir vine), 10 g of Du Zhong (eucommia bark), 10 g of Zhi Zi (Cape Jasmine fruit), 15 g of Niu Xi (achyranthes root), 8 g of Chai Hu (hare's ear root), 12 g of Bai Shao (white peony), 10 g of Dan Pi (cortex of tree peony root), and 10 g of Chuan Xiong (Szechuan lovage root).

• Formula two: Mix 10 g of Huang Qi (milk-vetch root), 10 g of ginseng, 12 g of Bai Zhu (white atractylodes rhizome), 12 g of Chuan Xiong (Szechuan lovage root), 6 g of ShengMa (bugbane rhizome), and 12 g of Bai Shao (white peony).

• Formula three: Combine 12 g of Dang Gui (Chinese angelica root), 12 g of Bai Shao (white peony), 10 g of Chuan Xiong (Szechuan lovage root), 12 g of Di Huang (Chinese foxglove), 8 g of Ju Hua (chrysanthemum flower), 8 g of Huang Qin (baical skullcap root), and 3 g of Gan Cao (licorice).

**Acupuncture:** Migraines are commonly treated with acupuncture. The frequency of treatments will depend on the individual condition. It is recommended that severe migraines be treated three times a week.

**Acupressure:** The Shuai Gu point is located on the head directly above top of the ear, 1½ inches past the hairline. Use your thumb to apply pressure to this point for one minute and then repeat. The Tai Yang point is situated at the temple, in the depression between the lateral end of the eyebrow and eyelid. Apply medium pressure to this point with the tip of your finger. The Yang Bai point is on the forehead, 1 inch above the eyebrow and in line with the pupil. Press this point for one to two minutes with the tip of your finger.

**Diet:** Sweet basil, radish, watermelon, banana, spinach, orange squash, green onion, taro rosemary, and spearmint are recommended foods. There are also several teas you can drink. Combine 6 g of peeled, ground apricot seeds and 6 g of chrysanthemum flowers with an adequate amount of water. Bring them to a boil, simmer for three to five minutes, and drink the liquid. You can also combine 10 g of chrysanthemum flowers with green tea. Infuse the tea in boiling water before drinking. Another recipe is to bring 6 g of dried tangerine peel to a boil, and then infuse with a few green tea leaves before drinking. Lastly, try making a tea with 15 g of chrysanthemum flowers and white sugar or honey.

## NATUROPATHY

 **Diet:** Be mindful of foods that can trigger migraines and eliminate them from your diet. The most common culprits are wheat, dairy, eggs, corn, citrus fruits, soy products, chocolate, wine, alcohol, pork, tea, and yeast. Additives such as monosodium glutamate (MSG) can trigger headaches, as can artificial flavorings and nitrates, which can be found in cold cuts and hot dogs. Avoid sugary foods and junk food at all cost, and cut out cold foods and drinks as they may trigger headaches. Instead, eat whole foods that are minimally processed and low in refined sugars. Constipation is linked to migraines, so guard against this by eating foods that are high in fiber, such as fresh vegetables and fruits, beans, and whole grains, and by drinking 8–10 glasses of water a day. Consuming good sources of calcium and magnesium, such as green leafy vegetables, beans, almonds, walnuts, and wheat germ, and foods high in omega-3 fatty acids, such as salmon, can also prevent migraines.

**Supplements:** Take 250 mg of magnesium three times a day as it has been shown to alleviate and prevent headaches. Take 50 g of vitamin B6 a day. It is partially involved in the synthesis of serotonin, a neurotransmitter that is deficient in those that suffer from migraines. Take 400 mg of riboflavin (vitamin B2) a day, and 100 mg of 5-hytroxytrptophan (5-HTP) three times a day; both have been shown to be effective in preventing migraines.

Also take 5 g of fish oil a day for its anti-inflammatory effect and 1,000 mg of calcium a day to relax the nervous system and muscles.

**Herbs:** Feverfew has been shown to reduce the duration and frequency of migraines. Take 250–500 mg daily of a product standardized to contain parthenolides. White willow bark is an effective pain reliever and can be taken at 60–120 mg a day. Also take 1–2 g of ginger, or 1–2 ml of a tincture, three times a day for its anti-inflammatory benefits and ability to relieve pain. Do not take more than 1 g of ginger a day if you are pregnant.

---

**TIP:** TRY TO REDUCE STRESS

Massage the upper neck and back for a few minutes for instant relief, and take deep breaths to make sure your body is getting an appropriate amount of oxygen.

---

## HOMEOPATHY

The homeopathic remedies listed below can help to ease the acute symptoms of a migraine, shorten the duration of an episode, and reduce the general feeling of toxicity that can linger after a migraine has resolved. Recurrent, severe migraines will benefit most from constitutional treatment by an experienced homeopathic practitioner, who will be able to prescribe at a deeper level to discourage acute attacks of migraine from developing.

**Nux vomica:** If migraine has developed in response to stress and pressure, too little sleep, too much alcohol, and/or too much junk food, try Nux vomica. It can also be helpful to treat rebound migraines have are triggered by an over-reliance on painkillers or sleeping tablets. As well as feeling sick and hungover after waking, sufferers are likely to be hypersensitive to noise and desire a quiet, peaceful environment to sleep off the pain and discomfort. Additional, classic symptoms include constipation and queasiness.

**Lachesis:** Consider this remedy when a migraine is predominantly on the left side of the head, or moves from above the left eye to the right. It is also appropriate for women who suffer from migraines mid-cycle (when ovulating) to the onset of a period. Symptoms include feeling aggravated when waking up, and bursting or constricting pains. The migraine may also be accompanied by disorientation or dizziness, which is more intense when the eyes are closed. An episode may be a response to overexposure to sunshine, and/or becoming overheated.

**Sulphur:** This remedy is especially helpful in easing an acute migraine that has been triggered by low blood sugar levels. Classic symptoms include a heavy, throbbing sensation in the crown of the head, where the brain feels tight and constricted, and dizziness and disorientation that are made worse by stooping or bending forwards. Eating a small snack at frequent intervals eases symptoms by balancing blood sugar levels.

---

**TIP:** REGULATE YOUR SLEEP PATTERNS

It is often easy to overlook the importance of regular, refreshing sleep, especially when life is demanding. Burning the candle at both ends can lead to stress-related migraines. To prevent this from occurring, avoid engaging in demanding mental work just before going to bed, and using caffeine and alcohol to stay awake. Instead adopt a regular sleep routine.

---

## HERBALISM

 Migraines can be very debilitating and, at times, difficult to treat. Symptoms associated with migraines include nausea, vomiting, dizziness, and tinnitus. In addition to adding herbs to your migraine repertoire, also consider identifying and avoiding potential food and environmental allergies, and take supplements of particular minerals (e.g., magnesium) and vitamins (e.g., B2 and B6) that are often found to be deficient in migraine sufferers.

**Butterbur root:** This herb has anti-spasmodic, analgesic, anodyne, and sedative effects. Clinical trials have shown butterbur to be very effective when taken daily to prevent migraines. Studies show that a 50–100 mg dose of butterbur standardized to 7.5% petasin and isopetasin twice a day is most effective. Possible side effects include itchy eyes, diarrhea, pruritis, and stomach upset. Make sure you buy products that are certified free of butterbur's toxic pyrrolizidine alkaloids (PAs), as they can cause liver and kidney damage.

**Feverfew:** Although recently discovered to treat and prevent migraines, the traditional use of feverfew is for healing colds, coughs, fever, and dyspepsia. The active constituents found in feverfew are sesquiterpene lactones such as parthenolide, which are thought to contribute to its anti-inflammatory action; flavonoids, which are antioxidant and heal and stabilize vascular tissue; essential oils; and small amounts of melatonin, which promotes the release of growth hormone, the body's natural rejuvenator. Clinical studies have shown feverfew to effectively treat and reduce the frequency of migraines when 100 mg of the dried herb, standardized to contain at least 0.6 mg of parthenolide, is taken twice daily. You can also take 1–2 ml of 1:5 dried plant tincture per day. Side effects are rare, but include mouth ulcers (from fresh leaves), indigestion, and diarrhea.

# MUSCLE CRAMPS

## DIAGNOSIS

A muscle cramp is the result of an involuntarily contracted muscle that does not relax. Any of the body's muscles can cramp, but it is particularly common in the legs and feet, and the calf muscle tends to be the most affected. When a muscle involuntarily contracts, it is called a spasm, which becomes a cramp when the spasm is sustained. It is a common condition, and most people experience it at one time or another. Cramps generally arise after exercise, or due to an imbalance of body fluids, hormones, or salts (the "electrolytes" calcium, magnesium, and potassium), or because of dehydration. Poor circulation can also trigger cramps, as can some medications. Although not dangerous in themselves, in some cases cramps may be a symptom of an underlying condition.

Most muscle cramps can be stopped if the muscle is stretched. If a cramp occurs in your leg, straighten the leg and point the toes upward, while gently rubbing the cramped area to help the muscle relax. For a calf cramp, put weight on the affected leg and bend the knee slightly. For a thigh cramp, keep both legs straight and lean forward at the waist (while supporting yourself). A cold pack can also be used to relax tense muscles. Following a cramp, a warm towel or heating pad can also alleviate pain or tenderness.

## SYMPTOMS

- Muscle spasm, leading to a rigid sensation
- Pain in the affected area

## TREATMENT GOAL

To ease the pain and discomfort of cramps and to prevent them from occurring. It is also important to get a correct diagnosis for the cause of the cramps to determine whether there is an underlying condition. The most common and usually the most effective treatment for leg cramps is daily stretching of the affected muscles.

## CONVENTIONAL MEDICINE

Muscle cramping is not a medical disease in itself but a symptom of another condition. The first step in conventional medicine is to make an accurate diagnosis and rule out a serious disease.

**Diet and supplements:** Deficient amounts of electrolytes in the body, particularly magnesium, calcium, and potassium, can lead to cramps. These deficiencies can usually be corrected by modifying your diet to include foods that are high in these nutrients, but magnesium supplements may also be needed. Keeping the body hydrated is also essential in the prevention of muscle cramping.

**Castor oil:** A castor oil pack is sometimes helpful in easing muscle cramps. Apply castor oil to a washcloth, warm it in the microwave, and place it on the affected area for 15 minutes. This can reduce the pain of muscle cramping and may help stop the cramping itself.

**Muscle relaxants:** These may be used if a doctor has determined that cramping is due to an injury and is short term. Muscle relaxants may also be necessary if the cramping is due to a neuromuscular condition. Plants such as valerian may also provide some relief for chronic cramping.

## TRADITIONAL CHINESE MEDICINE

**Herbs:** The herbs called for in the following formula are available from Chinese pharmacies or online. Combine 10 g of Yan Hu Suo (corydalis rhizome), 12 g of Bai Zhu (white atractylodes rhizome), 15 g of Fuling (poria), 10 g of Mu Xiang (costus root), 8 g of Zhi Ke (bitter orange), 5 g of Gan Cao (licorice), and 3 g of Sha Ren (cardamom) in a glass or ceramic pot. Add 3 cups of water, bring to a boil, and simmer for 30 minutes. Strain the liquid and drink 1 cup twice a day.

**Acupuncture:** Acupuncture can be used to treat cramps both during an episode or before and after to help dispel the underlying cause. For a chronic condition, you may need treatment once a week. A course of treatment is made up of 12 sessions and you may need one or more courses.

**Acupressure:** Pressing the Qi Hai and Zhong Wan points is recommended for easing cramps. Lie down and use your fingertip to press the Qi Hai point, located in the center of the lower abdomen, about 1 inch below the navel, as you inhale. Also use your fingertip to press the Zhong Wan points, found just to the left and right of the centerline of the upper abdomen, about 3 inches above the navel. Do not press these points too hard.

**Diet:** Licorice, spearmint, and peppermint tea are very helpful in treating cramps. You can also try crushing 30 g of lychee seeds and boiling them in water with 6 g of fresh ginger or dried orange peel. Drink 1 cup of the tea once a day to help relieve the pain.

## NATUROPATHY

**Diet:** Follow a high-nutrient diet based on whole foods such as fresh vegetables, fruit, and grains. This sort of nutritional regime decreases inflammation and strengthens the liver. If you eat animal protein make sure it is antibiotic and hormone free. Eat cold-water fish such as salmon, mackerel, and herring, along with flaxseeds and walnuts, as they are a good source of essential fatty acids, which help in reducing inflammation. You can also sprinkle 1 tbsp of high-fiber ground flaxseeds on your cereal. Add some wheat germ and/or brewer's yeast to two of your meals a day. Avoid hydrogenated oils, and trans-fatty acids. These foods promote inflammation and worsen symptoms. Avoid alcohol as it dehydrates and throws out blood sugar levels, all of which aggravate cramping symptoms.

**Supplements:** Take 250 mg of magnesium twice a day as it is a natural muscle relaxant. Calcium works synergistically with magnesium to promote muscle and nerve relaxation and can be taken at 500 mg twice a day. Potassium deficiency can lead to muscle cramping, so protect against this by taking up to 300 mg a day. If taking blood pressure medication, potassium should be taken under medical supervision. B vitamins become depleted when undergoing stressful events, which causes muscle cramping in some people. Take a 50 mg complex every day.

**Massage:** Have a massage that involves deep kneading to help relax muscles and improve circulation. Use a combination of rosemary, rose, and germanium oil in an essential oil solution and add these to a base oil, such as almond or apricot oil. Gently massage the oil into the affected area to improve circulation.

## HOMEOPATHY

The following remedies can be helpful in shortening the duration and easing the severity of a recent bout of cramps. More established conditions are best treated by an experienced homeopathic practitioner who will prescribe to eradicate the underlying cause.

**Arnica:** This is the main homeopathic remedy to consider to ease cramps that have come on after over-exertion, especially in anyone who is unused to exercise and has over-done it as a result.

**Nux vomica:** If cramps (especially those that come on at night) are associated with high stress levels, poor, disturbed sleep, a hangover, or nausea, consider this remedy. Symptoms include a general sense of muscle tension and spasm, and a short temper and irritability in response to stress and mental and physical tension.

**Veratrum album:** If cramps in the calves set in during or after a bout of vomiting and diarrhea caused by dehydration, try Veratrum album. This remedy is especially helpful if massaging the affected area brings relief, and walking makes symptoms worse.

## HERBALISM

Herbal medicines can be used to ease cramps by improving circulation, restoring nutrients, and relieving muscle tension.

**Anti-spasmodic tincture:** Cramp bark is astringent and drying, and excellent at relieving cramping muscles due to tension and overuse. Khella, part of the parsley family, is used to treat mild forms of angina. These anti-spasmodic and pro-circulatory benefits extend to spasming muscles throughout the body. Black cohosh is a bitter herb used for the treatment of muscle cramps as well as menstrual cramps. Black cohosh also acts as a mild sedative, an anti-inflammatory, a circulatory stimulant, and a digestive stimulant. Greater celandine, a bitter and cooling herb, aids digestion and acts as an anti-inflammatory and anti-spasmodic. Celandine is especially indicated for relief of headaches due to shoulder and neck muscle spasm. Chamomile is a wonderful herb for the relief of nervous tension and irritability. Chamomile gently sedates while inhibiting inflammation and spasm in muscles. Combine tinctures of all these herbs in equal parts and take 2–3 ml every three hours.

**Alfalfa:** This herb contains potent anti-inflammatory properties. Infuse 1 tsp of this cooling herb in a cup of water and drink or take 30 drops of a 1:1 tincture three times daily. Due to alfalfa's high vitamin K content, do not take it with blood-thinning medications.

**Kava root:** This herb is used to relieve insomnia, stress, anxiety, and spasms related to these conditions. This sharp and pungent-tasting herb also acts as a mild pain reliever and anti-inflammatory. Decoct 1 tsp of root in 1 cup of water and drink or take 30 drops of 1:1 tincture twice daily, but only under the guidance of a medical herbalist because of recent reported liver toxicity in certain individuals.

# MUSCLE PAINS

## DIAGNOSIS

Muscle aches and pains (also known as myalgia) are common in the body's soft tissues and can involve one or several muscles, as well as ligaments, tendons, and fascia (the soft tissues that connect muscles, bones, and organs). Muscle pain is most frequently related to tension or stress, overuse, muscle injury from exercise or physically demanding work, or injury from sprains and strains. In these situations, the pain tends to involve specific muscles and starts during or just after the injurious activity. The cause of the pain is usually obvious.

However, muscle pain can also be a sign of conditions that affect your whole body, such as an infection (including the flu) and disorders that affect connective tissues throughout the body (such as lupus). One common cause of muscle aches and pain is fibromyalgia, a condition that involves tenderness in your muscles and surrounding soft tissue, sleep difficulties, fatigue, and headaches. Muscle pain may also be due to electrolyte imbalances, such as too little potassium or calcium, or be caused by certain drugs, including statins for lowering cholesterol and ACE inhibitors for lowering blood pressure.

## SYMPTOMS

- An area of acute tenderness
- Localized pain
- Inactivity due to not being able to move or use a particular part of the body
- Disturbed sleep
- Fatigue

## TREATMENT GOAL

It is important to isolate the cause of the muscle pain and treat the condition accordingly. Once the cause has been identified, treatment is focused on relieving symptoms, resolving the underlying condition, and restoring full mobility to the affected area.

## CONVENTIONAL MEDICINE

Treatment of muscle pain involves first ruling out any serious underlying diseases and relieving symptoms. Medical evaluation should be sought if symptoms persist.

**Exercise:** Although it is important to rest the sore muscle, weight-bearing exercises, which strengthen the muscles and bones, are usually beneficial.

**Compresses:** If muscle pain is caused by an injury, apply ice for 15–20 minutes three times a day. If cramping occurs in association with pain, warm, moist heat can also be applied. You can also try applying warm castor oil on a washcloth for 20 minutes twice daily to relieve pain.

**Supplements and herbs:** Magnesium is helpful when taken orally in the form of magnesium aspartate or topically by taking an epsom salts bath. Valerian is a natural muscle relaxant and can be used in conjunction with magnesium. Bromelein is also sometimes helpful in relieving chronic muscle soreness.

**Medications:** Acetaminophen, non-steroidal anti-inflammatory drugs (NSAIDs), and muscle relaxants can be used as needed.

## TRADITIONAL CHINESE MEDICINE

**Herbs:** Make a decoction using 12 g of Chi Shao (red peony root), 12 g of Bai Shao (white peony root), 15 g of Huang Jing (Siberian Solomon seal rhizome), and 12 g of Bai Zhu (white atractylodes rhizome). Combine these herbs with 3 cups of water and bring to a boil. Simmer for 30 minutes, strain the liquid, and drink 1 cup twice a day. These herbs are available from Chinese pharmacies or online.

**Acupuncture:** Depending on the severity of pain, acupuncture sessions (which are very helpful for pain conditions) may be needed twice or three times a week. An experienced practitioner will provide advice on the frequency of treatment.

**Acupressure:** Press the Shou San Li, Susanli, Yang Lin Qian, Yin Lin Quan, and San Yin Jiao points with the tip of your finger for one minute, release the pressure, and repeat. The Shou San Li point is located on the back of the forearm, about 2 inches below the elbow on the outer muscle. The Susanli point is on the lower leg, about 1 inch to the outside of and 3 inches below the kneecap. The Yang Ling Quan point is on the outside of the leg, in the depression about 2 inches below the bottom of the knee. The Yin Lin Quan point is on the inside of the lower leg, about 3 inches below and 3 inches to the inside of the knee. The San Yin Jiao point is located in the center of the inside of the leg, about 3 inches above the anklebone.

**Diet:** Eat black soybeans regularly to relieve muscle cramps. Also eat green onions, purslane, taro, honey, lychees, spearmint, squash, and bitter gourds to help with the pain. Also try drinking 30–60 g of hawthorn fruit wine before bed to manage pain.

## NATUROPATHY

**Diet:** Eat an anti-inflammatory diet that cuts out refined sugars, hydrogenated oils, and gluten, a common allergen that can cause inflammation. Instead, eat lean protein, such as organic grass-fed beef, lean poultry, fish, and raw nuts. Salmon, mackerel, and walnuts have high levels of essential fatty acids (EFAs), specifically omega-3 fatty acids, which have anti-inflammatory properties. Flaxseed also has high levels of EFA and contains high amounts of fiber. Sprinkle it onto your cereal, or add it to shakes or juices. Also eat foods that are high in magnesium, such as green vegetables, kelp, cashews, and almonds, and flush out toxins by drinking a fresh glass of water every couple of hours.

**Supplements:** A high-quality multivitamin will provide the proper nourishment to help heal damaged tissue. Follow the dosage instructions on the label. Take 4,000–8,000 mg of methylsulfonylmethane (MSM) in divided doses for its natural anti-inflammatory effects and ability to help with pain. Fish oil reduces inflammation, therefore relieving pain. Take 4–6 g a day, but allow two to three months to see the full benefits. Take one to two protease enzyme capsules on an empty stomach to reduce inflammation and ease pain. Magnesium has been shown to relax nerves and muscles. Take 250 mg of the glycinate or aspiatate form three times a day, as these tend to be the most tolerable forms. Also take 100 mg of 5-hytroxytrptophan (5-HTP), a precursor used by the brain to produce serotonin, which helps reduce pain, three times a day. Vitamin C and E also have anti-inflammatory benefits. Take 1,000 mg three times a day and 400 IU a day respectively.

**Herbs:** Take 500 mg of bromelain three times a day for its natural anti-inflammatory effects. Cayenne cream can deplete the nerves of a neurotransmitter that transmits pain messages to the brain. Try applying the cream to the affected area two to four times a day. Take a white willow product standardized to contain 240 mg of salicin to relieve pain, or take 5 ml of a tincture three times a day. Ginger, taken at 2–4 g or 1–2 ml of tincture three times a day, has anti-inflammatory benefits and relieves pain. Do not take more than 1 g of ginger a day if you are pregnant. Take 300–500 mg of valerian in pill form, or 1 ml of tincture three times a day, to relax the nerves. Black cohosh is a good hormone balancer and can also be taken to relax muscle spasm. Take 40 mg of a 2.5% triterpene glycoside extract twice a day. You can also massage arnica oil into the affected area to relieve muscle pain and tenderness.

**Hydrotherapy:** Take warm showers, especially in the morning when pain tends to be worse. This is a pleasant way to relax your muscles.

## HOMEOPATHY

Any of the following homeopathic remedies can help speed up recovery from an episode of acute muscle pain that is attributable to an obvious cause, such as straining an underused muscle during exercise.

### TIP: STRETCH BEFORE EXERCISING

If you are beginning a new exercise regime, always make a point of building up your program slowly and steadily. Remember that cold muscles are more prone to injury, so take plenty of time to do some gentle stretching before exercising. This is especially important when exercising in cold weather or cool, air-conditioned rooms.

**Arnica:** Use this remedy to treat sore, aching muscles that feel bruised or exhausted. It is equally appropriate for easing soreness in muscles after remedial massage, chiropractic, or osteopathic treatment.

**Aconite:** This remedy can help to ease pain and discomfort in muscles that feel worse when exposed to cold air. It can also be useful for treated the early stages of muscle pain that is related to not warming up sufficiently in chilly surroundings.

**Bryonia:** If muscle pains have set in as a result of a distressing, tickly, cough that refuses to be productive, use Bryonia. The physical effort of coughing causes the muscles of the chest wall to become strained and painful. Classic symptoms include pain that is aggravated by even the slightest movement, and relieved by resting in one position as much as possible.

**Gelsemium:** This is a strong candidate for relieving muscle aching and heaviness that is related to a nasty bout of flu. As well as feeling feverish and shivery, sufferers are characteristically exhausted and just want to lie down and sleep off the symptoms.

## HERBALISM

 Muscle pain is commonly caused by tearing the muscle fibers or part of the muscle tendon (known as muscle strain), creating inflammation, broken vessels (bruising), and occasionally nerve irritation. Sore muscles may also result from trauma or conditions such as fibromyalgia, a type of rheumatism that affects the muscles and ligaments but not the joints. Herbs are generally used to relieve muscle inflammation and spasm, while encouraging the healing of the tissue. For topical anti-inflammatory relief, refer to Back Pain (p. 604).

**Blue and black cohosh:** These herbs decrease spasm and guard the injured muscle. Use blue cohosh when the muscle pain has an achy, heavy quality, but do not use it if there is a history of the heart condition angina. Not to be confused with blue cohosh, black cohosh is also quite effective for relief of muscle pain and spasm, especially in conjunction with arthritic or rheumatic conditions. The fatty acids and antioxidant flavonoids it contains also heal traumatized and inflamed tissue. Combine tinctures of both herbs in equal parts and take 3 ml of a 1:2 tincture or 100 mg of dried root per day.

**Cramp bark:** A more appropriate name for this herb is "anti-cramp bark," as it is used to relieve pain and spasm. Use it for muscle pain that is worse in the evening and when lying on the affected area. Decoct either 1 tbsp of bark per cup of water or take 30 drops of a tincture every 30 minutes as needed throughout the day. The berries and leaves of this plant are toxic and should not be consumed.

# NECK PAIN

## DIAGNOSIS

Pain in the neck is a common condition that affects most people at some time in their lives. Two of the main triggers are sitting for long hours at a computer and falling asleep in an awkward position. It can also be triggered by injury, such as whiplash (p. 973), a mechanical or muscular problem, a trapped nerve in one of the discs between the vertebrae, osteoporosis, or arthritis of the neck. Problems can range from mild discomfort to severe, burning pain that makes daily tasks impossible. Acute pain comes on suddenly and is intense, such as a crick in the neck, while chronic pain can last for more than three months.

Neck pain and stiffness is often the result of muscle strain, but it can be a symptom of a variety of more serious illnesses, so it is always a good idea to get a medical assessment. It can be associated with conditions such as meningitis, encephalitis, spinal cord injuries, and some types of cancer, so it is important to rule out these conditions. Often, there is no obvious cause for neck pain. Those with weak neck muscles are more prone to neck problems and, in such cases, an exercise program to strengthen the neck is often a good idea.

## SYMPTOMS

- General pain located in the neck area
- Stiff neck
- Pain in the shoulder or between the shoulder blades
- Headache
- Tense muscles in the neck
- Sore muscles in the neck
- Tingling sensation in the arms

## TREATMENT GOAL

Conventional and complementary therapies focus on identifying the cause of the pain and ruling out any serious complications or conditions. Treatment is also aimed at relieving symptoms of pain and discomfort, and restoring the full range of motion in the neck.

## CONVENTIONAL MEDICINE

Neck pain can be caused by muscular strain, neck bone and disc problems, a thyroid problem, or an infection. Conventional treatment is dependent on the cause of the pain. If trauma is associated with the neck pain, then X-rays are usually needed to rule out fracture.

**To treat muscular strain:** Muscle strain is the most common form of neck pain. Any muscle can be strained and pain will increase when you make any movement that involves the muscle. Treatment is predominantly rest. Applying ice for 15–20 minutes three times a day, and taking non-steroidal anti-inflammatory drugs (NSAIDs) is also helpful. When the muscle is healed, it is important to perform strengthening exercises to avoid further strain.

**To treat cervical disc syndrome:** Aching pain in the neck and shoulder is often associated with cervical disc syndrome, where inflammation around the cervical bones, discs, and nerves causes pain. This is associated with degenerative disc disorder, trauma, or injuries where the neck is overextended. This is usually treated by rest and taking NSAIDs.

**To treat a disc herniation:** Neck pain that extends into the arms or shoulders with effects on the muscles is usually caused by a disc herniation, swelling around the nerves, and trauma to the bones. It is treated by taking NSAIDs as well as steroids. Surgical intervention is often needed to decompress the nerves.

## TRADITIONAL CHINESE MEDICINE

**Herbs:** In general, there are no specific herbs that treat neck pain. However, you should consult a doctor of traditional Chinese medicine for advice on herbs that may be appropriate for your individual condition.

**Acupuncture:** When treating neck pain, an acupuncture session will generally last for 30 minutes, and a typical course of treatment will consist of 12 sessions. For severe pain, treatment may go on for a longer time. Consult an experienced practitioner to determine the frequency and number of sessions that are appropriate for your condition.

**Acupressure:** Press the Da Zhui points to help relieve neck pain. The Da Zhui points are on the back, in the depression below the seventh cervical vertebra (at the base of neck). Sit or lie on your stomach and have someone apply pressure to this point with the tip of their finger for one to two minutes.

**Dietary therapy:** Eat green onions, purslane, taro, and bitter gourd to help ease the pain. Peppermint, spearmint, watermelons, bananas, and radishes are also helpful. Try making a tea by boiling 20 g of cinnamon stick and 30 g of fresh ginger in enough water to cover the ingredients. Boil the herbs until only half the liquid left and drink the tea.

## NATUROPATHY

See the naturopathy section on muscle pains (p. 669) for advice on diet, supplements, and herbs. The techniques below can also help you to relieve neck pain.

**Hydrotherapy:** Relieve neck pain with an ice massage. Freeze water in a plastic cup, remove the ice, and after rubbing your neck with your hand to prime the area, rub the ice on your neck for 5–15 minutes. (Wear a glove or mitt to protect your hand from the cold.)

**Imagery:** Picture your neck pain as a ball that has a particular size, shape, color, and texture. It may be as small as a marble or as large as a basketball. Allow the ball to grow larger and larger. As it does, the pain may momentarily increase. Now let the ball shrink so that it is smaller than its original size, but do not let it disappear. As the intensity of the pain changes, allow the ball to change color, too. Now imagine that the ball turns into a liquid that flows down your arm, drips on the floor, and reforms into a ball. Now kick or throw the ball out into space. Watch it disappear. Practice this technique for 10 minutes twice a day and whenever the pain flares up.

**Massage:** A good massage can release trigger points, relieve stress, and help subdue neck pain. Triggers points are knots that form in muscle tissue. They can be felt as nodules or bumps of tightness within a muscle. Find a qualified massage therapist in your area for a consultation regarding treatment. You can also have someone give you a massage with arnica oil mixed with lavender oil and a massage oil. These oils relieve pain and relax the muscles.

## HOMEOPATHY

The homeopathic remedies suggested below can help to treat a mild to moderate bout of neck pain that has recently developed in response to an obvious trigger. More severe or established problems with neck pain fall outside the remit of self-prescribing and should be assessed by a doctor of conventional medicine.

**Aconite:** Consider this remedy to treat neck pain that has been triggered by sitting in a draft of cold air, especially if you have been sitting in an awkward position. When this remedy is helpful, symptoms come on quite suddenly, often waking the patient from sleep.

**Nux vomica:** Use this remedy to treat a recent episode of neck pain that has developed in response to feeling stressed, tense, and irritable. Pains may be more noticeable on the right side, and when moving around first thing in the morning.

**Rhus tox:** This remedy may be helpful in treating stiffness and pain in the neck that follows on from straining tight muscles. Classic symptoms include discomfort that is most noticeable after resting, and eased by moving around during the day, and/or taking a warm shower.

## HERBALISM

Neck pain due to tightness of the muscles in the shoulders or in the neck is best treated with a combination of muscle stretching, deep tissue massage, herbal anti-inflammatories and anti-spasmodics, and possibly by correcting vertebrae that are out of alignment.

**Anti-inflammatory and anti-spasmodic herbal blend:** Jamaican dogwood is indicated for muscle pain and spasm combined with nervous irritability and nerve pain, making it an excellent choice to treat neck pain. Jamaican dogwood demonstrates analgesic and sedative properties, relieving pain while soothing the nerves. This herb is potentially toxic and should only be used in low doses. Take 5 drops of tincture twice a day in combination with other treatments to relieve spasms such as cramp bark, black haw, and black cohosh.

**Hot and cold compress:** If your neck has been injured in the last 24–48 hours, place ice on the neck and shoulders for three to five minutes, or for as long as can be tolerated, at regular intervals throughout the day. After two to three days, alternate compresses with hot and cold towels. Begin immediately applying this anti-inflammatory and pain relieving salve to initiate healing. You can also combine equal parts of arnica, rue, calendula and St. John's wort with a beeswax and canola or olive oil base and apply as often as needed to the neck.

**TIP: IMPROVE YOUR POSTURE**
Look in a mirror to see if your shoulders are hunched over and your neck is bent forward. Your head weighs about 10 lb and if it is not properly balanced over your shoulders it may lead to neck pain. See a qualified chiropractor for help with posture. Also, find out about postural therapies such as Feldenkrais and Alexander technique. They can help you move your body with greater ease and less strain.

# NEURALGIA

## DIAGNOSIS

Neuralgia is a type of nerve pain that is often described as a burning or shooting sensation. There are several types that affect different parts of the body. The most common forms are trigeminal neuralgia and post-herpetic neuralgia.

Trigeminal neuralgia affects the face. The trigeminal nerve extends from the brain to supply sensation to the face, scalp, teeth, mouth, and nose. The cause of trigeminal neuralgia is often unknown, but is sometimes attributed to pressure on the nerve from nearby blood vessels. Symptoms include severe face pain, which can at times be so intense that the sufferer calls out in agony. A simple action such as swallowing or brushing the teeth can trigger the pain. The frequency of attacks is variable but pain can sometimes strike several times a day. Once the condition has been diagnosed, individual triggers must be identified and avoided.

Post-herpetic neuralgia is associated with the virus that causes chickenpox and shingles. With this condition the area where the chickenpox or shingles rash was located becomes painful after the scabs have resolved. Post-herpetic neuralgia can last from a few weeks to several months.

## SYMPTOMS

- Stabbing, burning, or lancing pains
- Pains may last from a few seconds to over a minute
- Pains are brought on by touching a trigger point, or activities such as chewing or brushing the teeth

## TREATMENT GOAL

It is necessary to identify and avoid triggers as much as possible. Treatment also aims to develop ways of managing the pain when an attack occurs.

## CONVENTIONAL MEDICINE

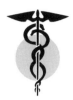

Neuralgia can have many causes and ultimately treatment depends on identifying the source of the pain. This may involve an in-depth assessment from a neurologist or general practitioner. Some conditions that may cause neuralgia are metabolic disease such as diabetes or vitamin deficiency, inflammatory disease such as swelling around the nerves, infections, tumors, a reaction to medication, and toxins such as pesticides.

**Medication:** There are numerous medications used to treat this condition. A category of drugs called tricyclic antidepressants can be used. Paxil, a newer antidepressant, is also used to treat neuralgia. A class of drugs called anti-eleptics, which includes carbamazepine (Tegretol®), gabapentin (Neurontin®), topiramate (Topamax®), and lamotrigine (Lamictal®) are often prescribed. Analgesic pain-relieving drugs may be used as well. Tramadol, morphine, and oxycodone are sometimes needed to treat the serious pain of neuralgia. Topical anesthetics such as a lidocaine patch can also ease symptoms.

**Other types of therapy:** Patients may need to begin counseling since psychological issues can make neuralgia worse. Also, physical therapy may be helpful, as well as stress reduction techniques.

## TRADITIONAL CHINESE MEDICINE

**Herbs:** According to traditional Chinese medicine theory, the numbness, tingling, and pain of neuralgia are caused by poor circulation. To treat this mix 12 g of Huang Qi (milk-vetch root), 12 g of Fang Fen (ledebouriella root), 12 g of Qiang Huo (notopterygium root), 12 g of Chi Shao (red peony root), 10 g of Chen Xiang (aloeswood), 12 g of Dang Gui (Chinese angelica root), 8 g of fresh ginger, and five pieces of Da Zhao (Chinese jujube). Place these herbs in a ceramic or glass pot and add 3 cups of water. Bring to the boil and simmer for 30 minutes. Strain the liquid and drink 1 cup twice a day. The herbs listed above are available from Chinese pharmacies or online.

**Acupuncture:** Treatment can be effective by increasing the circulation of energy and blood to nourish nerve endings. Consult a practitioner regarding a treatment plan and prognosis. A typical course of treatment will consist of sessions once a week for 12 weeks. You may see an improvement following the first few sessions if your condition is not severe and relatively recent; otherwise, longer-term treatment may be needed, since chronic neuralgia is difficult to heal.

**Acupressure:** Gently massage the area that is numb and aching. Press the Xue Hai, Yin Lin Quan, and Jie Xi points to treat the upper extremities, and the Qu Chi and Wai Guan points to treat the lower extremities. The Xue Hai point is on the inside of the leg in the depression just above the knee. The Yin Ling Quan point is in the depression on the inside of the lower leg about 3 inches below the kneecap. The Jie Xi point is found on the crease between the foot and the leg, in the depression between the tendon of the big toe and the smaller toes. With the elbow flexed, you will find the Qu Chi point on the outside of the elbow at the lateral end of the crease. The Wai Guan point is on the top side of the lower arm, about 1 inch above the center of the wrist. Apply pressure to these points for one to two minutes at a time.

**Diet:** Eat foods that help circulation, such as spinach, bamboo shoots, ginger, and green onions. Eat fresh fruits such as pears, cranberries, blueberries, and bananas. Beef, egg, milk, mung beans, red beans, peach kernel, and safflower are also recommended.

## NATUROPATHY

**Diet:** Eat foods that are high in B vitamins, which are healing to the nervous system. These include wheatgerm, brewer's yeast, eggs, and whole grains. Brightly colored fruits and vegetables such as squash, carrots, berries, and oranges have high amounts of bioflavonoids and vitamins C and A, which will help resolve inflammation and blisters of the skin, and increase the efficiency of the body's immune system. A freshly pressed green vegetable juice a day will give you essential nutrients to alkalinize the body and boost immunity. Avoid meat, fried foods, sugar, chocolate, and sodas, which suppress the immune system and interfere with the healing process.

**Supplements:** Take 1,200 IU of natural vitamin E (mixed tocopherols and tocotrienols) a day to help treat neuralgia, and 400 IU a day to help prevent it. Vitamin C helps to support the immune system and reduces stress damage to nerves. Take 1,000 mg four times a day. Also take 30 mg of zinc a day to help support the immune system. Take 200 mg of selenium a day to help with viral infections, and 500 mg of L-lysine twice a day to help with healing. B vitamins are essential for nerve health. Take 100 mg three times a day. Vitamin B12 injections, administered by a qualified practitioner, are also essential to help the body recover more quickly and reduce pain associated with neuralgia. Proteolytic enzymes are thought to benefit cases of neuralgia caused by the herpes zoster virus by decreasing the body's inflammatory response and regulating immune response to the virus. Take 2–3 capsules on an empty stomach twice a day.

**Herbs:** Take 500 mg of olive leaf extract four times a day for its potent anti-viral benefits. Lomatium root, which can be taken at 500 mg four times a day, is used for immune support and anti-viral effects. St. John's wort also has anti-viral properties. Take 300 mg or 4 ml of tincture three times a day. Capsaicin cream is available in two strengths: 0.025 and 0.075%. Both preparations are indicated for use in neuralgia and should be applied sparingly to the affected area three to four times daily. Treatment should continue for several weeks as the benefit may be delayed. Capsaicin creams are approved over-the-counter drugs and should be used as directed. You may feel a burning or stinging sensation when this cream is first applied, but the pain will subside.

> **TIP:** DO NOT SCRATCH
>
> Keep blistered areas clean using soap and water. This will help prevent any bacterial infections from developing. Although it may be difficult, do not scratch. Scratching increases the risk that the blisters will become infected from dirt under the fingernails.

## HOMEOPATHY

The following remedies can help ease a recent, mild to moderate episode of neuralgia. More severe and/or established symptoms are best treated by a homeopathic practitioner, possibly in combination with conventional treatment.

**Aconite:** Consider this remedy if symptoms of facial nerve pain have been triggered by exposure to cold, biting winds. Signature symptoms in the affected area include a feeling of being pierced with hot wires, and/or a sensation that icy water is traveling along the pathway of the affected nerves. There may also be a feeling of crawling on the surface of the skin of the face.

**Arsenicum album:** This is a possible option for easing symptoms of neuralgia that are associated with very high anxiety levels, which are likely to be the most severe during the night and in the early hours of the morning. Neuralgic pains lodge in the area around the right side of the face, especially around the right eye socket. There may also be a sensitive, sore scalp, and discomfort is aggravated by exposure to cold, and temporarily eased by warmth.

**Lachesis:** This remedy can also be useful to treat neuralgic pains that have been triggered by exposure to cold winds, especially if the pains are more intense on the left side, and worse on waking from sleep. When this remedy is helpful, pains are most likely to be at the back of the head, and soreness is intensified from the pressure of the pillow when lying down.

**Colocynthis:** If neuralgic pains are spasmodic in nature, coming in waves and affecting one side of the face in the area of the jaw and/or around the eye socket, use Colocynthis. Pain and discomfort are temporarily eased by applying pressure and heat. Resting is more uncomfortable than being on the move.

**Mag phos:** This remedy is called for when symptoms are similar to those described for Arsenicum album, such as night-time aggravation, and pain on the right-side that is eased by warmth. However, pains are not burning in nature, and symptoms may come on after an excessive amount of mental effort, resulting in poor concentration and exhaustion.

## HERBALISM

**St. John's wort:** Nerve irritation and pain may respond to a few drops of St. John's wort, either blended with ½ tsp of olive oil and directly applied to the affected area on the face, or in a warm compress applied to the area. Some practitioners find St. John's wort more successful if the symptoms are described as stinging, burning, or shooting. This wonderful nerve tonic can be helpful whenever there is nerve injury or irritation, especially when this pain leads to nervous exhaustion, inability to sleep, and a depressed mood. For internal use, take 30 drops of a 1:1 tincture or 300 mg of a standardized extract three times daily. This herb may cause photosensitivity with long-term use, and may react with medications, so consult a doctor before taking St. John's wort orally if you are taking pharmaceutical medications.

**Chili pepper:** This can be applied topically to provide pain relief. Capsicum, found in chili pepper, is available in health food stores in cream or ointment formulation. Most preparations contain 0.025–0.075% capsaicin and can be applied to the affected area three to four times daily. Capsicum causes very few side effects, the most prevalent being a slight burning and itching of the application area. This treatment may make symptoms worse for one to three days until improvement occurs. If your neuralgia still is not better after a week of therapy, discontinue use and consult your herbalist.

**Nerve tonics:** There are a variety of other herbs that can be helpful for neuralgia; these generally fall into the category of nerve, or nervine, tonics. These plants are usually taken orally for long periods of time to help restore optimal activity of nerves and decrease symptoms of neuralgia, among other disorders. Plants such as skullcap, damiana, and ashwaganda are examples of useful nerve tonics.

# OSTEOPOROSIS

## DIAGNOSIS

Osteoporosis or brittle bone disease is a condition characterized by loss of bone density, where the amount of bone tissue in the body is below what is considered normal for a person of a particular sex and age. As a result, the bones become weak and take on the texture of honeycomb. Fractures can occur in areas where there is a greater percentage of weakened bone, such as the wrists, the hip joint, and in the vertebrae of the lower spine. Hip and wrist fractures usually result from falls, whereas fractures of the spine tend to occur spontaneously when a weakened vertebra eventually crumbles under the stress of having to support the body.

Osteoporosis is a widespread problem. One in two women and one in five men over the age of 50 will suffer a fractured bone as the result of osteoporosis. It is, however, normal for bones to get weaker each year after the age of about 30. Various factors are known to trigger osteoporosis, and many of them are unavoidable. Contributory factors include getting older, a family history of osteoporosis, being female, going through menopause/estrogen loss, and being underweight. Lifestyle factors play a role, such as lack of exercise, a poor diet that is lacking in calcium, smoking, and regularly drinking alcohol. Other triggers include the use of steroid drugs, an overactive thyroid gland, chronic liver or kidney disease, and vitamin D deficiency.

## SYMPTOMS

- A fractured or broken bone can be the first indication of problems
- Bending forward into a hunched position
- Shortening of the spine due to fractured vertebrae

## TREATMENT GOAL

If you think you may have osteoporosis or are at risk of it, have your bone density measured. Treatment aims to prevent further deterioration and protect against complications such as fractures and broken bones.

## CONVENTIONAL MEDICINE

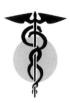

Prevention is the most important goal. Risk factors such as poor nutrition should be identified and corrected wherever possible.

**Exercise:** Engage in physical activity on a daily basis. Performing weight bearing exercises, which work your bones and muscles, is especially important.

**Vitamins and supplements:** Increase your intake of vitamin D3 (cholecalciferol) to about 400–1,000 IU daily. Also take 45 mg of vitamin K2 and 1,800 mg of calcium hydroxyapetite a day. In postmenopausal women, minimal amounts of natural estrogen and natural progesterone may be helpful. However, estrogen should be avoided if breast cancer has been diagnosed in the past or if a strong family history exists.

**Medication:** The medications alendronate, raloxifend, and risedronate are approved for the treatment of osteoporosis for the prevention of bone loss. A bone density test should show that bone loss has stopped after one year of beginning medication.

## TRADITIONAL CHINESE MEDICINE

**Herbs:** The herbs called for in the formulas below are available from Chinese pharmacies or online. For either formula, make a decoction be combining the ingredients in a ceramic or glass pot. Add 4 cups of water, bring the mixture to a boil, and simmer for 30 minutes. Strain the liquid and drink 1 cup twice a day. Take the formulas for one to three months.

• Formula one: This combination will benefit bones by nourishing the blood and improving circulation. Mix 10 g of Shan Zhu Yu (Asiatic cornelian cherry fruit), 12 g of Dang Gui (Chinese angelica root), 15 g of Di Huang (Chinese foxglove), 15 g of Dan Shen (salvia root), 12 g of Gou Ji Zi (wolfberry), 12 g of Ji Shen (jilin root), and 15 g of Ji Xue Teng (milletia root).

• Formula two: These herbs tonify kidney energy, which is important for bone health according to Chinese medicine theory. Mix 30 g of Long Gu (fossilized bone), 30 g of Mu Li (oyster shell), 12 g of Sang Ji Sheng (mulberry mistletoe stem), 12 g of Huai Niu Xi (achyranthes root), 15 g of Shu Di Huang (Chinese foxglove cooked in wine), 12 g of Shan Zhu Yu (Asiatic cornelian cherry fruit), 15 g of Shan Yao (Chinese yam), 15 g of Fuling (poria), and 12 g of Zi Xie (water plantain rhizome).

**Acupuncture:** A practitioner will be able to identify your condition in terms of whether you have insufficient kidney energy, or some other disorder, by Chinese medicine differentiation. He or she will probably recommend several courses of treatment. Typically, one course consists of 12 sessions. You may also benefit by taking herbal medicine along with receiving acupuncture.

**Acupressure:** Press the Xuan Zhong point, found on the outside of the lower leg, about 3 inches above the anklebone. Take a seat and apply pressure to the Xuan Zhong point on each leg with the tip of your finger or thumb. Apply pressure for one to two minutes and repeat a couple of times a day.

**Diet:** Eat foods that strengthen the kidneys, such as black sesame seeds, string beans, sword beans, wheat, kidney, plums, mutton, chives, dill seed, tangerines, walnut, pork, clove, and fennel. Also eat foods that are rich in vitamin B, tonify the blood, and strengthen bones, including red beans, kidney beans, soybeans, spinach and other dark green vegetables, fish, seafood, lamb, chicken, beef, and pork. It is recommended that you eat bone soup for natural calcium intake. To make it, use any meat bones, add water, salt, and a few drops of vinegar and cook on a slow heat. Either drink the broth or use it in your cooking.

## NATUROPATHY

**Diet:** Eat plenty of sea vegetables, green leafy vegetables (except spinach), soybeans, nuts, molasses, and unsweetened cultured yogurt. These foods contain high levels of calcium and other nutrients important in the absorption of calcium. Spinach, which contains oxalic acid, a substance that interferes with the absorption of calcium, should be avoided. Vitamin K is known for coagulation and bone formation, and can be found in high amounts in green vegetables such as collard greens, kale, and romaine lettuce. Processed sugars contribute to osteoporosis and should be cut out of your diet wherever possible. Moderate your levels of caffeine and alcohol consumption, as they contribute to bone loss. Unlike the popular belief, milk and milk products are not the best sources of calcium. This is largely due to intolerances to lactose and casein, which can lead to problems with absorption. Unsweetened yogurt is the exception.

**Supplements:** Calcium has been shown to be effective in helping to build bone mass. For optimum nutrition, the recommended calcium intake is between 1,000–1,500 mg per day, depending on your age, dietary intake, and other health conditions. Use the forms that most easily absorbed by the body, such as calcium citrate, malate, chelate, or hydroxyappatite. Vitamin D has also been shown to be effective in building bone mass by improving intestinal calcium absorption and reducing excretion of calcium in the urine. Your daily intake should be approximately 400 IU a day for prevention and 800–1,200 IU per day if you already have osteoporosis. Vitamin K reduces bone loss and low levels have been associated with fractures. Take 2–10 g a day—a smaller amount for prevention and a higher amount if you have osteoporosis. Do not take vitamin K if you are on anticoagulant medications. Ipriflavone has been shown to help bone strength when combined with calcium and vitamin D. Take 600 mg a day with food. Take 250–350 mg of magnesium twice a day as it is required for proper calcium metabolism. Fish oils can also improve calcium absorption and deposition into bones when taken at 4 g a day. Boron is a mineral that activates vitamin D and supports estrogen levels of effective calcium metabolism. Take 3–5 mg daily. Vitamin C, among its many other healthy functions, synthesizes collagen, an important component of bone. Take 340 mg a day of strontium, which has been shown to increase bone density when taken with calcium. Finally, take 2–3 capsules of betaine hydrochloric acid with each meal to improve stomach acid, which aids in the absorption of calcium.

## HOMEOPATHY

Due to its chronic nature and the complications that can accompany this condition, such as fractures, osteoporosis requires professional medical management. Homeopathic treatment can play a positive role in helping patients who suffer from poor bone density, but for the most successful outcome this support needs to come from an experienced practitioner. The practical suggestions below can help to discourage the condition from escalating.

**Diet:** If you suspect that your bone density is at risk, avoid foods that have a reputation for aggravating osteoporosis. These include alcohol, coffee, salt, and preserved meats. Instead, eat plenty of oily fish (especially sardines and salmon), green leafy vegetables, small amounts of dairy foods, and soy products. This is especially important for women, as bone density begins to be lost from around the age of 35.

**Lose weight sensibly:** Avoid crash diets that may be nutritionally challenging, since not only do such diets appear ineffective in the long term, but extreme fluctuations of weight can also leave you more vulnerable to problems with bone density. This is especially the case if your periods stop as a result of drastic weight loss over a significant period of time.

**Exercise:** Regular weight-bearing exercise has been shown to play an important role in guarding against osteoporosis, especially when performed up to three or four times a week. Pursue this with regular walking, weight training, running, cycling, swimming, and dancing sessions for maximum variety.

**Calcium:** If you take a calcium supplement, bear in mind that vitamin D and magnesium promote its absorption by the body.

## HERBALISM

**Red clover:** There is evidence that red clover could be useful for osteoporosis. Its benefits are probably due to compounds called isoflavones (sometimes referred to as phytoestrogens) that have hormonal activity. Red clover can be ingested as a tea (made from 1–2 g and taken once to three times daily) or ½ dropper full of an alcohol or glycerin tincture can be taken three times a day. However, the most effective preparation of red clover appears to be capsules of a semi-purified leaf extract where the standardization to the percentage of isoflavones is listed specifically on the bottle. Some caution should be taken if you are also on medications that can thin the blood, and some people can react to red clover by developing a skin rash.

**Horsetail:** The presence of minerals like silica, potassium, and manganese has prompted people to consider the use of horsetail extract for osteoporosis treatment and prevention. There is some animal research to suggest the importance of silica in bone growth, and clinical trials suggest that horsetail may slightly increase bone density. In theory, horsetail may cause vitamin B1 (thiamine) to become depleted.

# REPETITIVE STRAIN INJURY

## DIAGNOSIS

Repetitive strain injury (RSI) is mainly caused by work that involves performing small repetitive tasks and movements, such as typing on a keyboard. It affects the musculoskeletal system, particularly the neck, shoulders, arms, and hands. Tenosynovitis (inflammation of the tendon sheath) of the wrist associated with typing or operating a word processor is the most common repetitive strain injury. Appropriate work furniture can help prevent injuries by keeping the back and hands in the correct position and as relaxed as possible. RSI can be painful, and may eventually result in the loss of function in a limb. A variety of movement is important: while you are working, flex your fingers, stretch your arms, and do exaggerated backward shoulder rolls. Take regular breaks to stretch, walk around, and shake tension out of your arms. Stretch your fingers and press your palms together. Early detection and treatment is essential as chronic RSI is often irreversible.

## SYMPTOMS

- Pains in the neck, shoulders, arms, and hands
- Localized tenderness in the affected area
- Tingling sensation like pins and needles
- Aching
- Stiffness
- Muscle spasms
- At the outset, symptoms may only be experienced towards the end of the day
- Eventually they may progress, and affect the sufferer all day

## TREATMENT GOAL

Prevention through correct exercises and using the right equipment at work is essential to RSI treatment. Conventional and complementary therapies aim to relieve any pain and discomfort and discourage RSI from developing into a chronic condition.

## CONVENTIONAL MEDICINE

**Rest and ice:** Initial treatment is to immobilize the affected area and rest it from the trigger activity. However, a shoulder should not be immobilized as it may become "frozen." Applying ice to the affected site for 15–20 minutes is often helpful.

**Exercise:** Exercise or physical therapy may serve to strengthen the surrounding tendons and prevent recurrence of RSI. Ergo dynamic training should be carried out to learn different postures to avoid further strain. Hydrotherapy may also be a particularly effective form of physical therapy. Lifestyle changes to improve fitness in general are helpful.

**Medication:** Non-steroidal anti-inflammatory drugs (NSAIDs) such as Motrin® are commonly used for pain relief. Steroid injections into the area of the injured tendon in combination with lidocaine can also cause notable pain relief.

**Supplements:** Fish oil can be used in amounts of about 4 g a day to reduce inflammation, as can ginger root in the amount of 1 g a day.

**Surgery:** Surgical procedures may be helpful for chronic pain, but it is not appropriate for all cases of RSI. The benefits depend on the individual injury and the area of the body that is affected. Splints and assistive devices and supports may be necessary, and therapeutic ultrasound may be helpful for healing if chronic pain is present.

## TRADITIONAL CHINESE MEDICINE

**Herbs:** Take Du Huo Ji Shen Wan pills to strengthen the soft tissue and prevent recurring injury. To treat existing pain, try taking Yuan Hu Suo Zhi Tong Pian or Shan Qi Shen Pian pills for relief. All of these patent Chinese herbal pills are available from Chinese pharmacies or Chinese medicine clinics.

**Acupuncture:** Treatment not only helps to relieve pain, but also heals injured tissues and prevents recurrence by strengthening damaged and weakened tissues. Acupuncture is very effective in treating RSIs. Consult a practitioner for advice, but a course of treatment consisting of 12 sessions is usually suggested, beginning with treatment once or twice a week. Progress will be evaluated during these sessions.

**Acupressure:** Press the acupressure points around the injured area. Usually you can press each point for one to two minutes twice a day.

**Diet:** Eat a balanced diet that includes fresh vegetables and fruits such as pears, cranberries, blueberries, and bananas. Mung beans, red beans, bamboo shoots, and purslane are also recommended.

## NATUROPATHY

**Diet:** An anti-inflammatory diet is essential in helping an RSI to heal. Eat anti-inflammatory foods such as deep-water fish, which are a rich source of the polyunsaturated fats called omega-3 fatty acids. Originally praised for their heart-healthy actions, the omega-3s have also been shown to fight inflammation. All fish contain omega-3s, but the cold-water varieties—such as salmon, sea bass, tuna, trout, and mackerel—contain especially high amounts of these beneficial fats. Pineapple contains bromelain, a powerful enzyme that has been shown to have an anti-inflammatory effect on muscle and tissue. Bromelain breaks down fibrin, a blood-clotting protein that can impede circulation and prevent tissues from draining properly. It also blocks the production of certain compounds that cause swelling and pain. Apples and onions are high in quercetin. With its proven anti-inflammatory properties, quercetin can help reduce inflammation in the joints and muscles. Include anti-inflammatory spices such as turmeric and ginger in your meals and drink eight glasses of water a day to flush clean your system of waste material and metabolites that increase inflammation and inhibit the healing process. Whole grains, fresh fruit, and vegetables should be a staple for providing the muscles with all the nourishment they need to assist in the healing process.

**Supplements:** Proteolytic enzymes destroy free radicals, which inhibit healing, and proteins involved in the inflammatory process. Take three tablets or capsules between meals. Vitamin C is required for the formation of connective tissue and to combat free radicals. Essential fatty acids such as flaxseed and fish oil reduce inflammation and promote tissue healing. Take 5 g of fish oils a day or 1–2 tbsp of flaxseed oil. Take 1,500 mg of glucosamine sulfate a day to provide the raw material for the body to manufacture ligaments and tendons.

**Herbs:** Ginger has anti-inflammatory properties that help with pain. Try taking 100–200 mg of the standardized extract in pill form three times a day. You can also take ½–¾ tsp of fresh powdered ginger every four hours or up to three times a day. Try drinking several cups of ginger tea a day. It is available in prepackaged bags or can be prepared by steeping ½ tsp of grated ginger root in 8 oz of very hot water for 5–10 minutes. A cup of tea, when steeped for this amount of time, can contain about 250 mg of ginger. Alternatively an 8 oz glass of ginger ale, which can be drunk several times a day, contains approximately 1 g of ginger. However, be sure to select products that are made with real ginger. Ginger is also available in crystallized form; eat two 1-inch-square, ¼-inch-thick pieces a day to obtain about 500 mg of ginger. Do not take more than 250 mg of ginger four times a day during pregnancy without consulting your obstetrician.Bromelain also has natural anti-inflammatory effects; take 500 mg three times a day between meals. Also take 1,500 mg of boswelia three times a day for its strong anti-inflammatory properties. Make sure this product contains 60–65% boswellic acids. Arnica oil reduces swelling and pain and can be applied to the injured area twice a day. White willow bark is a natural pain reliever without the side effects of over-the-counter aspirin. Take 30–60 mg a day of an extract standardized to salicin.

---

**TIP:** IMPROVE YOUR POSTURE

Good body positioning is essential in preventing RSI. Nature did not intend for the body to sit for long periods, and sitting over a keyboard tends to force the head down and weaken the neck muscles. The best position for typing is with your feet flat on the floor, your ribs centered over the pelvis, and your head balanced on top of your spine, so that your ears, shoulders, and hips are in alignment. Also remember to take regular breaks. Sitting combines awkward positioning and poor posture with static loading (holding still while tightening muscles) and is unnatural to the body. Mix sit-down work with rest and stretching for the best results.

---

## HOMEOPATHY

Established and severe symptoms associated with this condition are best treated by an experienced practitioner, rather than attempting to manage the injury through home prescribing. The following practical suggestions may also be helpful in easing the condition.

**Yoga:** There is some evidence to suggest that practicing yoga regularly may be helpful in relieving some of the symptoms of RSI. In addition, yoga is a very helpful therapy for stress-relief. Since high levels of stress and tension may aggravate symptoms of RSI, regular yoga may bring benefits on both physical and psychological levels.

**Evaluate your work station:** Postural issues may also have an effect on RSI, and it is worth considering how healthy your workstation is, especially if you work for extended periods of time at a computer. Issues to consider include the height of your chair versus your desk, whether you need to use a foot and/or hand rest, and the maximum amount of time you can safely spend engaged in one activity at a time.

## HERBALISM

 **Arnica:** the topical use of arnica flowers calms the swollen and inflamed tissue associated with RSI. After icing the site for three to five minutes, place a poultice or oil of arnica on the affected area, and repeat this several times daily. Create a poultice by infusing 2–3 g of the whole plant or flower heads in 150 ml of hot water for 15 minutes. Place gauze or bandages in the infusion and wrap the injured area. You may also create arnica oil by adding 1 part of chopped up arnica flowers to five parts of vegetable oil. Arnica should not be placed over open wounds or taken internally.

**Rue:** This is an effective topical treatment for RSI. Rue oil, when combined with arnica in a cream or lotion (this combination can be purchased in herbal medicine stores), or added to an arnica poultice or oil as described above, improves circulation to the inflamed area and heals inflammation of the soft tissues. It should only be used topically.

**Castor oil:** This oil can be massaged into the affected area, or applied to a washcloth which is then wrapped around the injury. The washcloth should be wrapped with a thin plastic wrap to contain the oil and is covered with a hot towel for 20–30 minutes. The castor oil pack can also be placed on the site before going to bed and, once well covered, left on all night to decrease inflammation.

**Anti-inflammatory oils:** There are several essential oils that can be rubbed either singly or in combination over the site of an RSI. These oils soak into the tissue and relieve inflammation. For example, peppermint essential oil contains menthol, which desensitizes nerves that conduct pain messages to the brain, leading to a decrease in pain. Camphor yields a cooling oil that acts locally as a counter-irritant and numbs sensation, thereby relieving pain. Camphor is safe when used in the short-term in lotions or ointments of low concentrations (0.1–11%) on intact skin. Wintergreen and arnica oils are other topical treatments that can be massaged onto the area of an RSI.

# RHEUMATIC FEVER

## DIAGNOSIS

Rheumatic fever is an inflammatory disease that can affect many connective tissues of the body, especially those of the heart, joints, skin, and occasionally the brain. The exact cause is unclear, but it is linked to streptococcal infection, and symptoms usually appear within five weeks after an untreated case of strep throat (see p. 304). Most cases of strep throat, however, do not lead to rheumatic fever, even in untreated cases. Permanent heart damage that results from rheumatic fever is called rheumatic heart disease. The heart is usually affected to some degree, and there can be lasting damage to the valves. There is no cure, but it can be prevented by promptly treating strep throat with antibiotics. This condition mostly affects children, although adults can also get it. Often it is so mild that children do not know that they have it, and only discover that they have rheumatic heart disease later in life. It is now a more rare condition as the streptococcal bacteria that causes it is much less common. Once someone has had rheumatic fever they are vulnerable to subsequent infections.

## SYMPTOMS

- Streptococcal infection is the triggering mechanism
- Arthritic pains
- Irregular jerking movements of limbs
- Rash
- Heart valve problems leading to breathlessness and palpitations

## TREATMENT GOAL

The goals of treatment are to reduce symptoms, monitor cardiac function, and provide prevention guidelines.

The main treatment for rheumatic fever is anti-inflammatory drugs such as aspirin. In severe cases, corticosteroid drugs are prescribed.

**Antibiotics:** A 10-day course of penicillin is prescribed as a first line of treatment. Alternatively, erythromycin can be used by those who are allergic to penicillin. Long-term prophylaxis is necessary following this full-dose treatment.

**Other medication:** Aspirin is usually used to relieve joint pain if there is no inflammation of the heart. Corticosteroids are prescribed if significant inflammation of the heart is present.

**Treatment in the acute phase:** During the acute phase of the illness it is necessary to take plenty of bed rest. If any damage to the heart valve occurs then a different antibiotic must be used before other procedures to prevent bacterial endocarditis, an infection of the inner heart or heart valves. This is necessary because the antibiotics used to prevent the recurrence of acute rheumatic fever are inadequate for preventing bacterial endocarditis.

## TRADITIONAL CHINESE MEDICINE

**Herbs:** Combine 12 g of  Huang Bai (Phellodendron), 12 g of Cang Zhu (black atractylodes rhizome), 12 g of Zhi Mu (anemarrhena rhizome), 8 g of Gui Zhi (cinnamon), 12 g of Bai Shao (white peony), 12 g of Hu Zhang (bushy knotweed root and rhizome), and 30 g of sweet rice. Place these herbs in a ceramic or glass pot and add 3 cups of water. Bring to the boil and simmer for 30 minutes. Strain the liquid and drink 1 cup twice a day. Take this formula for five to seven days for relief of symptoms, but consult a TCM practitioner for the longer-term. These herbs are available from Chinese pharmacies on online.

**Acupuncture:** Treatment has proven to be effective for rheumatic fever. One course of acupuncture will consist of 12 treatments, and a practitioner will determine whether treatment should be once or twice a week. A practitioner will also be able to advise on further courses as he or she evaluates your progress.

**Acupressure:** Press the Qu Chi, Hegu, and Tai Chong acupressure points. With the elbow flexed, the Qu Chi point is found on the outside of the elbow at the lateral end of the crease. The Hegu points are located on the back of the hands in the depression between the thumb and the first finger. The Tai Chong points are on the instep of the feet in the depression between the first and second toe, at the base of the big toe. Press these points with the tip of a finger for one minute. It may help to relieve some of the fever, but its effect is mild. It is recommended that you consult a traditional Chinese medicine doctor.

**Diet:** Foods that clear heat and dampness such as honeysuckle flower, purslane, mung beans, crab, lotus root, celery, spinach, lettuce, and hyacinth flowers are recommended. Avoid shrimp, beef, lamb and chili peppers, since they may interfere with your herbal treatment and increase heat in your body. Eat balanced meals that include fresh food rather than frozen food. In addition, make sure you drink enough water every day.

## NATUROPATHY

See a doctor for treatment of rheumatic fever as it can be potentially life threatening. The recommendations below may be helpful as a complementary therapy.

**Diet:** You or your child should drink plenty of fluids in the form of water, tea, and soup. Miso and chicken soup are the most beneficial. Eliminate dairy and refined carbohydrates from your diet. These will increase mucus accumulation and decrease your immunity.

**Supplements:** The primary interest is to boost the immune system so that the body can fight the infection as effectively as possible. Vitamin C can help prevent rheumatic fever in those who have a streptococcal infection as it increases the strength of the immune system. Take 500 mg every two hours. Children under the age of 12 should have children's vitamin C and follow the dosage instructions on the label. Take 200,000 IU of beta carotene a day to help increase the strength of the immune system. Vitamin A also stimulates the immune system; take 50,000 IU a day for one week, but do not take this if you are pregnant. Zinc increases immunity. Adults can take 30 mg a day, and children should take 10–15 mg a day.

**Herbs:** Goldenseal contains an ingredient called berberine that has antibiotic properties against different stains of streptococcus bacteria. Take 350–500 mg a day or 3 tsp of a tincture a day. Echinacea can be taken at 150–300 mg a day to boost immune activity. You can also take two to four tbsp of a tincture.

**Hydrotherapy:** Sit on a chair and place your feet in a bucket of warm water for 15 minutes. Dry them and put whave been placed in cold water and wrung out. Cover the cotton socks with a pair of wool socks and leave them on overnight. This diverts blood flow to the feet and away from the upper body, thus reducing fever.

## HOMEOPATHY

This condition has potentially serious complications and is best treated by conventional medical attention. Homeopathy can be helpful in a complementary context to strengthen the constitution of the patient. If your child is already receiving homeopathic treatment and this condition develops, a practitioner may suggest using one of the following acute homeopathic remedies alongside conventional treatment to make the patient more comfortable. It must be stressed that this situation calls for professional medical treatment, and is not suitable for home-prescription.

**Aconite:** If symptoms of fever come on quickly and dramatically, often developing in sleep and waking the patient in a state of great distress, restlessness, and anxiety, Aconite can be helpful. Pain and inflammation in the joints magnify the general state of upset and fear as there is a marked sensitivity to, and intolerance of, pain.

**Pulsatilla:** This remedy may be used to treat pains that shift from one joint to another. Lying in bed in a warm, stuffy room generally makes the patient feel worse, while contact with fresh, cool air helps. When this remedy is well indicated, patients are tearful and clingy, and respond well to lots of sympathy, attention, and affection.

**Mercurius:** If sweating at night produces an unpleasant smell, and joint pains cause particular distress, making it difficult to get comfortable in bed, Mercurius may be used. It is not appropriate to take this remedy in the feverish stage of illness, but tends to be well indicated in the late stage of an acute condition.

**Dulcamara:** Symptoms that respond to this remedy often come on, or are aggravated after, exposure to cold, damp conditions. The joints are red, swollen, painful, and tender to the touch. Joint pain prompts patients to repeatedly change position to get comfortable, and the pain may alternate with bouts of exhausting diarrhea.

## HERBALISM

This is a serious condition that needs to be immediately treated conventionally with antibiotics and other medication, depending on any complicating conditions, until the patient is stable and improving. Herbs have a limited role, and are primarily used in symptomatic treatment of the pain associated with arthritis (see p. 598) and fever (see p. 545).

**Willow:** Aspirin is an effective treatment of the fever and arthritis that can be associated with rheumatic fever. Willow bark, from which aspirin was originally derived, is a "natural" alternative that has the same effect, though a large quantity of willow needs to be ingested to equal effective doses of aspirin. Willow contains mildly anti-inflammatory salicylate compounds, which are responsible for helping with the symptoms of rheumatic fever. In addition to Salix alba, there are many other species of willow that have medicinal effects with specific varieties and concentrations of the active medicinal compounds. A tea can be made from high-quality willow bark (at least 7% total salicin compounds). Boil 1 heaped tsp of powdered root bark per cup of water and strain prior to drinking. Several cups of this tea should be ingested daily, but given that the concentration of active compounds in willow bark is quite low, most people will have to supplement willow with anti-inflammatory medication. The more finely ground the bark, the better the extraction of the active compounds. As with aspirin itself, there is the possibility of bleeding problems and stomach upset with repeated use of willow bark, and it should not be used by children with rheumatic fever due to concerns about Reye's syndrome that occurs with aspirin and Streptococcal infections.

# RHEUMATOID ARTHRITIS

## DIAGNOSIS

Rheumatoid arthritis is an aggressive inflammatory condition that affects the fingers, thumbs, wrists, knees, and feet. The tissue that surrounds the joint, called synovial fluid, allows for smooth movement between the bones. Rheumatoid arthritis develops when this fluid becomes damaged, causing inflammation, pain, and swelling of the joints. This inflammation can eventually destroy the joint, eating away at the cartilage and bone. It may involve many areas of the body, making you feel generally unwell, and in some severe cases it can affect the whole body and have crippling results.

No one knows what triggers the inflammation, but it is thought to be an "autoimmune disease" in which the immune system creates antibodies that fight against the body's tissues. It is unclear why this occurs, but it is a common illness that affects millions of people and tends to run in families. It can develop at any age, but usually starts in middle age. The severity of attacks is extremely variable and ranges from a single episode to severe disability.

## SYMPTOMS

- Acutely painful, hot, swollen joints
- Inflammatory skin nodules
- Puffy joints
- Fatigue, weakness, fever, and flu-like aches and pains
- Pains typically located in fingers, wrists, elbows, knees, and ankles
- Pain can be continual or variable
- Morning stiffness
- Occasionally, eye problems

## TREATMENT GOAL

Conventional and complementary treatments focus on developing a therapeutic lifestyle plan that looks at nutrition, exercise, rest, and medication, particularly the new drugs being developed to treat this condition. These factors can help to slow the rate of joint damage and minimize pain and inflammation.

## CONVENTIONAL MEDICINE

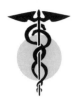

**Medication to treat pain:** Drugs used to treat rheumatoid arthritis are pain relievers such as acetaminophen and non-steroidal anti-inflammatory drugs (NSAIDs). NSAIDs have the added benefit of reducing inflammation as well as pain. Corticosteroids are given orally to treat severe or aggressive disease. Local infections of the joint can be used when there is swelling and loss of motion.

**Medication to control the disease:** Other classes of drugs are used to modify and control the disease. These drugs include methotrexate, sulfasalazine, leflunomide, hydroxycholoroquine, azathioprine, etanercept, and infliximab. Adalimumab is a newly approved rheumatoid arthritis disease-modifying drug that is given subcutaneously (under the skin). These drugs are strong and have side effects that are significant, but they are generally effective. They should not be used if pregnancy is a possibility, or if liver disease is present.

**Physical therapy:** Hydrotherapy (also called balneotherapy) is effective for soothing pain and is one of the oldest treatments for rheumatoid arthritis. It is often used in conjunction with other treatments. Thermotherapy is the application of heat or cold to sore joints, which can ease pain. Exercise is also usually recommended by a physiotherapist. A light daily routine to improve joint mobility, muscle strength, aerobic capacity, and function is ideal.

**Diet and supplements:** If you are overweight and suffer from rheumatoid arthritis, weight loss is important. Follow an anti-inflammatory program that excludes dairy and processed foods, avoids excess gluten and sugar, and includes the herbs ginger, curcumin, and turmeric. Doses of 600 mg of curcumin three times a day on an empty stomach are also effective. Fish oil is a natural anti-inflammatory and may be helpful at doses of 4 g daily. Selenium and vitamin E should also be supplemented at 400 IU a day and 400 mcg a day respectively.

## TRADITIONAL CHINESE MEDICINE

**Herbs:** Combine 12 g of Chuan Xiong (Szechuan lovage root), 12 g of Tao Ren (peach kernel), 12 g of Qiang Huo (notopterygium root), 12 g of Du Huo (pubescent angelica root), 12 g of Dan Gui (Chinese angelica root), 15 g of Niu Xi (achyranthes root), 12 g of Du Zhong (eucommia bark), 15 g of Bai Zhu (white atractylodes rhizome), and 15 g of Chi Xiao Dou (adzuki bean). Make a decoction by placing the herbs in a ceramic or glass pot and adding 3 cups of water. Bring the mixture to the boil, simmer for 30 minutes, and drink 1 cup twice a day. You may take this formula for five to seven days to relieve symptoms. However, consult a doctor of traditional Chinese medicine for longer-term use. You can purchase the herbs from Chinese pharmacies or online.

**Acupuncture:** Treatment can be affective in relieving the pain and discomfort of rheumatoid arthritis. It can also can help you to reduce your dosage of anti-inflammatory medication. Depending on the severity of the condition, a practitioner may recommend acupuncture once or twice a week.

**Acupressure:** The Yang Lin Qian point is generally used for joint pain and inflammation. This point can be pressed once a day as a complementary therapy to acupuncture and herbal remedies. The Yang Ling Qian point is on the outside of the lower leg, parallel to the knee in the depression on the head of the fibula. You can also press the painful area with gentle pressure. However, if you have severe inflammation of the joints, first consult a doctor.

**Diet:** Eat food that is neutral and good for clearing dampness and heat. Some suggestions include apricot, beetroot, Chinese cabbage, carrots, corn, duck, grapes, and beef liver. Avoid food that is overly warm from the perspective of Chinese medicine, such as asparagus, brown sugar, butter, chives, ginger, and red or green peppers. Also, avoid food that is too cold in its properties, such as bamboo shoots, bananas, clams, grapefruit, and muskmelon.

## NATUROPATHY

**Diet:** An anti-inflammatory diet is essential for the relief of pain. Deep-water fish, such as salmon, sea bass, tuna, trout, and mackerel, are rich sources of the polyunsaturated fats called omega-3 fatty acids and have anti-inflammatory properties. Eliminate the top food allergens from your diet such as wheat, dairy, corn, and soy, as they increase inflammation in the joints. Vegetables from the nightshade family, including tomatoes, aubergine, potatoes, and peppers, also increase inflammation and should be avoided. Blueberries, cherries, and hawthorn berries are rich sources of flavonoids, particularly proanthocyanidins. These flavonoids exhibit membrane and collagen stabilizing, antioxidant, and anti-inflammatory actions as well as many other actions that are beneficial in the treatment of rheumatoid arthritis. Low levels of vitamin E have been found in the joint fluid of rheumatoid arthritis patients. The antioxidant properties of vitamin E are thought to protect joint cells from free radical damage. Food sources high in Vitamin E include broccoli, almonds, avocados, mangoes, peanuts, sunflower seeds, and Brazil nuts.

**Supplements:** A good-quality multivitamin/multimineral will provide the proper nourishment to prevent joint destruction. Follow the dosage instructions on the label. Glucosamine sulfate reduces knee pain and rebuilds cartilage. Usually it is combined with chondroitin sulfate. Take 1,500 mg daily of glucosamine with 1,200 mg of chondroitin. Methylsulfonylmethane (MSM) has natural anti-inflammatory benefits and contains the mineral sulfur, an important component of cartilage. Take 4,000–8,000 mg daily. Take 500 mg of niacinamide, which has been reported to help arthritic patients, three times a day. Higher dosages should be supervised by a doctor. Take 250 mg of sulfur four times a day as it is important for cartilage structure. Vitamin C is beneficial in collagen synthesis repair, a major component of bone. Take 1–3 g a day. Protease enzyme breaks down protein molecules that promote inflammation. Take 2–3 capsules between meals.

**Herbs:** Take 500 mg of bromelain three times a day for its natural anti-inflammatory effects. Cayenne cream can deplete the nerves of a neurotransmitter that transmits pain messages to the brain. Try applying the cream to the affected area two to four times a day. Devil's claw helps with arthritic pain in the joints. Take 1,500–2,500 mg three times a day, but do not take it if you have a history of gallstones, heartburn, or ulcers. Take a white willow product standardized to contain 240 mg of salicin to relieve pain, or take 5 ml of a tincture three times a day. Take 1,000 mg of yucca root, which has been traditionally used for arthritic pain, twice a day. Ginger has anti-inflammatory benefits and relieves pain. Take 1–2 g or 1–2ml of tincture three times a day, but do not take more than 1 g of ginger a day if you are pregnant. Dimethyl sulfoxide (DMSO) is a sulfur-containing substance derived from wood pulp. It may relieve pain, stiffness, and inflammation in the joints and in the body in general. Talk to your doctor about this option. Celery seeds help clear uric acid from the joints of gout and arthritis sufferers. Boil 1 tsp of seeds in 1 cup of water for 15 minutes, strain, and sip. Dandelion dispels uric acid. Take 3 capsules daily, or 1 tbsp of juice or 1 cup tea twice daily for four to six weeks to reduce the frequency and intensity of pain, and to strengthen the connective tissue. Parsley juice is effective in combating and flushing out uric acid from the tissue, which eases painful limbs and joints. Take 1 tsp of parsley juice three times daily for six weeks. Wait three weeks before repeating.

## HOMEOPATHY

This is a chronic condition that results when the small joints of the body becoming inflamed, stiff, and painful. Homeopathic treatment can play a significant role in treatment by providing a complementary route for reducing pain, inflammation, and stiffness. However, treatment should be given by an experienced homeopathic practitioner to see the best results. Some self-help strategies are suggested below, but it must be emphasized that these are stop-gap measures only, and should not be relied upon in the long-term.

**Bryonia:** This remedy can be helpful for reducing heat, swelling, and stiffness in joints that respond obviously well to rest and are aggravated by even the slightest movement. Joint pains can be accompanied by a generally "toxic" feeling with associated symptoms of frontal headache and constipation. Applying pressure and support to the tender joints gives some relief, while light touch feels uncomfortable.

**Apis:** If the affected area is rosy-pink, puffy, and swollen, and acutely sensitive to contact with heat in any form, try Apis. Contact with cool air or cool compresses gives temporary relief from stinging pains and discomfort.

**Ledum:** This is a potentially helpful acute remedy to relieve pain in a joint that has been subject to a steroid injection. Symptoms include a numb, cool sensation in the affected area that is relieved by applying a cool compress, or bathing in cool water.

**Rhus tox:** This is one of the leading remedies for rheumatism and arthritis. It is appropriate if stiffness in the joints is relieved by moving around, applying hot compresses, or soaking in warm water. The body feels restless and there is a constant need to move around to find a comfortable position. Symptoms may come on after overexertion or getting cold and/or wet.

> **TIP: SWIM**
> Try to keep the joints as mobile as possible. Swimming is an ideal form or exercise, as the buoyancy of the water provides gentle support for any affected joints.

## HERBALISM

**Boswellia:** The boswellic acids in this herb act to inhibit enzymes that lead to the production of inflammation-causing compounds. Research on the effectiveness of treating rheumatoid arthritis with boswellia has been mixed, although one study showed that the use of boswellia can lessen the need for conventional medication in some people, of course depending on the extent and severity of the condition. Standardized extracts of boswellia can be purchased in stores that sell herbal medicines; to treat rheumatoid arthritis, approximately 3,600 mg of such an extract should be taken, divided three times per day. Some people experience stomach upset or heartburn when taking boswellia extracts orally. Ointments and creams that contain boswellia can also be purchased and applied topically to swollen and painful joints; sometimes, dermatitis can develop with these products.

**Ginger:** This herb contains compounds that can exert significant anti-inflammatory effects by inhibiting certain inflammatory prostaglandins, which are components of the blood that can worsen symptoms of rheumatoid arthritis. These effects are partly due to compounds in ginger called shogaols, present in both fresh ginger rhizome and powdered, dried ginger (the latter may also be sold in capsule form). Typical capsules contain 500 mg of dried ginger, and a usual dose is 1–3 g per day. A tea of fresh ginger rhizome can be made by chopping 1 g of the rhizome and steeping it in about 150 ml of boiling water for 10 minutes, covered so as to contain the volatile compounds. Strain and drink 1 cup three times daily. There are theoretical concerns about ginger's potential for thinning the blood, and ginger may also stimulate bile flow, causing problems if gallstones are present, and lower blood sugar. Do not take more than 1 g of ginger a day if you are pregnant.

**Turmeric:** This powerful anti-inflammatory agent is possibly as effective as anti-inflammatory medications such as ibuprofen or acetaminophen in controlling some of the symptoms of rheumatoid arthritis. One of its isolated phytochemicals, curcumin, is often used for conditions such as rheumatoid arthritis in doses of 400–600 mg three times daily, though many practitioners prefer to use whole turmeric for the added effect of other compounds. Powdered turmeric root is often dosed at 0.5–1 g two or three times daily, and it may take several weeks for symptoms to improve. It is probably easiest to simply incorporate this amount of turmeric regularly into your cooking. It is also possible to purchase turmeric extract standardized to its curcuminoid content; the dose will depend on the exact product purchased. Some people experience some stomach upset with turmeric, and care should be taken with any medications or supplements that thin the blood.

**Green tea:** The daily consumption of green tea can help to decrease inflammation and pain in rheumatoid arthritis, primarily through the actions of its compounds, called polyphenols, which are similar to the compounds in red wine and dark chocolate. Three to four cups of green tea a day can help with symptoms; decaffeinated tea should work just as well. You can also take green tea extracts standardized to the polyphenol percentage. These standardized extracts should be taken as directed on the label.

# SCIATICA

## DIAGNOSIS

Sciatica is a common condition in which pain radiates along the sciatic nerve, located in the lower spine. When this nerve becomes irritated it causes pain in the lower back, which then travels to the buttocks and down into the leg, foot, and toes. It can start suddenly or be triggered by exertion or injury. The pain may be continuous or only be felt when in certain positions. Typically the symptoms are only felt on one side of the body. Sciatica is generally caused by the compression of a nerve root in the lumbar spine, which can be triggered by a herniated disc, spinal stenosis, infection, or a fracture. Risk factors include a sedentary lifestyle, gardening, sports (particularly if they are not played consistently), being overweight, and wearing high heels. Improving your general muscle tone and fitness is the best way to strengthen and protect your back.

Usually the pain goes away without treatment but this will depend upon the severity of the condition. It is wise to rest in bed for up to 48 hours and then to get up and move about as soon as you can. Prolonged rest probably worsens recovery.

## SYMPTOMS

- Numbness down one side of the body
- Tingling
- Pain in the lower back, buttocks, and legs
- Throbbing pains
- Sharp, shooting pains
- Weak legs
- Occasionally, problems with bladder or bowel function

## TREATMENT GOAL

Symptoms of sciatica usually begin to feel better within one week of the initial injury. Treatment involves easing the pain and restoring mobility to the affected area. Exercise and other lifestyle changes can be adopted to prevent against further attacks.

## CONVENTIONAL MEDICINE

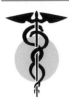

Conservative treatment should be attempted first, as 95% of patients improve without resorting to more complicated treatment. Rest for 48 hours. Serious possible causes, such as cancer, infection, or severe trauma, should also be excluded.

**Medication:** Use non-steroidal anti-inflammatory drugs (NSAIDs) for pain relief and to reduce inflammation. Corticosteroids, including prednisone, may be helpful for short-term use, and muscle relaxants such as cyclobenzaprine (Flexeril®) and carisoprodol (Soma®) may also be helpful in managing pain. However, caution should be exercised, as these drugs are sedating and may be addictive.

**Steroid injections:** Epidural steroid injections may give good short-term relief, and repeated injections into the epidural space around the spinal cord may be necessary.

**Surgery:** Surgical intervention is sometimes needed in people who have severe symptoms that do not respond to the above treatments.

**Lifestyle modifications:** If you are overweight and suffer from sciatica, begin a weight-loss program to help ease symptoms. Nutrition should be based on a high-protein diet, with plenty of whole grains, fruits, and vegetables. Cut out processed foods and sugar, and drink plenty of water. Exercise is important but heavy lifting, twisting, bending, and exposure to vibrations should be limited.

## TRADITIONAL CHINESE MEDICINE

**Herbs:** The following decoction can be taken to relieve sciatic nerve pain and keep the condition from worsening. Combine 12 g of Ji Shen (jilin root), 15 g of Niu Xi (achyranthes root), 12 g of Du Huo (pubescent angelica root), 12 g of Ru Xiang (frankincense), 8 g of Huang Hua (*flos carthami tinctorii*), 15 g of Bai Shao (white peony), 12 g of Yan Hu Suo (corydalis rhizome), 5 g of Gan Cao (licorice), and 10 g of Huang Bai (phellodendron) in a ceramic pot. Add 3 cups of water, bring to a boil, and simmer for 30 minutes. Strain the liquid and drink 1 cup twice a day. You may take this formula for five to seven days. These ingredients can be purchased from Chinese pharmacies or online.

**Acupuncture:** A practitioner will generally recommend treatment twice a week. To treat an acute condition, sessions once a day are necessary. You may see some relief following the first treatments.

**Acupressure:** While lying down so that the painful side is facing up, have someone press the Huan Tiao and Yang Lin Qian points with deep and strong pressure for one to three minutes, once or twice a day. The Yang Ling Quan point is on the outside of the lower leg, parallel to the knee, in the depression on the head of the fibula. The Huan Tiao point is on the outside of the thigh in a depression just behind the top of the femur.

**Diet:** Food that is easy to digest is recommended during an acute episode. Foods that are cooling such as spinach, lettuce, apples, barley, tofu, loquat, mandarin oranges, mangoes, and peppermint are also good.

## NATUROPATHY

**Diet:** Extra weight and constipation can aggravate sciatica. Sciatica sufferers should eat a diet that will enable them to lose weight if necessary and have regular bowel movements. Eat light, frequent meals throughout the day. Big, heavy meals slow digestion and decrease overall gastric function within time. Apples, fresh vegetables, and whole grains have high fiber levels. Eat several portions a day to relieve constipation. Stay hydrated by drinking eight glasses of water a day, as dehydration aggravates sciatic pain. Eat foods that are high in essential fatty acids, such as walnuts, salmon, and flaxseeds to help relieve constipation and reduce inflammation.

**Supplements:** Vitamin C helps with inflammation and strengthens connective tissue in your lower back. Take 1,000 mg three times a day. Take 2 protease enzymes on an empty stomach between meals twice a day to reduce inflammation and help with pain. Take 2,000 mg of methylsulfonylmethane (MSM), a natural anti-inflammatory that also alleviates pain, three times a day. Take 250 mg of magnesium twice a day as it also alleviates muscle spasm. Glucosamine sulfate is helpful for sciatica caused by a herniated disc. Take 1,500 mg a day.

**Herbs:** Take 500 mg of bromelain three times a day for its anti-inflammatory effects. White willow relieves pain in the lower back and throughout the body. Products should be standardized to contain 240 mg of salicin or take 5 ml of a tincture three times a day. Ginger has anti-inflammatory benefits and relieves pain. Take 1–2 g or 1–2 ml of a tincture three times a day. Dimethyl sulfoxide (DMSO) is a sulfur-containing substance derived from wood pulp. It may relieve pain, stiffness, and inflammation in the lower back. Talk to your doctor about whether this is appropriate and about dosage options. Curcumin, the yellow pigment of turmeric, has a significant anti-inflammatory action. Curcumin has been shown to be as effective as cortisone or phenylbutazone in certain models of inflammation. Curcumin also exhibits many beneficial effects on liver functions. The typical dosage of curcumin is 400–600 mg three times a day.

> **TIP:** TRY VERTEBRAL AXIAL DECOMPRESSION (VAX-D)
> VAX-D may reduce pain and improve function in patients with chronic lower back pain and sciatic pain. The procedure is thought to alleviate pain and enhance healing by relieving pressure within the discs, and promoting the in-flow of oxygen, fluids, and nutrients to the spinal column. Some chiropractors, naturopathic doctors, or osteopaths may have this type or equipment.

## HOMEOPATHY

 The following homeopathic remedies can be helpful in providing complementary pain relief for a mild, recent attack of sciatica. However, any mechanical problem that has caused the sciatica will also need to be dealt with by the appropriate therapist, whether an orthodox medical, chiropractic, or osteopathic practitioner. More established, chronic conditions should be referred to an experienced homeopathic practitioner.

**Hypericum:** This remedy can ease shooting, sharp pains that can develop into burning, tingling sensations that radiate into the affected leg. Pains may be restricted to the left side, and can be set off by a fall that has jarred the base of the spine. Pain and discomfort may be aggravated by damp, cold conditions and sharp, jarring movements, while massage or lying on the belly may give temporary relief.

**Kali carb:** When this remedy is indicated there may be a general sense of weakness in the affected leg, with tearing pains radiating from the hip, down the thigh to the knee. Throbbing, stabbing pains are likely to be made more intense when lying on the affected side.

**Dioscorea:** Consider this as a possible option for right-sided sciatic pain that burns and shoots down the affected leg. Pain and discomfort trigger feelings of anxiety and shakiness, while firm pressure, stretching, or standing gives some temporary relief.

**Colocynthis:** Try this remedy when shooting pains extend from the top of the leg to the foot on the affected side. Classic symptoms that respond well to this remedy include sharp pains that are followed by a numb sensation. The latter can be temporarily eased by applying pressure to the affected area. Exposure to cold drafts makes the pain and discomfort more troublesome.

Applying arnica cream to the affected area may soothe aching pains, while hypericum cream or oil may help ease shooting pains. For maximum effect, apply when the skin is warm either after a bath or shower. The muscles will be relaxed by the heat and the warm skin will absorb creams or oils more readily.

## HERBALISM

Inflammation of the sciatic nerve, or sciatica, can occur anywhere along the length of the nerve and causes a variety of symptoms. The underlying cause needs to be addressed, following recommendations from your doctor. Herbs can be used to calm the pain and inflammation, providing relief until the situation resolves. See Back Pain (p. 604) for other herbal treatments relevant to sciatica.

**Anti-inflammatory herbs:** See Arthritis (p. 598) and Rheumatoid Arthritis (p. 696) for details about anti-inflammatory herbs such as turmeric, ginger, green tea, and Indian frankincense. These herbs act on some of the same physiological systems as pharmaceutical medications, though they may not act as quickly.

**Willow:** This plant contains mildly anti-inflammatory salicylate compounds. There are many species of willow that have medicinal effects, with specific varieties and concentrations of the active medicinal compounds. Willow bark is used to relieve pain related to muscle and joint inflammation, and can help with the symptoms of sciatica. A tea can be made from high-quality willow bark (it should contain at least 7% total salicin compounds). Boil 1 heaped tsp of powdered root bark per cup of water. Several cups of this tea should be ingested daily, but given that the concentration of active compounds in willow bark is quite low, most people have to supplement willow with anti-inflammatory medication. The more finely ground the bark, the better the extraction of the active compounds. As with aspirin itself, there is the possibility of bleeding problems and stomach upset with repeated use of willow bark.

# SHIN SPLINTS

## DIAGNOSIS

A shin splint is pain and inflammation in the tissues that connect muscles to the front and side of the shins. A tough membrane encases the muscles, which cannot expand readily as the muscle bulk enlarges. It is a condition that generally affects people who are fit and do a lot of high-impact sports such as running and tennis, or any other sport that takes place on a hard surface and bulks up muscles. The muscles involved are those responsible for lifting the foot, and typically jumping and running might bring on the pain, especially during periods of intense training and vigorous exercise. Stretching before beginning any sporting activity helps prevent this condition.

RICE (rest, ice, compression, and elevation) therapy and anti-inflammatory drugs will usually relieve acute pain. Physiotherapy can also help to ease symptoms. Mild cases tend to settle in a few weeks, and it is very important to have a break from sport when shin splints occur to rest your legs. If you continue to train with shin splints, you might cause permanent damage to the muscles. If the problem is a recurring one, you may eventually need an operation to split the membrane to allow your developing muscles to expand.

## SYMPTOMS

- Pain on the front of the shin
- Swelling
- Redness

## TREATMENT GOAL

Treatment involves identifying triggers and easing painful symptoms. Techniques, particularly stretching, can be adopted to prevent episodes from occurring.

## CONVENTIONAL MEDICINE

**Rest:** Shin splints, also known as medial tibial stress syndrome, is initially treated by relative rest. This implies a reduction in normal activity, not a cessation of activity. Cycling, swimming, or walking or running on terrain or at a pace that does not precipitate pain is encouraged. Generally, a rest of 7–10 days is sufficient to allow healing to the extent that some of the original training can be resumed. Ultrasound and whirlpool therapy seems to be of value as adjunct therapies.

**Medication:** Anti-inflammatory medication (non-steroidal anti-inflammatory drugs) is helpful in easing pain.

**Exercise:** Stretching the Achilles tendon is often suggested, as tight Achilles tendons have been noted to be more prominent in runners who develop shin splints. Achillies tendon stretching prior to running is strongly recommended. It may be helpful to have your runner's gait assessed to identify any mechanical problems. Those with excess foot pronation (flat feet) are particularly prone to shin splints.

## TRADITIONAL CHINESE MEDICINE

**Herbs:** Try using Wan Hua oil, Chinese medicine oil for external use. Apply the oil to the shin twice a day. It can help reduce the pain and promote local circulation.

**Acupuncture:** Consult an experienced practitioner regarding how frequently you should receive treatment and for how long. The number and length of sessions will depend on your particular condition. It usually takes three to six treatments to relieve the pain, but each case is different.

**Acupressure:** The Yang Lin Qian and Susanli points are recommended. The Yang Lin Quan point is on the outside of the lower leg, parallel to the knee, in the depression on the head of the fibula. You will find the Susanli point on the lower leg, about 1 inch to the outside of and 3 inches below the kneecap. Take a seat and apply moderate pressure to these points for one minute and repeat.

**Diet:** Eating balanced meals is strongly encouraged. Eat fresh food instead of frozen food and make sure you drink plenty of water. Avoid shrimp, beef, lamb, and chili pepper, since they may interfere with your herbal treatment and increase heat in your body.

## NATUROPATHY

See Sciatica (p. 702) for guidelines on anti-inflammatory supplements and herbs that can help with shin splints. Below is some advice on how to protect against this type of injury.

**Wear the right shoes:** Prevention is the most effective way to treat shin splints. Athletes, especially runners who are overpronators, tend to suffer shin splints most. Overpronation occurs when the feet roll inward too much. To avoid this, it is important to get the right shoes and/or the right insole. Features should include a rigid plastic collar that wraps around the shoe heel for support and controls excess pronation, and a rear-heel area made of solid rubber and a dual density midsole with the firmer material on the inside edge. Shock-absorbing insoles can help reduce the impact transmitted through the foot to the lower leg, particularly when running on hard surfaces for long periods of time. Orthotic insoles are firm insoles designed to correct biomechanical dysfunction such as overpronation. They will usually have strong arch support. Off-the-shelf orthotic insoles are available and suitable for many, although for the perfect fit a podiatrist can make them specifically for your feet. Go to a professional sports store for help on getting the correct running shoe, and see a podiatrist regarding an appropriate insole.

**Warm up:** Warm up before any physical activity even if it is moderate. A thorough and correct warm-up will help to prepare the muscles and tendons for any activity. Without a proper warm-up the muscles and tendons will be tight and stiff. There will be limited blood flow to the lower legs, which will result in a lack of oxygen and nutrients for the muscles.

**Stretch:** Stretch before and after any physical activity. Stretching will allow your muscles to remain flexible and flexible muscles are extremely important in the prevention of lower leg injuries. When muscles and tendons are flexible and supple, they are able to move and perform without being over stretched. If, however, your muscles and tendons are tight and stiff, it is quite easy for those muscles and tendons to be pushed beyond their natural range of movement.

## HOMEOPATHY

Ideally, this condition is best treated by a practitioner who has knowledge of physiotherapy as well as homeopathy. The advice given below is included to give an idea of what homeopathic support has to offer in terms of speeding up recovery, rather than encouraging self-help prescribing. Consult a practitioner regarding an appropriate frequency and duration of treatment.

**Ruta:** This is the remedy of choice for treating symptoms of shin splints, including pain, stiffness, and limited movement. Discomfort tends to be worse when resting, and when walking outside. However, walking for a limited amount indoors tends to provide relief, as does contact with warmth.

**Calc phos:** If Ruta has initially helped, but has not resolved the situation completely, Calc phos may be useful. Classic symptoms include pain in the affected limb that responds negatively to wet weather and movement. The injured area generally feels cold and numb. Rest, however, provides some relief, as does exposure to warmth.

---

**TIP:** RUN ON SOFT SURFACES

If shin splints are a recurring problem, avoid jogging or running on hard surfaces such as sidewalks, as the impact is likely to trigger injury. Run on grassy, soft surfaces whenever possible to protect your body's shock absorbers.

---

## HERBALISM

 **Arnica:** The "micro-tears" between the muscle and bone of the shin is essentially a repetitive strain injury of the lower leg. The inflammation and pain that occurs with shin splints will respond to similar herbs as those recommended for RSI. Start by icing the site for three to five minutes, and then apply a poultice of arnica flowers with about 1 tsp of rue oil added. These herbs should only be used topically. They can be applied several times per day and a castor oil pack, described below, can be used in between application and at night. For more details about arnica and rue, please see Repetitive Strain Injury (p. 686).

**Castor oil:** This oil can be massaged directly into shins, or you can soak a washcloth in the oil and wrap it around the lower leg. This washcloth should be covered with a thin plastic wrap to contain the oil, and a heated towel can be placed over the area for 20–30 minutes. The castor oil pack can also be placed on the site before going to bed, and, well-covered with plastic wrap, left on overnight to decrease inflammation and reduce pain.

# SHOULDER PAIN

## DIAGNOSIS

Shoulder pain is usually an indication that bones, tendons, or ligaments have been damaged. It can be associated with a range of conditions, some mild and others more serious. If the shoulder pain begins after an injury and is accompanied by swelling, bruising, or bleeding and you have difficulty moving your shoulder, you may have dislocated or fractured it. Seek emergency medical attention immediately. If the shoulder pain started after a sports activity and is accompanied by pain in the joint when you move your arm, you may have tendonitis (see p. 721) or bursitis (see p. 613). Shoulder pain can also be a symptom of a more chronic condition, such as rheumatoid arthritis (see p. 696), osteoarthritis (see arthritis, p. 598) and osteoporosis (see p. 681). It may also be a result of pain from an irritated nerve in the neck that radiates to the shoulder.

**DANGER:** If shoulder pain is accompanied by breathlessness, dizziness, and tingling in the chest or arms, it could indicate you are suffering from angina or even having a heart attack. Seek emergency medical assistance.

## SYMPTOMS

- Pain in or around the shoulder
- Pain in the joint
- Pain may be accompanied by swelling, bruising, or bleeding
- Breathlessness, dizziness, and tingling in the chest or arms may indicate a serious heart condition

## TREATMENT GOAL

If you are not sure what is causing the pain, see your doctor to establish what is wrong so that the condition can be treated accordingly.

## CONVENTIONAL MEDICINE

The treatment of shoulder pain is dependent on the cause. Seek an evaluation by a doctor: if pain in the shoulder follows a trauma of any kind so that a serious injury, if present, can be treated; if pain occurs along with another chronic illness, such as diabetes or cancer; if there is a loss of muscle function or sensory changes in the arm or hand; or if the shoulder is red, warm, swollen, and very painful, as this may be linked to septic arthritis.

**To treat chronic pain:** Chronic shoulder pain that develops over a period of time is often due to a condition called rotator cuff syndrome, in which the rotator cuff tendons and surrounding bursa become inflamed. This is also known as shoulder impingement syndrome, swimmer's shoulder, tennis shoulder, and painful arc syndrome. It is important to rest from the activity that has caused the pain—usually for two weeks but sometimes longer. Non-steroidal anti-inflammatory drugs (NSAIDs) can also be used to help with the pain. It is recommended that the patient have physical therapy so that the shoulder does not become frozen and to strengthen muscle groups. The use of steroid injections is debatable, but if the above measures do not help, they are sometimes given. If all of the above fails, shoulder surgery is recommended.

## TRADITIONAL HERBAL MEDICINE

**Herbs:** Since shoulder pain can be a secondary condition, and there are varying degrees of pain, it is best to consult a doctor of Chinese medicine for specific advice about which herbal medicine to take. You can also use patent external herbal medicine, such as Wan Hua oil. Apply it to the painful area twice a day.

**Acupuncture:** Treatment is very effective for shoulder pain. Depending on the severity of the pain, a ½ hour treatment once, twice, or three times a week may be required. A typical course of treatment will consist of 12 sessions. You may experience some relief with each acupuncture session, but in some cases it may take a while before the pain is eased. A doctor of traditional Chinese medicine will be able to evaluate and recommend a treatment plan for your particular condition.

**Diet:** Eating balanced meals that include fresh food is important for your general health. In addition, drink adequate amounts of fluid daily. Avoid shrimp, beef, lamb, and chili pepper, since they may interfere with your herbal treatment and increase heat in your body.

## NATUROPATHY

**Diet:** Shoulder pain can be caused by several factors, but in most cases inflammation is involved, causing pain and discomfort throughout the body. Eat an anti-inflammatory diet that cuts out refined sugars, hydrogenated fats, and glutens. Gluten is a protein found in some grains, especially wheat, that has been shown to be an allergen to many people, causing inflammation. Other common allergens include soy, dairy, egg, and corn. Eat salmon, mackerel, and walnuts for their high levels of essential fatty acids, which have anti-inflammatory properties. Also eat fruit and vegetables high in vitamin C and bioflavonoids. These substances strengthen ligaments and tendons, decreasing the occurrences of injuries. Such foods include berries, citrus fruits, green leafy vegetables, and carrots. A whole food diet consisting of whole grains and fresh fruit and vegetables would provide the essential nutrients to sustain healthy extremities.

**Supplements:** A high-quality multivitamin will provide the proper nourishment to prevent deterioration in the joints. Follow the dosage instructions on the label. Glucosamine sulfate reduces shoulder pain and rebuilds cartilage and ligaments. Usually it is combined with chondroitin sulfate. Take 1,500 mg daily of glucosamine with 1,200 mg of chondroitin. Methylsulfonylmethane (MSM) has natural anti-inflammatory benefits and contains the mineral sulfur, which can also be beneficial for shoulder pain. Take 4,000–8,000 mg daily. Take 4–6 g of fish oil a day to reduce inflammation and provide lubrication to the shoulder joints, but allow two to three months to see significant effects. If shoulder pain is linked to arthritis try taking 500 mg of niacinamide three times a day, as it has been clinically reported to help arthritic patients. Higher dosages should be supervised by a doctor. Also take 250 mg of methionine four times a day for arthritic shoulder pain. It is a sulfur-containing amino acid that has been shown to have benefits in arthritic patients. Vitamin C is beneficial in collagen synthesis repair, a major component of bone. Take 1–3 g a day. Also take 1–2 protease enzyme capsules on an empty stomach to reduce inflammation.

**Herbs:** Take 500 mg of bromelain three times a day for its anti-inflammatory effects. Cayenne cream depletes the nerves of a neurotransmitter that transmits pain messages to the brain and can be applied to the affected area two to four times a day. Devil's claw helps with pain in the knee and shoulder joints. Take 1,500–2,500 mg three times a day, but do not take it if you have a history of gallstones, heartburn, or ulcers. White willow relieves pain in the joints and throughout the body. Products should be standardized to contain 240 mg of salicin or take 5 ml of a tincture three times a day. You can also take 1–2 ml of tincture three times a day. Dimethyl sulfoxide (DMSO) is a sulfur-containing substance derived from wood pulp. It may relieve pain, stiffness, and inflammation in the joint and in the body in general. Talk to your doctor about the dosage and appropriateness of this option.

## HOMEOPATHY

The following remedies are appropriate to treat shoulder pain that has developed recently in response to an obvious trigger, such as overly vigorous exercising or a minor accident where the shoulder remains fully mobile, but bruised. For treatment of chronic or severe pain and stiffness in the shoulder, consult a homeopathic practitioner.

**Arnica:** If pain and stiffness in the shoulder has set in as a result of overuse, or exposure to cold and damp weather, try Arnica. The affected area feels bruised and achy, and sudden, jarring movement aggravates shooting, sharp pains that radiate from the shoulder.

**Chelidonium:** This remedy may be helpful in treating right-sided shoulder pain that settles around the shoulder blade. The neck muscles may feel stiff, and the affected area feels bruised, sore to the touch, and heavy.

**Rhus tox:** If shoulder pain settles in the muscles, making them sore and stiff when initially moved, take Rhus tox. Gentle movement (provided it does not go on for too long) eases the discomfort and stiffness, as does taking a warm bath or shower. The stiffness and discomfort may have been brought on by exposure to cold and damp conditions, or from too much exercise.

**Sanguinaria:** This is predominantly a remedy for sharp pains and stiffness that affect the right shoulder. The discomfort intensifies when turning or raising the arm, and is temporarily relieved when sleeping and lying on the back or on the left side.

**TIP:** USE ARNICA CREAM
If there is bruising or minor muscle strain in the shoulder (but the skin remains intact), Arnica cream may be helpful if massaged into the affected area after a warm bath or shower.

## HERBALISM

Shoulder pain can have many different causes, each of which has different conventional and herbal treatments; you should consult your doctor to determine exactly why your shoulder is painful. For shoulder pain that results from muscle irritation or strain, see Muscle Cramps (p. 663) and Muscle Pain (p. 667) for helpful herbs such as cramp bark and black haw. Effective topical treatments for muscle problems are discussed in detail in the section on back pain (p. 604). For shoulder pain due to arthritis in the joint, consider taking devil's claw, turmeric, ginger, green tea, and Indian frankincense, as discussed in the sections on arthritis (p. 597) and rheumatoid arthritis (p. 696). Devil's claw is most effective when taken in higher doses—3–6 g of powdered herb or 600—1,200 mg of 5:1 powdered extract per day. Powdered turmeric root is often recommended at 0.5–1 g two or three times daily. Ginger can be ingested as a tea or you can take two capsules of 500 mg of dried ginger one to three times per day. Do not take more than 1 g of ginger a day if you are pregnant. Drink 3–4 cups of green tea a day and take a total of 3,600 mg of boswellia as a standardized extract divided into separate doses two to three times daily.

> **TIP:** STRETCH AFTER YOUR WORKOUT
> Shoulder pain often results from repetitive motion, whether it is caused by your job or by playing a sport such as tennis. One of the best ways to remedy this problem, and help prevent it in the future, is to perform a full range of stretching and strengthening exercises to compensate for the repetitive movements.

# SPRAINS

## DIAGNOSIS

A sprain occurs when you stretch or tear a ligament, a strong band of tissue that connects one bone to another to support your joints. The ankle and wrist are particularly vulnerable to sprains and are the most commonly affected parts of the body. Sprains generally result from a sports injury or a fall. They cause pain, swelling, and bruising in the affected joint, and the skin around the injury often turns blue. This occurs when the small blood vessels and fibers in the flesh burst, causing blood to enter the surrounding tissue. When this happens the injured area must be kept still or the bleeding may become worse. If you suffer a sprain, rest the affected joint for one or two days, but it is then important to start moving again to reduce the amount of scarring formed in the damaged area. When the pain and swelling have subsided, start exercising the injured part of the body gently. As with any activity, warm up slowly and begin with stretching exercises.

## SYMPTOMS

- Pain and tenderness
- Swelling
- Redness or bruising
- Loss of mobility in affected area

## TREATMENT GOAL

Consult a doctor to confirm that you do have a sprain. Conventional and complementary therapies can help to reduce the pain and discomfort and speed up recovery from an injury.

## CONVENTIONAL MEDICINE

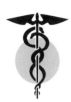

**Use the RICE therapy:** The mainstay of treatment for a sprain is rest, ice, compression, and elevation (RICE). Elevate the affected joint whenever possible, and apply ice to the injury for 20 minutes three times a day. An Ace wrap (an elastic bandage) can be wrapped around the injury to provide support and compression. Most sprains heal completely with conservative treatment.

**Splints and crutches:** In the past mild sprains were sometimes put into a cast and immobilized, but this is now associated with injuries that require longer healing times. Plaster splinting is now reserved for more severe sprains, and usually remains on for three weeks. Crutches are used until a few steps can be taken without pain.

**Medication:** The pain caused by a sprain can be managed by using non-steroidal anti-inflammatory drugs (NSAIDs), such as ibuprofen and acetaminophen. If this does not take care of the pain, opioid analgesics (such as hydrocodone and oxycodone) can be used. Once swelling has subsided and you can begin to put weight on the affected joint, begin to exercise gently. Motion exercises and muscle strengthening are both important, and can be supervised by a physiotherapist if necessary.

**Surgery:** Severe sprains that do not respond to conservative management are treated with surgical repair.

## TRADITIONAL CHINESE MEDICINE

**Herbs:** Apply Wan Hua oil to the sprained area twice a day. It helps reduce pain and promotes local circulation. You can find this at Chinese medicine pharmacy. You can also take Du Huo Ji Shen Wan or Yuan Hu Zhi Tong pills in combination with acupuncture and/or external herbal medicine.

**Acupuncture:** This can be used to treat pain and swelling. Treatment may consist of sessions two or three times a week. You may experience relief after the first session.

**Acupressure:** Lie on your stomach and have someone press the Cheng Shan and Cheng Jin points on the back of your legs for one minute, then release and repeat. When the leg is stretched with the toes pointing out, the Cheng Shan point is in the depression between the muscles on the back of the leg. The Cheng Jin point can be found about 4 inches below the bend in the back of the leg.

**Diet:** As general practice, eat a well-balanced diet that includes plenty of fruits, vegetables, and grains. Drink plenty of water as part of your daily routine. Have fresh food, but avoid shrimp, beef, lamb, and chili peppers since they may interfere with your herbal treatment and increase heat in your body.

## NATUROPATHY

**Diet:** Follow an anti-inflammatory diet to help with the healing process. Cold-water fish, such as salmon, sea bass, tuna, trout, and mackerel, contain high amounts of omega-3 essential fatty acids, which have been shown to fight inflammation. Pineapple contains bromelain, a powerful enzyme that has been shown to have anti-inflammatory effects on muscle and tissue. Bromelain also breaks down fibrin, a blood-clotting protein that can impede circulation and prevent tissues from draining properly. It also blocks the production of certain compounds that cause swelling and pain. Apples and onions are high in quercetin, a flavonoid that can help reduce inflammation in the joints and muscles. Include anti-inflammatory spices such as turmeric and ginger in your meals, and drink at least eight glasses of water a day, to flush out waste material and metabolites from the system, which increase inflammation and inhibit the healing process. Whole grains, fresh fruit, and vegetables should be a staple in your diet to providing the muscles with all the nourishment they need to assist in the healing process.

**Supplements:** Proteolytic enzymes destroy free radicals, which inhibit healing, and proteins involved in the inflammatory process. Take three tablets or capsules between meals. Vitamin C is required for the formation of connective tissue and to combat free radicals. Essential fatty acids such as flaxseed and fish oil reduce inflammation and promote tissue healing. Take 5 g of fish oils a day or 1–2 tbsp of flaxseed oil. Take 1,500 mg of glucosamine sulfate a day to provide the raw material for the body to manufacture ligaments and tendons. Take 50,000 IU of beta-carotene per day to make collagen, which can help repair connective tissue. Take 15–30 mg of zinc a day to help you heal faster, along with 2 mg of copper to avoid copper deficiency.

**Herbs:** Ginger has anti-inflammatory properties that help with pain, and is available in many different forms. You can take ginger as a standardized extract in pill form, 100–200 mg every four hours up to three times a day; as a fresh powder, ½–¾ tsp every four hours up to three times a day; or raw, ¼–½-inch (peeled) slice of ginger every four hours up to three times a day. Ginger tea is available in prepackaged bags or can be prepared by steeping ½ tsp of grated ginger root in 8 oz of very hot water for 5–10 minutes. A cup of tea, when steeped for this amount of time, can contain about 250 mg of ginger. Do not take more than 1 g of ginger a day if you are pregnant. Take 500 mg of bromelain three times a day for its natural anti-inflammatory effects.

Turmeric makes the effect of bromelain stronger, has anti-inflammatory properties, and is a strong antioxidant. Take 250–500 mg of turmeric three times a day between meals. Boswellia also has strong anti-inflammatory properties. Take 1,500 mg three times a day, but make sure it is a product that contains 60–65% boswellic acids. White willow bark is a natural pain reliever. Take 30–60 mg a day of an extract standardized to salicin.

> **TIP:** USE CASTOR OIL
> To relieve pain and swelling, apply castor oil directly to the skin and cover it with a clean, soft cloth and plastic wrap. Place a heated towel over the pack and leave it on for 30–60 minutes. For the best results, repeat for three consecutive days.

## HOMEOPATHY

The remedies below can play a complementary role in speeding up recovery from a mild to moderate sprain, provided the necessary first aid measures have been taken. To treat a severe sprain that requires a plaster cast and even surgery, consult an experienced homeopathic practitioner.

**Arnica:** If an injury has been sustained, Arnica can help the body deal with the systemic shock. In addition, it will help ease pain and encourage the re-absorption of blood from engorged tissues.

**Bryonia:** If Arnica has been initially helpful in reducing pain and swelling, but has ceased to improve the situation any further, try Bryonia. The pain and distress is aggravated by movement of any kind, and there is an obvious improvement when keeping the affected limb firmly supported and rested.

**Rhus tox:** This remedy can help to relieve the pain and stiffness of a sprain that has passed the initial stage of trauma. Unlike the symptoms that respond well to Bryonia, pain and stiffness is made much worse by resting, and is eased by gentle movement for a limited period of time. It can also be used to follow Arnica appropriately.

**Ledum:** If a sprain is stiff, painful, and hot, but not red in appearance, try using Ledum. Pain and discomfort is soothed and relieved by cool applications, and aggravated by becoming warm, especially in bed at night.

**Ruta:** This remedy can follow either Bryonia or Rhus tox to support the final stage of recovery from an established sprain. It is appropriate if stiffness and pain lodges in one area, as though a nail were sticking into the affected joint. Ruta can treat sprains that affect the wrists, knees, and/or ankles.

## HERBALISM

**Compresses:** Apply ice to acute sprains for three to five minutes as often as can be tolerated within the first 24–48 hours after the injury. On the third day, begin contrasting hot compresses (apply for three minutes) with ice packs (apply for 30 seconds). Arnica, which has anti-inflammatory action, can be applied in a gel or lotion form with the ice to assist tissue healing and decrease swelling and pain. The arnica should be continued for several days, even when you make the transition to ice alternating with heat. You can also make an arnica poultice (see Repetitive Strain Injury, p. 686).

**Essential oils:** Prior to applying ice or heat, massage a few drops of essential oil of wintergreen or peppermint, commonly available in small vials from stores that sell herbal medicines, into the sprain. These oils penetrate the skin and have anti-inflammatory action; in particular, the peppermint oil deadens the pain sensation transmitted by nerves, providing comfort as the sprain heals. Any oil or plant product applied topically has the potential to cause skin irritation in some people. If redness, itchiness, or blistering occurs, cease using the oils and check with a medical herbalist or your doctor for guidance.

**Rue:** Another plant that is specifically indicated for strains, sprains, and joint inflammation is rue, which is cooling to the touch. Rue oil, when combined with arnica into a cream or lotion (this can be purchased in herbal medicine stores), or added to an arnica poultice or oil as mentioned above, improves circulation to the inflamed area and heals inflammation of the soft tissues. It should only be used topically.

**Pain relief:** Some herbs with pain-relieving properties include meadowsweet, turmeric, and cayenne. Combine equal parts of these herbs, except cayenne, which should only make up 2–5% of the blend. Infuse 1 tbsp of this mixture per cup of water and drink every three to four hours as needed for pain relief.

> **TIP:** USE ARNICA CREAM
> Apply arnica cream to the affected area as soon as possible after the injury has been sustained to ease bruising and swelling. But do not use this cream if the surface of the skin has been broken, since it may cause inflammation at the edges of the wound or be absorbed systematically.

# TENDONITIS

## DIAGNOSIS

Tendonitis is the painful inflammation of a tendon, a sinew-like tissue that joins muscles to bones. When a tendon becomes inflamed, the action of pulling the muscle is irritating, causing pain and making movement difficult. The most common cause of tendonitis is the overuse of a particular muscle. This can occur through exercise, particularly when a new exercise program is begun, or the level of exercise is increased. As the tendon is unused to this increased movement it can become inflamed. The risk of tendonitis also increases with age, as muscles begin to lose their elasticity and range of movement. The symptoms of tendonitis usually subside after a few days, but they can last for up to six weeks in more severe cases. The areas of the body that are prone to tendonitis include the Achilles tendon, shoulders, and wrists.

## SYMPTOMS

- Restricted movement in the affected area
- Tenderness and pain
- Swelling
- Weakness

## TREATMENT GOAL

Pain management is the primary goal of both conventional and complementary therapies. Once the pain has eased, treatment involves increasing the range of motion and building strength in the tendons to protect against further injuries.

## CONVENTIONAL MEDICINE

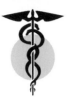

**Rest and ice:** Initial treatment is to immobilize the affected area and rest it from the trigger activity. However, a shoulder should not be immobilized as it may become "frozen." A sling, heel pads, or splints may be used at the discretion of the doctor to keep the area stable. Applying ice to the affected site for 15–20 minutes is often helpful.

**Exercise:** Once the initial pain has subsided, begin an exercise program to restore the range of motion and strengthen the tendons. Hydrotherapy, or water aerobics, is a good form of exercise to restore muscle function, as the buoyancy of the water supports the body. Physical therapy is recommended to strengthen tendons and prevent recurrence.

**Medication:** Non-steroidal anti-inflammatory drugs (NSAIDs) can used to relieve pain as needed. Steroids are sometimes injected into the joint associated with the tendonitis.

**Ultrasound therapy:** High-power focal ultrasound therapy, also known as shock-wave therapy (a non-invasive treatment in which high-energy shock waves are passed through the skin to the affected area), can have positive effects if small calcium deposits have developed in the tendon. Therapeutic ultrasound without focal pulses can be used to treat pain and swelling with or without calcifications.

## TRADITIONAL CHINESE MEDICINE

**Herbs:** Consult a doctor of Chinese medicine for a particular herbal medicine that can reduce the pain and inflammation. The herbs recommended will depend on the particular condition. In some cases, you may only need acupuncture treatment.

**Acupuncture:** Treatment can reduce the pain and prevent tendonitis from recurring. The number of treatment sessions will vary depending on the severity of the condition. You may experience some relief shortly after treatment begins.

**Acupressure:** Consult your doctor before performing acupressure to treat your condition. Treatment may not be suitable for your condition.

**Diet:** No specific foods are recommended for tendonitis; however, maintain a well-balanced diet to promote good health. Eat fresh food and drink adequate amounts of water daily. Avoid shrimp, beef, lamb, and chili peppers. They may interfere with your herbal treatment and increase heat in the body.

## NATUROPATHY

Inflammation is the cause of pain and discomfort in cases of tendonitis. See Sprains (p. 716) for guidelines on an anti-inflammatory diet as well as supplements and herbs that can help ease the pain of tendonitis by reducing inflammation. Below are some suggestions of other types of therapies that can relieve the pain.

**Prolotherapy:** With this treatment, a solution of simple compounds (usually dextrose or calcium carbonate) is injected at the point of the injury. This triggers an inflammation response that increases the blood supply and delivers the nutrients necessary to promote the growth of new cells and repair damaged connective tissue. Consult a naturopathic practitioner who practices prolotherapy regarding treatment.

**Massage and hydrotherapy:** Massage may be helpful in relieving pain and improving range of motion. Find a qualified massage therapist who has experience with tendonitis. Apply ice to the area for the first 48 hours and then try contrast hydrotherapy, alternating hot and cold applications. Soak the affected part for three minutes in hot water, then 30 seconds in cold water.

**Ultrasonography (phonophoresis):** This type of therapy involves using high-frequency sound to heat an area and increase the blood supply. This treatment can be offered by a chiropractor or sports injury clinic.

**TENS:** Transcutaneous electrical nerve stimulation (TENS) electricity can be used to control pain. This treatment can be offered by a chiropractor or at any sports injury clinic.

## HOMEOPATHY

The following homeopathic remedies can be helpful in providing complementary support to ease the pain and distress of a recent, mild to moderate episode of tendon inflammation. However, more severe examples of this problem, such as those involving the Achilles tendon, will require professional homeopathic assessment and treatment.

**Ruta:** Consider using this remedy if the affected area feels broken, achy, sore, and bruised internally. Inflamed tendons in the ankle joint are tender enough to cause temporary lameness. This may lead to a feeling of general weakness in the legs, with a tendency for the knees to give way when going up and down stairs.

**Bryonia:** If inflammation and pain are obviously aggravated by even the slightest movement, and clearly eased by keeping the affected area as still and rested as possible, use Bryonia.

**Rhus tox:** This remedy can be helpful if the affected area feels hot and inflamed, and if tearing pains are noticeably troublesome and distressing when trying to rest and sleep at night. Symptoms temporarily improve with gentle movement, and by taking a warm bath or shower.

## HERBALISM

 As with many musculoskeletal problems such as shin splints and repetitive strain injuries, arnica and rue are good topical treatments to combat the inflammation, leading to pain relief and healing of the damaged tissues.

**Arnica and rue:** Start by icing the site for three to five minutes then apply a poultice of arnica flowers with about 1 tsp of rue oil added. These herbs should only be used topically, and can be applied several times per day. In between applications and at night, a castor oil pack would be useful (see below). For more details about arnica and rue, see Repetitive Strain Injury (p. 686).

**Castor oil:** This oil can be massaged into the inflamed area. Alternatively, soak a washcloth and apply it to the site, covering it with plastic wrap and an elastic bandage to hold it in place. Allow 30–60 minutes to let the castor oil soak in to the tissues. You can also apply the oil before going to bed and leave it on overnight. The fatty acid profile of castor oil acts to promote the formation of compounds in the blood and tissue with which it comes into contact, calming the pain, redness, swelling, and inflammation associated with the tendonitis.

**Comfrey:** Comfrey can be used topically to relieve pain and fight the inflammation associated with tendonitis. Comfrey is cooling and moisturizing and acts as a mild analgesic and potent anti-inflammatory. Use a poultice of fresh or moistened roots and leaves by mashing them into a paste (add water if needed). Place the poultice onto the affected tendon when you are not using the other treatments described above.

# TENNIS ELBOW

## DIAGNOSIS

Tennis elbow is the common name for inflammation and pain that results from overstraining the muscles of the forearm, particularly the muscles used to straighten the fingers. Symptoms begin on the outside of the elbow, but can eventually spread to the upper arm as well as down the outer side of the forearm. The condition occurs when the tendon that connects the muscle in the forearm to the elbow becomes irritated, usually from overstraining or overuse. Common triggers include repetitive movements with the elbow bent while holding tightly onto something, such as a racquet or a tool. Despite the name, it is more common to develop this condition while gardening or doing household tasks than while actually playing tennis. The overuse of the muscle causes tiny tears in the tendon, resulting in irritation, inflammation, and swelling in the area. Tennis elbow often heals spontaneously, but in a few cases the pain can last for years. If the arm is not rested sufficiently after the initial injury occurs, further, more serious tearing of the tendon can result. Tennis elbow most frequently affects middle-aged people, and women seem to be affected more than men.

## SYMPTOMS

- Pain on the outer side of the elbow
- Pain around the projection of the bone on the outer elbow
- Pains radiating up and down the arm
- Feeling of weakness in the wrist

## TREATMENT GOAL

To bring relief of pain and swelling in the elbow, and restore full mobility to the arm.

## CONVENTIONAL MEDICINE

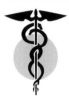

The medical name for tennis elbow is lateral epicondylitis. Symptoms can last for a couple of weeks to years, but the average recovery time is six to 12 weeks. It is necessary to avoid the activity that has caused the problem for as long as pain continues.

**Ice packs:** Apply ice to the affected elbow for 20 minutes three times a day for the first two days following the onset of pain. Ice can also be used thereafter whenever soreness develops.

**Medication:** Non-steroidal anti-inflammatory drugs (NSAIDs) such as Motrin®, ketoprofen (Orudis®), and naproxen (Naprosyn®) can be taken. Steroid injections are a controversial treatment for tennis elbow, although some people use them.

**Elbow strap:** It may be helpful to support the tendons by using an elbow strap, but is not necessary for recovery.

**Surgery:** Surgery may be recommended for severe symptoms that do not respond to the above treatments.

## TRADITIONAL CHINESE MEDICINE

**Herbs:** Consult a practitioner of traditional Chinese medicine for herbal remedies to reduce pain and inflammation. The herbs used depend on the individual condition. In some cases, you may only need acupuncture treatment.

**Acupuncture:** A practitioner may recommend sessions once or twice a week, beginning with one course of treatment. A course consists of 12 sessions, each lasting 30 minutes. You may see results right away, but continue having regular treatment to achieve the best long-term results.

**Acupressure:** Press the Zhou Jian and Zhou Liao points with gentle pressure. The Zhou Jian point is in the depression on the tip of the elbow when the elbow is flexed. With the elbow bent at 90 degrees, the Zhou Liao point is in the depression on the humerus (upper arm bone) on the thumb side of the elbow.

**Diet:** There no specific foods recommended to treat tennis elbow. However, it is always good practice to eat a well-balanced diet consisting of plenty of fresh fruits and vegetables, and to drink adequate amounts of fluid every day. Avoid shrimp, beef, lamb, and chili peppers, as they may increase heat in your body and interfere with treatment.

## NATUROPATHY

See Knee Pain (p.649) for advice on how to reduce inflammation, the common cause of elbow pain, through diet, supplements, and herbs. Suggestions for techniques that can help to prevent tennis elbow from occurring include bracing and strapping, modifying equipment, taking extended rests, and even learning new routines for repetitive activities.

**Warm up:** A thorough and correct warm up will help to prepare the muscles and tendons for any activity to come. Without a proper warm up the muscles and tendons will be tight and stiff. There will be limited blood flow to the forearm area, which will result in a lack of oxygen and nutrients for the muscles. This is a sure-fire recipe for a muscle or tendon injury.

**Increase flexibility:** Flexible muscles and tendons are extremely important in the prevention of most strain or sprain injuries. When muscles and tendons are flexible and supple, they are able to move and perform without being over stretched. If, however, your muscles and tendons are tight and stiff, it is quite easy for them to be pushed beyond their natural range of movement. When this happens strains, sprains, and pulled muscles occur.

**Check your swing:** If you play tennis and have tennis elbow, you probably have a poor backhand technique. Instead of leading with your elbow on your backhand you should get your racquet in front when you hit a backhand shot. Take tennis lessons if you need help finding and treating the problem.

## HOMEOPATHY

The following remedies, as well as those suggested for tendonitis (p. 721) and sprains (p. 716) can be used as stop-gap measures for relieving pain. For more comprehensive treatment for an underlying, recurrent problem, it's best to consult a homeopathic practitioner.

**Ruta:** Consider using this remedy if the affected area feels broken, achy, sore, and bruised internally. Inflamed tendons are tender enough to cause temporary lameness, and stiffness and pain lodge in one area, as though a nail were sticking into the affected joint.

**Bryonia:** If inflammation and pain are obviously aggravated by even the slightest movement, and clearly eased by keeping the affected area as still and rested as possible, use Bryonia.

**Rhus tox:** This remedy can be helpful if the affected area feels hot and inflamed, and if tearing pains are noticeably troublesome and distressing when trying to rest and sleep at night. Symptoms temporarily improve with gentle movement, and by taking a warm bath or shower.

## HERBALISM

Tennis elbow, essentially a repetitive strain injury of one of the tendons of the elbow, responds well to many of the same herbs used for other musculoskeletal conditions such as sciatica (p. 702), bursitis (p. 613), tendonitis (p. 721), repetitive strain injury (p. 686), and pain in different joints. Consult these sections for additional treatment options to those mentioned below.

**Apply ice:** Begin treatment by applying ice to the elbow at the site of pain, especially after activity or when the elbow is particularly painful. Place ice on the area for 20–25 minutes (or as long as can be tolerated) every two to three hours, making sure to keep a thin barrier between the ice and skin so as not to cause frostbite. As with shin splints, a poultice of arnica flowers with about 1 tsp of rue oil added can also be used in between ice treatments. Create a poultice by infusing 2–3 g of the whole plant or flower heads in 150 ml of hot water for 15 minutes. Place gauze or bandages in the infusion and wrap the injured area. For additional benefit, add a few drops each of wintergreen and peppermint essential oils to the arnica and rue. These oils penetrate the skin and have an anti-inflammatory action; in particular, the peppermint oil deadens the pain sensation transmitted by nerves, providing comfort as the tennis elbow heals. Discontinue use if the skin becomes irritated.

**Anti-inflammatory tincture:** Many people find it helpful to take anti-inflammatory herbs orally to assist in the healing of conditions like tennis elbow. Create a wonderful blend of anti-inflammatory herbs by purchasing tinctures of licorice, which naturally prolongs the life of the body's natural steroid, cortisol; yucca, a cooling and astringent anti-spasmodic and anti-arthritic herb; meadowsweet, which inhibits pro-inflammatory chemicals and contains small amounts of the salicylate compounds found in aspirin; and turmeric, which improves circulation, is high in antioxidants, vitamins, and minerals, and inhibits inflammation. Combine these tinctures in equal parts and take about ½ tsp of the blend three times daily until your tennis elbow is healed. If you not wish to take alcohol-based tinctures, most stores that sell herbal medicines offer glycerin-based tinctures as an alternative, which are just as effective.

# PERSONAL
# COMPLAINTS

# CHLAMYDIA

## DIAGNOSIS

Chlamydia is a sexually transmitted disease (STD) caused by the bacteria Chlamydia trachomatis. This infection can be contracted through unprotected oral, vaginal, or anal sexual contact with an infected partner. It is one of the most common STDs, and is preventable and treatable. It often presents no symptoms in men or women, unless it leads to complications, and many people are unaware that they even have the disease. In women, the infection can cause cystitis, urethritis, a change in vaginal discharge, or abdominal pain. More seriously, it can damage the fallopian tubes and possibly lead to infertility. In men, chlamydia can cause discharge from the urethra and mild irritation at the tip of the penis that tends to subside within a few days. More serious complications include inflammation of the testicles, which can create problems in the tubes through which sperm travels and also potentially lead to infertility. Chlamydia can also lead to pelvic inflammatory disease (PID) in women if not treated. Younger people (under 25) who are sexually active with multiple partners seem to be most at risk.

## SYMPTOMS

### IN WOMEN (SOMETIMES)
- Cystitis
- A change in vaginal discharge
- Mild lower abdominal pain

### IN MEN (SOMETIMES)
- Urethral discharge from the penis
- Mild irritation of the penis, which often goes away

## TREATMENT GOAL

This condition is easily preventable by practicing safe sex. If the disease is contracted, then both conventional and complementary therapies aim to eliminate the bacteria and prevent further infection.

## CONVENTIONAL MEDICINE

**Prevention:** This is the best strategy for treating chlamydia. Always have protected sex by using condoms.

**Antibiotics:** If you do become infected, conventional medical treatment is to prescribe antibiotics. A first line of treatment is to take a one-time dose of 1 gm of azithromycin orally. This is usually given on site at the time of diagnosis. All sexual partners should also be treated to avoid reinfection. Alternately 500 mg of erythromycin can be taken four times daily for seven days. Those who are allergic to these medications, can take ofloxacin or levofloxacin as seven-day treatments. If infection occurs during pregnancy, ampicillin or erthromycin should be used. Ofloxacin and doxycycline cannot be used in pregnancy. Patients should be tested for the STD after treatment to make sure the infection is gone.

## TRADITIONAL CHINESE MEDICINE

**Herbs:** Consult a TCM practitioner for comprehensive herbal treatment for chlamydia.

**Acupuncture:** Consult with a doctor of traditional Chinese medicine regarding acupuncture treatment for chlamydia. The doctor evaluating your condition can determine the number of treatments needed.

**Diet:** Eat a well-balanced diet that includes fresh food and make sure you drink plenty of water. Shrimp, beef, lamb, and chili pepper should be avoided as they may interfere with your herbal treatment and increase heat in your body.

## NATUROPATHY

Seek the help of a holistic practitioner who can provide you with the proper treatment, whether drug based or complementary. Untreated chlamydia can cause long-term complications.

**Diet:** A diet that supports the immune system is appropriate. Include whole foods, fresh fruit and vegetables. Brightly colored foods and green leafy vegetables are helpful due to their high nutrient levels and bioflavonoids (plant chemicals with many health-supporting properties).

**Supplements:** Immune-supporting nutritional supplements are highly important in the treatment of chlamydia infection. Take a multivitamin/multimineral as directed on the container; 1,000 mg of vitamin C four times a day; 400 IU of vitamin E a day; 200,000 IU of beta carotenes a day; and 30 mg of zinc picolinate a day.

**Herbs:** Herbs that contain the natural antibiotic berberine are best suited to treat chlamydia, but should not be used if you are pregnant. Take 6–12 ml of a goldenseal tincture, or 250 mg in pills from a solid extract, three times a day. Take 250–500 mg of Oregon grape root extract three times per day, standardized to berberine or total alkaloid levels (approximately 5%). Continuous use should not exceed three weeks. Also take 2,000 mg of barberry in solid extract form three times a day.

> **TIP: MAKE A NATURAL DOUCHE**
> Add 3 drops each of lavender and tea tree essential oil—both have antimicrobial properties and lavender gives the douche a pleasant smell—to 3 cups of warm water and 2 tbsp of yogurt (packed with some healthy probiotics, which are important for the overall health of the vaginal area). Put the ingredients into a douche bag and slosh it around to mix them well. Use the douche once a day. If the problem does not clear up within five days, consult your doctor.

## HOMEOPATHY

This condition requires prompt conventional diagnosis and treatment, but homeopathy can provide complementary support once an initial conventional treatment has been given. In particular, the remedies listed below may be helpful if vaginal discharge is present. However, they are listed to give an idea of the range of potential remedies available to a practitioner, rather than to encourage self-prescribing.

**Sepia:** This remedy is helpful if there is a general sense of feeling depressed, flat, and exhausted. Possible localized symptoms include bloating and distention of the belly. If a discharge is present, it is likely to smart and be yellow-tinged in appearance. There may also be an uncomfortable itchy sensation in the vulva.

**Pulsatilla:** If you feel emotional and weepy, Pulsatilla may be helpful. Localized symptoms include a cloudy discharge that is watery or thick and bland in texture. This triggers vaginal soreness that tends to be most troublesome when you are warm in bed, and pre-menstrually.

**Borax:** If vaginal discharge resembles uncooked egg white and feels very irritating and possibly corrosive, Borax may help. The discharge may also irritate the top of the thighs. There may also be heat and inflammation in the vagina.

## HERBALISM

 This is a serious infection with the potential to cause severe complications, especially in women. For that reason, it is extremely important to treat chlamydia infections with antibiotics as soon as possible; treatment should also be given to sexual partners. Herbs have a role only as adjunctive therapies, such as helping with urinary discomfort, until the antibiotics rid the body of infection. As well as the herbs listed below, see Urinary Tract Infection (p. 484) for other herbs that could be helpful for some of the symptoms associated with chlamydia.

**Cleavers:** The above-ground parts of cleavers have many helpful effects on the urinary system. It contains antioxidants, tannins, coumarins, and many other compounds that make it effective for kidney stone prevention, prostate problems, painful urination, and lingering symptoms from chlamydia infection. Purchase a tincture from a store that sells or makes herbal medicines, and take a ½ dropper (30 drops) twice a day until your symptoms have improved.

**Marshmallow:** This herb can soothe the urinary tract. To treat urinary symptoms of Chlamydia, use a tincture of marshmallow root, available from herbal medicines stores. The dose will depend on the severity of symptoms, but an average dose is one dropper full (60 drops) three times daily.

# FIBROIDS

## DIAGNOSIS

Fibroids are non-cancerous growths of tissue that develop in the muscular wall of the uterus. They vary in number (although seldom develop singly) and size (they can be as small as a pea, or grow to be as large as a melon). The exact cause of fibroids is unknown, but they are stimulated by the female hormone estrogen, and tend to shrink after menopause. They are rare in women under 20, and tend to affect women in their 30s and 40s. Afro-American women are also more at risk of developing fibroids.

There are four different types of fibroid, which are classified according to where they develop in the uterus. Submucosal fibroids grow on the inside of the womb; intramural fibroids grow within the uterine wall (the wall of the womb); subserosal fibroids grow on the outside of the womb on the lining between the uterus and the pelvic cavity; and pedunculated fibroids are stalk-like growths that are attached to either the inside or outside wall of the womb.

Many women with fibroids have no symptoms, while others experience heavy bleeding, pain, and/or incontinence. If fibroids become too large they can put pressure on other organs such as the bladder and the bowel, a condition known as compression syndrome. This can lead to backache, hip pain, and constipation.

## SYMPTOMS

- Often, no symptoms are present
- Painful periods
- Heavy periods
- Irregular periods
- Bowel or bladder discomfort
- Frequent urination/constipation
- Hip and back pain
- Infertility, if the fibroid is blocking the fallopian tube
- Miscarriage, if the fibroid is pressing on the cervix

## TREATMENT GOAL

Most fibroids do not require treatment. If the fibroids are causing complications, they may need to be removed. Conventional and complementary therapies focus on relieving the discomfort of symptoms.

## CONVENTIONAL MEDICINE

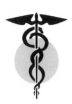

Conventional medical treatment involves reducing heavy bleeding, and relieving pain and pelvic discomfort. If a woman is approaching menopause, watching and waiting may be the extent of the treatment, as fibroids tend to shrink after this time due to reduced estrogen. If the fibroids are small and not causing significant symptoms such as anemia and pain, it is best to wait until they shrink on their own.

**Medication:** Non-steroidal anti-inflammatory drugs (NSAIDs) such as ibuprofen and mefenamic acid can help ease pain and, to an extent, the amount of heavy bleeding. Aminocaproic acid treatment, given either intravenously or orally, reduces heavy bleeding by affecting clotting. However, it should be used with caution in people with a history of thrombosis. Progesterone, when taken for 21 days of a woman's menstrual cycle, can also have an effect on bleeding; synthetic medroxyprogesterone or natural progesterone can be used. Oral doses should be used with caution in patients with a history of depression, and those with a history of progesterone receptor positive breast cancer should not take progesterone. Oral contraceptive agents may be used to reduce fibroid size, but in some women, they actually increase fibroid size as they increase synthetic estrogen in the body. However, they do reduce menstrual loss and regulate the timing of periods. Anti-gonadotropin agents, such as danazol, can be used to abolish ovulation, thus suppressing menstruation.

**Surgery:** Surgical procedures include a hysterectomy, where the uterus is removed, an endometrial ablation, which destroys the layer of cells that lines the uterus, a myomectomy to remove fibroids, and a laparoscopic myomectomy, which is key hole surgery to remove fibroids. Uterine artery embolization is a new non-surgical procedure that is rapid and has a good success rate.

**Lifestyle modification:** Many women who have fibroids have an excess of estrogen present in the body. Fat cells make more estrogen, so lifestyle changes that promote weight loss can help to decrease the chance of fibroids developing.

## TRADITIONAL CHINESE MEDICINE

**Herbs:** Use herbs that are proven to remove blood stagnation and dispel phlegm, which are associated with fibroids according to traditional Chinese medicine. Combine 15 g of Xuan Shen (ningpo figwort root), 12 g of Chi Xiao Dou (adzuki bean), 15 g of Niu Xi (achyranthes root), 15 g of Dan Shen (salvia root), 12 g of Bai Jie Zi (white mustard seed), 12 g of Dang Gui

(Chinese angelica), 12 g of Xiang Fu (nut grass rhizome), and 3 g of Gan Cao (licorice). Place the raw herbs in a ceramic or glass pot and add 3½ cups of water. Bring to the boil and simmer for 30 minutes. Strain the liquid and drink 1 cup twice a day. These herbs are available from Chinese pharmacies or online.

**Acupuncture:** Treatment can be used to shrink fibroids. Consult a doctor of traditional Chinese medicine who will evaluate your particular case according to the principles of Chinese medicine to determine the best approach. One course of treatment consists of 12, 30-minute acupuncture sessions. The practitioner will determine the frequency of sessions required, depending on the condition and prognosis.

**Acupressure:** Press the Xue Hai, Feng Shi, Susanli, and San Yin Jiao acupressure points. The Xue Hai point is on the inside of the leg, at the depression just above the knee. Locate the Feng Shi point along the outside of the leg, at the tip of the fingers when the arm is hanging straight down at the side of the body. The Susanli point is found on the lower leg, about 1 inch to the outside of and 3 inches below the kneecap. The San Yin Jiao point is located on the inside of the leg, about 3 inches above the anklebone.

**Diet:** Eat food that is helpful for blood circulation like black soybeans, brown sugar, chestnuts, peaches, and sweet basil.

## NATUROPATHY

**Diet:** Fibroids are affected by hormones, which are in turn affected by diet. Base your diet around whole grains, fruit, vegetables, fish, beans, and fermented soy products. It is important to eat organic products as much as possible because some of the chemicals used to fumigate foods mimic estrogen activity. If you have heavy periods, eat foods that have high amounts of iron such as blackstrap molasses, liver, and organic, grass-fed beef. Drink eight glasses of water a day to help flush out impurities. Soy products and flaxseeds are good sources of phyto-estrogens, which are thought to help prevent fibroids. Avoid sugar, alcohol, caffeine, and foods that contain hydrogenated fats to avoid inflammation. These foods also depress your immune system.

**Supplements:** A high-potency multivitamin supplement supplies nutrients important in estrogen metabolism. Take them as directed on the label. B-complex vitamins are also necessary for estrogen metabolism. Take 100 mg twice a day. Take 400 IU of vitamin E to helps with inflammation. Essential fatty acids (EFAs) also help decrease inflammation and are nourishing to the female reproductive system. Take a daily combination of 2 tbsp of flaxseed oil a day, 500 mg of fish oils, and 300 mg of borage oil, all good sources of EFAs.

**Herbs:** Chasteberry balances estrogen/progesterone levels. Take 240 mg of a standardized extract that contains 0.6% aucubin. Do not use this herb if currently taking a contraceptive pill. Take 300 mg of indole-3-carbinol a day, a substance found in cruciferous vegetables such as broccoli that helps estrogen metabolism. D-glucarate is a plant chemical that assists the liver in estrogen breakdown. Take 500 mg a day. Drink 3 cups of red raspberry tea a day to help with uterine inflammation and pain.

**Hydrotherapy:** Regular sitz baths, where only the hips and buttocks are soaked in water or saline solution, will improve circulation to the pelvic region and help ease pain. You can add 10 drops of warming oils, such as rosemary or marjoram essential oils, to the bath to increase blood flow and relieve pain.

---

**TIP:** USE PROGESTERONE CREAMS

Under the supervision of a doctor, apply progesterone creams to the abdomen, thighs, neck, and arms to balance estrogen, regulate the menstrual flow, and relieve pain. An appropriate dose is ½ tsp applied twice a day to your skin, but do not apply the cream during the week of your menstrual flow.

---

## HOMEOPATHY

The following can be helpful short-term remedies to ease moderately heavy bleeding and pain that occur on an occasional basis as a result of fibroids. Severe and/or recurrent problems should be treated by a homeopathic practitioner.

**Lachesis:** If menstrual pain is accompanied by a clotted flow that is dark in color, try Lachesis. Cramping pains are relieved as soon as menstrual bleeding begins. Sufferers also experience mood swings and disturbed sleep from mid-cycle until the beginning of a period.

**Phosphorus:** To treat menstrual bleeding that is not heavy, but continues for an extended period and is bright red in color, use Phosphorus. Those who respond well to this remedy are anxious and fearful, but are calmed by reassurance and attention.

**Silica:** If heavy periods are combined with waves of icy coldness that travel through the body, use Silica. Menstrual cramps and pains are sharp and cutting in nature, and are aggravated when passing water. Classic symptoms include a profound sense of weakness and feeling stressed, nervous, and strung out when unwell.

## HERBALISM

There are many herbs traditionally used to help with one of the main symptoms of fibroids, uterine bleeding. These herbs have a variety of effects to control abnormal blood flow.

**Dong Quai:** The root of Dong Quai may help to normalize female hormones that contribute to the abnormal bleeding associated with uterine fibroids. Water extracts, alcohol tinctures, and standardized extracts all have slightly different activities, the nuances of which would be best assessed by a medical herbalist. See Hot Flashes (p. 749) for more information about Dong Quai.

**Beth root:** Beth root can be effective in stopping uterine bleeding. Make a tea of beth root from 2–4 g of the herb and drink daily; you can also take 60 drops of tincture three times a day to control excessive uterine bleeding. This herb should not be used if you have heart troubles, or are pregnant or lactating. Sometimes beth root can cause stomach upset, nausea, and vomiting. Beth root is sometimes combined with other herbs for this condition, such as Canadian fleabane tincture or oil.

**Ragwort:** Ragwort tincture has a traditional reputation as a uterine tonic that could help with symptoms associated with fibroids, but it can be quite toxic when taken internally. It is best to avoid any species of Senecio ragwort. Consult a medical herbalist about other plants that are useful uterine tonics.

# HERPES

## DIAGNOSIS

Genital herpes is an infection caused by the herpes simplex virus, which infects the skin and mucous membranes of the genitals. It is one of the most common sexually transmitted diseases (STDs). It enters the body through a break in the skin and once you are infected it is possible for the virus to lie dormant in your system for months, and in some cases even years. During this time you will not have any symptoms. Stress can activate the virus, leading to an outbreak. After an initial phase of tenderness in the genital area, a rash of blisters appears. The blisters burst and turn into small ulcers, which crust over after two to three weeks. There are two types of herpes simplex virus that attack both skin and mucous membranes. HSV-1, the most common type, usually appears as cold sores on the mouth and lips, while HSV-2 affects the genitals. Genital herpes develops very differently in different people. Some people experience just a few attacks or none at all, while others will have regular outbreaks. Episodes do tend to decline with age.

## SYMPTOMS

- Prickling sensation in the genital area
- Redness and small watery blisters on the genitals
- Pain, itchiness, and burning
- Fever, aches and pains, and fatigue
- Discomfort during urination

## TREATMENT GOAL

Herpes is a preventable STD that can be avoided by practicing safe sex. Condoms reduce the risk of becoming infected or passing on the virus. If infection does occur, treatment involves resolving the infection and reducing the occurrence of further outbreaks.

## CONVENTIONAL MEDICINE

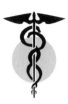

**Medication:** The first drug of choice to treat herpes is acyclovir, which is used for both initial and recurrent episodes. The recommended dosage is five times a day for seven to 10 days to treat the first episode, and for five days to treat recurrent episodes. Usually a slow but steady improvement is seen. To treat viruses that are resistant to acyclovir, valcyclovir can be used. Famcyclovir is another option, and requires fewer daily doses. Some of these medications may also be used at lower doses to suppress the herpes virus and keep it in remission.

**Local pain relief:** Apply cool compresses of Burrow's solution four to six times a day to relieve local discomfort and promote healing. Additional measures include applying lidocaine gel, taking cool baths, and taking simple pain relievers.

**Prevention:** Avoid high-risk sexual behavior, fatigue, and stress to help keep herpes in remission. Some studies show that taking lysine supplements is also helpful.

## TRADITIONAL CHINESE MEDICINE

**Herbs:** The herbs listed below are available from Chinese pharmacies or online.
• To treat simplex Type 1 herpes or cold sores: Take Chuang Xin Lian Pian, a Chinese patent herbal pill. It contains the herbs Chuang Xin Lian and Bu Gong Yin, which have antiviral effects to clean heat toxins.
• To treat simplex Type 2 herpes or genital herpes, or herpes zoster or shingles: You can take the Chuang Xin Lian Pian herbal pill for this type of condition as well, or try washing the genital area with the following external formula. Mix 15 g of Ku Shen (sophora root), 15 g of She Chuang Zi (cnidium seed), 15 g of Huang Bai (phellodendron), 12 g of Xia Ku Cao (common selfheal fruit-spike), 15 g of Ma Zhi Xian (dried purslane), and 15 g of Ban Lan Gen (isatis root) in a ceramic pot. Add 3½ cups of water and bring to a boil. Simmer for 30 minutes and strain the liquid. Soak the area in the decoction for 15 minutes twice a day.

**Acupuncture:** Needles are usually applied around the area where the herpes occurs, although some other points may also be selected. Consult a practitioner, who will make a Chinese medicine prognosis to determine a treatment plan. To treat acute conditions, especially acute stages of shingles, you may need treatment as often as once a day. Chronic herpes is typically treated by a 12-session course of acupuncture, performed once or twice a week. You may experience pain relief and less outbreaks of the virus, and treatment may also prevent herpes from recurring.

**Diet:** Eating foods that clean heat from the body may help this condition. Examples of such foods include mung beans, watermelon, purslane, towel gourd, crab, grapefruit, pears, red beans, cucumber, cabbage, watermelon, and tofu. Generally, light, fresh food is recommended such as celery, spinach, aubergine and wax gourd. Avoid ginger, chilies, mustard greens, oranges, shrimp, baked potatoes, cheese, and mutton because they are pungent, irritating, and increase heat in the body, which may make the condition worse. Also avoid acidic, sweet, and greasy foods.

## NATUROPATHY

**Diet:** Consume foods that are high in the amino acid L-lysine, such as legumes, fish, turkey, chicken, and vegetables. Foods high in vitamin C and bioflavonoids such as peppers, broccoli, berries, and carrots help to heal the skin. Avoid foods high in the amino acid L-arginine such as almonds, peanuts, chocolate, and whole wheat, as they can stimulate herpes replication. Eliminate sugar and foods that contain sugars and hydrogenated fats; these suppress the immune system and interfere with the healing process. Acidic foods, such as tomatoes and citrus fruits, may aggravate symptoms during outbreaks and should be avoided.

**Supplements:** L-lysine, which has been shown to help with acute outbreaks of herpes, can be taken as a supplement at a dosage of 1,000 mg three times a day, or take 500 mg twice a day as a preventive measure. Take 1,000 mg of vitamin C with 500 mg of bioflavonoids three to four times a day for their ability to improve immune function and decrease the duration of the infection. Zinc reduces the severity of herpes and increases immune function. Take 30 mg daily with 3 mg of copper. Topical zinc sulfate can also be applied to the affected area two to three times a day. Taking 100 mg of B-complex vitamins twice a day can help to treat frequent herpes cold sore outbreaks. It is also important to supply the gut with friendly bacteria to promote immune function. Take 4 billion active organisms 30 minutes after a meal.

**Herbs:** Lemon balm has been shown to help resolve the herpes virus and to heal cold sores. Apply a lemon balm cream, available from health food stores, to the affected area three times a day. Take 500 mg of lomatium root four times a day for its anti-viral and immune-enhancing properties. An anti-viral compound in St. John's Wort, called hypericin, helps kill herpes simplex and several other viruses to help heal sores.

Brew a strong tea made from the herb, and, after it cools, dab it on the affected area. You can also take 300 mg three times a day of an extract standardized to contain 0.3% hypericin.

## HOMEOPATHY

The following remedies can be used as short-term, complementary therapies alongside conventional treatment to ease the discomfort and distress of an acute flare-up of herpes. For more extensive support, consult an experienced homeopathic practitioner, rather than trying to handle the situation through self-help measures alone.

**Natrum mur:** Consider using this remedy if the affected area feels dry and sore, leading to smarting, burning sensations. Symptoms tend to emerge when feeling emotionally stressed or physically run down, are sensitive to contact with heat, and soothed by contact with cool air and cool bathing.

**Rhus tox:** If the affected area feels sore and itchy, causing particular distress and restlessness at night, try Rhus tox. Cold and damp conditions can also trigger, or aggravate burning and itching sensations.

**Petroleum:** This can be a helpful remedy for herpetic eruptions that lead to violent itching, burning, and irritation. Sores may appear on the perineum, and between the scrotum and the thighs. Clothing and movement make the irritation more intense, while exposure to warm air may feel soothing.

## HERBALISM

 It is difficult to definitively treat a herpes infection, as it involves a virus that lives in a particular nerve, occasionally causing an "outbreak," or blister and pain in the skin served by that nerve. Herbs can, however, help with the skin symptoms, and facilitate the resolution of the pain and blisters.

**Black walnut tree:** The leaves of black walnut trees are used medicinally for their astringent, tonifying, antiseptic, hemostatic, and wound-healing properties. These medicinal actions make the walnut leaves a wonderful treatment for healing the skin symptoms of a herpes outbreak. Make a strong decoction by boiling 1 oz of cut or powdered leaves in 2–3 cups of water for 10 minutes. Strain the liquid, soak a cloth in the decoction, and apply it to the affected area for 10–15 minutes.

**Aloe vera:** To treat the blisters associated with a herpes outbreak, simply take the gel from a fresh cut leaf and apply it directly to the affected area. If fresh leaves are not available, there are a variety of gels and lotions containing aloe vera that can be purchased at your local health food store.

**Licorice:** Licorice root extracts, in creams, lotions, or ointments, can help provide pain relief and decrease healing time. Licorice, which has anti-viral properties, is a demulcent that coats and soothes the skin. Interestingly, whole licorice or one of its compounds, glycyrrhizin, works against the herpes virus, but only when used topically; when ingested, glycyrrhizin is metabolized to an ineffective compound. Look for topical products with glycyrrhizin, often combined with anti-viral medicines such as idoxuridine. A synthetic form of glycyrrhizin, carbenoxolone, has also been used topically to treat herpes lesions.

# HIRSUTISM

## DIAGNOSIS

Hirsutism is the abnormal growth of hair in women. It is usually classified as hair growth in a male pattern, for example thick hair on the face, chest, and stomach—areas where most women would not normally expect to grow hair. This condition usually first appears during puberty. It is not a disease and is rarely caused by a serious illness, but it can be very distressing. For the majority of women who suffer from hirsutism, it is an inherited condition that results in a higher sensitivity to the male hormone testosterone, which is naturally produced in all women. Although sufferers produce normal amounts of testosterone, their increased sensitivity causes hair to grow more quickly and thicker. However, there are also certain medical conditions that can make hair growth in females excessive. The most common of these is polycystic ovary syndrome (PCOS), where an excess of androgenic hormones causes hairiness. If left untreated, this condition can lead to problems with infertility. Hirsutism can also be an indication of problems with hormones and thyroid function, and some women find they suffer from hirsutism after menopause. It is advisable to consult with a doctor to determine the cause of the excess hair and treat the underlying condition as necessary.

## SYMPTOMS

- Thick hair on the face, chest, and/or stomach
- More hair growth than usual on the arms and legs

## TREATMENT GOAL

To determine the reason for the excessive hair growth and treat any underlying conditions. If the excess hair is causing emotional distress, cosmetic hair-removal methods should be explored.

## CONVENTIONAL MEDICINE

 A woman who has hirsutism that progresses gradually, and who has normal menstruation and a family history of the condition, does not usually need laboratory evaluation. If this is not the case, or if abnormalities show up in preliminary tests, further testing is necessary to diagnose the cause and determine treatment. Diagnosis generally involves testing the adrenal glands, the thyroid, and the sex hormones. Scans of the adrenal glands and ovaries are taken if androgen-secreting tumors are suspected. It is important to identify any potentially dangerous underlying cause.

**Reducing male hormone secretion:** If a pathological condition is not found, treatment involves reducing the production of the male hormone androgen, or blocking the effects of these hormones, to reduce hair growth. Treatments to block or shut down the male hormones include oral contraceptives; however, some of these contain androgenic hormones and should not be used. Other anti-androgen drugs such as spironolactone can also be used. If hirsutism is a result of PCOS, the drug metformin is used.

**Cosmetic solutions:** Since these treatments take about six months to bring results, methods of hair removal should be explored. These include tweezing, shaving, waxing, laser treatment, and electrolysis. Laser treatment and electrolysis are the only permanent methods of hair removal.

**Diet and supplements:** Those who suffer from hirsutism and are overweight may benefit from weight loss. Also reduce the amount of hormone-laden dairy and meat products in your diet. Saw palmetto, a natural herb that blocks, to an extent, the action of androgen hormones, may also be helpful.

## TRADITIONAL CHINESE MEDICINE

 **Herbs:** Hirsutism is secondary condition that may be related to other, more serious disorders. As such there are no herbal formulas recommended for self-use in this situation. Consult a doctor of Chinese medicine for an individual diagnosis and treatment.

**Acupuncture:** Consult a practitioner for specific recommendations. Acupuncture sessions once or twice a week may be given, beginning with one course of 12 sessions.

**Diet:** Eat a well-balanced, healthy diet of fresh fruit and vegetables and drink an adequate amount of fluids every day. Avoid shrimp, beef, lamb, and chili peppers since they increase heat in your body.

## NATUROPATHY

**Diet:** A correct diet is probably the single most important naturopathic treatment for hirsutism and its causes. Hirsutism has been linked to insulin resistance, so follow a low-carbohydrate diet to reduce insulin levels, improve insulin resistance, and help you lose weight if needed. When consuming starches, consume mostly whole grains, such as brown rice as opposed to white rice. Increase your consumption of omega-3 fats, one of the essential fatty acids. Omega-3 fats are found in cod liver oil, and in fatty fish such as salmon, sardines, and mackerel. Eliminate trans-fatty acids from your diet. A trans-fat is unsaturated liquid oil that has been chemically transformed into a saturated fat so that it will be a solid instead of a liquid. Margarine, partially hydrogenated oils, and deep fried foods are examples of products containing trans-fats. Trans-fatty acids cause a fatty, sluggish liver making it more difficult to metabolize hormones that may be causing hirsutism. When eating red meat, choose beef that is grass-fed and organic. You can also eat other lean meats such as chicken and turkey that contain less saturated fat. Limit the amount and type of simple carbohydrates you eat. A diet that is high in refined carbohydrates will lead to an excessive insulin response, which can in turn stimulate androgen (male hormone) production that contributes to hirsutism. The best carbohydrates to consume are whole grains, nuts, seeds, fruit, and vegetables.

**Supplements:** Chromium encourages your liver to produce a substance called glucose tolerance factor (GTF), which increases the effectiveness of insulin. Take 200–400 mg of chromium picolinate a day. Vitamin B3 (niacin) is a component of glucose tolerance factor, vitamin B5 (pantothenic acid) helps to control fat metabolism and improves the response to stress, and vitamin B6 balances hormone levels. It is best to take 50 mg of a B-complex vitamin that contains all the above B vitamins three times a day. Inositol increases the effectiveness of insulin in people with PCOS, reduces male hormone levels, and restores normal periods. Although inositol can be found in a B-complex vitamin, a total of 500 mg should be taken twice a day.

**Herbs:** Chaste tree vitex seems to have anti-androgenic properties that inhibit hirsutism. Take 1–4 ml of a 1:2 dried plant tincture or 500–1,000 mg of dried berries daily. Saw palmetto inhibits the action of testosterone in men and in women. Take 160 mg twice a day.

## HOMEOPATHY

This complaint is often linked to conditions that involve hormone imbalance such as PCOS. This embarrassing problem can also arise after menopause has occurred, as a result of plummeting levels of the female sex hormone estrogen. Situations such as these are best treated by an experienced homeopathic practitioner. He or she will take your mental, emotional, and physical health into account to select a remedy to stimulate and balance your system. As a result, you should find that you cope with this distressing problem better emotionally, and the quantity of hair produced may also decrease. Remedies are outlined below to give an idea of some choices practitioners may make, rather than to encourage self-prescription.

**Sepia:** This remedy is particularly appropriate for treating unwanted hair that grows leading up to and following menopause, when there is a predominance of androgen (male hormone) produced. Symptoms include low libido, exhausting hot flashes, and a general state of mental and emotional indifference that may be combined with an overwhelming feeling of being unable to cope.

**Thuja:** If excess hair growth is confined to the upper lip, and combined with greasy, unhealthy-looking skin that tends to develop warty growths, Thuja may help. The texture of hair on the head is likely to be poor and greasy, and there may be a history of adverse reactions to vaccinations.

**TIP:** AVOID PLUCKING
Always avoid the temptation to tamper with heavy hair growth on the face by plucking or other forms of temporary hair removal. This can encourage hair to grow back even more strongly. Instead, consult a well-trained beauty therapist who has had some experience in more sophisticated forms of permanent hair removal.

## HERBALISM

**Asian or Korean ginseng:** These herbs can be helpful in treating hirsutism by balancing hormone levels through their action on the hypothalamus, pituitary, and adrenal glands; these three organs are usually tightly regulated so that hormones, especially cortisol, stay within narrow ranges. A tonic herb like Asian ginseng may help the body normalize the hormones that are either abnormally low or high, accounting for some of the physiological changes associated with hirsutism. Asian ginseng, like the other ginseng species, is very expensive and as such can be subject to adulteration by other, cheaper plants. For this reason, use a standardized extract, or buy ginseng only from reputable suppliers. A standardized extract of Asian ginseng, G115, has been studied extensively in medical research and the recommended dose is 100–200 mg a day. This can be purchased in most stores or pharmacies that sell herbal medicines. A tincture of Asian ginseng is often dosed at 60–180 drops daily. Water-based infusions or decoctions of Asian ginseng may be effective, though many of the important phytochemicals are not soluble in water; standardized extracts and alcohol or glycerin tinctures are usually the most efficacious. Take herbal tonics of Asian ginseng daily for three weeks, followed by one week of a ginseng "holiday," and repeat as necessary. Asian ginseng may cause a decrease in blood sugar, so people with diabetes taking oral hypoglycemic medication or insulin, should be careful. Also, Asian ginseng may raise or lower blood pressure, so people with blood pressure abnormalities should monitor their blood pressure closely when they begin ginseng therapy. To aid hirsutism, it is necessary to take ginseng for four to six months, checking in regularly with a medical herbalist to assess progress and make any necessary changes.

**Herbs with possible hormonal effects:** See Osteoporosis (p. 681) and Hot Flashes (p. 749) for details on the use of red clover, black cohosh, and Dong Quai. These herbs have a variety of compounds that may have effects similar to the body's own progesterone or estrogen, helping to counteract the hormone abnormalities that lead to hirsutism. As with Asian ginseng, above, or any other treatment for hirsutism, treatment should be continued for at least four to six months and should not take the place of conventional medical treatment or diagnosis. Red clover can be ingested as a tea (made from 1–2 g of herb and taken once to three times daily) or as an alcohol or glycerin tincture (30 drops taken three times a day), though the most effective preparation of red clover appears to be capsules of a semi-purified leaf extract where the standardization to the percentage of isoflavones is listed specifically on the bottle. For black cohosh, use extracts standardized to the triterpene glycoside compounds, usually dosed at 40 mg twice daily. Dong Quai is usually taken as 4–5 g daily of a water-based extract standardized either to the ferulic acid content or other compounds such as ligustilide.

# HOT FLASHES

## DIAGNOSIS

A hot flash is the sudden unpleasant sensation of burning heat spreading across the face, neck, and chest. It is a side effect of menopause (see p. 774) that affects many women, some long before menopause actually begins (this period is known as the perimenopause). A hot flash is triggered by a lack of estrogen, which causes irregularities in the body's cooling system. This can result in extreme discomfort, and disturbed sleep, particularly if flashes are accompanied by drenching night-time sweats. There is great variation in both the degree and the persistence of symptoms between different women. Some have no symptoms whatsoever, whereas others have severe problems that make a huge impact on their lives and last for years, sometimes even into old age. Generally, however, the number of hot flashes women experience will subside over time.

## SYMPTOMS

- Sudden changes in body temperature
- Redness and blushing in the face, neck, and chest
- Increased sweating, particularly at night in bed

## TREATMENT GOAL

To relieve the distress and discomfort of hot flashes, and develop techniques for coping with episodes. Hormone replacement therapy (HRT) is effective at relieving hot flashes following menopause; however, HRT is not recommended for use for longer than five years. Discuss this treatment option with your doctor.

## CONVENTIONAL MEDICINE

**HRT:** Treating hot flashes involves stabilizing hormones during the menopausal period. Hormone replacement therapy (HRT), which involves increasing the levels of female hormones in the body, is the most effective way of achieving this, but it is currently a controversial form of treatment.

Recent trials have shown that the use of combined synthetic estrogen-progestin therapy in postmenopausal women increases the risk of cardiovascular disease, stroke, breast cancer, venous thromboembolism, and probable dementia in women aged 65 years of age or older. Newer bio-identical hormones, which are natural, do not seem to share the same risk as synthetic hormones, but extensive tests have not yet been done. The severity of the hot flashes and other menopausal symptoms should be weighed against the risks of hormone therapy. In any case, the lowest amount of the most bio-identical hormone should be used to treat hot flashes. Estrogen should be combined with progesterone, rather than used by itself.

**Other medication:** Anti-depressant drugs, the selective serotonin reuptake inhibitors (SSRIs) drugs in particular (including Prozac®, Zoloft®, and Lexapro®), can be helpful in reducing episodes of hot flashes. Natural treatments such as vitamin E, taken at a dose of 400–800 IU daily, and black cohosh extract standardized to 5% triterpene glycosides, taken at 40 drops daily, are also recommended. Soy phyto-estrogens as well as the phyto-estrogens found in celery, parsley, whole grains (flax in particular), and alfalfa are weak estrogens that may be helpful. Plant medicine that contains estrogens includes Dong Quai, licorice root, chaste berries, and black cohosh.

## TRADITIONAL CHINESE MEDICINE

**Herbs:** Combine 15 g of Shen Di Huang (Chinese foxglove), 12 g of Shan Zhu Yu (Asiatic cornelian cherry fruit), 15 g of Shan Yao (Chinese yam), 15 g of Fuling (poria), 12 g of Ze Xie (water plantain rhizome), 12 g of Dan Pi (cortex of tree peony root), 12 g of Di Gu Pi (cortex of wolfberry root), 12 g of Nan Sa Shen (glehnia root), and 5 g of Gan Cao (licorice). If hot flashes are accompanied by heavy sweating, add 12 g of Fu Xiao Mai (wheat), and 15 g of Bai Shao (white peony root). Place the herbs in a glass or ceramic pot and add 3 cups of water. Bring the mixture to the boil and simmer for 30 minutes. Strain the liquid and drink 1 cup twice a day. The raw herbs are available from Chinese pharmacies or online.

**Acupuncture:** Hot flashes are one of the more common conditions treated with acupuncture. Consult a practitioner who can recommend the number of sessions you will need based on a traditional Chinese medicine diagnosis. A typical course of treatment will consist of 10–12 sessions.

**Acupressure:** Press and release the Hegu point, located between your index finger and thumb, 10 times on each hand and repeat. The Fu Liu point is on the inside of the leg, beside the ankle, in the depression 1 inch directly above the Achilles tendon. Place your index fingers on the depressions in each leg and apply gentle to moderate pressure, pressing and releasing 10 times. Press these points once or twice a day to treat both acute and chronic conditions.

**Diet:** Generally, light, fresh food is recommended, including turnips, celery, spinach, aubergines, purslane, and wax gourd. Add foods to your diet that tonify yin and clear out excessive heat, such as peppermint, mung beans, red beans, watermelon, string beans, black sesame, and sword beans. Foods to be avoided are ginger, chilies, mustard greens, and mutton, because they are pungent, irritating, and increase heat in the body, which may make hot flashes worse.

## NATUROPATHY

**Diet:** Eat two to three servings of foods that contain phytosterols, such as whole grains, legumes, fresh vegetables and fruits, as they have hormone-balancing effects. Phyto-estrogens, estrogen-like compounds found in plant food, should be consumed as often as possible. Have one to two servings a day of miso, flaxseeds, or tofu. For example, 1–2 tbsp of ground flaxseeds can be sprinkled on cereal or salads, or added to smoothies. When eating meat, choose the organic, hormone-free variety to avoid hormone imbalances.

**Supplements:** A high-quality multivitamin can be helpful in nourishing your body to keep your hormones balanced. Follow the dosage directions on the label. Take 100 mg of B-complex vitamins three times a day, as they have been shown to relieve hot flashes. Vitamin C has also been shown to help relieve hot flashes and help women through menopause. Take 1,000 mg three times a day. Evening primrose oil is excellent for promoting the production of estrogen and alleviating hot flashes. Take 1 tbsp of the oil three times a day. Take 30 mg of pregnenolone, which is involved in making estrogen and progesterone, twice a day. Vitamin E complex may also help reduce hot flash symptoms. Take 400 IU a day.

**Herbs:** Take 80 mg of of black cohosh twice a day, which studies show alleviates hot flashes. Chaste berry has been used historically for prevention of hot flashes. Take 160–240 mg of a 0.6% aucubin extract daily. Hops can help reduce anxiety and tension, which are common menopausal symptoms, and have hormone-balancing effects. Take 250 mg three times a day. Soy protein powder has been shown in some studies to reduce hot flashes. Try mixing 60 g a day in a smoothie. Also take 4–6 g of sage a day, as it may help with controlling night sweats associated with hot flashes.

**TIP: STOP SMOKING**
Smoking can aggravate hot flashes and lead to premature menopause, so think about giving up if you smoke.

## HOMEOPATHY

 As concerns about using hormone replacement therapy over an extended period of time become more prevalent, many women are considering using complementary therapies such as homeopathy to manage menopause symptoms. Homeopathic remedies can be effective in reducing the frequency, severity, and duration of hot flashes, which is one of the most troublesome and common problems associated with menopause. Remedies can be used on their own, or as complementary treatments to conventional support. The remedies listed below can provide short-term relief for mild to moderate, infrequent hot flashes. Consult an experienced homeopathic practitioner to treat severe, recurring episodes.

**Belladonna:** If hot flashes come on swiftly and dramatically, triggering bright red, hot patches on the affected area, consider using Belladonna. Skin also remains dry, no matter how overheated and flashed it becomes. Belladonna is also appropriate if sufferers feel irritable and cranky when feeling hot and bothered.

**Aconite:** This is also helpful for flashes that come on very quickly and dramatically, but those people helped by this remedy are more vulnerable to feelings of terror and panic than irritability. Flashes emerge and fade quickly, but cause a great deal of emotional distress that manifests as trembling, shaking, and palpitations.

**Glonoin:** If hot flashes affect the whole body, and are often triggered or aggravated by hot, sunny weather, use Glonoin. Feeling hot and bothered is made worse by wearing tight clothing.

**Phosphorus:** This remedy is helpful for burning hot flashes that are triggered by feeling anxious or excited, and that are eased by washing the face in cool water. Symptoms tend to be the most intense in the evening.

**Sepia:** If draining, exhausting, pulsating, sweaty flashes that sweep up the body are accompanied by feelings of anxiety, and preceded by a feeling of weakness, use Sepia. Signature symptoms include lowered emotional, mental, and physical energy levels that improve after aerobic exercise, which stimulates the circulatory system.

**TIP:** WEAR LAYERED CLOTHING
Wear light layers that can be discarded as necessary with the minimum amount of fuss. Also avoid wearing anything tight or restrictive around the neck, such as a scarf or polo neck sweater.

## HERBALISM

**Black cohosh:** The rhizome of black cohosh is well-known for treating menopausal and pre-menstrual symptoms. The most convincing studies have been on extracts standardized to the triterpene glycoside compounds, which are usually dosed at 40 mg twice daily. Most, but not all, of these clinical trials have shown a reduction in the frequency and severity of hot flashes. Black cohosh can also be taken as a decoction or tincture. To make a decoction, boil about 100 mg of the rhizome in 8 oz of water for 10 minutes, strain the herbs, and split the liquid into three amounts. Drink one of these in the morning, at noon, and at night. Or, take 30–60 drops of tincture twice a day for optimal effect. There have been conflicting results about how black cohosh helps with hot flashes; it may act on several of the female hormones, although it is uncertain whether or not the levels of estrogen it contains are high enough and it is not recommended for women recovering from or at high risk of breast cancer. New research is surfacing constantly, so check with a medical herbalist if you have any questions about the hormonal effects of black cohosh.

**Dong Quai:** The root of Dong Quai has traditionally been used by women suffering from hot flashes. There is conflicting data about how Dong Quai helps with hot flashes, but it may be through mild estrogen or progesterone effects, and because of this there is still some concern over the use of Dong Quai by women recovering from or at risk of breast cancer. One research trial found that taking 4–5 g daily of a water-based extract standardized to the ferulic acid content of Dong Quai did not lead to a decrease in the frequency and severity of hot flashes. Extracts may also be standardized to other compounds such as ligustilide and combined with other herbs such as chamomile; the latter seemed to help alleviate hot flashes. Care should be taken if you are also taking blood-thinning medications.

# IMPOTENCE

## DIAGNOSIS

Impotence (also known as erectile dysfunction) is the inability to get or keep an erection to allow for satisfactory intercourse. An erection occurs when blood is pumped into the penis, making it hard, and generally results when a man becomes sexually aroused. Men who suffer from erectile dysfunction are unable to get an erection at all, cannot get an erection that is firm enough for penetration, or cannot stay erect once penetration is achieved. It is a common problem that occurs in men of all ages. It can be caused by a variety of reasons, but is generally due to a mixture of psychological and physical factors. In some cases, there is a problem with the blood vessels that carry blood into the penis. In younger males, the most common cause of impotence is anxiety about having sex, or drinking too much alcohol. Middle-aged men tend to have erectile dysfunction as a result of stress, tiredness, relationship issues, and other major life events that trigger an emotional response, such as loss of work or the death of a close friend or family member. Sometimes being overweight, unfit, and smoking can also lead to problems, and the condition tends to become more common in men as they get older.

## SYMPTOMS

- Inability to attain an erection
- Inability to sustain an erection

## TREATMENT GOAL

Treatment involves first determining the cause of impotence, whether due to emotional or physical factors, or a combination of both. Conventional and complementary therapies focus on treating the cause, relieving psychological distress, and preventing further problems.

## CONVENTIONAL MEDICINE

The treatment of erectile dysfunction is dependent on a diagnosis of the cause. Possible treatment options are described below.

**Medication:** The most common drugs used are sildenafil (Viagra®), vardenafil (Levitra®), and tadalafil (Cialis®), all of which help sustain erection by increasing tissue levels of nitric oxide, a vasodilating chemical. These drugs should not be used by patients who are also taking nitrates to treat angina because of the potential for life-threatening low blood pressure. The lowest possible dose should be used first, as these drugs may have serious cardiac side effects in those who are already at risk. Intracavernosal alprostadil is a medication that is injected into the sides of the penis to treat impotence. This too has some potential cardiac effects and should not be used without a thorough evaluation.

**Modify your lifestyle:** Stop smoking, cut down on alcohol, exercise regularly, take adequate rest, and lower your stress levels. Exercises that may help improve erectile dysfunction include pelvic floor muscle exercises (also called Kegel exercises). These involve strengthening the same muscles one would use to stop the flow of urination. Exercises should be performed at least twice a day. Taking supplements of L-arginine, an amino acid that can increase blood vessel dilation, may also be helpful to treat cases of erectile dysfunction.

**Mechanical instruments:** A vacuum constriction device is a mechanical instrument that can be used to maintain an erection. It is relatively effective. If all of the above measures fail, surgery may be performed to insert a penile prosthesis, an artificial support for the penis.

## TRADITIONAL CHINESE MEDICINE

**Herbs:** According to traditional Chinese medicine, the common causes of impotence are kidney deficiency, spleen deficiency, and liver Qi stagnation. The herbs called for to treat these causes are available from Chinese pharmacies or online. To prepare any of the formulas below, place the raw herbs in a glass or ceramic pot and add 3½ cups of water. Bring to the boil, simmer for 30 minutes, and strain. Drink 1 cup twice a day.

• To treat kidney deficiency: TCM considers kidney energy to be important for the reproductive system. If kidney energy is low, you may have impotence accompanied by dizziness, tiredness, and lower back pain. This formula can tonify your kidneys and treat impotence. Mix 10 g of Rui Gui Zhi (inner bark of Saigon cinnamon), 15 g of Shu Di Huang (Chinese foxglove cooked in wine), 12 g of Shan Zhu Yu (Asiatic cornelian cherry fruit),

15 g of Shan Yao (Chinese yam), 15 g of Fuling (poria), 12 g of Zi Xie (water plantain rhizome), 12 g of Dan Pi (cortex of tree peony root), 12 g of Gou Ji Zi (wolfberry), 12 g of Du Zhong (eucommia bark), and 12 g of Ba Ji Tian (morinda root).

• To treat spleen deficiency: Symptoms include impotence accompanied by poor digestive function, loose stools, and fatigue. Combine 10 g of ginseng, 15 g of Bai Zhu (atractylodes rhizome), 15 g of Fuling (poria), 15 g of Shan Yao (Chinese yam), 12 g of Yuan Zhi (Chinese senega root), 12 g of Wu Wei Zi (schisandra fruit), and 5 g of Gan Cao (licorice).

• To treat liver Qi stagnation: Impotence is accompanied by depression, low motivation, loss of interest in life, and/or stress. Mix 12 g of Chai Hu (hare's ear root), 15 g of Bai Shao (white peony root), 15 g of Bai Zhu (atractylodes rhizome), 15 g of Fuling (poria), 5 g of Bo He (field mint), 6 g of Gan Cao (licorice), 12 g of Xiang Fu (nut grass rhizome), and 12 g of Gou Ji Zi (wolfberry).

**Acupuncture:** In most cases, acupuncture is an effective therapy for this condition. Consult a doctor of Chinese medicine for an evaluation to determine the underlying cause of the impotence. You may need 30-minute sessions once or twice a week to deal with the underlying cause. One full course of treatment consists of 12 sessions. A practitioner will determine the need for further courses, and may recommend Chinese herbal medicine along with acupuncture treatment.

**Acupressure:** The Guan Yuan point is in the center of the abdomen, about 3 inches below the navel. The Tai Xi point is on the inside of the leg, in the depression between the Achilles tendon and the anklebone. Press these points with your fingertip for one to two minutes, release, and repeat. Repeat this two or three times a day.

**Diet:** To treat impotence, eat foods that strengthen kidney and yang energy, such as black sesame seeds, string beans, wheat, caraway seeds, chives, tangerines, walnuts, plums, chicken, egg yolk, shrimp, dates, lamb, and pork.

## NATUROPATHY

**Diet:** Follow a diet high in vitamin E, which is essential for dilating blood vessels and improving circulation. Foods high in vitamin E include wheat germ, leafy green vegetables, almonds, avocado, and whole grains. Pumpkin seeds and sunflower seeds should be added to salads for their high zinc concentration, important for prostate health. Do not overeat before sexual intercourse, as this draws blood to your digestive tract, which may interfere with a healthy erection. Limit the amount of hydrogenated fats in your diet, found in margarine, baked foods, junk foods, and refined vegetable oils, as they can contribute to blocked arteries, which will impede with proper blood flow to the penis. Drink alcohol moderately, as over-consumption can lead to impotence.

**Supplements:** If tests show that your levels of DHEA, a steroid hormone, are low, take 50 mg daily under your doctor's supervision. Vitamin B3 or niacin is required to improve blood flow. Use the no-flush niacin found in most health food stores and take 250 mg three times a day. Zinc promotes health for the prostate and helps with testosterone synthesis. Take 30 mg twice a day, plus 3 mg of copper to avoid deficiency.

**Herbs:** Panax ginseng improves energy, sexual function, and libido in men. Take 100 mg three times a day of a product standardized to 4–7% ginsenosides. Ginkgo biloba has been shown in some research to benefit sexual function and increase circulation. Take 120 mg twice a day of the standardized form of 24% flavone glycosides and 6% of the terpene lactones. Take 500 mg of potency wood, which has been historically used in South America to increase sexual vigor, three times a day. Also take 500 mg of pucture vine, which may increase testosterone levels and is a folk remedy for improving libido and erectile function, three times daily. Damiana, a traditional remedy for increasing libido and potency, can be taken at 400 mg three times a day, and yohimbe, which increases blood flow to the penis during an erection, can be taken at 10 mg three times a day under a doctor's supervision. This latter herb should be avoided if patients have high blood pressure, a heart condition, kidney disease, or psychological disorders.

## HOMEOPATHY

Men who are experiencing established problems with achieving and maintaining an erection are likely to be under a great deal of psychological pressure, which can itself contribute to further problems. Due to the complex nature of this condition, it is best treated by a homeopathic practitioner who will prescribe at a constitutional level. The following lifestyle recommendations can provide further support in improving the situation.

**Avoid alcohol:** If stress levels are high, it may be tempting to drink alcohol as a way of relaxing. However, bear in mind that this can have a negative effect on achieving an erection. Alcohol, as well as caffeine and some prescription drugs, may restrict efficient blood flow.

**Relaxation techniques:** Make it a priority to address high stress levels. Psychological tension and anxiety are known to contribute to a significant number of cases of erectile dysfunction where a physical cause has been ruled out. Consider taking up relaxation techniques, meditation, or yoga.

**Counseling:** If unresolved tensions exist within a relationship, counseling may help by allowing sensitive issues to be aired and discussed in a neutral environment.

## HERBALISM

**Yohimbe:** The bark from this West African tree contains several alkaloids, including yohimbine, which have a long history of use as aphrodisiacs, useful for combating impotence. This herb may work for different types of impotence, whether psychological or physiological, and has effects on specific receptors relevant to libido and impotence. Most tablets have about 5 mg of yohimbine, and 5–10 mg can be taken 10–15 minutes before sexual intercourse. Other sources recommend more regular doses of 5.4 mg tablets three times daily. The many side effects of this herb include problems sleeping, agitation or anxiety, rapid heartbeat, headache, high blood pressure, tremor, and severe heart problems. Stop taking the herb and consult a medical herbalist if any of these occur. In addition, yohimbe may interact with heart medications, anti-depressants, and caffeine.

**Pygeum:** The bark of this African plum tree has been extensively studied for its use in prostate troubles, but there are also reports of improvement in cases of impotence. A standardized extract of pygeum can be purchased and taken at 50 mg twice a day. This extract contains phytochemicals such as beta-sitosterol and n-docosanol that may help to increase testosterone through changes in prolactin levels. Alternatively, 100 mg of the raw herb can be ingested daily as a tea, or 60 drops of tincture can be taken twice daily. Some people experience stomach upset with this plant. If this occurs decrease the dose, stop taking the herb completely, or check with a medical herbalist for advice.

# INFERTILITY

## DIAGNOSIS

Infertility is the inability to reproduce. Although fertility peaks in your 20s, if you are healthy you can be fertile well into your 40s. There is no denying, however, that the likelihood of becoming pregnant decreases with age. By the time a woman is 35 years old she is half as fertile as she was at 21, and after the age of 35 a woman's chance of conceiving falls by about 5–10% a year. Age, however, is far from being the only factor that contributes to this condition. In women, medical problems that can lead to infertility include damaged fallopian tubes, pelvic inflammatory disease, polycystic ovary syndrome (PCOS, see p. 790), and endometriosis. Hormonal disturbances in the thyroid, pituitary, and adrenal glands may also cause complications. Problems with the uterus such as fibroids (see p. 734) and scarring from previous surgery can also have an impact on fertility levels. In men, infertility is linked to sperm count. Male fertility is dependent on producing an adequate amount of sperm that has proper motility (efficient movement) and that is not deformed or abnormally shaped. Occasionally, men can suffer from retrograde ejaculation, where the sperm travels backwards after ejaculation. Other problems can stem from sexually transmitted diseases, hormonal disorders, inflammation of the testicles, impotence, and complications from previous surgery. Stress and other lifestyle factors can also contribute to infertility in both men and women.

## SYMPTOMS

### IN WOMEN
- Inability to fall pregnant
- Irregular or non-existent periods
- Excessive hair growth
- Pelvic pain

### IN MEN
- Swollen testes
- Descended testes

## TREATMENT GOAL

The first step is a complete fertility evaluation for you and your partner to isolate the root of the problem. Treatment then focuses on resolving the underlying condition and introducing lifestyle changes to increase your chances of conceiving.

## CONVENTIONAL MEDICINE

Various laboratory tests can be taken to evaluate hormone levels and ovulation to identify a reason for an inability to conceive. An evaluation may also involve tests such as an ultrasound, which show if the pelvic organs are present and look normal.

**Clomid:** If ovulation is irregular or non-existent, clomid treatment is used to induce ovulation. It is taken orally for five days starting on the third day of menstruation. Side effects are hot flashes, emotional instability, headaches, and disturbed sleep. If clomid does not work, gonadotropin, a natural hormone, is available. If the patient does not fall pregnant after three months of treatment, she is usually referred to an endocrine specialist.

**Invitro fertilization:** IVF involves retrieving eggs from a woman's ovaries and then introducing sperm into the egg. The fertilized egg is cultured for three to five days and then reintroduced into the uterus. The Centers for Disease Control report on assisted reproductive technology shows a success rate to be 30–50%.

## TRADITIONAL CHINESE MEDICINE

**Herbs:** Although there are many causes of infertility, the most common according to traditional Chinese medicine are kidney deficiency, blood deficiency, and Qi blood stagnation. You may try taking one of the following formulas, but it is best to first consult a practitioner of traditional Chinese medicine for an evaluation and appropriate formula. To prepare the formulas below, place the raw herbs in a glass or ceramic pot and add 3½ cups of water. Bring to a boil, simmer for 30 minutes, and then strain. Drink 1 cup twice a day. These herbs are available from Chinese pharmacies or online.

• To treat kidney yang deficiency: Symptoms include cold hands and feet, low libido, delayed periods, and fatigue. Mix 10 g of Rui Gui Zhi (inner bark of Saigon cinnamon), 15 g of Shu Di Huang (Chinese foxglove cooked in wine), 12 g of Shan Zhu Yu (Asiatic cornelian cherry fruit), 15 g of Shan Yao (Chinese yam), 15 g of Fuling (poria), 12 g of Zi Xie (water plantain rhizome), 12 g of Dan Pi (cortex of tree peony root), 12 g of Gou Ji Zi (wolfberry), 12 g of Du Zhong (eucommia bark), and 12 g of Ba Ji Tian (morinda root).

• To treat kidney Yin deficiency: Symptoms include difficulty conceiving, trouble sleeping, hot flashes, constipation, dizziness, or ringing in the ears. Combine 15 g of Shu Di Huang (Chinese foxglove cooked in wine), 12 g of Shan Yu (Asiatic cornelian cherry fruit), 15 g of Shan Yao (Chinese yam), 12 g of Ze Xie (water plantain rhizome), 12 g of Dan Pi (cortex of tree peony root), 15 g of Niu Zhen Zi (privet fruit), 15 g of Xuan Shen (ningpo figwort root), 15 g of Bai Shao (white peony root), and 3 g of Gan Cao (licorice).

• To treat Qi and blood stagnation: Symptoms include difficulty conceiving, irregular menstruation, cloudy blood flow or dark blood with large clots, strong menstrual cramps, and premenstrual mood swings. Mix 12 g of Chai Hu (hare's ear root), 15 g of Bai Shao (white peony root), 15 g of Bai Zhu (white atractylodes rhizome), 15 g of Fuling (poria), 5 g of Bo He (field mint), 6 g of Gan Cao (licorice), 12 g of Xiang Fu (nut grass rhizome), and 12 g of Gou Ji Zi (wolfberry).

**Acupuncture:** Acupuncture has proven to be effective in treating many cases of infertility. Consult a practitioner of traditional Chinese medicine who will make a diagnosis of the cause and advise on how best to treat it with acupuncture. Herbal formulas may also be recommended.

**Acupressure:** Press the Guan Yuan point, found on the midline of your abdomen, about 3 inches below the navel. The Di Ji point is on the inside of the lower leg in the depression between the tibia and fibula, the two bones in the lower leg, about 3–4 inches below the knee. Press these points for one to two minutes. Repeat twice a day.

**Diet:** Eat food that is good for the blood, such as spinach, beef, chestnuts, sweet basil, peaches, black soybeans, fish, carrots, black beans, black sesame seeds, red beans, and radishes. You should also eat food that is cooling, such as watermelon, green vegetables, tofu, and Chinese jujube dates. Avoid hot, spicy food such as chili peppers, garlic, beef, and lamb.

## NATUROPATHY

**Diet:** Eat wholesome foods that nourish your hormones and your body as whole. A typical wholesome diet consists of drinking plenty of water and eating fish, whole grains, and fresh fruit and vegetables. Use cold-pressed nut oil for a cooking base or to add to a salad, as it contains healthy levels of vitamin E, which helps to nourish the endocrine system—the system responsible for hormone production. Wheat germ also has high levels of vitamin E and can be added to smoothies and salads. Snacking on pumpkin seeds can be helpful, especially for men, because their high zinc content nourishes the prostate gland—the gland that produces the most semen. Avoid fried, processed foods, sugar, and white flour as they tend to depress the body and deplete nutrients. Wherever possible eat organic, hormone-free food. Other meats have chemicals that mimic estrogen, a hormone that, in excess, decreases fertility in men and women.

**Supplements:** A good-quality multivitamin provides a base of nutrients that are important for fertility. Follow the dosage instructions on the bottle. Vitamin C has been shown to be helpful in treating both men and women for fertility. Take 1,000 mg two to three times a day. Also take 400 IU of vitamin E a day, which has been shown in some studies to be helpful for fertility. Men should take 4 g of L-arginine a day as it has been shown to increase sperm quality, and 1,500 mg of L-carnitine twice a day to help with sperm motility. Selenium also improves sperm motility, and can be taken at 100 mcg twice a day. Women can take 100 mg of PABA three times a day; it has been shown to help treat infertility by improving the effects of estrogen. Zinc improves prostate and sperm health. Take 30 mg twice a day with 3 mg of copper to avoid copper deficiency.

**Herbs:** Chaste berry acts on the pituitary gland to stimulate the hormones involved in ovulation. A women should take 240 mg of a 0.6% of aucubin extract each morning. False unicorn root stimulates the ovaries and restores hormonal balance. A typical dose of false unicorn is 1–2 g three times daily. Drink 3 cups of stinging nettle seed tea (made from a handful of seeds boiled in 1 quart of water) a day, or add 1 tsp of seeds to every meal for their estrogen-like phyto-hormones. Panax ginseng helps with sperm motility and sperm count. Men should take a product standardized to ginsenosides at 300 mg daily.

**TIP:** AVOID SAUNAS, HOT TUBS, AND TIGHT-FITTING UNDERWEAR
Testicles are set apart from the rest of the body because they need to be kept cool for healthy sperm production. Men with fertility issues should avoid overheating the testicles in saunas and hot tubs, and wearing tight-fitting underwear.

## HOMEOPATHY

The causes of infertility can be diverse and complex in nature, and are best treated by an experienced homeopathic practitioner. Ideally treatment should begin for both partners after the appropriate medical tests have been carried out to determine if a mechanical impediment to conception exists. This will allow a homeopath to prescribe as appropriately as possible to treat individual situations. The basic lifestyle changes suggested below may also help increase the chances of conception.

**Avoid alcohol:** Alcohol has been shown to have a negative effect on fertility levels for both men and women. Couples who are trying to conceive may benefit from cutting it out completely.

**Stop smoking:** Cigarette smoking has a similar negative effect on fertility. Both partners should make an effort to give up.

**Reduce stress:** Difficulty conceiving can increase stress levels significantly, which, paradoxically, can further contribute to infertility. If one or both partners lead a high-stress lifestyle, explore methods of stress reduction. This can make conception more likely to occur, and will benefit your health in general.

**Use an ovulation kit:** Although keeping track of when you ovulate should not dominate your thoughts, knowing precisely when ovulation will occur is essential to increasing your chances of conceiving. Use an ovulation kit, or take your temperature each day before getting out of bed. A rise in temperature of up to 0.5–1°F accompanied by a mucus-like vaginal discharge, suggests that ovulation is taking place.

## HERBALISM

**Red clover:** An infusion of dried red clover flowers can be used to enhance fertility in women, as the phyto-estrogens in red clover can help to regulate the menstrual period. Steep 1 oz of dried flowers in 1 quart of hot water for several hours. Ingesting 1 cup of this infusion one to three times daily for several weeks, or even months, may be necessary for any benefit to appear in fertility.

**Dong Quai:** The root of Dong Quai, through its volatile oils and furanocoumarin compounds, may help to normalize female hormones that contribute to abnormal menstrual cycles, making it difficult to become pregnant. Water extracts, alcohol tinctures, and standardized extracts all have slightly different activities, the nuances of which would be best assessed by a medical herbalist. Some sources recommend that you boil 3–5 g of root or ingest 4–6 ml of tincture per day. Research trials have studied 4–5 g daily of a water-based extract standardized to the ferulic acid content of Dong Quai, while other extracts may be standardized to other compounds such as ligustilide. Care should be taken when using this herb if you are also taking anti-coagulant medications.

**Chaste tree:** This herbs effects on the female reproductive tract may also help with infertility. It is most often dosed at ½ –1 g of the herb three times daily. It may cause an increase in vaginal bleeding, and you should discontinue use if this occurs. See Premenstrual Syndrome (p. 799) for more information on chaste tree.

**Tribulus:** Tribulus been used to enhance fertility in both males and females. Extracts of tribulus may alter blood hormone levels, and improve sperm activity. The tablets for infertility contain 250 mg of this herb, and for men, one tablet is taken three times daily for one to two months, and, for women, one tablet is taken three times daily at certain times of the menstrual cycle (either days 1–12, or 5–14). Further research is necessary to establish definitive use for infertility. Sometimes, extra vaginal bleeding occurs with the use of these tablets, as does insomnia, and decreased blood sugar. Discontinue use if any of these occur.

# LOW LIBIDO

## DIAGNOSIS

Our libido (sex drive) is the biological force connected with sexual arousal. It is associated with the hypothalamus part of the brain and is influenced by various hormones and chemicals. Loss of libido is a fairly common problem. It can occur in both men and women, but tends to affect women more. There is no such thing as a "normal" libido, as everyone's sex drive level is different. Sex drive is influenced by many factors and tends to fluctuate. Each of us has an individual drive that develops according to circumstances and life stages. Although sex is a part of most adults' lives, it is a more important factor for some than it is for others.

In women, libido can be affected by changes in hormonal levels, menstrual cycle, pregnancy, childbirth, perimenopause, and menopause. Some women may also experience pain and discomfort during sex, which can contribute to a low libido. In men, a low sex drive may be associated with prostate problems, the disorder known as hyperprolactinemia, where too much of the hormone prolactin is produced by the pituitary gland, and low testosterone levels.

Psychological factors that affect both sexes, such as stress, emotional worries, fatigue, depression, and low self-esteem, also influence sex drive. Poor health and certain illnesses or conditions can have a negative impact, as can some medications. Some people can develop an aversion to sex suddenly, while others may experience long-term problems, which may be linked with sexual abuse or childhood hang-ups.

## SYMPTOMS

- Disinterest in, or aversion to, sex
- High stress
- Depression

## TREATMENT GOAL

It is important to determine whether a low libido is caused by a physical or psychological condition. Conventional and complementary therapies aim to treat the cause and restore the sex drive.

## CONVENTIONAL MEDICINE

Before treating low libido, a doctor will evaluate a person's medical history, social situation, and life stressors, both past and present, to determine a cause. Low libido may be secondary to another problem, such as premature ejaculation, inability to reach orgasm, anxiety, depression, or sexual aversion disorder, in which a person (usually a woman) is repulsed by the sexual act. In this case the underlying cause should be treated, either through psychotherapy or conventional medicine.

**To treat low hormone levels:** Low androgen levels, which occur during menopause and in andropause (male menopause) are a common cause of low libido. If this is the case, androgen hormones can be prescribed, usually as testosterone and DHEA, a steroid hormone. In women, low estrogen and progesterone can also be associated with a low libido. These hormones can be evaluated and administered in a natural or synthetic form. Thyroid levels should also be evaluated, as low thyroid function can also be a factor.

## TRADITIONAL CHINESE MEDICINE

**Herbs:** According to traditional Chinese medicine, low libido is due to kidney deficiency, spleen deficiency, or liver Qi stagnation. The formulas below can treat each different cause. To prepare a decoction, place the raw herbs in a ceramic pot, add 3½ cups of water and bring to the boil. Simmer for 30 minutes and strain. Drink 1 cup twice a day. All the herbs required are available from Chinese pharmacies or online.

• To treat kidney deficiency: If your kidney energy is low, you may have a low sex drive accompanied by dizziness, tiredness, and lower back ache. The following herbal formula can tonify your kidney. Mix 10 g of Rui Gui Zhi (inner bark of Saigon cinnamon), 15 g of Shu Di Huang (Chinese foxglove cooked in wine), 12 g of Shan Zhu Yu (Asiatic cornelian cherry fruit), 15 g of Shan Yao (Chinese yam), 15 g of Fuling (poria), 12 g of Zi Xie (water plantain rhizome), 12 g of Dan Pi (cortex of tree peony root), 12 g of Gou Ji Zi (wolfberry), 12 g of Du Zhong (eucommia bark), and 12 g of Ba Ji Tian (morinda root).

• To treat spleen deficiency: If low libido is accompanied by poor digestive function, loose stools, and fatigue, you may have spleen deficiency. Mix 10 g of ginseng, 15 g of Bai Zhu (white atractylodes rhizome), 15 g of Fuling (poria), 15 g of Shan Yao (Chinese yam), 12 g of Yuan Zhi (Chinese senega root), 12 g of Wu Wei Zi (schisandra fruit), and 5 g of Gan Cao licorice).

• To treat liver Qi stagnation: If a low sex drive is accompanied by depression and/or stress, low motivation, and loss of interest in life, you may have liver Qi stagnation.

Combine 12 g of Chai Hu (hare's ear root), 15 g of Bai Shao (white peony root), 15 g of Bai Zhu (white atractylodes rhizome), 15 g of Fuling (poria), 5 g of Bo He (field mint), 6 g of Gan Cao (licorice), 12 g of Xiang Fu (nut grass rhizome), and 12 g of Gou Ji Zi (wolfberry).

**Acupuncture:** Consult a practitioner who will begin with a course of treatment, made up of 12, 30-minute sessions over 6–12 weeks. The acupuncturist will then evaluate your progress to determine whether further courses are needed.

**Acupressure:** Guan Yuan and Shan Yin Jiao acupressure points are recommended. The Guan Yuan point is on the midline of your abdomen, about 3 inches below the navel. The Shan Yin Jiao point is in the center of the lower leg, about 3 inches above the anklebone. Use the tip of your finger to press these points with moderate pressure for one to two minutes. Repeat a couple of times a day.

**Diet:** To improve a low libido, eat food that will increase kidney energy and help you to relax. Such foods include chamomile, peppermint, Chinese jujubes, black sesame seeds, string beans, sword beans, wheat, and chicken livers.

## NATUROPATHY

**Diet:** Various foods and spices have been traditionally used as aphrodisiacs in different cultures, including avocado, bananas, cucumbers, chocolate, basil (sweet basil), chili peppers, honey, garlic, ginger, figs, licorice, nutmeg, pine nuts, and oysters. They are thought to increase sexual desire either because of their appearance (if it is similar to a sexual organ), aroma, or their chemical components. However, there has been little or no research to support most of these claims. If low libido is linked to impotence, see p. 754 for further diet recommendations.

**Supplements:** Take 50 g of B-complex vitamins three times a day; they calm the nervous system, reduce anxiety about sexual experiences, and are involved in the synthesis of hormones involved in sexual function and desire. Semen contains large amounts of zinc, which is a fundamental requirement for healthy male sexuality, and is needed for the production of testosterone. Men should take 30 mg twice a day plus 3 mg of copper, as zinc can inhibit the body's ability to absorb copper.

**Herbs:** Ginkgo biloba is a powerful antioxidant that enhances circulation and increases the supply of oxygen to the brain and sexual organs. The standard dosage of ginkgo is 40–80 mg three times daily of a 50:1 extract standardized to contain 24% ginkgo-flavone glycosides. Take 500–1,000 mg of horny goat weed, which, as the name implies, is a natural aphrodisiac that helps restore sexual desire in men and women. Maca root is used throughout the world to increase energy, libido, stamina, and sexual performance in men and women. A recommended dose is 500–1,000 mg three times a day. Damiana, a nervous system stimulant that acts as an aphrodisiac and a tonic for the reproductive organs, is traditionally used to promote energy and increase libido in women. Take 2–4 g two to three times daily, or as directed on the label. Sarsaparilla contains steroidal saparins thought to mimic the action of some human hormones. To use it as a tonic for sexual functioning and also as a rejuvenator, drink a tea two or three times a day. To make sarsaparilla tea, soak 1–4 g of chopped or shredded dried root for 10 minutes in about 8 oz of hot water and then strain before drinking. You can also take 2–3 tsp of an alcohol-based liquid extract up to two or three times a day.

**TIP:** EXERCISE
Research shows that exercise is linked to sexual vitality. Bike riding, running, weight-lifting, tennis, swimming, or other similar sports help to regain much needed energy.

## HOMEOPATHY

A flagging libido can occur at any time. A short-term problem of this kind is not a cause for concern. However, a significant, prolonged reduction in libido can be a sign of an underlying chronic condition. In such cases, consult an experienced homeopath who can help to balance the body's energy reserves on all levels, emotional as well as physical.

**Lycopodium:** If a low libido is related to diminished self-confidence and high levels of anxiety, consider using Lycopodium. Sufferers may adopt a domineering or sarcastic manner to camouflage feelings of insecurity. Burning sensations in the vagina during and after intercourse may also play a part in dampening libido in women, while anxiety about maintaining an erection can undermine the libido in men.

**Sepia:** If there is a general sense of exhaustion that makes sex feel like yet another demand that has to be satisfied, take Sepia. The genital area may also feel hypersensitive, sore, and irritated. Even if there is no physical discomfort, feeling emotionally low and depressed may lower libido. In women, this remedy is indicated if a low sex drive occurs after childbirth, or while going through menopause.

**Staphysagria:** This remedy may be helpful if low libido follows invasive tests, examination, or surgery to the genital area. Patients may feel violated or the affected area may be hypersensitive, with lingering sharp, stinging pains. It is also helpful for those who experience recurrent cystitis after intercourse. Emotional stress may make symptoms more intense, while rest and warmth feel comforting.

**Graphites:** This remedy is likely to be helpful if a low libido is causing you to avoid sexual activity. Physical symptoms, such as a dry, uncomfortable feeling in the vagina, or premature ejaculation, may also have a negative effect on libido.

## HERBALISM

**Damiana:** The leaves of damiana, also called Mexican damiana, old woman's broom, or rosemary, have traditionally been used as a male reproductive tonic, probably acting on the sex hormones to improve sexual desire and function. However, it may cause liver toxicity and seizures in some people. Nonetheless, some people use 30 drops of a tincture two to three times daily, or drink 2–4 g of the herb in a tea, split up throughout the day, in order to boost libido. This plant should either be avoided completely or used under the direction of an experienced medical herbalist.

**Yohimbe:** This herb has a history of use as an aphrodisiac, and has effects on specific hormone receptors relevant to libido and impotence. It is most commonly taken in pill form (tablets contain 5.4 mg of yohimbine) three times daily. This plant may cause problems with sleeping, agitation or anxiety, a fast heartbeat, headaches, high blood pressure, tremors, and severe heart problems. If any of these side effects occur, stop taking yohimbe and consult a medical herbalist for guidance. In addition, this herb may interact with heart medications, anti-depressants, and caffeine. This plant should be used under the direction of an experienced medical herbalist.

# MASTITIS

## DIAGNOSIS

Mastitis, an inflammation and infection of the breast, is a common problem in women. It generally occurs between the ages of 18 and 50 and affects both those who are breastfeeding and those who are not. In breastfeeding women, mastitis is most likely to occur during the first six weeks of breastfeeding, although some women develop it during the weaning process. A course of antibiotics will clear the infection in a matter of days, and patients can continue breastfeeding. If, however, mastitis follows on from other problems, such as sore nipples or blocked ducts, this is usually an indication of an incorrect feeding technique. If you suspect that you are developing an infection, consult a doctor as soon as possible. It is important that you continue to breastfeed/express because if you do not drain the infected milk from the breast an abscess may develop, in which case you will need to go to a hospital to have it drained.

In non-breastfeeding women, the most commonly affected site is the area close to the nipple. Most women who get this type of infection are in their 20s and 30s and most of them are smokers. It is thought that one of the toxins in cigarette smoke damages the ducts in the breasts, causing infection. Antibiotics can be taken to clear up the infection.

## SYMPTOMS

- Sore breasts and engorgement, with pain, swelling, and tenderness
- Cracked nipples
- High temperature, aches and pains, and sweats
- Blockage or a lump in the breast
- Occasionally, breast stops producing any milk

## TREATMENT GOAL

Mastitis is generally a temporary condition and in most cases is linked with breastfeeding. Treatment involves identifying the cause of the infection, resolving symptoms, and preventing infection from recurring, for example, by correcting breastfeeding technique or stopping smoking.

## CONVENTIONAL MEDICINE

This infection of the ductal glands occurs most frequently in the first two to four weeks after having a baby. It also seems to be aggravated when mothers begin to nurse their babies less frequently.

**Prevention:** Several factors contribute to mastitis and should be avoided. These include maternal fatigue and stress, poor feeding technique, and trauma to the nipple. Often, hospital staff can give immediate postnatal advice on how to avoid these complications. If a staphylococcal infection is present in the home or community, particular care should be taken to avoid it. It is also important to support the breast properly, drink plenty of water, and practice good hand washing and hygiene.

**Antibiotics:** Staphylococcus is the most common organism that causes mastitis, but it can also be caused by streptococcus. Antibiotics are prescribed to treat these infections, and mothers should continue nursing and get plenty of bed rest until their energy returns. The antibiotics used include dicloxacillin (a penicillin type of drug) and erythromycin for those allergic to penicillin. It is necessary to continue treatment for a full seven days. About 80% of patients recover fully after treatment. An abscess will develop in 10% of patients, and infection recurs in the remaining 10%. Specific antibiotics are dicloxacillin and, erythromycin for those allergic to penicillin.

## TRADITIONAL CHINESE MEDICINE

**Herbs:** Although conventional medicine is unclear about what causes mastitis, traditional Chinese medicine considers it to be related to a patient's mental and emotional health, liver and kidney energy deficiency, and blood stagnation. The following formulas can be used to treat each cause. The herbs listed are available from Chinese pharmacies or online. To make a decoction, add the herbs to 3 cups of water in a ceramic pot. Bring the liquid to a boil and simmer for 30 minutes. Strain the liquid and drink 1 cup three times a day for three to five days.

• To treat mastitis associated with stress: Mix 10 g of Chai Hu (hare's ear root), 10 g of Gui Zhi (cinnamon), 10 g of Yu Jin (turmeric tuber), 12 g of Bai Shao (white peony root), 6 g of Chuan Xiong (Szechuan lovage root), 15 g of Dan Shen (salvia root), 10 g of Xiang Fu (nut grass rhizome).

• To treat liver and kidney deficiency: Symptoms include mastitis associated with fatigue or insomnia. Herbs that help tonify liver and kidney energy are suitable for this type of condition. Mix 15 g of Guo Ji Zi (wolfberry), 12 g of Tu Si Zi (Chinese dodder seed), 15 g of Shu Di Huang (Chinese foxglove root cooked in wine), 12 g of Han Lian

Cao (eclipta), 12 g of Wu Wei Zi (schisandra fruit), and 15 g of He Shou Wu (fleece flower root).

- To treat blood stagnation: Mix 10 g of Tao Ren (peach kennel), 12 g of Chi Shao (red peony root), 10 g of Chuan Xiong (Szechuan lovage root), 12 g of Dan Shen (salvia root), and 8 g of Hong Hua (*flos carthami tinctorii*).

**Acupuncture:** Long-term treatment (sessions once a week for three to six weeks) is usually required to improve symptoms. Treatment can be combined with herbal formulas.

**Acupressure:** Press the Qu Chi, Hegu, Xue Hai, and San Yin Jiao for one to two minutes two to three times a day to improve circulation. With the elbow flexed, the Qu Chi point is located in the depression on the outside of the bend. The Hegu point is located on the back of the hand between the thumb and first finger. The Xue Hai point is on the inside of the leg in the depression just above the knee. The San Yin Jiao point is located on the inside of the leg, about 3 inches above the anklebone.

**Diet:** Peaches, sweet basil, chives, hawthorn fruit, celery, liver, loquat, persimmons, pineapple, duck, grapes, lotus, yam, and tangerines are recommended for this condition.

## NATUROPATHY

If the mastitis does not improve or gets worse after following the recommendations below for 24–48 hours, contact your doctor. You may need antibiotic treatment.

**Diet:** Drink an 8 oz glass of water every two waking hours to help flush out the infection. Use unrefined, cold-pressed flaxseed oil daily as a dressing on salads, on a baked potato, or incorporated into any dish that does not need to be heated to a high temperature. This oil contains the essential fatty acids omega-6 linoleic acid and the more rare omega-3 alpha-linolenic acid. These two fatty acids, which the body cannot manufacture itself, are needed to prevent hormone imbalances, thus reducing the risk of mastitis. Cold-water fish (such as salmon, mackerel, sardines, and halibut) also contain high levels of omega-3 fatty acids. Add at least two to three cloves of raw garlic a day to meals. It acts as a broad-spectrum antibiotic, and does not cause the side effects that orthodox antibiotics do, such as yeast infections or thrush.

**Supplements:** Take 3,000–5,000 mg of vitamin C a day. It increases the body's production of white blood cells, which the body uses to defend against infection and impede the growth of viruses and bacteria. Bioflavonoids enhance the effectiveness of vitamin C as well as improve the body's absorption of this vitamin. Take 500–1,000 mg three times daily. Also take 400 IU of vitamin E with mixed tocopherols daily as it is a powerful antioxidant that helps destroy free radicals, which inhibit healing. By protecting the cells, vitamin E promotes immune system efficiency. Colloidal silver is another potent natural antibiotic. Take 1 tsp a day orally or use it topically around the nipple.

**Herbs:** Herbs can be used to increase circulation, reduce inflammation, and relieve pain due to mastitis. Ground fenugreek seeds can be applied as a hot pack to increase protein absorption and promote blood building. Fenugreek is also very beneficial as a tea. Add 1 cup of boiling water to 3 tsp of fenugreek seeds and drink 1–3 cups daily. Calendula has antiseptic and anti-inflammatory properties and is soothing to dry skin. Apply the cream to sore nipples and after every feed. St. John's wort oil can also be rubbed on dry, cracked nipples to relieve pain, but clean the breast thoroughly before breastfeeding. Combine 2–4 oz each of aloe vera, marshmallow, and slippery elm in powder form and mix this with 6 oz of cold, boiled water to make a thin paste. Apply this to sore nipples to alleviate pain and promote healing. Also try using dandelion as a compress to soothe sore nipples. Boil about 1 oz of minced dandelion root in 2–3 cups of water until only half the liquid remains. Soak a cloth in the remaining liquid and use it as a compress.

> **TIP:** USE HOT AND COLD COMPRESSES
> Between feedings, use a cold compress on the breast to help relieve any inflammation. Before breastfeeding your baby, place a warm, wet washcloth over the affected breast for about 15 minutes. Try this at least three times a day to increase milk flow in the breast. Massaging the affected breast may also increase milk flow.

## HOMEOPATHY

The following homeopathic remedies may be helpful if they are taken at the first sign of mastitis. However, symptoms that continue to progress without improvement require prompt conventional medical attention. If orthodox drugs are required to manage the situation, bear in mind that homeopathic support may still be used as a complementary measure.

**Belladonna:** This remedy is helpful when used at the first sign of inflammation, when the affected area looks red and feels hot to the touch. Pain and discomfort are made more intense by jarring movements, and when lying flat. Sufferers may be uncharacteristically irritable and grouchy.

**Phytolacca:** If mastitis is accompanied by a general sense of achiness and swollen, tender glands, use Phytolacca. Classic symptoms include shooting pains that seem to radiate in all directions, or from the breast to the armpits, and the affected area of the breast has a reddish purple tinge. When this remedy is helpful sufferers feel feverish and tired.

**Bryonia:** Symptoms that call for this remedy include strong pain and distress from even the slightest movement. Inflammation and pain are often the result of low-grade dehydration. Firm pressure reduces discomfort, as does resting in one position and drinking plenty of fluids.

**Graphites:** If symptoms affect the left side, and the left breast feels inflamed and hard, try Graphites. Excruciatingly sensitive nipples show signs of cracking, and pain and discomfort make it difficult to rest during the night, which leads to feeling drowsy and out of sorts during the day.

**TIP:** USE A BREAST PUMP
When breastfeeding, ensure that each breast is thoroughly drained after each feed. If your baby does not feed regularly enough to accomplish this, use a breast pump in between feeds.

## HERBALISM

**General advice:** In addition to using herbs to treat the infection and move lymph, apply heat to the affected area either with heating pads or by taking a hot shower. Continue to breastfeed; the infection will not harm the baby, and moving milk through the inflamed duct will help heal the infection. Drinking large amounts of water daily is also recommended.

**Topical treatment:** Apply 20–30 drops of poke root, a potent lymphagogue that encourages lymph movement from swollen gland and infected tissue, and 20–30 drops of thyme oil, a powerful antimicrobial, to the affected area of the breast. Cover the oils with a heating pad for 20 minutes and repeat four to five times per day. They should be washed off just before the baby breastfeeds.

**Antimicrobial formula:** If antibiotics are needed, try this potent antimicrobial blend of herbs to fight infection. Goldenseal root has demonstrated antibacterial activity. Oregon grape is also astringent, and is antimicrobial as well as anti-inflammatory. Garlic is antibacterial and improves immune function. Thyme is especially useful against staph infections. Cleavers is a gentle, nourishing lymphagogue. Combine equal parts of each herb and drink an infusion made from 1–2 tsp per cup of water, three to four times daily.

# MENOPAUSE

## DIAGNOSIS

Menopause marks the end of menstruation and a woman's reproductive years. There is no definitive age at which this occurs. On average it tends to happen around the age of 51, but there have been cases where periods have stopped in women in their 20s, while other women will continue to menstruate until their late 50s or early 60s. Lifestyle factors have an impact on when menopause begins. For example, it is thought that women who smoke generally experience menopause earlier than women who do not. The perimenopause, the period leading up to menopause where periods start to become irregular, generally starts when a woman is in her 40s. Menopause can go on for many years, but once a woman has not had a period for one year she is considered to be "postmenopausal."

Menopause is triggered when the ovaries no longer respond to the controlling hormones released by the pituitary gland. As a result, the ovaries stop releasing an egg each month and no longer produce the female sex hormones estrogen and progesterone. It is this decline of function in the ovaries and fall in hormone levels that give rise to the symptoms of menopause. Symptoms vary from woman to woman. Many only notice that their periods become irregular. Others, however, suffer from heavy bleeding, hot flashes, disturbed sleep, and emotional instability.

## SYMPTOMS

- Irregular periods
- Hot flashes
- Disturbed sleep, often with night sweats
- Emotional distress
- Vaginal dryness
- Dry skin
- Weight gain
- Low libido

## TREATMENT GOAL

To alleviate the symptoms of the menopause by adjusting hormone levels and introducing lifestyle changes. This should help to limit the physical and emotional impact that menopause can have on many women's lives.

## CONVENTIONAL MEDICINE

Menopause is a normal life transition, so there is no necessary medical treatment. It is possible, however, to ease symptoms through lifestyle modification and hormone replacement. For treatment of hot flashes, see p. 749.

**Lifestyle modifications:** A high-fiber, low-fat diet and reducing your intake of dairy and processed foods is recommended. Perform an aerobic exercise for 20 minutes every day to help with the weight gain that tends to occur with menopause. Stress-reduction techniques are also recommended.

**Hormone replacement:** Balancing the hormones can help the emotional challenges associated with menopause, as well as other troubling symptoms such as vaginal dryness, skin dryness, and low libido. Synthetic hormones have been shown to be detrimental to a woman's overall health, and they are now rarely recommended by doctors. Many doctors instead advocate the use of natural estradiol and estriol as well as progesterone and/or testosterone and DHEA, a steroid hormone. Blood levels can be taken to determine the amount of hormone needed and a pharmacist can make up an exact prescription. These hormones have not been studied to the same extent as synthetic hormones. They are thought to be safer due to their bio-identical compounding (they match the natural hormones of the body) and low dosage. Frequently, selective serotonin reuptake inhibitors (SSRIs) drugs such as Prozac® and Lexapro® are also prescribed to treat emotional difficulties, and may also alleviate hot flashes.

## TRADITIONAL CHINESE MEDICINE

**Herbs:** The herbs listed below are available from Chinese pharmacies or online. To prepare a formula, place the herbs in a ceramic pot and add 3 cups of water. Bring to the boil, simmer for 30 minutes, and strain the liquid. Drink 1 cup twice a day.

• To treat perimenopause: Mix 15 g of Shen Di Huang (Chinese foxglove root), 10 g of Shan Zhu Yu (Asiatic cornelian cherry fruit), 15 g of Shan Yao (Chinese yam), 15 g of Fuling (poria), 12 g of Zi Xie (water plantain rhizome), 12 g of Dan Pi (cortex of peony root), 12 g of Niu Zhen Zi (privet fruit), and 12 g of Wu Wei Zi (schisandra fruit).

• To treat kidney Yang deficiency: Symptoms may include chills, dizziness, cold hands and feet, and loose stools. Combine 15 g of Shu Di Huang (Chinese foxglove cooked in wine), 12 g of Shan Zhu Yu (Asiatic cornelian cherry fruit), 15 g of Shan Yao (Chinese yam), 12 g of Tu Si Zi (Chinese dodder seed), 12 g of Du Zhong (eucommia bark), 8 g of Ru Gui Zhi (inner bark of Saigon cinnamon), and 12 g of Dang Gui (Chinese angelica root).

• To treat Qi stagnation: Symptoms include depression, loss of interest in life, and stress. Mix 12 g of Chai Hu (hare's ear root), 15 g of Bai Shao (white peony root), 15 g of Bai Zhu (white atractylodes rhizome), 15 g of Fuling (poria), 5 g of Bo He (field mint), 6 g of Gan Cao (licorice), 12 g of Xiang Fu (nut grass rhizome), and 12 g of Gou Ji Zi (wolfberry).

**Acupuncture:** Consult a practitioner who will perform an evaluation and diagnose your condition. You may need 30-minute treatment sessions once or twice a week depending on your particular condition.

**Acupressure:** The Hegu and Fu Liu acupressure points may help to reduce hot flashes and perspiration. The Hegu points are located on the back of the hands in the depression between the thumb and the first finger. The Fu Liu point is on the inside of the leg, beside the ankle, in the depression 1 inch directly above the Achilles tendon. Use the tip of your fingers to press these points with moderate pressure for one to two minutes.

**Diet:** Eat a nutritious diet of fresh fruits and vegetables and grains to maintain good health. It is also important to drink plenty of water every day. You can also try making a soup by cooking 10 g of cinnamon twigs and 100 g of lean pork. Drink the soup slowly.

## NATUROPATHY

Menopausal symptoms are related to falling levels of estrogen and progesterone, and the recommendations below may help to boost the levels of these hormones in the body.

**Diet:** Eat two to three servings of foods that contain phytosterols, which have hormone-balancing effects. These include whole grains, legumes, and fresh vegetables and fruits. Phyto-estrogens, estrogen-like compounds that also have hormone-balancing effects, should be consumed as often as possible. Have one or two servings a day of miso, flaxseeds, or tofu, unless you are allergic to soy products. You can sprinkle 1–2 tbsp of ground flaxseeds, which also lower cholesterol, over cereal or salad, or add it to a smoothie. If eating meat, choose the organic, hormone-free kind to avoid hormonal imbalances.

**Supplements:** A high-quality multivitamin can nourish your body to keep hormones balanced. Follow the directions on the label. Take 1,000 mg of calcium and 500 mg of magnesium, both of which are essential for bone health. B-complex vitamins and vitamin C may all help to relieve hot flashes. Take 100 mg and 1,000 mg respectively three times a day. Take 1 tbsp of evening primrose oil three times a day. It can also help to relieve hot flashes and is excellent for the production of estrogen. Pregnenolone, which is involved in making estrogen and progesterone, can help with hormone imbalances. Take 30 mg twice a day.

**Herbs:** Take 80 mg of black cohosh twice a day; studies show that it alleviates hot flushes. Chaste berry has historically been used to prevent of hot flashes. Take 160–240 mg of an 0.6 % aucubin extract daily. Take 40 mg of red clover twice a day, as it has been shown to reduce some of the symptoms of menopause. Hops, taken at 250 mg three times a day, can help to reduce anxiety and tension, which are common menopausal symptoms, and has hormone-balancing effects. Soy protein powder has been shown in some studies to reduce hot flashes. Take 60 g a day mixed into a smoothie. Also take 4–6 g of sage a day to help control night sweats associated with hot flashes.

> **TIP:** EXERCISE
> Weight-bearing exercises are essential in avoiding demineralization of bone that occurs during menopause, which leads to osteoporosis. Weight-lifting, jogging, and brisk walking can all be helpful.

## HOMEOPATHY

Homeopathic treatment can provide invaluable support in easing distressing but common symptoms such as sleep disturbance, hot flashes, night sweats, mood swings, fatigue, and poor mental focus and concentration. Homeopathy treats the whole person, and is equally effective in treating the emotional traumas that a difficult menopause can involve. Some women benefit from solely using these remedies, while others use them in a complementary way until they are ready to reduce their conventional treatment. The remedies below provide a general overview of some of the most helpful homeopathic strategies that practitioners will utilize when treating symptoms.

**Calc carb:** If menopausal symptoms include the feeling that the whole body system has slowed down, take Calc carb. Weight gain may be noticeable, coupled with persistently low energy levels. Hot flashes are likely to be come on with the least amount of physical effort, followed by a cold, clammy sensation.

**Natrum mur:** Symptoms that call for this remedy include dry mucous membranes, particularly of the vagina. The skin is also likely to show signs of major dryness and sensitivity as a result of hormone changes. Emotionally, sufferers tend to bottle up their feelings, resulting in low moods and depression.

**Sepia:** If menopause brings on exhaustion associated with feeling emotionally, mentally, and physically drained, take Sepia. The libido is very low and patients tend to feel irritable and emotionally flat, and find it difficult to rise to the challenges of everyday life. Flashes, which are likely to be a major symptom, sweep upwards from the torso to the head, leading to profuse sweating that feels immensely draining.

**Pulsatilla:** If changeableness is the key symptom of menopause, use Pulastilla. Moods are especially affected, and there is an underlying tendency to be uncharacteristically emotional and weepy. Although sufferers feel chilly, sweats break out on the face due to waves of heat that are aggravated by being in stuffy, warm surroundings, and when trying to sleep at night.

**TIP:** WEAR APPROPRIATE NIGHTWEAR

If night sweats are a major issue, avoid wearing nightwear that is made from synthetic materials as it tends to hold in heat. Opt instead for natural fibers that allow air to circulate and the skin to sweat freely when the body needs to cool down.

## HERBALISM

**Black cohosh:** This herb is recognized for its ability to reduce or eliminate menopausal symptoms such as hot flashes, insomnia, fatigue, depression, irritability, and mood swings. Black cohosh also acts as an anti-spasmodic, anti-inflammatory, digestive stimulant, mild sedative, and blood pressure lowering agent by relaxing blood vessels in the extremities. Clinical studies show that black cohosh standardized to 1% triterpene glycosides (Remifemin® and Menofem®) does indeed reduce symptoms of menopause in a similar manner to low-doses of estrogen replacement. Most importantly, these effects occur without increasing the lining of the uterus or estrogen levels in the body. The recommended dose is 40 mg per day of a standardized extract or 4–8 ml of a 1:5 tincture. Black cohosh is not recommended for women who have a history of breast cancer.

**Dong Quai:** This herb has been shown to decrease symptoms of menopause. Boil 1 tsp of root or take 3 ml two times daily. Do not take this herb if you are also taking anti-coagulant medications.

**Liver and adrenal tonic:** Because adrenal and liver stress exacerbates the symptoms of menopause, combine equal parts of the following herbs to support adrenal function and repair and detoxify the liver: licorice, wild yam, Dong Quai, black cohosh, milk thistle, burdock, and bupleurum. Add cinnamon and spearmint to taste. Boil 1 tbsp of the bark per cup of water and drink three times daily.

# MENSTRUAL DISORDERS

## DIAGNOSIS

The average menstrual cycle is about 28 days and for most women menstruation takes place once a month. However, no two women are alike, and there can be great variation among cycles in different women. Menstrual disorders include absent periods, irregular and light periods, and heavy periods.

Amenorrhea (absent periods) can happen for a number of reasons. The most common include pregnancy, early menopause, extreme weight loss or gain, taking a contraceptive pill, recreational drug abuse, stress, hormonal imbalances, and polycystic ovary syndrome (PCOS). Oligomenorrhea, or irregular or light periods, occurs when your period begins every 35 days. Periods that are light and infrequent are a fairly common occurrence during the teenage years and the years leading up to menopause. For some women, irregular periods are the norm, and are not a cause for alarm. Oligomenorrhea can also be an occasional condition triggered by stress, changes in diet, travel, illness, or a strict exercise regime. Irregular periods are not a medical problem as such; however, they can be linked to more serious conditions, such as polycystic ovaries. Menorrhagia, or heavy periods, occur when more than the usual amount of blood is lost. They are also common in teenage girls and women approaching menopause. This condition can be caused by pelvic inflammatory disease, fibroids, and endometriosis. Occasionally, a particularly heavy period can actually be a miscarriage, in which case you may need to have a surgical procedure known as dilation and curettage (D&C).

## SYMPTOMS

- Irregular or absent periods
- Heavy or light periods
- Abdominal pain

## TREATMENT GOAL

Treatment of menstrual disorders depends on the type and cause of the condition.

## CONVENTIONAL MEDICINE

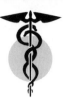 Treatment involves first ruling out serious causes of menstrual disorders. These include abnormalities of the uterus such as fibroids (see p. 734) and polyps, both of which would generally be treated surgically. Certain sexually transmitted diseases, such as chlamydia, can also cause abnormal bleeding, as can intra-uterine contraceptive devices. Some types of cancer, as well as disorders of the urinary system and rectum, can cause spotting, and these will need to be ruled out. A doctor will carry out a detailed history and a physical examination of the pateint to make sure the above conditions do not exist before determining a treatment plan.

**Diet:** Good nutrition is essential to regulating menstrual disorders. Eliminate processed foods and sugar from your diet as much as possible and instead eat plenty of fresh fruit and vegetables, flaxseed, and soy products. Also take adequate amount of vitamins and minerals, particularly the B vitamins. Stress reduction is also important in regulating menstrual disorders.

**Balancing hormones:** If menstrual disorders are linked to a hormone imbalance, current medical treatment involves progesterone, which is given either as a shot or as a daily oral dose for 15 days. Taking one oral contraceptive pill four times a day for five days, followed by a one tablet of a low dose of estrogen once a day for 21 days, usually relieves heavy bleeding. Following this, oral contraceptive pills are used to establish a normal menstrual cycle. For women with menstrual disorders who want to become pregnant, antiprostaglandins (which relieve discomfort and make flow lighter) and hormones like GnRH (which stimulates the secretion of sex steroids) and hMG can be used.

**To regulate bleeding:** Progesterone agents can be used for 12 days to induce bleeding, which occurs when the progesterone is discontinued. Depo Provera is an intramuscular shot that can be given every three months to regulate bleeding.

**To treat severe bleeding:** If the bleeding is life threatening, conjugated estrogen (Premarin®) is given intravenously every four hours in a maximum of three doses until the bleeding stops. For prolonged bleeding that is not life threatening, Premarin® is given orally in a dose of 1.25 mg daily for 24 days, and progesterone (Provera®) is added for the last 10 days. Alternatively, oral contraceptive pills can be taken to regulate a heavy period.

**To treat light bleeding:** Light periods can be regulated by taking an oral contraceptive pill. Taking progesterone (Provera®) may also be helpful.

**Surgery:** Various surgical treatments can be used to correct menstrual disorders. Dilation and curettage, which involves the scraping of the lining of the uterus, endometrial ablation, which destroys the layer of cells that lines the uterus, and a hysterectomy, where the uterus is removed, are among the surgical treatments that can be used to correct menstrual disorders.

## TRADITIONAL CHINESE MEDICINE

**Herbs:** The herbs listed in the formulas below are available from Chinese pharmacies or online. To prepare a formula, place the ingredients in a ceramic pot and add 3 cups of water. Bring the mixture to the boil and simmer for 30 minutes. Strain the liquid and drink 1 cup twice a day.

• To treat liver Qi and blood stagnation: If you have irregular menstruation, cramping, and your menstrual bleeding is dark, and you are experiencing symptoms of depression, and/or are under stress, you may have liver Qi and blood stagnation. Mix 12 g of Chai Hu (hare's ear root), 15 g of Bai Shao (white peony root), 15 g of Bai Zhu (white atractylodes rhizome), 15 g of Fuling (poria), 5 g of Bo He (field mint), 6 g of Gan Cao (licorice), 12 g of Xiang Fu (nut grass rhizome), 12 g of Chi Shao (red peony root), and 12 g of Dang Gui (Chinese angelica root).

• To treat kidney deficiency: Symptoms include fatigue, cold hands and feet, insomnia, headaches, and dizziness. Mix 15 g of Shen Di Huang (Chinese foxglove root), 10 g of Shan Zhu Yu (Asiatic cornelian cherry fruit), 15 g of Shan Yao (Chinese yam), 15 g of Fuling (poria), 12 g of Zi Xie (water plantain rhizome), 12 g of Dan Pi (cortex of peony root), 12 g of Niu Zhen Zi (privet fruit), and 12 g of Wu Wei Zi (schisandra fruit).

**Acupuncture:** Consult a practitioner and be prepared to answer questions about your menstrual history and general health. A practitioner will make a diagnosis and explain the cause of your menstrual disorder according Chinese medicine. You may then be advised to have least one course of treatment, which consists of 12 sessions over 6–12 weeks.

**Acupressure:** Press the Xue Hai, Feng Shi, Susanli, and San Yin Jiao acupressure points. The Xue Hai point is on the inside of the leg in the depression just above the knee. Locate the Feng Shi on the outside of the leg at the end of the fingers when the arm is hanging straight down at the side. The Susanli point is found on the lower leg, about 1 inch to the outside of and 3 inches below the kneecap. The San Yin Jiao point is located in the center of the inside of the leg, about 3 inches above the anklebone.

**Diet:** Eat food that promotes blood circulation such as black soybeans, sugar, chestnuts, peaches, and sweet basil. Eat a healthy, well-balanced diet that includes fresh vegetables and fruits, and whole grains, and drink plenty of water.

## NATUROPATHY

**Diet:** More than one study has reported less menstrual pain and a reduction of heavy bleeding when the amount of omega-3 fatty acids, which are found in oily fish such as salmon, sardines, and mackerel, and in walnuts and flaxseeds, is increased in the diet. Some research has shown that limiting salt may help minimize bloating. Foods high in thiamine have been found to be helpful in all sorts if menstrual ailments. Thiamine is found in almost all foods, but the best source is pork. Other good sources of thiaminee are dried fortified cereals, oatmeal, and sunflower seeds.

**Supplements:** Take 100 mg of vitamin B1 (thiamine) a day to help relieve menstrual cramps. Calcium seem to be deficient in patients with menstrual problems especially those with amenorrhea (absent periods). Take 750 mg a day of the citrate form of calcium and 500 mg of magnesium to help your body absorb it. You can also take 400 IU of vitamin E a day to help with menstrual problems. Do not take more than this as it may cause excess bleeding.

**Herbs:** Chaste tree is known to benefit female hormonal health and relieve PMS. Take 40 drops of a tincture or 180 mg in capsule form of a standardized extract.

## HOMEOPATHY

Menstrual disorders are often recurring, so treatment from a homeopathic practitioner tends to bring the best result. However, the remedies listed below can be helpful in establishing hormone balance, especially when combined with positive changes in lifestyle. Symptoms of this kind may respond positively to self-help measures, but if an improvement does not occur within a maximum of four monthly cycles, seek professional treatment.

**Pulsatilla:** If irregular, frequently late periods are accompanied by severe symptoms of premenstrual syndrome (PMS), use Pulsatilla. Breasts are tender and enlarged, and premenstrual headaches also tend to develop. There is also likely to be a persistent sense that a period is about to start, long before it actually does.

**Lachesis:** When this remedy is indicated, the menstrual flow is heavy, dark, and clotted, and severe symptoms of PMS build from the point of ovulation and slightly subside once a period begins. Palpitations, feeling faint, and hot flashes often accompany heavy periods. Mood swings, anxiety, disturbed sleep, and left-sided premenstrual headaches may also occur.

**Kali carb:** If heavy periods are accompanied by lower back pain and fluid retention, try Kali carb. Because the menstrual flow is heavy, there may also be symptoms of anemia, such as feeling chilly and tired, or appearing pale. The areas affected by pain feel cold to the touch, and sufferers are emotionally withdrawn as a result of feeling exhausted and drained.

**Ipecac:** If heavy menstrual bleeding is accompanied by severe, persistent nausea, use Ipecac. The flow itself is likely to alternate between being steady and being very heavy. The heavy flow can cause patients to feel dizzy and faint.

## HERBALISM

**Light-flow formula:** Dong Quai improves blood flow to the uterus and soothes symptoms of PMS such as cramping and bloating. However, do not use it during menstruation or with blood-thinning medications. Ginger also stimulates blood flow to the pelvic region. Licorice promotes hormonal balance through its support of the liver and adrenals. Mugwort is a bitter digestive, uterine, and liver tonic that brings the menstrual cycle back into balance, while stimulating the uterus. Black cohosh has phyto-estrogenic properties that stimulate uterine movement. Raspberry leaf is a wonderful, nourishing uterine and pelvic tonic that is high in vitamins and minerals. Combine equal parts of these dried herbs and drink an infusion made from 1 tsp per cup of water, or take 2 ml of a combined tincture, twice a day.

**Heavy-flow formula:** Black haw root and stem bark relieve uterine and intestinal spasm, thereby reducing painful menstruation and flow. Chaste tree berries, which are astringent and drying, normalize the menstrual cycle by regulating the secretion of hormones from the pituitary gland. Cramp bark calms uterine spasm and relieves cramping. Partridge berry, also known as squaw vine, improves uterine tone, decreases cramping, and reduces flow. Yarrow improves uterine tone and reduces excessive menstrual bleeding. Combine equal parts of these dried herbs and drink an infusion made from 1 tsp per cup of water, or take 2 ml of a combined tincture in water, twice a day.

**Infrequent-flow formula:** Chaste tree is considered to be a "progesteronic" herb and typically increases the ratio of progesterone over estrogen in the body by increasing luteinizing hormones released from the pituitary gland. This increase in progesterone typically normalizes menstruation. Nettle nourishes the body and is considered to be a woman's tonic. Lady's mantle is an astringent uterine tonic that helps to normalize irregular cycles. Wild yam is another progesteronic herb, which is useful for treating spotting, reducing uterine spasms, and supporting the liver. Dandelion supports the liver to conjugate and excrete excess estrogens from the body, thereby normalizing menstrual function. Combine equal parts of these dried herbs and drink an infusion made from 1 tsp per cup of water, or take 2 ml of a combined tincture, three times a day or during the last half (after ovulation) of the menstrual cycle. This combination of herbs will help to create a regular cycle when taken consistently over a period of four to six months.

**TIP:** GUARD AGAINST ANEMIA

Heavy, frequent periods can trigger problems with iron-deficiency anemia, and it may be helpful to have a blood test to determine whether you are at risk. Free-range, organic eggs, green leafy vegetables, oatmeal, molasses, nuts, seeds, fish, and whole meal cereals are all good sources of iron. Avoid drinking tea with meals, and instead have a glass of orange juice or a portion of vitamin-C-rich fruit with a meal to help your body absorb iron.

# PERIOD PAINS

## DIAGNOSIS

Many women experience uncomfortable cramping pains (known as dysmenorrhea) at the time of their period. It is a common problem and not generally a cause for concern. These pains are caused by contractions in the muscle of the uterus that result from the release of prostaglandins, which are hormones produced by the lining of the womb. For most women, the pain is not so severe that it interferes with their daily lives or requires any special attention. However, some women experience such severe pain that it affects their daily routine, or forces them to stay in bed for a couple of days. Lifestyle changes can help to improve symptoms. Try to eat a healthy, balanced diet, take daily exercise, get plenty of sleep, and avoid stressful situations. If period pains are more than an inconvenience, it is wise to consult your doctor, who may wish to perform a pelvic examination to rule out any underlying conditions, such as pelvic inflammatory disease, endometriosis, or fibroids (see p. 734).

## SYMPTOMS

- Cramping sensations in the abdomen
- Pain in the lower back
- Dragging pains
- Heavier blood loss than usual
- Headaches
- Dizziness and fainting

## TREATMENT GOAL

Conventional and complementary therapies focus on isolating the cause of the pain to rule out a serious underlying condition. Treatment involves relieving symptoms of pain and discomfort to prevent period pain from interfering with daily routines.

## CONVENTIONAL MEDICINE

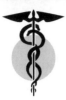

A thorough medical history is taken and a physical examination performed to make sure there a serious disease is not causing the pain. An ultrasound is also usually carried out to check for fibroids or cysts. Once it has been established that there is not a serious problem, therapies can be initiated.

**Compresses:** Applying warm compresses to the abdomen can be helpful in relieving pain. Add castor oil to a warm washcloth and place it over the painful area.

**Diet:** A dairy-free diet has reportedly helped relieve menstrual cramping.

**Medication:** Taking non-steroidal anti-inflammatory drugs (NSAIDs) such as ibuprofen (Motrin®) or naproxyn (Naproxyn® and Alleve®) two days before a period begins until the second day of bleeding can help to ease pain. Taking oral contraceptive pills may also help.

**TENS machine:** Transcutaneous electrical nerve stimulation (TENS) has been shown to have some effect. A TENS machine gives out tiny pulses of electrical energy which prevent pain signals from reaching your brain.

**Surgery:** If all else fails, a procedure called laparoscopic presacral neurectomy, which involves interrupting nerve tissue that goes to and from the uterus, may be effective.

## TRADITIONAL CHINESE MEDICINE

**Herbs:** The herbs listed below are available from Chinese pharmacies or online. To prepare a formula, place the herbs in a ceramic pot with 3 cups of water. Bring the mixture to a boil, simmer for 30 minutes, and strain. Drink 1 cup twice a day.
• To treat period pains associated with strong mood swings: Mix 12 g of Dang Gui (Chinese angelica root), 12 g of Chuan Xiong (Szechuan lovage root), 12 g of Chi Shao (red peony root), 10 g of Zhi Ke (bitter orange), 12 g of Yan Hu Suo (corydalis rhizome), 12 g of Xiang Fu (nut grass rhizome), 12 g of Dan Pi (cortex of tree peony root), and 3 g of Gan Cao (licorice).
• To treat sharp pains in your lower abdomen and cold hands and feet: Symptoms also include feeling chilly and looking pale. Mix 10 g of Wu Zhu Yu (evodia fruit), 12 g of Dang Gui (Chinese angelica root), 12 g of Chuang Xiong (Szechuan lovage root), 10 g of ginseng, 10 g of Gui Zhi (cinnamon), 8 g of Xiao Hui Xiang (fennel fruit), 10 g of Ai Ye (moxa), and 3 g of Gan Cao (licorice).

**Acupuncture:** Consult a doctor of traditional Chinese medicine regarding treatment. It is helpful to begin sessions before your period starts. You can have acupuncture treatment for both acute and chronic conditions. In chronic conditions, treatment regulates your circulation or rebuilds your internal balance by tonifying some of the deficient organs or reorganizing the disordered energy. Patients may need to undergo treatment for a few months depending on the severity of the condition.

**Moxibustion:** Moxibustion is a method of burning Moxa, a slow-burning herb, on the skin or on acupuncture needles. It should be performed by an experienced practitioner. In this case, the practitioner will place and ignite a small Moxa cone on various locations. When the cone burns to near the bottom it will be removed and extinguished. The whole procedure uses three to six cones. The local skin will feel warm and look reddish.

**Acupressure:** Press the Xue Hai, Feng Shi, Susanli, and San Yin Jiao acupressure points. The Xue Hai point is on the inside of the leg in the depression just above the knee. Locate the Feng Shi point along the outside of the leg at the end of the fingers when the arm is hanging straight down at the side. The Susanli point is found on the lower leg, about 1 inch to the outside of and 3 inches below the kneecap. The San Yin Jiao point is located in the center of the inside of the leg, about 3 inches above the anklebone.

**Diet:** Drink a sufficient amount of water every day. Eat fresh fruits and vegetables, and food that promotes blood circulation such as black soybeans, brown sugar, chestnuts, peaches, and sweet basil. Eat less fatty and greasy food since they create stagnation that will worsen the pain.

## NATUROPATHY

**Diet:** Constipation is often linked to menstrual pain. Eat a high-fiber diet to guard against this. Vegetables, fruits, whole grains, nuts, seeds, and beans all contain high levels of fiber. Ground flaxseeds, also high in fiber, can be sprinkled on salads and cereals. If you eat meat, stick to organic, hormone-free beef and chicken to avoid hormonal imbalances in your body. Diets low in inflammatory foods are essential for the relief of pain with periods. These foods include hydrogenated fats, sugar, processed carbohydrates, wheat, and dairy products. Also eat oily fish such as salmon, sardines, and mackerel, and flaxseed to obtain omega-3 fatty acids, which can help reduce inflammation. Drink at least eight glasses of water a day, and cut down on the amount of alcohol and caffeine you consume to protect against dehydration, which contributes to period pain.

**Supplements:** Take 50 mg of vitamin B6 a day, as it has been shown to help with pre-menstrual syndrome (PMS) and painful periods. Magnesium is required for the metabolism of estrogen, and also works synergistically with vitamin B6 to reduce pain; take 250 mg a day. Muscles that are calcium-deficient tend to be hyperactive and therefore might be more likely to cramp, so take 1,000 mg of the citrate form of calcium a day. Niacin has been shown to be helpful in treating menstrual cramps as it dilates the blood vessels to improve blood flow to the contracting uterus. Take 100 mg every three hours during episodes of menstrual cramping, and 100 mg a day for prevention, but make sure you use the non-flushing type of niacin. Vitamin C appears to work synergistically with niacin in people suffering from painful periods. Take 3,000 mg a day with 1,500 mg of bioflavonoids, which help the body to absorb vitamin C and also have other general health benefits. Take 400 IU a day of a natural vitamin E with a blend of mixed tocopherols to relieve menstrual pain and breast tenderness. Evening primrose can counter the inflammatory hormones causing pain. Take 2,000–3,000 mg of evening primrose oil with 200–300 mg of gamma-linolenic acid (GLA) a day.

**Herbs:** Black cohosh has a history as a folk medicine for relieving menstrual cramps. Take 250 mg three times a day of a dry powdered extract. Tinctures can also be taken at 2–4 ml three times per day. Blue cohosh has also been used traditionally for easing painful menstrual periods. Blue cohosh, which is generally taken as a tincture, should be limited to no more than 1–2 ml taken three times per day. False unicorn was used in the Native American tradition for a large number of women's health conditions, including painful menstruation. Generally, false unicorn root is taken as a tincture at 2–5 ml three times per day. It is typically taken in combination with other herbs that support the female reproductive organs.

## HOMEOPATHY

If you experience severe period pains, consult a homeopathic practitioner regarding treatment that can reduce the pain each month, as well as help with other symptoms. These may include tender breasts, bloating, fatigue, food cravings, and mood swings. The acute homeopathic remedies listed below can help as a stop-gap measure and as complementary support in providing pain relief.

**Belladonna:** If violent, abrupt pain that feels similar to labor contractions is accompanied by a bright red flow and some clotting, use Belladonna. Sufferers also tend to be irritable and short-tempered.

**Arsenicum album:** Use this remedy if exhausting period pains are associated with a profound sense of chilliness, restlessness, nausea, diarrhea, and possibly vomiting. There may also be severe anxiety and a fear of feeling ill. Applying a hot water bottle to the abdomen feels soothing and provides temporary relief.

**Colocynthis:** If waves of cramps come on and then subside rapidly, consider using Colocynthis. The pain may leave you feeling weak and cause you to instinctively double over to try and get comfortable. Firm pressure provides some relief, but it is usually difficult to find a comfortable position.

**Cimicifuga:** When this remedy is helpful, period pains become proportionally more severe and distressing as the flow increases. Symptoms include flitting, shock-like pains that often radiate from the belly down to the thighs. Walking around, moving your bowels, and warmth provide some temporary relief.

**Lachesis:** To ease period pains that are most severe immediately preceding the onset of a period, use Lachesis. The flow tends to be dark in color, and large clots are usually present. Cramping pains build in intensity from around mid-cycle until the onset of a steady flow. Other symptoms include premenstrual left-sided headaches, migraines, disturbed sleep, night sweats, hot flashes, palpitations, and anxiety.

## HERBALISM

Painful menstruation is typically caused by excessive uterine tone and spasm. Elevated pro-inflammatory chemicals (prostaglandins and leukotrienes) are commonly found in uterine tissue of women with this condition. Many herbal medicines can reduce uterine tone and spasm quite effectively.

**Cramp bark:** This is a wonderful uterine and intestinal antispasmodic. Clinical studies have shown that two active constituents, scopoletin and viopudial, have a strong antispasmodic effect on uterine tissue. Cramp bark also has anti-inflammatory properties, can calm the nerves, and may help to lower blood pressure. To treat moderate to severe cramps, take 30 drops of tincture every 15 minutes, or 1 tsp per hour.

**Lady's mantle:** This herb is high in tannins, which account for its astringent effect on the uterus, and is ideal for treating heavy menstrual bleeding. Flavonoids within this herb also provide anti-inflammatory and nutritive properties to the uterus. Drink an infusion made from 2 tsp of dried herb in 1 cup of water, or take 30 drops of tincture, three times daily.

**Motherwort:** This herb relieves painful uterine cramping, as well as heart palpitations and high blood pressure brought on by stress. Take 1 tbsp of the above-ground parts, or 2 ml of a tincture three times daily. The best results are seen when this herb is taken in the long term.

# POLYCYSTIC OVARY SYNDROME

## DIAGNOSIS

Polycystic ovary syndrome (PCOS) is a condition where multiple cysts develop from follicles on the ovaries. These follicles, which emerge around the egg, result from the influences of stimulating hormones from the brain. They are small and immature, and generally do not exceed ¼–½ inch in size and rarely grow to maturity. Problems begin when the eggs fail to be released.

PCOS is a common hormonal disorder among women. As some sufferers rarely ovulate, they can have a problem conceiving. One of the main symptoms is irregular periods or going for weeks without a period. There seems to be a tendency for PCOS to run in families. It is also more likely to develop if there is a family history of diabetes (especially Type 2), or if there is early baldness in the men in the family. Women are also more at risk if they are overweight. Symptoms vary greatly from one woman to another, and treatment is customized for the individual case. If fertility is an issue, there are some very successful treatments available that your doctor will be able to tell you more about.

## SYMPTOMS

- Absent, infrequent, or heavy periods
- Hirsutism (increased hair on the face and body, see p. 744)
- Infertility linked with infrequent ovulation
- Obesity
- Acne
- Deepening voice
- Recurrent miscarriage

## TREATMENT GOAL

To establish whether or not you have PCOS, blood tests to check hormone levels, glucose and thyroid function tests, and ultrasound examination can be carried out. If any of the symptoms are an issue, then further advice and treatment, and possibly specialist referral, is needed. Of particular relevance is fertility treatment, via the stimulation of ovulation, reduction of insulin resistance, and dealing with the removal of excess body hair.

## CONVENTIONAL MEDICINE

Treatment of polycystic ovary syndrome is weight loss, if obese. Often Type 2 diabetes is concomitant with PCOS and it too should be treated if the condition is present.

**Diet and exercise:** Eat a high-fiber, low-dairy diet. It is also important to do 20 minutes of aerobic exercise daily.

**Hormone suppression:** Oral contraceptives can be used to decrease the androgens (male hormones) that are usually elevated in those with PCOS. Spironolactone is an androgen receptor antagonist that can be added to the oral contraceptive pill. Steroids (glucocorticoids) can also be used to suppress male hormones. Flutamide is another such drug, which can be used in the same manner.

**To increase fertility:** Metformin, an oral anti-diabetic agent, can be used to promote fertility. Clomifene also be used. A surgical procedure called an ovarian wedge resection, which involves removing part of the ovarian tissue so that less hormones are produced, is an option if all other means have failed and fertility is desired.

## TRADITIONAL CHINESE MEDICINE

**Herbs:** According to traditional Chinese medicine, polycystic ovary syndrome is caused by blood stagnation. The following herbs, available from Chinese pharmacies or online, can help to remove blood stagnation to treat this condition. Mix 12 g of Chi Shao (red peony root), 12 g of Huai Niu Xi (achyranthes root), 12 g of Dan Shen (salvia root), and 15 g of Ji Xue Teng (millettia root) in a ceramic pot and add 3 cups of water. Bring the mixture to a boil, simmer for 30 minutes, and strain. Drink 1 cup two to three times a day. Do not use this formula if you have heart disease or a blood disorder.

**Acupuncture:** Treatment can promote circulation in the body. Usually, long-term, regular treatments are recommended to achieve the best results. Consult a doctor of Chinese medicine about your individual condition.

**Acupressure:** Press the Xue Hai, Susanli, and San Yin Jiao acupressure points. The Xue Hai point is on the inside of the leg in the depression just above the knee. The Susanli point is found on the lower leg, about 1 inch to the outside of and 3 inches below the kneecap. The San Yin Jiao point is located in the center of the inside of the leg, about 3 inches above the anklebone.

**Diet:** Eat food that promotes blood circulation such as black soybeans, brown sugar, chestnuts, peaches, and sweet basil. Eat a well-balanced diet that includes plenty of fresh fruit and vegetables and whole grains, and drink plenty of water.

## NATUROPATHY

Polycyctic ovary syndrome is characterized by increased levels of androgens, such as testosterone, and insulin resistance. The recommendations below can help to correct the hormone and insulin levels in the body.

**Diet:** A correct diet is probably the most important naturopathic treatment for PCOS. Follow a low-carbohydrate diet to reduce insulin levels, improve insulin resistance, and help you lose weight if needed. Starches in your diet should be mostly from whole grains, such as brown rice as opposed to white rice. Increase your consumption of omega-3 fatty acids, found in cod liver oil and oily fish such as salmon, sardines, and mackerel. Eliminate products that contain trans-fatty acids from your diet, including margarine and deep fried foods. Trans-fatty acids are unsaturated liquid oils that have been chemically transformed into saturated fats so that they will be solids instead of liquids. They cause a fatty, sluggish liver, making it more difficult to metabolize hormones that may be causing PCOS. If you eat red meat, opt for beef that is grass fed and organic, as it contains less saturated fat. You can also eat other lean meats such as chicken and turkey. Saturated fat interferes with the metabolism of some hormones that cause PCOS. Also limit the amount and type of simple carbohydrates you eat. A diet high in refined carbohydrates will lead to an excessive insulin response, which in turn can stimulate androgen (a primarily male hormone) production, which contributes to PCOS. The best carbohydrates to consume are whole grains, nuts, seeds, vegetables, and fruit.

**Supplements:** Chromium encourages your liver to produce a substance called glucose tolerance factor (GTF), which increases the effectiveness of insulin. Take 200–400 mg of chromium picolinate a day. Vitamin B3 (niacin) is also a component of glucose tolerance factor. Vitamin B5 (pantothenic acid) helps to control fat metabolism and improves the response to stress. Vitamin B6 balances hormone levels. Take 50 mg of a B-complex vitamin that contains all of the above B vitamins three times a day. Inositol increases the effectiveness of insulin in women with PCOS, reduces male hormone levels, and restores normal periods. Although inositol can be found in a B-complex vitamin, a total of 500 mg should be taken twice a day.

**Herbs:** Chaste tree seems to have anti-androgenic properties that inhibit PCOS. Take 1–4 ml of a 1:2 dried plant tincture or 500–1,000 mg of dried berries daily.

## HOMEOPATHY

PCOS is a complex chronic problem that can give rise to multiple, severe symptoms. It is best treated by a practitioner, but the following lifestyle changes may help to reduce symptoms.

**Lose weight:** Being significantly overweight appears to aggravate symptoms of PCOS, partly by stimulating the secretion of androgens. The latter are male hormones that can lead to common and distressing symptoms of PCOS, such as facial hair. For advice on how to healthily lose unwanted pounds see Obesity (p. 459).

**Diet:** PCOS can increase the risk of developing Type 2 diabetes, so make an effort to keep blood sugar levels as stable as possible. Avoid eating foods that are high in refined carbohydrates such as white bread, white rice, and any foods that are a source of white sugar. Instead, opt for foods that release energy slowly and that are high in fiber, such as organic brown rice cakes with a protein topping, fresh, raw vegetable crudites, and a small amount of fresh fruit.

## HERBALISM

As well as taking herbal medicines for PCOS, begin a weight-loss program if necessary, eat a whole-food diet, and replace vitamins and minerals commonly deficient in those with PCOS, such as vitamin B6 and magnesium.

**Hormone-balancing formula:** Elevated testosterone, DHEA, and estrogens, combined with deficient levels of progesterone, result in polycystic ovaries, hirsutism (male-pattern hair growth), and irregular or absent menstruation. To elevate progesterone levels, which normalizes the menstrual cycle and stimulates shedding of the uterine lining (menstruation), combine the following dried herbs in equal amounts: chaste tree berry, Siberian ginseng root, squaw vine leaves, cramp bark, ladies' mantle leaf and flowers, and wild yam root. Drink an infusion made from 1 tbsp per cup of water, steeped for 10 minutes, or take 3 ml of a combined tincture in water, three times daily.

**Saw palmetto:** Due to the elevated levels of testosterone associated with PCOS, saw palmetto is indicated for women who have this condition. Saw palmetto prevents the conversion of testosterone to DHT (dihydrotestosterone), a more potent form of testosterone, and prevents the binding of DHT to testosterone receptor sites. The overall result is a decrease in symptoms of hyperandrogenism, which includes male-pattern hair distribution, acne, balding, and a deepening voice. Take 160 mg of this herb twice daily.

# PREGNANCY

## DIAGNOSIS

Pregnant women commonly suffer from a range of symptoms that cause discomfort and pain. Some women are lucky and experience few or no symptoms, while others suffer from everything from morning sickness to edema.

Lower back pain is common during pregnancy, as women tend to lean backwards to compensate for the weight of the growing fetus, putting strain on the back muscles. Constipation can develop when the hormone progesterone, produced during pregnancy, slows the intestinal muscles in the digestive tract so that food is not processed as quickly as usual. Progesterone can also lead to heartburn as it relaxes the muscle at the base of the esophagus, allowing food and digestive enzymes to wash into the gullet, causing a burning sensation. Pregnant women may also feel uncomfortably full as the fetus grows larger and puts pressure on the intestinal tract. Nearly half of all pregnant women are affected by hemorrhoids, which can develop when the fetus presses down on the veins in the rectum. Another common complaint is morning sickness, which can in fact occur at any time during the day. It frequently affects women during the first 12 weeks of being pregnant, but some women experience symptoms for a longer period. Pregnant women may also experience edema (water retention), leading to swollen ankles and fingers, as the volume of fluid in the body increases during pregnancy.

If any of the above symptoms are severe, consult your doctor for advice on how best to treat them.

## SYMPTOMS

- Missed period
- Nausea (morning sickness)
- Tender breasts
- Frequent urination

## TREATMENT GOAL

Many of the complaints of pregnancy can be relieved through conventional and complementary measures. Treatment involves making mothers more comfortable, while ensuring the health of the fetus.

## CONVENTIONAL MEDICINE

Conventional medical care during pregnancy involves the early identification of risk factors, and educating and counseling women on necessary diet and lifestyle modifications. Fetal growth is also measured regularly, and the reproductive system is assessed to identify any abnormalities. The following histories are taken: medical history, focusing on any existing illnesses; obstetric history, identifying risk factors in any previous pregnancies; and family and genetic history. Toxin exposure is also evaluated. A physical examination may be performed, including height and weight checks and a Pap smear and pelvic examination if it is due. Screening for sexually transmitted diseases is also carried out. Other infectious diseases are evaluated through blood testing, including Hepatitis B, rubella, and HIV. Blood testing is done to check for blood type and Rh factor, antibodies, and a complete blood count (CBC). Urinalysis and culture is also done at the initial prenatal visit and urine is checked at each visit for protein and glucose levels.

**Modify your lifestyle:** The most critical period of fetal development is day 17 to 56 after conception, which is usually before the first prenatal visit. Preconception care involves eating a diet that includes five portions of fruit and vegetables a day, and that is rich in protein, complex carbohydrates, and monounsaturated fats. Folic acid supplementation of 1 mg a day is recommended preior to conception and throughout pregnancy to reduce risk of neural tube defects in the infant. About 60–100 oz of water should be consumed daily. Approximately 19–21 lb should be gained throughout a pregnancy. Consuming around 2,200 calories a day will usually achieve this, depending on an individual's metabolism and energy level. Pregnant women should take a folic acid supplement and a multivitamin. Vitamin A levels should not be excessive but it is necessary to take 100% of the recommended daily allowance. Pregnant women should stop drinking alcohol, taking drugs, and smoking.

**How often should I see a doctor?** Consult a doctor as soon as pregnancy is suspected. You will need to see a doctor for an ultrasound examination, which can be done in the first trimester. Genetic testing is also carried out, and an amniocentesis, which involves testing the amniotic fluid from the womb, can be performed to check for any abnormalities if necessary. It is generally indicated if a pregnant woman is older than 35. It is common to see a doctor once during weeks six to eight of a pregnancy, once during weeks 10–12, and once during weeks 16–20. A visit is also necessary during weeks 24, 28, 32, and 36, and then weekly visits should continue from week 38 through to week 41. Each visit involves taking your weight and blood pressure, monitoring the fetal heartbeat, and measuring fundal height (a measurement of the womb). Urine screening is also done to check for bacteria, and protein and glucose levels.

## TRADITIONAL CHINESE MEDICINE

**Herbs:** Whether or not herbal remedies are appropriate depends on your specific condition. Consult a practitioner of Chinese medicine for advice.

**Acupuncture:** Treatment can help to relieve morning sickness, and help prevent a miscarriage. Consult a TCM practitioner that has a lot of experience in dealing with pregnancy issues before beginning a course of acupuncture.

**Diet:** A well-balanced, healthy diet is important. Drink plenty of water daily and eat fresh vegetables and fruits. Bitter melon, watermelon, mung beans, radishes, and celery are beneficial foods. Also, eat food that nourishes the blood such as black sesame seeds, red beans, black beans, spinach, fish, and carrots. In addition, you should consider foods that are cooling, such as green vegetables, tofu, and Chinese jujube dates. Avoid food that has heat and warmth properties, such as hot chili peppers, beef, garlic, and lamb. Also avoid deep-fried food, and eat less fatty and greasy foods since they create more heat.

## NATUROPATHY

**Diet:** Pregnant women should consume 2,200 calories a day, obtained from lean meats such as chicken and fish, vegetable proteins such as beans and tofu, and whole grains, fruits, and vegetables. Eating an adequate amount of protein (about four servings or 74 g a day) is crucial to keeping you healthy and helping the proper development of the fetus. Eat four servings of calcium from green vegetables, almonds, and sea vegetables, as calcium is essential for bone health and the general health of the fetus. It is okay to eat chocolate or salty snacks, which are often craved during pregnancy, as long as they do not become a staple part of your diet. Drink water regularly throughout the day to stay hydrated and provide fluids for the amniotic sac and other tissues that are important for proper fetal development.

**Supplements:** Take a prenatal vitamin, following the dosage instructions on the bottle along with the suggestions of your doctor. Take 800 mcg of folic acid a day and 17 mg of niacin a day, particularly during the first trimester. Vitamin A consumption should not exceed 10,000 IU or it may cause birth defects. However, it is essential to take some vitamin A to prevent lung defects in the fetus and to avoid pre-eclampsia, a condition that involves swelling, sudden weight gain, headaches, and changes in vision, in the mother. Vitamin C plays a major role in the formation of collagen, a major protein found in the connective tissue, cartilage, and bone. It also helps with nerve health, healthy gums, and teeth. Take 75–250 mg a day.

**Herbs:** If there is any doubt than a herb should be taken during pregnancy, do not take it. The following herbs, however, are safe. Raspberry leaf is considered to be the most widely used, safest pregnancy tonic. It contains an alkaloid called fragrine, which helps tone the uterus and pelvic floor muscles. This herb also contains vitamins C and E as well as iron and calcium. Regular use during pregnancy is said to help prevent miscarriage, ease morning sickness, facilitate an easier labor, and assist in the production of plentiful breast milk. Make a light decoction by simmering a small handful of the dried or fresh herb in 2 cups of water for a few minutes and steeping the herb for 15 minutes. Drink 1 cup daily. Nettle is a nutritional powerhouse, containing every vitamin and mineral needed for human growth. Regular use of a nettle infusion during pregnancy ensures a plentiful supply of nutrients, helps reduce hemorrhoids, helps prevent postpartum hemorrhage, eases leg cramps and muscle spasms, and nourishes the kidneys. Nettle is also a wonderful herb for lactation as it promotes a rich supply of breast milk. Many women use nettle to nourish themselves after pregnancy. Its high mineral content has been used traditionally to support women postpartum by nourishing the nervous system and stabilizing hormone levels. Make a decoction by simmering 1 tbsp of herb or rhizome for every cup of water for 20–30 minutes. Drink 1–2 cups two or three times a day. Follow instructions on the packets for other products.

## HOMEOPATHY

Homeopathic treatment can help to ease common problems such as morning sickness, constipation, hemorrhoids, varicose veins, or heartburn. Since the conventional medicines on offer are strictly limited because of concern over potential side effects, homeopathic treatment is a particularly attractive option as remedies are highly diluted. To treat severe cases of the conditions mentioned above, seek advice from an experienced homeopathic practitioner, who will also be able to recommend remedies to support recovery following the birth. The remedies given below are some of the most commonly indicated homeopathic remedies, but should not be self-prescribed during pregnancy.

**Nux vomica:** This is one of the primary remedies for treating a system that feels generally "toxic" as a result of constipation. The urge to move your bowels is followed by the sense that the bowel has not been completely emptied. You may feel that nausea would be relieved after vomiting, but it may be difficult to do so. All symptoms are aggravated by high levels of stress and tension.

**Pulsatilla:** If you feel faint very easily, are extremely queasy and sensitive to rich, fatty foods, and have persistent heartburn, try Pulsatilla. Overheated, stuffy surroundings make symptoms worse, while taking a gentle stroll in the fresh air helps. Varicose veins are also likely to be troublesome, often aching in the evening and when trying to rest at night.

**Sepia:** This remedy can be immensely helpful if pregnancies have occurred in quick succession, leaving the mother feeling drained, exhausted, and unable to cope. Symptoms include a profound sense of mental, emotional, and physical fatigue, leading to moods swings between irritability and indifference. Morning sickness may be especially severe, and there is a high sensitivity to odors.

## HERBALISM

**Nausea remedies:** Clinical studies show that ginger is effective in relieving nausea during pregnancy. Take 250 mg or drink an infusion made from 1 tbsp of dried root per cup of water up to four times daily, but do not exceed more than 1 g daily. Peppermint and spearmint soothe the stomach and relieve gas. Infuse 1 tsp of leaves per cup of water and drink as needed.

**Varicose vein remedies:** Varicosities are a result of increased pressure within the veins. To relieve this pressure, elevate and massage the legs, get plenty of exercise and change sitting positions frequently. Onions, which are high in vitamin C and quercitin (a powerful antioxidant), and garlic, which is rich in antioxidants, are anti-inflammatory and support vascular tissue health. Dark leafy greens such as spinach and spring greens and beets are rich in B vitamins and promote liver health and regular bowel movements, lessening venous congestion. Also apply witch hazel topically, which is astringent and cooling, to varicose veins to reduce swelling and pain.

**Heartburn remedies:** Powdered slippery elm bark coats the stomach, neutralizes acid in the stomach, and relieves gas. Mix a little honey with 1 tsp of powder in 1 cup of water and drink.

**Mother's cordial:** This formula, used by herbalists for centuries, is made specifically for the last two weeks of pregnancy to prepare the uterus for an easier delivery. It should not be taken at any other time during pregnancy. These herbs strengthen the uterus, relieve unproductive spasms, and soothe nervous agitation. Mix a dried herb formula made from 40% squaw vine, 30% cramp bark, 20% blue cohosh, and 10% false unicorn. Drink an infusion made from 1 tsp of this formula per cup of water, three times daily.

# PREMENSTRUAL SYNDROME

## DIAGNOSIS

Premenstrual syndrome (PMS) affects around 50% of menstruating women. It involves various physical and/or psychological changes in the body that precede a period, starting from ovulation (two weeks before a period starts) and stopping within a day of the onset of bleeding. Common symptoms include mood swings, depression, cravings, cramping, and water retention. The symptoms are mild for the majority of women, but a small proportion (around 5–10%) experience symptoms that are so severe that they disrupt everyday life. Some women suffer from one or two symptoms, while others experience all of them.

The cause of PMS is uncertain. Symptoms such as bloating, tender breasts, and headaches are thought to be linked to the fluctuating levels of female hormones that occur just before menstruation. Lower-than-normal levels of serotonin, a chemical in the brain, may explain some of the non-physical symptoms such as irritability, depression, and mood swings. A diagnosis is based upon the type of symptoms and when they occur in a cycle. Symptoms tend to be noticeably worse in the week leading up to a period, and usually disappear as soon as a period starts.

## SYMPTOMS

- Fatigue
- Mood swings and/or irritability
- Loss of confidence and weepiness
- Poor memory and difficulty concentrating
- Cravings for sweet/salty foods
- Tender breasts
- Bloating
- Weight gain
- Headaches, sometimes severe

## TREATMENT GOAL

Treatment depends upon the nature of the symptoms and their severity. Conventional and complementary therapies focus on relieving acute symptoms and developing long-term strategies for dealing with symptoms, such as making lifestyle changes.

## CONVENTIONAL MEDICINE

The choice of therapy when treating PMS is largely determined through trial and error, beginning with the simple therapies and moving on if one fails. Most commonly, B-vitamins, evening primrose oil, and oral contraceptives are used to suppress the menstrual cycle.

**Lifestyle modifications:** Losing weight and stopping smoking, when applicable, are primary lifestyle modifications that can alleviate PMS. Other strategies include daily exercise and limiting your caffeine and alcohol intake. Diets that are high in lignans (found in flaxseed and soy), fiber, and whole grains, low in fat, and free from processed foods and dairy products seem to alleviate symptoms.

**Supplements:** Supplements that have shown promise in helping PMS are magnesium aspartate dosed at 400 mg daily, calcium hydroxyapetite at 1,500 mg daily, and vitamin B6 at 50 mg daily. Chaste tree (which should not be used if you are trying to become pregnant), rhodolia root, licorice, ground flaxseed, and St. John's wort can also help to relieve symptoms.

**Medication:** Generally oral contraceptives and antidepressants (selective serotonin reuptake inhibitors, SSRIs) are prescribed. Progesterone and/or estrogen can also alleviate symptoms when administered transdermally (through the skin). Other medications, such as non-steroidal anti-inflammatory drugs for pain relief, bromocriptine for breast tenderness, and beta blockers and anxiolytics for anxiety, are used as needed for severe symptoms.

## TRADITIONAL CHINESE MEDICINE

**Herbs:** The herbs listed in the formulas below are available from Chinese pharmacies or online. To prepare a formula, place the raw herbs in a ceramic pot and add 3 cups of water. Bring the mixture to a boil, simmer for 30 minutes, and strain. Drink 1 cup twice a day.

• To treat Qi stagnation: Symptoms include irritability, mood swings, and tender breasts. Mix 10 g of Chai Hu (hare's ear root), 15 g of Bai Shao (white peony), 12 g of Dan Gui (Chinese angelica), 12 g of Chuan Xiong (Szechuan lovage root), 15 g of Fuling (poria), 15 g of Bai Zhu (atractylodes rhizome), 6 g of Bo He (field mint), and 12 g of Xiang Fu (aromatic madder).

• To treat Qi stagnation and spleen deficiency: Symptoms include those above plus stomach bloating, diarrhea, and swelling. Add 5 g of Chen Pi (tangerine peel), 15 g of Shan Yao (Chinese yam), 25 g of Yi Yi Ren (seeds of Job's tears), and 10 g of Mu Xiang (costus root) to the ingredients above. Take this formula for one to three months, and consult a doctor of Chinese medicine if your condition does not improve.

• To treat blood stagnation: Symptoms include headaches, disturbed sleep, cramps, and dark bleeding. Combine 12 g of Chuan Xiong (Szechuan lovage root), 12 g of Chi Shao (red peony root), 15 g of Dan Gui (Chinese angelica root), 12 g of Yuan Hu (corydalis rhizome), 15 g of Niu Xi (achyranthes root), and 12 g of Dan Pi (cortex of tree peony root).

**Acupuncture:** Consult a practitioner regarding treatment. In some cases, you may only need acupuncture a week before your period, but it is most common to have treatment once a week for a few months or longer. Acupuncture can relieve symptoms, even after you have stopped regular treatments.

**Acupressure:** Pressing the Di Ji and Shan Yin Jiao acupressure points may help reduce some PMS symptoms. The Shan Yin Jiao point is on the inside of the leg, about 3 inches above the center of the anklebone. The Di Ji point is on the inside of the lower leg in the depression about 3 inches below the knee. Apply pressure to these points with the tip of the finger for one to two minutes, and repeat twice a day.

**Diet:** Eat foods that are light and neutral, including apricots, beef, beetroot, black sesame seeds, Chinese cabbage, castor beans, celery, duck, grapes, honey, beef, liver, oysters, pineapple, and soybeans.

## NATUROPATHY

**Diet:** Reduce your intake of sugar, red meat, and salt. These foods cause hormones to fluctuate and will augment common PMS symptoms including bloating and swelling of the hands and feet, tender breasts, and dizziness. When you do eat red meat, make sure it is organic, grass-fed beef as this will not interfere with estrogen levels in the body. Keep insulin and blood sugar levels balanced by eating frequent small meals throughout the day. Imbalanced insulin levels aggravate PMS and promote mood swings and tension. Restrict or eliminate caffeine, which can aggravate anxiety, depression, and tender breasts. The most common sources of caffeine are coffee, chocolate, soft drinks, and some pain-relieving pills. Increase your intake of fruits, vegetables, beans, nuts, and seeds. They contain fiber and nutrients that may help balance blood sugar, regulate bowel movements, and provide nourishment. Avoid alcohol, especially during the first two weeks before your period. Its dehydrating effects worsen PMS symptoms and blood sugar levels.

**Supplements:** Take 50 mg of vitamin B6 a day to assists in the production of progesterone to counterbalance estrogen. Take 250 mg of magnesium twice a day; it benefits women with cramps, mood swings, depression, fatigue, breast tenderness, and water retention, and is involved in prostaglandin metabolism and vitamin B6 activity. Evening primrose oil contains gamma-linolenic acid (GLA), which is involved in the metabolism of hormone-like substances called prostaglandins that regulate pain and inflammation in the body. Take 2,000–3,000 mg of an oil that includes omega-3 fatty acids such as flax oil or fish oil. Calcium may be beneficial for women with premenstrual cramps and moodiness. Take 500 mg of calcium citrate, the most easily absorbed form of the supplement, twice a day. Also take 15 mg of zinc a day as part of a multivitamin, as it has been shown to be low in women with PMS. Take 400 IU of vitamin E mixed tocopherol, which may reduce breast tenderness and relieve PMS. D-glucarate assists in the metabolizing of estrogen and can be taken at 500 mg twice a day, while indole 3 carbinol helps in the breakdown of estrogen in the liver and can be taken at 300 mg a day.

**Herbs:** One of the main causes of PMS is estrogen dominance—which occurs when estrogen levels are too high. One way of treating PMS is to decrease estrogen levels by increasing progesterone. Licorice is believed to lower estrogen levels while simultaneously raising progesterone levels. Take 500–1,000 mg of the freeze dried form a day, or 1–2 tsp of a tincture a day. Chaste tree berries are highly regarded for all menstrual problems, especially those associated with premenstrual syndrome. Do not take it if you are on birth control medication, as it can potentially decrease the effects, otherwise take 240 mg of a capsule standardized to 0.6% aucubine, or 1 tsp twice a day of the tincture. Passionflower relaxes the nervous system and improves some PMS symptoms. Take 300 mg two to three times a day. Milk thistle improves liver function, important in the metabolism of hormones. Take 250 mg three times a day an 80–85% silymarin extract.

## HOMEOPATHY

The following homeopathic remedies can be helpful in easing mild to moderate, infrequent symptoms of PMS. More established, severe problems are best treated by an experienced homeopathic practitioner.

**Lycopodium:** If PMS symptoms are associated with a craving for sweet foods and a bloated stomach, use Lycopodium. Leading up to a period there may be a noticeable amount of gastric disturbance that alternates between constipation and diarrhea. Sufferers also tend to experience mood swings and feelings of anxiety, irritability, and lack of confidence.

**Natrum mur:** If there is mild to moderate depression and emotional withdrawal before a period, try Natrum mur. Symptoms may also include fluid retention, cravings for salty foods and snacks, cold sores, dry, sensitive skin, and headaches or migraines that may come on before or after a period. Sufferers may also feel an aversion to displays of sympathy and affection.

**Lachesis:** When this remedy is well indicated, PMS symptoms build in intensity from mid-cycle until the onset of the period. Disturbed sleep, left-sided headaches, and mood swings that include anxiety, depression, and jealous outbursts all become most intense just before a period starts. Symptoms are then relieved as soon as the period starts.

**Sepia:** If PMS has a negative effect on optimism and motivation, and mental, emotional, and physical energy, try Sepia. Mood changes can occur very rapidly, from feeling irritable to complete indifference. When this remedy is well indicated symptoms are relieved by brisk, aerobic exercise.

**Pulsatilla:** If sufferers feel weepy, and PMS symptoms are eased after a good cry, Pulsatilla is a strong choice. Physical symptoms include pre-menstrual headaches that feel worse in hot, stuffy conditions, irregular periods, persistent indigestion, a sensitivity to rich, fatty foods, tender, enlarged breasts, and pre-menstrual thrush. All symptoms may become more intense following pregnancy or approaching menopause.

## HERBALISM

 An excess of estrogen is thought to contribute to the development of PMS symptoms. To rid the body of excess estrogen, herbal medicines are used to support the liver and digestion and to balance internal hormonal production.

**Liver support formula:** The liver is one of the main organs that removes internally and externally derived hormones (such as those found in birth control pills). If you have a poor diet, poor digestion, and excess hormones, the liver becomes overwhelmed and cannot detoxify the body as well as it should. The following herbs regenerate and heal the liver, improve the flow of bile (needed to break down fats), and encourage bowel movements. This is important because excess estrogen that is broken down by the liver must be moved out of the intestines in a timely manner, or it will be re-absorbed. Combine equal parts of dried dandelion leaf and root, yellow dock root, nettle, artichoke, and milk thistle. Decoct 1 tbsp of the combined herbs per cup and drink, or take 2–3 ml of a combined tincture three times daily.

**Reproductive tonic:** These following herbs support liver function, decrease uterine spasm, and stabilize emotions. Combine equal parts of the following dried herbs: chaste tree, wild yam, dandelion, Dong Quai, and cramp bark. Drink an infusion made from 1 tsp per cup of water or take 2 ml of a combined tincture three times a day one week before menstruation begins as a preventive measure. To ease symptoms, drink an infusion made from 2 tsp per cup of water, or take 2–4 ml of a combined tincture three to four times a day.

# PROSTATITIS

## DIAGNOSIS

Prostatitis is the inflammation of the prostate gland. It can occur as an acute or chronic condition. Acute prostatitis is commonly due to infection caused by bacteria that spreads from the urethra or bladder to the prostate. It is usually associated with lower urinary infection or with sexually transmitted diseases (STDs) such as gonorrhea or chlamydia. The main symptom is difficulty urinating, and the prostate can eventually become so swollen that it becomes impossible to pass urine. Contact a doctor immediately if this occurs.

Chronic prostatitis is rare and is usually associated with an infection elsewhere in the urinary tract. It is more common in older men and can follow an attack of acute prostatitis. The main symptoms are genital or pelvic pain that comes and goes over a period of weeks or months, and intermittent urinary problems such as a sudden urge to urinate. The term chronic pelvic pain syndrome (CPPS) is now often used instead of chronic prostatitis to describe this condition.

## SYMPTOMS

- Burning and discomfort when urinating
- Frequent urination
- Severe pain felt deep between the legs
- Fever
- Fatigue
- Pain in the lower back, scrotum, and rectum
- Discharge from the penis, if there is an STD present
- Problems with ejaculation

## TREATMENT GOAL

See a doctor to confirm that you have prostatitis. Treatment involves eliminating the bacteria that has caused the infection and relieving symptoms. Psychological therapy may also be needed to treat chronic conditions.

## CONVENTIONAL MEDICINE

**Antibiotics:** A broad spectrum of antibiotics such as Bactrim ® or ciprofloxacin is usually taken for four to six weeks to treat acute bacterial prostatitis. To treat chronic prostatitis, antibiotics are taken for an additional four to six weeks if a patient is asymptomatic, and for 12 weeks if he is symptomatic.

**Other medication:** If it is difficult to urinate, drugs such as doxazosin can be used to help improve urinary flow. Ibuprofen can also be taken to relieve pain and inflammation. Cernilton, which is a pollen extract, can help but may take several months to take effect.

**Prostate massage:** Chronic inflammation and swelling of the prostate can also occur with age. It is not caused by an infection, and repetitive prostate massage may help to relieve symptoms. Other lifestyle changes, such as cutting out caffeine and alcohol, may also help.

## TRADITIONAL CHINESE MEDICINE

**Herbs:** Mix 6 g of ginseng, 12 g of Mai Men Dong (ophiopogon tuber), and 6 g of Gan Cao (licorice). Place the herbs in a ceramic pot, add 2 cups of water, bring to the boil, and simmer for 30 minutes. Strain and drink.

**Acupuncture:** Treatment is based on an individual evaluation. Consult an experienced practitioner for an assessment and diagnosis.

**Acupressure:** Press the Nei Guan point, found on the center of the palm-side of the wrist, about 3 inches above the crease. The Susanli point is on the front of the lower leg in the depression about 3 inches below and to the left of the knee. Use the tip of a finger or thumb to press these points for one minute.

**Diet:** Drink plenty of water every day and eat fresh fruit and vegetables. Avoid hot chili peppers, beef, lamb, and deep-fried food since these create heat in the body.

## NATUROPATHY

**Diet:** Eat whole, fresh, unrefined, and unprocessed foods. Include fruits, vegetables, whole grains, soy, beans, seeds, nuts, olive oil, and cold-water fish (salmon, sardines, halibut, and mackerel) in your diet. Eating organic food helps to reduce your exposure to pesticides, herbicides, and hormones. Avoid sugar, dairy products, refined foods, fried foods, junk foods, alcohol, and caffeine. These foods wreak havoc on hormones that affect the prostate and increase inflammation. Use an elimination diet to determine whether you have any food sensitivities. Cut out a common allergen, such as wheat, dairy, corn, oranges, and soy, for three weeks and then reintroduce it at the end of the third week to see if any changes occur. Flaxseeds contain phyto-nutrients that balance estrogen levels. Grind 2–4 tbsp and add them to your food daily. You can also take 1 tbsp of flaxseed oil a day, although it is not as beneficial.

**Supplements:** Take 400 mg of bromelain three times a day in between meals for its anti-inflammatory properties. Also take 500–1,000 mg of vitamin C three times a day to enhance immune function, inhibit the growth of E. coli, and make the urine more acidic. Probiotics such as acidophilus should be taken if you are on antibiotics as it can replenish the beneficial gut flora that antibiotics can kill. Take a product that has at least 4 billion organisms daily. Also take 500 mg of quercetin twice a day for its anti-inflammatory properties. Selenium is an antioxidant, but may be more effective when taken with vitamin E. Take 200 mcg of selenium and 400 IU of vitamin E. Zinc is vital to the health of the prostate, which concentrates and secretes zinc, and also helps prevent infections. Take 100 mg daily along with 10 mg of copper for one month, then a preventive dose of 30 mg a day with 3 mg of copper.

**Herbs:** Bearberry acts as a diuretic and antiseptic for the urinary tract system. Take it standardized to arbutin at 250 mg of arbutin four times a day. Echinacea and goldenseal treat infections through their antiviral and antibacterial properties. Take 500 mg of the capsule or 4 ml of the tincture up to four times a day. Rye pollen extract has been used to improve symptoms of prostatitis, and can be taken as directed on the label.

## HOMEOPATHY

The following remedies can be used as a short-term, complementary measure to ease the pain and discomfort of a mild to moderate attack of prostatitis. However, severe and/or frequent attacks are best treated by an experienced homeopathic practitioner who will be aiming to treat at a deeper level.

**Nux vomica:** If symptoms have developed in response to "living in the fast lane" and escalating stress levels, use Nux vomica. Symptoms that are likely to respond to this remedy include spasmodic pains extending from the genitals to the thighs, with the right side often more affected than the left. Pain and discomfort feels more intense when lying on the back, and slight incontinence may occur when sneezing or coughing.

**Lycopodium:** If the need to urinate becomes more frequent and urgent when traveling, try Lycopodium. Urine may leak and/or dribble from the penis when feeling stressed and anxious, and may have a dark-colored and murky appearance. Cool compresses may give temporary relief from pain and discomfort.

## HERBALISM

There are four types of prostatitis: acute and chronic bacterial prostatitis, nonbacterial prostatitis, and prostatodynia (a painful prostate without inflammation).

**Prostate infection formula:** The following formula treats infection in the prostate and urinary tract. The herbs included fight bacterial infection in the urinary tract, soothe and decrease inflammation, and support the immune system in assisting the elimination of bacteria. Combine barberry, echinacea, buchu, goldenrod, uva ursi, corn silk, and usnea as dried herbs or tinctures. When combining these herbs, echinacea and barberry should comprise about 40% of the formula and corn silk and usnea around 10–15%. Equal parts of the remaining herbs should make up the rest of the formula. Herbal combinations can also be put together by a medical herbalist, or at a local herbal store. Drink an infusion made from 1 tbsp of the dried herbs per cup of water, or take 2 ml of the combined tincture every three hours, even throughout the night, for up to three days. Then reduce the dose to three to four times per day for up to 10 days.

**Inflamed prostate formula:** When the prostate is inflamed but not infected, herbs that reduce inflammation and congestion around the prostate are indicated. Non-bacterial inflammation of the prostate is thought to be affected by increased levels of DHT (dihydrotestosterone), a potent form of testosterone that can stimulate growth of the prostate. Saw palmetto and pygeum are both 5-alpha-reductase inhibitors, which prevent the conversion of testosterone to DHT. Pipsissewa is used to treat prostate and lymph congestion. Stinging nettle root is anti-inflammatory, anti-histamine, and pain relieving. Clinical studies show stinging nettles effectively relieve nonbacterial prostatitis. Cleavers is a gentle lymphagogue, moving congested lymph and swelling from the prostate. Combine equal parts of the above as dried herbs or in tincture form. Drink an infusion made from 1 tbsp per cup of water, steeped for five minutes, or take 3 ml of the combined tincture, twice daily. You can also take 160 mg of saw palmetto or 100 mg of pygeum twice daily.

# RECTAL BLEEDING

## DIAGNOSIS

There are many conditions that can lead to rectal bleeding. Contact your doctor if you notice bright red blood coming from the anus or in the stools after a bowel movement. If the blood is accompanied by rectal pain and itchiness, you may have an anal fissure (a tear in the lining of the anus) or hemorrhoids (see p. 413). If you have noticed a change in your bowel movements, for example, if they have become infrequent and stools are hard and dry, you may be constipated (see p. 346). Bleeding from the rectum can also be an indication of gastrointestinal disorders such as Crohn's disease and diverticulitis (see p. 372), particularly if it is accompanied by abdominal pain and mucus in the stools. Occasionally, rectal bleeding can also be symptom of cancer of the colon, especially if there is a history of this condition in your family, you have experienced previous problems, and you are over 45. Contact your doctor if symptoms persist.

## SYMPTOMS

- Blood coming from the anus
- Blood mixed with stools
- Itchiness around the anus
- Rectal pain

## TREATMENT GOAL

Treatment involves establishing the underlying cause of the bleeding and treating it accordingly.

## CONVENTIONAL MEDICINE

Most episodes of rectal bleeding are not serious. If the blood is bright red, it usually comes from the anus or rectum; darker blood indicates a source of bleeding higher up in the intestines or stomach. If you experience repeated or severe episodes of rectal bleeding, you should be examined by a doctor. This usually involves an anoscopy, which allows a physician to view the anus, and sigmoidoscopy, an internal examination of the colon, to rule out malignant diseases. Treatment again depends on the diagnosis.

**To treat a fissure:** Bleeding that occurs with a bowel movement and that is accompanied by pain, is usually caused by a fissure, or crack, in the skin around the anus. This is treated by preventing constipation (see p. 346) so that stools are softer and easier to pass.

**To treat hemorrhoids:** A hemorrhoid can sometimes cause bleeding during a bowel movement. See p. 413 for advice on how to treat hemorrhoids.

**To treat colitis:** Bleeding that is accompanied by diarrhea may be caused by colitis. See Colitis (p. 341) for treatment options.

## TRADITIONAL CHINESE MEDICINE

**Herbs:** The herbs listed below are available from Chinese pharmacies or online.
• To treat all kinds of rectal bleeding at all stages: Mix 10 g of Bei Mao Gen (wooly grass rhizome) and 5 g of Jin Yin Hua (honeysuckle flower). To make a tea, put the herbs into a teapot, add boiling water, and let them steep for five minutes.
• To treat chronic conditions: Do not use this formula if you have loose bowel movements or diarrhea. Mix 12 g of Han Lian Cao (eclipta), 15 g of Xuan Shen (ningpo figwort root), 15 g of Zhi Mu (anemarrhena rhizome), 12 g of Di Gu Pi (cortex of wolfberry root), 12 g of Dan Pi (cortex of tree peony root), and 12 g of Mai Men Dong (ophiopogon tuber). To make a decoction, place the ingredients in a ceramic or glass pot and add 3 cups of water. Bring the mixture to a boil, simmer for 30 minutes and strain the liquid. Drink 1 cup two to three times a day.

**Acupuncture:** An experienced acupuncturist will first diagnose the condition. According to traditional Chinese medicine, rectal bleeding is usually caused by severe heat in the lung meridian, stomach heat, liver stagnation, and spleen or kidney deficiency in some cases. Once the cause is identified, treatment can stop the bleeding and prevent a recurrence.

**Diet:** Include foods in your diet that are cooling such as purslane, mung beans, lotus, lettuce, mangoes, aubergines, spinach, pears, and cucumbers. Drink plenty of water every day and eat fresh fruits and vegetables. Avoid food that has warm properties, such as hot chili peppers, black pepper, beef, chicken, chives, spinach, cloves, ginger, red peppers, and lamb, as these will increase heat in the body. Also avoid deep-fried food, and eat less fatty and greasy food.

## NATUROPATHY

**Diet:** One of the most common causes of rectal bleeding is an inadequate fiber intake. Base your diet on whole foods like fresh vegetables, fruits, whole grains, beans, nuts, and seeds. Sprinkle ground flaxseeds on your cereal, homemade shakes, or salads. Flaxseeds contain high quantities of fiber and essential oils that help with bowel movements. Eat five or six light meals throughout the day rather than two or three large meals. If you try to eat too much fiber at one time this may put excess pressure on your intestines. Drink plenty of water, 8–10 glasses throughout the day, so that stools can pass more easily. This will also protect against dehydration, which can worsen hemorrhoids and other causes of rectal bleeding. Avoid trans-fatty acids and hydrogenated oils. They slow down the digestive system and contribute to inflammation.

**Supplements:** Bioflavonoids are a type of plant compound that stabilizes and strengthens blood vessel walls and decreases inflammation of the rectum and the whole body. They have been found to reduce anal discomfort, pain, and discharge during an acute hemorrhoid attack. The major flavonoids found in citrus fruits, which include diosmin, herperidin, and oxerutins, appear to be beneficial. Take 1,000 mg of a bioflavonoid complex three times a day. Also take 500 mg of vitamin C three times a day to strengthen the rectal tissue. Probiotics contain friendly bacteria that help improve digestion and constipation. Take a product that contains at least four billion live organisms of lactobacillus and bifidobacterium.

**Herbs:** A witch hazel compresses, in the form of a cream, distilled liquid, or medicated pad, should be applied topically to the anal area. You can also add 1 oz to a sitz bath. Witch hazel decreases the bleeding of the rectum by acting as an astringent. It also relieves pain, itching, and swelling associated with hemorrhoids. Butcher's broom has a long history of use for rectal bleeding. Butcher's broom extract has anti-inflammatory and vein-constricting properties believed to improve the tone and integrity of veins and shrink swollen tissue. Take a standardized extract that provides 200–300 mg of ruscogenins daily. Horse chestnut is often recommended when there is poor circulation in the veins, or chronic venous insufficiency. It relieves symptoms such as swelling and inflammation, and also strengthens blood vessel walls. Take 100 mg of a standardized aescin daily. Bilberry improves circulation and strengthens capillary walls. Take a standardized extract containing 25% anthocyanosides at 160 mg twice a day. Stoneroot reduces hemorrhoid swelling and improves rectal bleeding. Take 500 mg three times a day.

**Hydrotherapy:** Take two or three sitz baths daily. Sit in a warm bath with your knees raised for 5–15 minutes. You can also alternate between hot and cold sitz baths to gain relief and improve circulation. Sit in warm water for one minute and in cold water for 30 seconds.

## HOMEOPATHY

The following advice is only appropriate for treating mild rectal bleeding that is bright in color and has been triggered by an obvious acute problem, such as hemorrhoids. If you have no previous history of rectal bleeding, the condition must be assessed by a doctor. This also applies if a change in bowel habit occurs that cannot be explained by an obvious cause, such as a major change in fiber or water intake, and/or an escalation of stress and anxiety levels.

**Hamamelis:** If hemorrhoids bleed very easily and quite profusely, try Hamamelis. Pain in the affected area is likely to feel stinging or prickling, and there also tends to be a general sensation of tension in the hemorrhoids. Moving about, making sudden jolting or jarring movements, and contact with cold air aggravates symptoms and increases pain and discomfort.

**Nux vomica:** If hemorrhoids that bleed easily have been triggered or aggravated by ineffectual straining when constipated, use Nux vomica. When this remedy is indicated, the affected area is likely to feel very sensitive to touch, and sharp pains radiate up the rectum. Eating junk foods may have triggered problem, and rest and warmth feel soothing.

**TIP:** USE CALENDULA CREAM
If soreness has been caused by too much straining, apply calendula cream to soothe the sensitive area using a piece of clean toilet paper. Continue to use it until soreness has cleared up.

## HERBALISM

Rectal bleeding is usually due to hemorrhoids, but can also be caused by a more serious medical condition. Hemorrhoids are created by an increase in venous pressure, commonly as a result of constipation, diarrhea, pregnancy, prolonged sitting, or heavy lifting.

**Hemorrhoid and venous support suppository or salve:** Create a wonderful blend of astringent and tonifying herbs to support venous integrity throughout the body. Witch hazel bark, which is astringent and cooling, is indicated for venous congestion that results in hemorrhoids. Witch hazel contains tannins, quercitin, and gallic acid, which are anti-inflammatory, tonify lax tissues, and arrest bleeding. Butcher's broom strengthens and tonifies blood vessels, thereby reducing venous swelling, pain, and irritation. St. John's wort is helpful for relieving nerve pain associated with rectal bleeding. When used topically, St. John's wort alleviates inflammation and stops bleeding. Horse chestnut is anti-inflammatory, astringent, antispasmodic, and reduces swelling. Aescin, horse chestnut's main active constituent, reduces capillary permeability and improves venous tone, which results in smaller rectal veins and decreased pain. Calendula flowers speed the healing of connective tissue, possibly due to its anti-inflammatory and antioxidant properties. Add 1–2 oz each of the following powdered herbs to a base of 1 cup of olive oil or almond oil. Heat the herbs and oil in the oven at 100°F for four hours, stirring occasionally. Strain the herbs from the oil and add 1 oz of beeswax with added vitamin E and A over low heat. Either pour the oil into small containers to use as a salve, or into foil-shaped suppositories. Apply the salve topically or insert rectally once daily, usually in the evening.

**Venous support tea:** You can also combine the herbs listed above to drink as a tea to heal and improve the integrity and strength of the rectal veins from within. Drink an infusion made from 1–2 tsp of the combined herbs per cup of water, or take 2 ml of a combined tincture in water twice daily.

# STRETCH MARKS

## DIAGNOSIS

Also known as "striae," stretch marks are thin red or purple streaky lines on the skin that are triggered by changes in skin elasticity. They commonly appear on the abdomen, breasts, upper arms, thighs, and buttocks. They are usually a result of hormonal changes within the body, which cause the skin to become thinner. Although not everyone gets stretch marks, they generally occur when an individual gains weight rapidly, such as during pregnancy or puberty. During these times, the overlying skin is unable to keep up with the body's growth and becomes stretched. When the weight is then lost, the marks this stretching produces tend to become more noticeable. There are many different products on the market that claim to lessen the appearance of stretch marks, although there is little in the way of scientific evidence to support them. As time goes by, stretch marks do fade to a silvery white color, becoming lighter, less noticeable, and finer in appearance.

## SYMPTOMS

- Red or purple lines on the body
- Lines may fade over time

## TREATMENT GOAL

There is no cure or proven treatment for stretch marks. Wait to see how the marks fade over time before considering using any of the cosmetic products designed to improve their appearance. If worried, consult your doctor, who may be able to refer you to a dermatologist.

## CONVENTIONAL MEDICINE

Stretch marks are not a disease and are harmless. The appearance of marks tends to improve with time, and almost all adolescent stretch marks fade significantly.

**Retin A:** Medical treatment involves applying tretinoin (Retin A) twice a day. This generally results in significant improvement.

**Tri chloracetic acid (TCA):** This can be used in low doses of 15–20% to exfoliate the skin and peel away areas affected by stretch marks. This treatment is administered by a doctor in repeated monthly intervals until the desired firmness and color is achieved.

**Flash lamp pulse dye laser:** This device emits a tiny, but powerful, pulse of light that is absorbed by the pigment within the red blood cells. It shows some benefit in reducing the appearance of stretch marks.

## TRADITIONAL CHINESE MEDICINE

**Herbs:** It is not necessary to take herbs to treat this condition. If you have other complications associated with stretch marks, consult a doctor of Chinese medicine for advice.

**Acupuncture:** Treatment can be helpful for this condition. If you are pregnant, accupuncture can help you to make a faster recovery from labor and reduce the appearance of stretch marks as it helps your abdominal muscles regain some flexibility by increasing the flow of energy and blood circulation.

**Acupressure:** Use your palms to massage the abdomen in a clockwise circle for two minutes. Stop for 10 seconds and then massage in a counter-clockwise circle for two minutes. Repeat twice a day.

**Diet:** Drink plenty of water every day and include lots of fresh vegetables and fruits in your diet. Avoid food that has heat and warming properties, such as hot chili peppers, beef, and lamb. Avoid deep-fried food, and eat less fatty and greasy foods since they also create heat in the body. Bitter melon, watermelon, mung beans, tofu, radishes, and celery are all helpful foods to eat, as are foods that promote blood circulation throughout the body, such as black soybeans, brown sugar, chestnuts, peaches, and sweet basil.

## NATUROPATHY

**Diet:** Foods that are high in omega-3 fatty acids are especially important for healthy skin and for preventing and treating stretch marks. Salmon, mackerel, sardines, and other cold-water fish have high levels of omega-3 fatty acids, as do walnuts, flaxseeds, and flaxseed oil. Vitamin C is essential for collagen formation and skin health. Citrus fruits, such as oranges, tangerines, grapefruits, lemons, and limes, and berries, melons, kiwi, papaya, pineapple, watermelon, and most vegetables contain high levels of vitamin C. Vitamin E helps with all kinds of skin conditions, including stretch marks. Eat two servings of nuts and whole grains a day, which contain high levels of vitamin E. Sprinkle wheat germ, which is also high in vitamin E, on your cereal or mix it into shakes. Eat foods that are rich in zinc and silica as they are good for skin and help form collagen, the supporting fiber in the skin. Foods containing zinc include oysters, lamb, beef, spinach, and lentils. Whole grains, onions, and potatoes contain high levels of silica.

**Supplements:** A quality multivitamin is important to provide your body with all the essential nutrients for healthy, shiny skin. As mentioned above, vitamin C is important for healthy formation of collagen, and can be taken at 1,000 mg three times a day. Fish oils help with all kinds of skin problems, including stretch marks. Take 3,000–6,000 mg a day. Zinc increases immunity and helps all skin conditions and problems. Take 15–30 mg a day. Vitamin E strengthens the skin and heals stretch marks. For best results, use it internally and externally by taking 400 IU a day orally and massaging 3–6 drops of tincture into the affected site after showering.

## HOMEOPATHY

Stretch marks are a common cosmetic nuisance that can be triggered by noticeable or severe fluctuations in weight. It is a very common complaint following pregnancy and childbirth, and/or among those who "yo-yo" diet. The best treatment is prevention.

**Avoid fluctuating weight:** As well as producing stretch marks, fluctuations in weight can also cause cellulite to develop.

**Calc fluor tissue salts:** These have a reputation for possibly helping minimize problems with stretch marks.

**Dry skin body brushing:** This can generally improve skin texture, especially as part of a lifestyle that includes exercise to stimulate the efficient movement of lymphatic fluid.

Use a long-handled natural bristle brush, and brush the skin using firm, but gentle sweeping strokes that move from the feet up the legs, and up the arms in the same direction. Concentrate on the upper arms, thighs, and buttocks, but avoid any areas of broken, irritated, or inflamed skin.

**TIP:** MOISTURIZE

Ensure that the skin on your body is thoroughly moisturized, particularly if pregnant, and to keep it as supple as possible. Pay special attention to areas that are especially vulnerable, such as the upper arms, breasts, thighs, and abdomen. Vitamin E oil and creams that contain vitamin E have good reputations as moisturizers.

## HERBALISM

Stretch marks commonly occur when the body grows in a short period of time, for example, during pregnancy. One approach to stretch mark prevention is the application of oil, typically almond or olive oil, to the affected area daily. It is not known whether the oil or the increased circulation due to the massage prevents or decreases the appearance of stretch marks.

**Topical oil:** One study showed a decrease in the appearance of stretch marks in 30% of people through the daily topical application of an oil and herbal combination over a period of three to six months. Horse chestnut seeds, bark, and leaves contain an active ingredient, aescin, which tonifies and strengthens connective tissue. Horse chestnut is used internally to treat varicose veins, hemorrhoids, and chronic venous insufficiency. American ivy contains resins and tannins that give ivy its astringent and tissue-tonifying qualities. However, do not take American ivy internally as the berries and leaves cause nausea and vomiting. Bladderwrack, a brown seaweed, contains highly mucilaginous starches (polysaccharides) and antioxidants, and is high in minerals, especially iodine. Its ability to promote skin cell regeneration while breaking down scar tissue makes bladderwrack good for wound healing. Butcher's broom, a member of the lily family, tonifies and strengthens arteries and veins, thereby improving venous insufficiency, varicose veins, and circulation. This is possibly due to it high antioxidant flavonoid content, as well as its ability to narrow blood vessels. Blue-green algae, thermal plankton, soy protein, and methylxanthines (a form of caffeine) are also helpful. Combine 2 oz of almond oil or cream with 60–90 drops of tincture of the herbs listed and apply it to stretch marks once daily.

# SWEATING

## DIAGNOSIS

Sweating is necessary to control body temperature, and is regulated by the nervous system. In around 1% of the population, this system works at a very high level, causing inappropriate sweating to occur in specific areas of the body. This condition is known as hyperhidrosis. Regardless of which area of the body is affected, hyperhidrosis can be an embarrassing problem.

Hyperhidrosis is not a temporary problem. Those who have this condition sweat constantly, regardless of whether they are in a hot or cold environment. It is uncertain what triggers hyperhidrosis, but it has been linked to overactivity in the thoracic sympathetic ganglion chain, which runs along the vertebrae of the spine inside the chest cavity. This chain controls the glands responsible for perspiration, known as the apocrine and eccrine glands. Different parts of the body become affected depending on which part of the chain is overactive.

Excessive sweating can also be a symptom of an underlying condition, such as hyperthyroidism, psychiatric disorders, menopause, or obesity. These causes must first be ruled out before treatment can begin.

## SYMPTOMS

- Excessive sweating
- Sweating can occur in many different areas of the body. However, the palms of the hands are most commonly affected
- Other commonly affected areas include the soles of the feet, the armpits, the face, the head, the groin, and the back

## TREATMENT GOAL

To establish the cause of excessive sweating, whether due to hyperhidrosis or another condition. Treatment involves decreasing the amount of sweat produced, replacing any fluids and other nutrients lost through sweating, and easing any feelings of embarrassment brought on by this ailment.

## CONVENTIONAL MEDICINE

The following therapies can be used to treat primary hyperhidrosis. If excessive sweating is associated with another condition, it is necessary to treat the underlying cause.

**Antiperspirants:** The first choice of treatment should be the simplest and least invasive therapy. As such, antiperspirants are usually recommended as a first step. The most effective antiperspirant ingredient is aluminum chloride. Natural antiperspirants, although safer than aluminum chloride (as some people are worried about aluminum toxicity), are generally not as effective in treating hyperhidrosis.

**Iontophoresis:** If antiperspirants are ineffective, iontophoresis can be attempted, which involves applying a low intensity electric current. Sessions are about 20 minutes long and take place twice a week to relieve acute symptoms, and then once every two weeks as a preventive measure. This treatment can be carried out in a doctor's office or at home. It works well for sweating that occurs on the palms of the hands and soles of the feet, and moderately well on the armpits.

**Botox:** This can help to manage excessive sweating in the armpit area. It is injected at a low dose and lasts 6–12 months. Minimal side effects may occur.

**Surgery:** If the above treatments do not work, the sweat glands in the armpit area can be removed through a surgical procedure. Several surgeries may be needed. Other surgical procedures include a sympathectomy, which removes the nerves responsible for transmitting the signal to sweat. This can be an effective procedure for relieving excessive sweating in the face, head, armpits, and palms of the hands. The procedure can be performed using an endoscope, which is less invasive and requires a shorter recovery time.

## TRADITIONAL CHINESE MEDICINE

**Herbs:** Consult a doctor to identify the cause of sweating. A herbal formula may be prescribed by a practitioner of Chinese medicine depending on the cause of the condition.

**Acupuncture:** Excessive sweating may be a condition that is secondary to an internal imbalance. Acupuncture treatment will address these internal issues. An experienced practitioner will determine the length of treatment based on a consultation and diagnosis. It may last for a few weeks or a few months.

**Acupressure:** The Hegu and Fu Liu acupressure points are traditionally used to regulate perspiration. The Hegu point is located on the back of the hand in the depression between the thumb and the first finger. The Fu Liu point is on the inside of the leg and to the side of the ankle in the depression 1 inch directly above the Achilles tendon. Use the tip of your finger to press these points with moderate pressure for one to two minutes.

**Diet:** To treat excessive sweating, eat foods that are light such as wheat, rice, spinach, tomatoes, carrots, tofu, and soy milk. Foods that replenish Qi and the spleen are also recommended, such as Chinese yam, chicken, and duck. Avoid pungent foods such as green onions, garlic, and chili peppers.

## NATUROPATHY

**Diet:** Drink one 8 oz glass of water every two hours to replenish fluids lost through sweating. Sports drinks such as Gatorade® can be beneficial in replacing important electrolytes. Coconut milk is an ideal drink in a hot climate, in which people tend to perspire profusely, as it replaces sodium and liquid lost through sweating. It also replaces potassium and calcium, preventing the muscle cramps and weakness that can result from the loss of these minerals through heavy sweating. Drinking fresh-pressed juice from green vegetables (such as celery, cucumber, and parsley) is also an excellent way to replace lost nutrients. Lemons and limes possess a mildly astringent quality that tends to reduce perspiration. Make freshly squeezed lemon and lime juice and add 1 tbsp of honey to take away some of the tartness. Eat plenty of salads, fruits, and vegetables as they contain water and minerals.

**Supplements:** As mentioned above, it is important to replace the minerals, such as calcium and potassium, that are lost during sweating. A lack of calcium can cause muscle cramps, while potassium deficiency causes muscle weakness and constipation. Take a good multimineral/multivitamin to replace lost minerals, following the dosage instructions on the label. Also take 1,200 mg of calcium a day and 2,500 mg of potassium a day (if required to treat muscle weakness). If you have kidney disease, consult a doctor before taking potassium.

**Herbs:** Sage has a calming effect on sweat-producing nerves. Horsetail also provides essential minerals that are lost when sweating. Valerian root relaxes the nervous system, which can be helpful if anxiety triggers sweating. Mix 5 tbsp of sage leaves, 1 tbsp of horsetail, and 1 tbsp of valerian root and make a tea by boiling 1 tsp of this mixture in 1 cup of water. Bring it to a boil twice, strain the herbs, and drink 1 cup of the liquid daily, or as needed.

## HOMEOPATHY

Homeopathic treatment can be useful in treating chronic problems of excessive sweating. However, treatment is best carried out by an experienced homeopathic practitioner.

**Phosphorus:** If sweating occurs in response to feeling anxious, use phosphorus. Eating or drinking may also have an effect on a raised body temperature. Rinsing the hands in cool water helps, as does emotional reassurance.

**Aconite:** If symptoms of panic descend quickly and dramatically, making the sufferer feel petrified and sweaty, try Aconite. Symptoms include feeling sweaty, but although the head feels hot, the body continues to feel cool. Waves of heat and coolness course through the body when in the grip of panic.

**Arsenicum album:** This is helpful in situations where a cold, clammy, chilled sweat sets in as a result of panic and anxiety. It can also help ease sweating that is associated with nausea and vomiting. Although sufferers may sweat profusely, they feel incredibly chilly.

**Pulsatilla:** If hot flashes and night sweats are associated with hormonal changes, such as those that occur during menopause, Pulsatilla is a strong candidate. Symptoms include severe hot flashes and feeling faint, especially while in overheated, stuffy rooms. Night sweats also occur, making it impossible to get comfortable at night.

**Calc carb:** This remedy is suitable if profuse, cold, clammy sweats break out on the head, face, and scalp as a result of physical exertion when unfit, feeling emotionally stressed, or frightened. The feet may also tend to break out in a cold, sour-smelling sweat.

## HERBALISM

Several herbal medicines used to address excessive sweating tonify and treat the adrenal glands and liver. It is thought that additional stress placed on the adrenals and the liver by poor eating habits, medications, and chemical toxins in the environment create a tendency for the nervous system to overreact, leading to excessive sweating.

**Adrenal tonic formula:** The adrenal glands are responsible for secreting our "sex, sugar, and stress" hormones. When we experience a short-term stressful situation—for example, running late for an important meeting on an empty stomach—the adrenals kick in and secrete cortisol, our "stress" hormone, to get us through. When stress is high on a daily basis, the adrenals eventually become fatigued. The following adaptogenic herbs support the adrenal glands in times of stress. Licorice, a sweet, soothing root, extends the life of cortisol in our bodies by preventing its breakdown. Licorice is also a potent antiviral and antioxidant, and protects the liver. Gotu kola, a spicy, cooling plant, also spares cortisol and improves connective tissue integrity. It is adaptogenic, anti-inflammatory, a diuretic, and acts as a mild laxative. Ashwaganda increases vitality and also acts as an anti-inflammatory and mild sedative. Ginseng improves mental and physical stamina and is a wonderful herb specifically for adrenal fatigue. It also improves circulation, balances blood sugar, and is an antioxidant and antispasmodic. Combine ½ tsp of each loose herb or 1 ml of a tincture. Place 2 tsp of the mixed loose herbs in 1 cup of hot water and steep for 10–15 minutes before drinking. You can also take 4 ml of the combined tincture two to three times daily.

**Liver tonic formula:** The liver is responsible for breaking down the chemicals, hormones, and toxins we ingest or make within our body. Out exposure to pollution, medications, poor eating, and being stressed can overwhelm the liver. Create a liver regenerating and supportive formula by combining milk thistle, bupleurum, dandelion, and artichoke. Combine ½ tsp of each dried herb and add 1 cup of hot water. Let the herbs steep for 10 minutes before drinking. You can also combine 1 ml of each in tincture and take the blend three times daily.

# YEAST INFECTION

## DIAGNOSIS

A vaginal yeast infection is caused by the yeast fungus, Candida albicans. Yeast is tiny organisms that usually live in small numbers on the skin and inside the vagina. The acidic environment inside the vagina normally keeps yeast from growing. However, if the vagina becomes less acidic too much yeast can grow, causing an infection. The acidic balance in the vagina can be changed by menstruation, pregnancy, diabetes, some antibiotics, oral contraceptives, and steroids. Clothing (particularly underwear) that is too tight or made of materials such as nylon that trap heat and moisture can also lead to infections, as yeast thrives in this type of environment. Using scented sanitary products, and wiping from back to front after urinating, can upset the balance of bacteria in the vagina and trigger an infection.

Yeast infections are extremely common and will affect three out of four women at some point in their lives. Many women will also suffer from repeated infections, which become more common after menopause. Although they are uncomfortable, they are not usually serious and are easy to treat. However, it is important to consult a doctor to get an accurate diagnosis as other infections, such as some sexually transmitted diseases, can cause similar symptoms but require different treatments.

## SYMPTOMS

- Itchiness and burning in the vagina and around the vulva
- A white vaginal discharge
- Pain during sexual intercourse
- Swelling of the vulva
- Burning sensation when urinating

## TREATMENT GOAL

To identify the cause of the infection and treat it accordingly. Conventional and complementary therapies involve relieving symptoms and restoring the balance of bacteria in the vagina. It is important to identify the cause of the yeast infection to avoid recurrence, and to rule out diabetes as raised glucose levels can trigger candida overgrowth.

## CONVENTIONAL MEDICINE

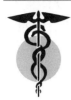

Conventional treatment of a vaginal fungal infection involves a proper diagnosis and pharmacological therapy. A diagnosis is usually made after a pelvic exam and swab. A yeast infection has a discharge that gives a typical pattern, and is easily identified under a microscope.

**Suppositories and creams:** Many women are familiar with the symptoms of a yeast infection and may opt to use an over-the-counter product such as miconazole (Monistat®) suppositories, which are taken for three to seven days. Alternative treatments include boric acid suppositories or tea tree oil suppositories, which are both made by a compounding pharmacist. Nystatin cream and suppositories can also be used. These have a cure rate of about 80% and cause few side effects. Clotrimazole, taken in the form of a 200 mg vaginal tablet, can be used for three to seven days as prescribed. Butoconazole, another cream, is usually used for three days and also has a good cure rate.

**Fluconazole:** Other pharmacologic therapy includes fluconazole, which is a pill that is taken in one dose. This can be associated with nausea, headaches, and stomach pain. Fluconazole (Diflucan®) can be used orally once a month for prevention.

**Oral probiotics:** The oral probiotics bifidus, acidophilus, and S. boullardii species are recommended to help prevent recurrence of a yeast infection, as is a diet that is low in processed food and sugar.

## TRADITIONAL CHINESE MEDICINE

**Herbs:** The herbs listed below are available from Chinese pharmacies or online. To make a decoction, combine the herbs from either formula in a glass or ceramic pot and add 3 cups of water. Bring the herbs to a boil, simmer for 30 minutes, and strain. Drink 1 cup twice a day.

• To treat yeast infection associated with a bloated abdomen, yellow or thick vaginal discharge, itchiness, and a thirst due to dampness and heat: Mix 12 g of Huang Qin (baical skullcap root), 15 g of Bai Zhu (white atractylodes rhizome), 15 g of Fuling (poria), 10 g of Zhi Zi (Cape Jasmine fruit), 10 g of Huo Xiang (agastache), and 10 g of Huang Bai (phellodendron).

• To treat yeast infection associated with fatigue, poor appetite, a bloated stomach, loose stools, and a clear vaginal discharge: These symptoms are considered to be related to spleen deficiency. Mix 12 g of Huang Qin (baical skullcap root), 12 g of Tai

Zi Shen (pseudostellaria), 15 g of Bai Zhu (white atractylodes rhizome), 15 g of Fuling (poria), 5 g of Chen Pi (tangerine peel), and 12 g of Fa Ben Xia (pinellia rhizome).

**Acupuncture:** An experienced practitioner will consult with you about your condition and will inquire about your health history as well as other ongoing health conditions. You may need acupuncture sessions once a week for 3–12 months, depending on your individual condition.

**Acupressure:** Press the Nei Guan and Shan Yin Jiao acupressure points for two to three minutes, once a day. The Nei Guan point is located in the center of the wrist on the palm side, about 2 inches below the crease. The Shan Yin Jiao point is in the center of the inside of the leg, about 3 inches above the anklebone.

**Diet:** Eat rice instead of wheat. Also include food in your diet that helps eliminate dampness, such as Daikon radishes, eggplant, celery, and cilantro. Avoid sweets and fatty, greasy food.

## NATUROPATHY

**Diet:** The following measures are part of a standard diet to control candida, which causes yeast infections. Eat chicken, eggs, fish, yogurt, vegetables, seeds, oils, and lots of raw garlic (garlic it has antifungal properties). Eliminate refined and simple sugars from your diet, and avoid added sugar of any kind, including white or brown sugar, raw sugar, honey, molasses, or grain sweeteners. Stevia is an allowed sugar substitute. Also avoid milk, alcohol, fruit or dried fruit, and mushrooms, which encourage fungal micro-organisms to grow. Avoid foods that contain yeast or mold, including all breads, muffins, cakes, baked goods, cheeses, dried fruits, melons, and peanuts. Take 1 tsp–1 tbsp of soluble fiber a day. Guar gum, psyllium husks, flaxseeds, or pectin can be mixed in an 8 oz glass of water and drunk twice a day on an empty stomach. Fiber helps to normalize bowel movements to expel fungal micro-organisms from the body, thereby preventing infections from developing.

**Supplements:** Take 1,000 mg of caprylic acid, a fatty acid that has been shown to have antifungal properties. Vitamin C, taken at 1,000 mg twice a day, helps to enhance immune functions. Also take a high-potency multivitamin to obtain many nutrients that will support immune function. Take a probiotic product that contains about four billion micro-organisms twice a day 30 minutes before each meal. These micro-organisms provide acidophilus and bifidus, which are friendly bacteria that prevent yeast overgrowth and fight candida. Also take 200 mg of grapefruit seed extract two to three

times a day for its anti-candida properties.

**Herbs:** Oregano oil is known for its strong antifungal properties. Take 5 drops of oil under the tongue, or mixed with a glass of water if you find the undiluted drops to be too strong. You can also take oregano in capsule form at 500 mg a day. Take 500 mg of garlic to fight fungus and boost the immune system. Undecylenic acid, a derivative from castor bean oil, has been shown to have strong antifungal activity. Take 200 mg three times a day. Drink 2 cups of Pau d'Arco tea a day for its strong antifungal properties. Barberry also contains antifungal and antimicrobial properties. Take 250–500 mg three times a day.

> **TIP:** WEAR APPROPRIATE CLOTHING
> Wear cotton underwear and loose clothes. This will help to keep the area dry and reduce irritation.

## HOMEOPATHY

The homeopathic remedies listed below can help to ease the severity and shorten the duration of a recent, mild to moderate vaginal yeast infection. A recurrent, severe, and/or established yeast infection should be treated by an experienced homeopathic practitioner.

**Borax:** To treat acute yeast infection symptoms that occur when ovulating (mid-cycle), take Borax. Symptoms include irritation and a swollen sensation in the vagina, with a thin discharge that may be bland or irritating.

**Kreosotum:** If symptoms include a smarting, burning sensation that travels deep into the vagina, Kreosotum may be appropriate. There may be a yellow discharge that eases symptoms, while sexual intercourse or being overheated is aggravating. Contact with cool air feels temporarily soothing, and eases irritation and burning.

**Natrum mur:** If symptoms of a yeast infection arise along with vaginal dryness, try this remedy. Persistent dryness and discomfort can alternate with the production of a thin, watery discharge. Symptoms tend to be more intense during or just after a period.

> **TIP:** AVOID SCENTED BATH PRODUCTS
> At the first sign of vaginal irritation, sensitivity, or itchiness, avoid using any bath products that are highly scented and/or contain harsh chemical detergents. Instead add a handful of sea salt, or a weak infusion of chamomile, to your bath.

Creams that act as a local anesthetic do not support the body in dealing with a yeast infection. They also potentially mask an infection that may not be due to yeast. It is also possible to develop a sensitivity to the cream, which can further aggravate symptoms.

## HERBALISM

 **Antifungal suppository:** To treat vaginal yeast infections, create an anti-fungal suppository. Add 5 drops each of garlic oil, thuja oil, and tea tree oil to a base of cocoa butter and vitamin A, which can then be put into a vaginal suppository. Insert one suppository into the vagina at night for seven days.

**Douche:** Make a vaginal douche by combining 2 tsp each of dried, chopped goldenseal root and lomatium root in 2 cups of hot water, and add 10 ml of vinegar. Let the mixture cool, and then douche with 1 cup of solution in the morning and 1 cup before bedtime. This treatment can be combined with vaginal antifungal suppositories.

# MIND
# AND
# SPIRIT

# ANXIETY

## DIAGNOSIS

Anxiety is something that most people experience at one time or another. It usually results from anticipating and worrying about an upcoming event, such as an exam, a presentation, a sporting event, or a job interview. Lifestyle factors such as including too much caffeine and sugar in your diet, poor nutrition, recreational drug use, exhaustion, and stress, and the side effects of certain medications can also cause anxiety.

Becoming anxious under pressure can sometimes be a positive thing, as it can lead to increased performance levels. For most people, anxiety is a short-term problem and tends to disappear after the anticipated event has passed. If anxiety occurs on a regular basis and threatens to overwhelm you, however, it becomes a bigger problem. The psychological effects of anxiety include fear, tension, irritability, and an inability to relax or concentrate. You may have an overwhelming desire to seek the reassurance of others, making you clingy and dependent. You may start to have a pessimistic outlook on life, and always assume that the worst is going to happen.

## SYMPTOMS

- Rapid breathing and lightheadedness
- Feeling shaky
- Sweating profusely
- Dry mouth
- Heightened senses
- Feeling alert
- Increased muscular tension can cause discomfort and headaches
- Pounding heart
- Butterflies in the stomach
- Nausea and sickness
- Repeated urge to move your bowels and urinate

## TREATMENT GOAL

Treatment first involves eliminating any possible physical causes of the symptoms. It is then important to identify the cause of the anxiety, relieve acute symptoms, and introduce any necessary lifestyle changes to improve quality of life.

## CONVENTIONAL MEDICINE

Conventional treatment involves relieving the acute symptoms of anxiety to improve the quality of life and prevent harm from occurring to the self or others.

**Diet and lifestyle modifications:** Avoid caffeine, alcohol, nicotine, and taking cold remedies that contain ephedrine (which can cause rapid heartbeat and trembling). The amino acid phenylalanine seems to decrease anxiety and can be taken as a supplement. Taking 300 mg of magnesium aspartate daily divided into three doses can also be beneficial. Blackcurrant oil may provide fatty acids, which also improve anxiety levels. Environmental stressors should be identified and avoided to whatever extent possible. In some cases it is more effective to try to modify your response to stressors, as they cannot always be controlled. There are many meditation and relaxation techniques available to help you deal with stress, such as yoga or T'ai chi.

**Benzodiazepines:** Pharmacological treatment of anxiety depends on the severity of the symptoms. To treat cases of incapacitating anxiety, benzodiazepine drugs are used in low doses for as short a time as possible. These include alprazolam, which is short-acting and highly addictive. It should not be used for more than four to six weeks at a time. Clonazepam is a longer-acting and therefore generally less addictive drug that may also be effective. Diazepam, or valium, is one of the more well known benzodiazepines.

**Other medication:** SSRIs (selective serotonin reuptake inhibitors) can be used to treat anxiety, as can the antidepressant venlafaxine. Buspirone is an anti-anxiety drug that is as effective as the benzodiazepines, but takes longer to work. It is approved for use in case of generalized anxiety disorder. Beta blocker drugs can be used to resolve the physical effects of anxiety, such as shaky voice and racing heart.

**Therapy:** Therapy is advisable if any of the above drugs need to be used to treat an anxiety disorder. Cognitive therapy, psychotherapy, and support groups are useful tools that can help you deal with anxiety issues.

## TRADITIONAL CHINESE MEDICINE

**Herbs:** The herbs listed in the following formulas are available from Chinese pharmacies or online. To make a decoction, combine the herbs of either formula in a ceramic pot and add 3 cups of water. Bring the mixture to a boil and simmer for 30 minutes. Strain the liquid and drink 1 cup twice a day.

- Formula one: Mix 10 g of Chai Hu (hare's ear root), 12 g of Bai Shao (white peony), 12 g of Bai Zhu (white atractylodes rhizome), 15 g of Fuling (poria), 5 g of Bo He (field mint), 12 g of Dang Gui (Chinese angelica), 5 g of Gan Cao (licorice), and 12 g of Zi Su Zi (perilla hips).
- Formula two: Mix 12 g of Tai Zi Shen (pseudostellaria), 15 g of Bai Zhu (white atractylodes rhizome), 15 g of Shan Yao (Chinese yam), 12 g of Yuan Zhi (Chinese senega root), 12 g of Suan Zhao Ren (sour Chinese jujube seed), 5 g of Chen Pi (tangerine peel), and five pieces of Da Zhao (Chinese jujube).

**Acupuncture:** A practitioner will analyze the patient's general health to determine the internal condition that may be contributing to the anxiety disorder. This underlying condition will then be treated. You may need acupuncture sessions once or twice a week for 6–12 weeks to make up one course of treatment. Needles will be inserted for 30 minutes at each session. A practitioner will recommend additional treatment courses if necessary.

**Acupressure:** Press the Nei Guan point, which is located in the center of the wrist on the palm side, about 2 inches below the crease. The San Yin Jiao point is located in the center of the inside of the leg, about 3 inches above the anklebone. Press these points for about one minute.

**Diet:** It is best to eat foods that are calming and nourishing, such as rice porridge, licorice (not the sweets since most do not have licorice in them), Chinese jujube, peppermint, chamomile, and chicken soup. Eat plenty of fresh vegetables and reduce the amount of coffee you drink. Fruits such as pears, cranberries, blueberries, and bananas are recommended. Mung beans, red beans, bamboo shoots, and purslane are also good. Avoid food that is rich and fatty.

## NATUROPATHY

**Relaxation movements:** T'ai chi is a form of stress reduction and exercise that involves specific body movements and deep breathing. Yoga can also help with relaxation and stress reduction. It primarily involves deep breathing, stretches and meditation.

**Biofeedback:** This type of therapy operates on the notion that we have the innate ability and potential to influence the automatic functions of our bodies through the exertion of will and mind. Stress and anxiety affects your muscles by causing them to tense and tighten. This, in turn, can produce other aches and pains, such as headaches or backaches. By helping you to become more attuned to your internal body functions, biofeedback teaches you to control certain unhealthy conditions. Muscle biofeedback equipment, for example, can measure the tension of your muscles and relay this information to you. By focusing on this information, your mind becomes less preoccupied with the problems causing stress, which in turn causes fewer messages to be sent from your brain to your muscles telling them to stay tense. You can use the information from the biofeedback instrument to make connections between the information and the way you feel. This increases your awareness of your own muscle tension and helps you learn to recognize tension when it first begins. Biofeedback training also teaches you ways to control the tension before other symptoms have a chance to develop. In order to use biofeedback effectively, you need to be trained by a biofeedback professional.

**TIP:** DRINK AN ANTI-ANXIETY TEA
Mix ½ oz of dried lavender, oats, linden flower, catnip, and lemon balm. Add 4 tsp of this mixture to 1 quart of boiling water. Let the herbs steep for about 10 minutes. Strain and drink the tea while it is warm. You can drink up to 6 cups a day after meals.

**Breathing exercises:** Deep breathing relaxes the mind, calms the nervous system, and improves mental focus and energy. Deep breathing requires imitating the breathing patterns of a child—they breath from the belly not the chest. To deep breath properly, find a comfortable, quiet area. Stand with your knees slightly bent or sit straight with your buttocks touching the back of your seat. Breath in through your nose to a count of five, hold for two seconds, and exhale to a count of five. While breathing in, your stomach, rather than your chest, should expand outward. When breathing out, your stomach should flatten.

**Aromatherapy:** Plant essential oils can be added to baths, massage oil, or infusers to relieve symptoms of anxiety. A few drops of essential oils in a base oil can be massaged into the scalp and temples before bed. Essential oils that are used for anxiety and nervous tension are: bergamot, cypress, geranium, jasmine, lavender, melissa, neroli, rose, sandalwood, and ylang-ylang. Lavender is the most common and forms the base of many relaxing blends.

**TIP:** EXERCISE
Exercise is perhaps the safest and most effective method of managing stress. Cardiovascular exercise combined with calming exercise, such as walking several times per week, can be very beneficial.

## HOMEOPATHY

The following remedies can help to relieve a single, mild to moderate episode of anxiety that has been triggered by an obvious cause. This might involve an emotional shock, a sharp escalation in stress and pressure, or anticipation regarding a stressful event (such as sitting an examination or going to a job interview). Established, severe, and recurrent anxiety symptoms are best treated by an experienced homeopath.

**Aconite:** This is a fantastic remedy for treating anxious, panicky feelings that wash over you very quickly and dramatically, making you feel terror-stricken. Symptoms are likely to be especially severe at night, waking you from sleep and making it very difficult to fall back asleep.

**Lycopodium:** If anticipatory anxiety particularly affects digestion, leading to tension in the stomach, try Lycopodium. The gut is also affected by bloating, noisy rumbling, and gurgling, and sufferers alternate between being constipated and having diarrhea. Although patients feel nervous and tense inside, they tend to look calm and confident on the outside. Alternatively, sufferers may be sarcastic, critical, and domineering.

**Nux vomica:** When this remedy is helpful, anxiety is accompanied by addictive behavior. This often involves relying on stimulants such as caffeine to keep going, and depressants such as alcohol to unwind. As a result, sleep patterns suffer, aggravating feelings of irritability and impatience. Additional symptoms include muscle tension, tension headaches, and constipation.

**Arg nit:** This can be a useful remedy for easing anticipatory anxiety that is associated with muscle trembling, palpitations, and talking nonstop when agitated. Emotional, mental, and physical restlessness are key symptoms, and sufferers tend to have loose stools or diarrhea when agitated or anxious.

**Gelsemium:** This remedy can ease anticipatory anxiety that causes sufferers to become withdrawn and preoccupied. When this remedy is most helpful, symptoms develop slowly and insidiously, until they reach a point where the anxious state has become draining and exhausting. This leads to symptoms of profound weariness, indifference, and apathy, often coupled with painless diarrhea.

**Arsenicum album:** This is especially helpful in relieving anxiety that develops in high achievers and perfectionists. Signature symptoms include waking up around 2 a.m. feeling anxious and struggling to go back to sleep, as well as nausea, diarrhea, and a sense of being prostrated, but unable to rest because of physical and emotional restlessness.

**Skullcap:** Historically, skullcap was used to cure people of hydrophobia, convulsions, mental agitation, and nervous system disorders including epilepsy. The sedative and antispasmodic properties of skullcap relieve restlessness leading to insomnia, nervous agitation, and fear, and have been shown to lower blood pressure related to anxiety. Skullcap's active constituents are antioxidant flavonoids, which are thought to induce brain-calming neurotransmitters, essential oils, lignans, and tannins, which give skullcap its astringent quality. Drink an infusion made from 1 tbsp of the aerial parts steeped 1 cup of water, take 3 ml of tincture, or take 1–2 g in capsule form up to three times daily. Large amounts of skullcap may cause drowsiness and should not be taken when driving or operating heavy machinery.

**Passionflower:** This herb relieves restlessness, insomnia, anxiety, and spasm within the muscles. Although not as potent as skullcap, clinical studies have shown passionflower to be effective at reducing symptoms of generalized anxiety disorder (GAD) and attention deficit hyperactivity disorder (ADHD). Recent studies have also shown some promising findings regarding passionflower's ability to relieve pain. The dried herb is used medicinally once the berries have matured. Drink an infusion made from 1–2 tsp of dried herb per cup of water or take 2–3 ml of a tincture three times daily.

**Hops:** As a tea or tincture, hops relieves anxiety, irritability, restlessness, and muscle tension. Drink an infusion made from 1 tbsp of dried strobiles (female parts) per cup of water or take 3 ml of a tincture three times daily. To treat insomnia, you may also place a packet of dried hops in your pillow to assist the onset of sleep.

# BED WETTING

## DIAGNOSIS

Bed wetting, also known by the medical term enuresis, can happen at any age but generally affects children. It mostly occurs in very young children, and they tend to grow out of it between the ages of two and five, but this of course varies from child to child. Accidents can still happen, and bed wetting is fairly common in children up to the age of six. However, if there is a frequent bladder control problem, it may indicate a physical or psychological problem that needs further evaluation.

In many cases of bed wetting, no cause can be identified. Often it is a genetic complaint, and someone else in the family may have experienced the same problem. It may have a medical cause, including a urinary infection such as cystitis, or diabetes. It may also be triggered by a psychological cause, such as the prospect of starting school or being affected by parents divorcing. Sometimes it can simply be explained by the fact that the child is a heavy sleeper and does not wake up when his or her bladder is full, or that they have not yet developed proper bladder control. Some children produce too little of the antidiuretic hormone (ADH), which controls the production of urine. In this case, a nasal spray containing desmopressin, which is available from a doctor, may help.

## CONSULT A DOCTOR IF:

- A child still wets the bed after the age of six
- A child suddenly starts wetting the bed
- A child's urine has a strong smell, or it hurts when he or she urinates
- A child starts to have accidents during the day

## TREATMENT GOAL

Do not make bed wetting a big issue. Encouragement is often the most helpful way to deal with the problem. Conventional and complementary therapies involve eliminating any underlying conditions that may be causing the bed wetting and introducing techniques that will support the child in overcoming this complaint.

## CONVENTIONAL MEDICINE

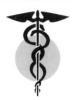

Bed wetting is rarely a psychological problem, but it can create psychological issues such as low self-esteem and family stress. A child who wets the bed should first be evaluated by a doctor to rule out any underlying conditions such as constipation, reflux, infection, and neurological problems.

**Motivational therapy:** This method of treatment involves positive reinforcement by rewarding dry nights with praise and using techniques such as sticker charts to record progress. This type of therapy has a cure rate of up to 70%. You can also try making children responsible for their actions in a non-punitive way, by getting them involved in changing the wet bed and helping with laundry. Shaming is to be avoided.

**Behavioral therapy:** When it is feasible, wake a child every four hours to go to the bathroom to encourage them to eventually wake up on their own. Have children imagine themselves waking up to go to the bathroom, and then waking up in a dry bed. The use of signal alarms can also help to modify behavior. This involves using a moisture-sensing device that is activated when a child begins to urinate, waking the child up so that she or he can go to the toilet. This is best used to treat a child over seven years of age.

**Medications:** Desmopressin, imipramine, and oxybutynin may be prescribed if a child does not respond to behavioral therapy. Desmopressin is an anti-diuretic; imipramine increases bladder capacity; and oxybutynin decreases bladder muscles contraction.

## TRADITIONAL CHINESE MEDICINE

**Herbs:** The herbs listed below are available from Chinese pharmacies or online. To make a decoction, combine the herbs of either formula in a ceramic pot and add 3 cups of water. Bring the mixture to a boil and simmer for 30 minutes. Strain the liquid and drink 1 cup twice a day.

• To treat bed wetting associated with tiring easily, cold hands or feet, a pale appearance, and lots of clear urine: Mix 10 g of Tu Si Zi (Chinese dodder seed), 10 g of Yi Zhi Ren (black cardamom), 10 g of Dan Shen (salvia root), 8 g of Wu Wei Zi (schisandra fruit), 10 g of Huang Qi (milk-vetch root), and 12 g of Shan Yao (Chinese yam). Give children under 12 years old ½ cup of the decoction twice a day.

• To treat bed wetting associated with yellow urine and being overly warm and sweating while asleep: Mix 8 g of Zhi Zi (Cape Jasmine fruit), 8 g of Huang Bai (phellodendron), 8 g of Chai Hu (hare's ear root), 8 g of Jin Qian Cao (lysimachia), 10 g of Qu Mai (aerial parts and flower of Chinese pink dianthus), 5 g of Gan Cao (licorice), and 8 g of Dan Pi (cortex of peony tree root). Give children under 12 years old ½ cup of the decoction twice a day.

**Acupuncture:** In most cases, treatment can reduce the frequency of bed wetting or stop it altogether after a few sessions. To treat young children, needles will not be left in but simply inserted and removed. In some cases acupressure might be recommended.

**Acupressure:** Use the Shen Shu, Shan Yin Jiao, and Guan Yuan points to treat bed wetting. The Guan Yuan point is on the midline of the abdomen, about 3 inches below the navel. The Shen Shu point is on the lower back below the second lumbar vertebra ½ inch lateral to the center, just below the top of hipbone. The Shan Yin Jiao point is on the inside of the leg about 3 inches above the center of the anklebone. Apply pressure or have another person apply pressure to these points with the tip of the finger for one to two minutes.

**Diet:** Foods that are nourishing for the kidney are recommended, such as chives, duck, plums, grapes, star anise, tangerines, egg yolks, string beans, black soybeans, wheat, and mutton.

> **TIP:** REGULATE BEDTIME
> Put children to bed at a regular time. Do not let children become overtired in the evening and avoid exciting activities before bed.

## NATUROPATHY

**Diet:** Many cases of bed wetting are caused by food allergens or intolerances to certain foods. Eliminate common allergens such as milk, wheat, and citrus fruits from the child's diet for two to three weeks to see if this leads to any improvement. A child who suffers from bed wetting should not consume any form of caffeine, including carbonated drinks, chocolate, or tea. Foods and drinks with caffeine will promote urination.

**Supplements:** Give your child a liquid calcium and magnesium formula, especially if he or she wets the bed due to nervousness, as this supplement helps relax the nervous system. Follow the instructions on the label.

**Massage:** According to practitioners of massage, applying pressure to various points on the body may help alleviate bed wetting. It can also help with bed wetting conditions that are caused by neurological problems.

**Hypnosis:** Hypnosis, when performed by a trained practitioner, may be successful in helping with this condition. Hypnosis trains the child to wake up and go to the bathroom when his or her bladder feels full. Hypnosis is less expensive, less time-consuming, and less dangerous than most approaches; it has virtually no side effects. Recent medical studies show that hypnotherapy can work quickly to bring improvement, sometimes within four to six sessions.

**TIP:** PRACTICE PREVENTION TECHNIQUES

Although preventing a child from wetting the bed is not always possible, parents can take steps to help the child to keep the bed dry at night. These include encouraging and praising the child for staying dry instead of punishing the child when he or she wets the bed, reminding the child to urinate before going to bed if he or she feels the need, and limiting the child's liquid intake at least two hours before bedtime.

## HOMEOPATHY

 This tends to be a chronic condition and is best treated by a homeopathic practitioner who will be able to provide support at a constitutional level. The remedies below may be helpful in treating an episode of bed wetting that has been caused by an obvious trigger in a child who is otherwise dry. If a positive response is not forthcoming after trying what seems to be a well-indicated remedy for four, or a maximum of five, days consult a homeopathic practitioner. Symptoms of bed wetting that set in after a child has been dry for some time should also be checked out by your family doctor to assess whether there is an underlying urinary tract infection.

**Lycopodium:** This remedy is appropriate if bed wetting occurs in an unconfident child (although on the surface he or she may seem extroverted and bossy) during a period of high anticipatory anxiety. Problems often revolve around undertaking any new challenge, although once things are underway, everything goes well. Bed wetting may also be more of a problem in an overheated or stuffy bedroom.

**Pulsatilla:** This remedy can be helpful where symptoms of bed wetting follow convalescence from an episode of measles, or getting wet and chilled. Lying on the back when trying to sleep makes the urge to urinate irresistible. Once bed wetting has occurred, the child feels emotionally upset and tearful and needs a great deal of comfort and affection.

## HERBALISM

Bed wetting occurs for many reasons, ranging from medical conditions such as diabetes to food allergies.

**Bed-wetting blend:** This herbal formula can be used in combination with other chosen therapies to address bed wetting. It is safe for children and should help to decrease nightly episodes. Corn silk tastes sweet and is soothing and healing to the urinary tract. Corn silk is also mildly diuretic and contains small amounts of antioxidant flavonoids and minerals. Stinging nettle leaf and root are anti-inflammatory, high in antioxidants and minerals, and slightly diuretic. St. John's wort has a mild sedating effect, ever so slightly calming the nervous system. St. John's wort is especially effective for bed wetting associated with nervous system conditions such as anxiety and depression. Plantain is slightly astringent, anti-inflammatory, and soothing to the urinary tract. Plantain is also high in vitamin K, beta-carotene and calcium, and other carbohydrates, making it a very nutritious addition. Oats are a gentle, calming herb that tonifies and rebalances the nervous system. Combine equal amounts of glycerin-based tinctures (these are better for children than alcohol-based tinctures) of these herbs to create a blend. Drink 10–20 drops of tincture diluted in water or juice in the morning and afternoon (twice daily).

# DEPRESSION

## DIAGNOSIS

It is normal to feel depressed or get a bout of the blues occasionally, but if these feelings start to interfere with your daily life and do not seem to subside, it could be a sign of clinical depression. This can be a life-threatening condition as it can cause people to lose the will to live and may potentially lead to suicide. Depression is certainly a common problem. At least one in every six people will admit to feeling depressed at some point in their life, and one in 20 become clinically depressed. There is no one single cause of depression; it varies very much from person to person and can be triggered by a combination of things. In many cases, depression is first triggered by an unwelcome or traumatic event, such as the death of a loved one. It can also be caused by various health problems. Occasionally people become depressed in response to certain foods or poor nutrition, a lack of physical fitness, or an illness.

## SYMPTOMS

- Restlessness and agitation
- Sleeping problems, including waking up early and feeling tired
- Excessive smoking and drinking alcohol
- Poor appetite and weight loss
- Memory loss
- Feeling irritable or impatient, and getting no pleasure out of life
- Loss of libido
- Low self-esteem
- Preoccupation with negative thoughts, and feelings of emptiness and despair
- Cutting yourself off from others emotionally
- Thinking about suicide

## TREATMENT GOAL

To establish the cause and severity of the depression, and identify and avoid triggers to relieve symptoms. Mild cases may benefit from simple lifestyle changes such as eating a balanced diet and getting regular exercise. Severe cases will require long-term psychological treatment.

## CONVENTIONAL MEDICINE

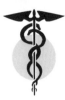

Conventional treatment of depression involves protecting the patient from self-harm, relieving the symptoms, and preventing recurrence. A combination of therapy that includes psychotherapy, nutrition, and lifestyle changes, plus medication as needed, works best.

**Diet and lifestyle modifications:** Complete a 30-minute exercise routine daily and eat a diet that is high in protein and low in processed food. Supplements that have been shown to help relieve depression include omega-3 oils (eicosapentaenoic acid, EPA, and docosahexaenoic acid, DHA, in a 3:2 ratio) taken at a dose of 4 g daily of EPA and DHA combined, and B-vitamins, particularly inositol, folate, and B12. Take a B-vitamin complex that provides about 1 mg of B12 and folate. SAM–e, a mood brightener, can be taken at 400 mg twice a day to increase the effects of the B-vitamin. Taking the supplements 5-hydroxytriptophan (5-HTP) at 150 mg daily and St. John's wort at 300 mg three times a day can also be tried. St. John's wort interacts with several medications, so always consult a doctor before using it.

**Medication:** SSRIs (selective serotonin reuptake inhibitors), of which there are a wide variety, may be prescribed to treat depression. Common side effects affect the gastrointestinal system, the libido, and the nervous system. Venlafaxine (Effexor®), a combined SSRI and norepinephrine reuptake inhibitor, can lift the mood. Side effects include anxiety and insomnia, as well as the inability to achieve orgasm. Other drugs used to treat depression include duloxetine and bupropion. Several other categories of antidepressant drugs exist and these tend to have more severe side effects.

**Other therapies:** Psychotherapy, cognitive behavioral therapy, and support groups are helpful options. Electroconvulsive therapy, which involves passing an electrical current through the brain, is still used for severe depression that does not respond to medication.

## TRADITIONAL CHINESE MEDICINE

Traditional Chinese medicine views depression as both a cause and a result of illness. Treatment for depression varies according to each individual patient's condition. Patients' physical conditions vary as well, and usually can be defined as excessive or deficient.

**Herbs:** The herbs listed below are available from Chinese pharmacies or online. To make a decoction, combine the herbs of either formula in a ceramic or glass pot and add 3 cups of water. Bring the mixture to a boil and simmer for 30 minutes. Strain the liquid and drink 1 cup twice a day.

• To treat excessive depression: Symptoms include feeling irritable and angry, a tightness in the chest, a bitter taste in mouth, and sighing. Mix 12 g of Chai Hu (hare's ear root), 15 g of Bai Shao (white peony), 10 g of Zhi Zi (Cape Jasmine fruit), 12 g of Dang Gui (Chinese angelica root), 12 g of Xiang Fu (nut grass rhizome), 12 g of Fuling (poria), and 5 g of Gan Cao (licorice).

• To treat deficient depression: Symptoms include fatigue, sleeplessness, decreased memory, and low motivation. Mix 12 g of Huang Qi (milk-vetch root), 10 g of Ren Shen (ginseng), 12 g of Bai Zhu (white atractylodes rhizome), 12 g of Fu Shen (poria spirit), 12 g of Yuan Zhi (Chinese senega root), 12 g of Suan Zhao Ren (sour Chinese jujube seed), and five pieces of Da Zhao (Chinese jujube).

**Acupuncture:** Treatment is often recommended in conjunction with herbal remedies, and may be given once or twice a week for one to three months depending on the particular condition. Consult a practitioner of Chinese medicine to determine the contributing factors, both physical and mental.

**Acupressure:** Press the Tai Yang and Nei Guan points. The Tai Yang point is situated at the temple, in the depression between the lateral end of the eyebrow and the eyelid. The Nei Guan point is in the center of the wrist on the palm side about 2 inches above the crease. Apply medium pressure to these points with the tip of your finger and repeat two to three times during the day.

**Diet:** Include foods in your diet that help you sleep and have calming effects, such as chamomile tea, peppermint, rice porridge, pears, and mandarin oranges. Eat a balanced diet and regular meals. Eat plenty of fresh vegetables to keep bowel movements regular.

## NATUROPATHY

**Diet:** Nutrition is essential for proper brain chemistry. Eat a well-balanced diet consisting of whole grains, organic vegetables, and lean protein. Consume fish such as salmon and mackerel for their high content of essential fatty acids (EFAs), specifically omega-3 fatty acids, which have been shown to be helpful in treating depression. Flaxseeds are a good source of fiber and also contain EFAs. Sprinkle 1 tbsp of ground flaxseeds on salads, yogurt, or cereal. Cut out simple, processed carbohydrates, hydrogenated oils, and saturated fats, which increase fatigue and sluggishness, and contribute to depression. Also avoid alcohol, which is a known depressant.

**Supplements:** Take a good multivitamin/multimineral, following the directions on the label, to obtain a good base of nutrients for brain chemistry function. S-adenosylmethionine (SAM–e) seems to increase the concentration of neurotransmitters in the brain that are involved in regulating mood. Take 200 mg of an enteric-coated form twice a day on as empty stomach. Fish oils have been shown in some preliminary studies to be beneficial for depression. The eicosapentaenoic acid (EPA) and docosahexaenoic acid (DHA) contained in fish oils, improve neurotransmitter function. Take 1,000 mg of of EPA/DHA a day. L-tyrosine is an amino acid that helps regulate brain function in depressed individuals. Take 500 mg a day, but do not take it in combination with other anti-depressive medications. Take 100 mg of 5-hydroxytryptophan (5-HTP), which is used by the brain to make serotonin, an important neurotransmitter in the regulation of mood, twice a day. Be sure to take it with 100 mg of a B-complex vitamin, as vitamin B6 is essential in the metabolism of serotonin, however, do not take it with pharmaceutical medications for depression.

**Herbs:** Ginkgo biloba improves blood flow to the brain. Take 60–120 mg twice a day. You can also take 1,000 mg of ashwagandha to improve stress hormone balance and relax the nervous system.

## HOMEOPATHY

Feelings that will respond well to the remedies suggested below are more appropriately described as the "blues," rather than a full-scale episode of moderate to severe clinical depression. The latter can be greatly helped by an experienced homeopathic practitioner. Depending on the severity of the symptoms, these remedies can be helpful as a first choice of treatment, or when used as a complementary measure alongside conventional treatment.

**Ignatia:** This remedy is helpful if depression follows a loss of any kind. This can include bereavement, a relationship break up, homesickness, or losing a loved job. Symptoms include rapid changes in mood, frequent sighing, and nausea, which is helped by eating a small amount.

**Natrum mur:** This remedy can help anyone who tries to keep a lid on their emotions and develops a low, depressed mood as a result. Symptoms include a strong dislike of breaking down in tears in public, and an equal distaste of receiving sympathy and physical displays of affection. The blues may have developed in response to a long-term emotional strain or loss.

**Sepia:** If depressed feelings are related to major fluctuations in hormone levels, such as those that develop post-natally, premenstrually, or during menopause, try Sepia. Classic symptoms include a feeling of being emotionally, physically, and mentally wiped out, and feeling aggressive one moment and totally indifferent the next. Although the idea of being in company is not appealing, being alone does not help either.

**Lachesis:** To treat premenstrual blues and mood swings that develop when ovulating and build in intensity until the onset of a period, use Lachesis. Classic symptoms include low, distressed, or anxious moods that are at their worst when you wake up. As a result, a real dislike and fear or going to bed may develop, and you may tend to stay up to avoid sleep for as long as possible.

**Pulsatilla:** This remedy can help to lift a mild bout of feeling blue that prompts you to feel much more emotional and weepy than is normally the case. Those who respond well to Pulsatilla feel much better after a good cry, and by being the object of attention and affection.

## HERBALISM

Many herbal medicines can be used to elevate your mood and restore vitality. That said, depression is a serious condition that should be monitored by a health professional. Herbal medicines should only be used in conjunction with treatments, such as counseling, that attempt to identify and treat any possible causes of the depression. Also be aware that many of these herbs should not be taken in high doses by those who are taking conventional medication for depression.

**St. John's wort:** Consider using this herb to treat depression associated with a sense of loss of connection with others, loss of self-worth, or depression due to chronic pain resulting in insomnia. Many clinical studies have demonstrated St. John's wort's effectiveness at relieving depression, while others have found it to be as effective as many of the pharmaceutical antidepressants, such as Prozac®, Zoloft®, and Paxil®. Its active constituents, hypericin and hyperforin, are thought to inhibit neurotransmitters in the brain, known as serotonin, dopamine, and norepinephrine. Small amounts of melatonin, the hormone responsible for sleep induction, have also been found within the herb. Take 300 mg three times daily, standardized to 0.3% hypericin content. St. John's wort is generally tolerated well; however, side effects include photosensitivity, photodermatitis, abdominal discomfort, and hypomania in those with bipolar disorder. Exercise caution if you are taking other medications as St. John's wort increases the liver's metabolism of many drugs. Do not take this herb with anti-coagulant medications.

**Rhodiola:** To treat mild depression, especially when combined with increased levels of daily stress and physical exhaustion, try rhodiola. Rhodiola is categorized as an adaptogen, recognized for its ability to improve physical performance, decrease fatigue and depression, and improve sleep. Rhodiola contains high amounts of antioxidant flavonoids, proanthocyanidins, catechins, and rosavin, one of the main active constituents thought to impart rhodiola's adaptogenic ability. Rhodiola increases neurotransmitters in the brain (serotonin, dopamine, and norepinephrine) which are known to elevate moods. Take a 100 mg dose a day standardized to 2% rosavin, and increase to 300 mg daily if needed. Higher doses (above 200 mg) may cause irritability and insomnia.

# FATIGUE

## DIAGNOSIS

It goes without saying that if you do not get enough sleep you will experience feelings of fatigue. When you have one or several nights of disturbed sleep, you will probably still be able to carry out simple tasks easily, despite feeling tired, but may find it difficult to concentrate. Over time, however, fatigue will also start to take its toll on your body physically. Lack of sleep aside, there are multiple other reasons for feeling tired, including a problem with blood sugar levels and adrenal exhaustion as a result of overdosing on stimulants such as caffeine when trying to counteract decreasing energy levels. Maintaining an even blood sugar level is crucial if you want to keep your energy levels consistent during the day. Stimulants such as caffeine, alcohol, and chocolate cause blood sugar levels to yo-yo wildly by triggering a quick burst of energy, which is then followed by a sharp dip in energy levels. In addition, stimulants lead to bursts of adrenalin being produced by your adrenal glands, which speed up everything in your body but ultimately lead to exhaustion as your body tries to cope with the demands being made of it. If you regularly get less than six hours of sleep a night, you will probably develop a sluggish metabolism, and your body will not be as efficient at turning glucose (sugars) in the blood into energy. Fatigue is often a first sign of nutritional deficiency. Regular feelings of fatigue can occasionally be a sign of a more serious condition, so consult a doctor if you experience serious, prolonged fatigue.

## SYMPTOMS

- Feeling tired
- Difficulty concentrating
- Increased appetite

## TREATMENT GOAL

It is important to identify the cause of fatigue, and rule out any potentially serious conditions. Treatment involves balancing nutritional levels in the body, developing stress-reduction techniques, and ultimately restoring quality of life.

## CONVENTIONAL MEDICINE

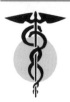

The first step is to make sure that there is not an underlying serious illness causing the fatigue. Blood tests are carried out to check that white blood cells and red blood cells as well as iron levels are normal. Liver and kidney function is evaluated and the adrenal and thyroid glands are also assessed, as problems with these glands are particularly associated with fatigue. Occasionally, fatigue can be linked to depression, so a doctor should evaluate for depression and treat it as needed.

**Sleeping aides:** Once any underlying conditions have been ruled out, fatigue is treated by ensuring that the patient gets an adequate amount of sleep. This can be achieved through medication, but most sleep aides have side effects and actually disrupt sleep. Ambien® or trazadone (Desyrel®), two sleep aides, may be prescribed, or alternatively, magnesium aspartate may be recommended at a dose of 270 mg at night, combined with 5-hydroxytriptophan (5-HTP) dosed at 150 mg.

**Lifestyle modifications:** Although patients often find it difficult to find the motivation to exercise, physical activity usually results in increased energy, particularly if you exercise in the morning. Avoid caffeine and follow a diet that is low in processed food. Eliminating simple sugars from the diet also helps to increase energy levels. Taking a B-vitamin complex supplement, along with folic acid and sub lingual B12 (taken under the tongue), can also be helpful. Try practicing stress reduction techniques such as massage and craniosacral therapy, which involves manipulating the skull to relieve tension.

## TRADITIONAL CHINESE MEDICINE

**Herbs:** The herbs listed below are available from Chinese pharmacies or online. To make a decoction, combine the herbs of either formula in a ceramic or glass pot and add 3 cups of water. Bring the mixture to a boil and simmer for 30 minutes. Strain the liquid and drink 1 cup twice a day.
• To treat Qi deficiency: Symptoms include fatigue associated with poor appetite, loose stools, and muscle weakness. Mix 10 g of ginseng, 12 g of Bai Zhu (white atractylodes rhizome), 15 g of Shan Yao (Chinese yam), 12 g of Huang Qi (milk-vetch root), 15 g of Fuling (poria), and 3 g of Gan Cao (licorice).
• To treat kidney and blood deficiency: Symptoms include fatigue associated with dizziness, a light headache, insomnia, and a poor memory. Mix 12 g of Ji Shen (jilin root), 15 g of Di Huang (Chinese foxglove), 15g of Dan Shen (Salvia Root), 15g of Shan Zhu Yu (Cornelian cherry fruit), 15 g of Shan Yao (Chinese yam), 15 g of Fuling (poria), 12 g of Sang Shen Zi (mulberry fruit-spike), and 12 g of Tu Si Zi (Chinese dodder seed).

**Acupuncture:** A well-trained acupuncturist will evaluate the patient, assessing his or her general health, and diagnose and treat the underlying condition that is causing fatigue. Generally, local points are used that promote circulation to reduce fatigue. You may have 30-minute sessions once or twice a week.

**Acupressure:** The Nei Guan and Susanli points are helpful for this condition. The Nei Guan point is found on the center of the wrist on the palm side, about 2 inches above the crease. The Susanli point is on the front of the lower leg in the depression about 3 inches below and to the left of the knee. Press these points with the tip of the finger or thumb for one minute.

**Diet:** Eat a well-balanced nutritional diet that includes fresh vegetables and fruits, such as pears, cranberries, blueberries, and bananas. Eating foods that nourish the blood is also helpful, such as black sesame seeds, red beans, black beans, spinach, fish, and carrots. Also eat foods that are cooling, such as watermelon, green vegetables, tofu, and Chinese jujube dates. Reduce your coffee intake and avoid food that is rich and fatty, or hot and spicy, such as chili peppers, garlic, beef, and lamb.

## NATUROPATHY

**Diet:** Follow a detox and cleansing diet for one to three weeks, avoiding all foods and chemicals that may be triggering symptoms. Wheat, dairy, corn, gluten-containing products (such as rye and oats), sugar, and fermented foods are some of the most common food allergens. Drink two to three freshly squeezed green vegetable juices and at least eight glasses of water a day. This will help strengthen all elimination organs including the liver, spleen, lymphatic system, and kidneys. If you have candidiasis avoid all types of sugar, including milk products and fruit, caffeine, alcohol, and refined carbohydrates such as white flour and white rice. After the cleansing diet, the excluded foods can be reintroduced into the diet systematically. Note any changes in your symptoms to identify any potential irritants. Eat two to four servings of leafy green vegetables a day. These foods are high in magnesium and other nutrients important for overall health. Blood sugar imbalance may cause or contribute to fatigue. Follow a whole food diet consisting of fruit and vegetables, whole grains, nuts, and seeds. Eat small regular meals that include some protein. This will help keep blood sugar levels stable.

**Supplements:** Beneficial bacteria found in probiotic products can improve digestion and strengthen the immune system by re-establishing a healthy microbial balance in the intestines. Take a product that contains four billion micro-organisms a day. Digestive enzymes (pancreatic or vegetable-derived enzymes) can supply your body with additional enzymes to digest fats, proteins, and carbohydrates. Products differ greatly;

some contain lactase to digest milk, others contain hydrochloric acid to assist the stomach, and still others contain ox bile to help with the emulsification and digestion of fats. A typical dose is one to two capsules two to three times a day, taken on an empty stomach. Vitamin C helps the immune system and nourishes the adrenal gland, which is responsible for secreting the hormones that affect wellbeing. Take 2,000 mg of the vitamin twice a day. Magnesium is essential for energy production, muscle function, nerve conduction, and bone health. Those who are lacking energy often have low magnesium levels, so take 400 mg a day. Coenzyme Q10 is essential for energy production, cell function, and helps with the repair and maintenance of tissues. Take 60–100 mg daily. L-carnitine converts fatty acids into energy, and some studies have found decreased carnitine levels in those who suffer from fatigue. Take 300 mg one to three times a day. Also take 100 mg of B-complex twice a day to help to reduce the effects of stress, which can lead to fatigue. Use a formula with extra B5 and B6 for maximum effect. Chromium, taken at 200 mcg a day, stabilizes blood sugar and insulin.

**Herbs:** Those who have chronic fatigue syndrome often have adrenal fatigue or weakness. Herbs that tonify the adrenal glands include licorice, which stabilizes levels of cortisol in the body. Take 1,000 mg two to three times a day, and take the de-glycyrrhizinated form if you suffer from high blood pressure. Ginkgo biloba improves circulation and memory. Take 60–120 mg twice a day of a standardized product containing flavone glycosides and 6% terpene lactones.

**Lifestyle modifications:** Identify stress triggers and learn to manage them through relaxation, meditation, and, if need be, counseling. Work to address the mental and emotional components of fatigue. Learn proper breathing techniques, and take part in regular, low intensity exercise. Get better sleep, as this can often improve sluggish, tired feelings.

## HOMEOPATHY

 The following strategies can be helpful in lifting a recent bout of fatigue that has followed an obvious cause, such as a lack of sleep, a sharp escalation of stress levels, or a poor diet. Chronic symptoms of fatigue that cannot be attributed to a cause are best addressed by a doctor, who will determine whether there is an underlying condition. If there is no underlying disorder, consult a homeopathic practitioner regarding treatment.

**Nux vomica:** Consider this remedy if you are feeling burnt out. It is particularly appropriate to treat disordered energy levels that have been triggered by too many late nights, a poor diet, coffee, and alcohol, and a lack of good-quality sleep. Psychological symptoms include irritability and a very short fuse, and a desire to relax in a calm and quiet environment.

**Sepia:** If there is a mental, emotional, and physical lack of energy, and an overwhelming feeling of being drained, flat and antisocial, try Sepia.

**Gelsemium:** To treat symptoms of persistent fatigue that linger after suffering a nasty bout of flu, use Gelsemium. Symptoms include a general sense of being physically and mentally drained and droopy, with a corresponding low-grade depression. The leg muscles in particular are likely to feel heavy and ache easily.

## HERBALISM

 Fatigue is commonly due to stress. However, there may be an underlying medical condition contributing to its development. Before self-treating, it is wise to seek advice from a doctor to rule out any underlying causes. Adaptogens, or tonics, are one group of herbal medicines commonly used to address fatigue. Adaptogens as a whole tend to improve energy, restore vitality, and allow greater resistance to stress by "tonifying" the adrenals, and immune and nervous systems.

**Siberian ginseng:** This is a bitter, warming herb used to improve symptoms of chronic fatigue, weakness, and debility. Current studies show that ginseng improves mental performance, increases physical work capacity, strengthens immune response, and improves stress adaptation. Begin dosing between 1–3 g per day of a capsule (standardized to 0.7 mg of eleutheroside E) or 2–6 ml of tincture per day. It is recommended that Siberian ginseng is taken for 6–12 weeks continuously, followed by a two to eight week break.

**Ashwaganda:** In Indian medicine, ashwaganda is used traditionally to restore vitality and as a mild aphrodisiac. Studies show ashwaganda has anti-inflammatory, adaptogenic, and immune-modulating properties, and is mildly sedating. Drink a decoction made by boiling 1 tbsp of dried root per cup of water or take 2 ml of tincture three times daily.

**Adaptogenic vitality formula:** Combine equal parts of astragalus, ginseng, devil's club, licorice, and gotu kola to create a herbal formula that restores energy and supports immune function. Drink a decoction made from 1 tbsp of the combined dried herbs.

# FEARS AND PHOBIAS

## DIAGNOSIS

A phobia is an intense, often irrational, fear of a situation, activity, or object. Those who suffer from phobias react to the object feared in a manner that is out of proportion to the actual threat posed by it, if indeed there is a threat at all. Sufferers experience feelings of real terror when exposed to the object of the phobia, and even though they know they are not in real physical danger, they are unable to convince themselves of it emotionally. It is clear that phobias are common and widespread, and generally fall into the following categories:

- Specific phobias often involve animals, particularly dogs, snakes, birds, insects (especially spiders and moths), or germs.
- Phobias about specific situations include agoraphobia (fear of being away from home), monophobia (fear of being alone), claustrophobia (fear of enclosed spaces), and a fear of the dark or heights.
- Social phobias can include a fear of meeting new people, going to parties, work situations, or eating in front of other people.
- Phobias may be about getting an illness, such as cancer.

## SYMPTOMS

- Feeling dread and terror
- Rapid heart beat
- Churning stomach
- Feeling dizzy and sick
- Shortness of breath
- Sweating and trembling
- Dry mouth
- Feeling confused and disoriented
- Feeling out of control and overwhelmed

## TREATMENT GOAL

Treatment focuses on helping people identify and deal with the cause of their distress, as well as developing coping strategies. Some people can trace their phobia back to their childhood and to a particular event, while others are unclear where the phobia originates.

## CONVENTIONAL MEDICINE

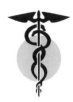

**Cognitive behavioral therapy:** The patient is first evaluated to rule out any anxiety-producing diseases such as hyperthyroidism. If no such disease is present, cognitive behavioral therapy is used to treat the phobia. This involves presenting the fear to the patient in a non-threatening way and in a controlled environment to encourage him to confront his fears and overcome them. The patient is usually asked to visualize his fear in an attempt to desensitize him to it. Gradual exposure to the feared object in this manner is then tested in a safe environment with a therapist present. Hypnotherapy may be tried to treat phobias, although evidence of success is stronger with cognitive therapy.

**Medication:** Benzodiazepines (drugs in the valium family) are often used to treat severe phobias that are unresponsive to cognitive behavioral therapy. These are addictive and should be used carefully while being monitored by a doctor. There are many side effects, most of which are related to depression.

**Lifestyle modification:** Meditation and other anxiety-relieving stress-reduction techniques are worth including in an overall treatment plan. Supplements such as B-complex vitamins, folate, blackcurrant oil, and magnesium aspartate are associated with a reduction of overall anxiety and as such may lead to a reduction of phobias.

## TRADITIONAL CHINESE MEDICINE

**Herbs:** The herbs listed below are available from Chinese pharmacies or online. To prepare a formula, place the raw herbs in a glass or ceramic pot and add 3 cups of water. Bring the mixture to a boil and let it simmer for 30 minutes. Strain the liquid and drink 1 cup twice a day.
• Formula one: Mix 12 g of Chai Hu (hare's ear root), 15 g of Bai Shao (white peony root), 18 g of Fuling (poria), 12 g of Suan Zhao Ren (sour Chinese jujube seed), 30 g of Zhen Zhu Mu (mother of pearl), and 30 g of Dai Zhe Shi (hematite).
• Formula two: Mix 15 g of Zhi Mu (anemarrhena rhizome), 15 g of Di Huang (Chinese foxglove), 12 g of Shan Zhu Yu (Asiatic cornelian cherry fruit), 15 g of Shan Yao (Chinese yam), 12 g of Zi Xie (water plantain rhizome), 15 g of Fuling (poria), 12 g of Dan Pi (cortex of tree peony root), 12 g of Sang Shen Zi (mulberry fruit-spike), and 12 g of Sang Ji Shen (mulberry mistletoe stem).

**Acupuncture:** The treatment approach is to focus on the causes of the condition. One course of treatment consists of 10–12 30-minute sessions. Consult an experienced practitioner for a diagnosis and treatment plan.

**Acupressure:** In a sitting position, apply moderate pressure to the Shen Men, Shan Yin Jiao, and Tai Xi points with the tip of your finger for one to two minutes. The Shen Men point is on the inside of the wrist, just above the crease in the first depression close to the base of the thumb. The Shan Yin Jiao point is on the inside of the leg, about 3 inches above the center of the anklebone. The Tai Xi point is on the inside of the leg in the depression between the inside of the anklebone and the Achilles tendon.

**Diet:** Eat food that is gentle and that strengthens the immune system, such as green vegetables, aubergine, radishes, mung beans, bitter melon, purslane, and pears. Drinking green tea is helpful since it has a gentle cleansing effect. Items that have a calming effect can help with sleep, such as chamomile tea, peppermint, rice porridge, pears, and mandarin oranges. Avoid seafood, and fatty and spicy food.

## NATUROPATHY

**Emotional freedom techniques (EFT):** A person affected with any kind of phobia requires professional help. This method is an "emotional form of acupuncture." The practitioner taps his fingertips on acupuncture meridian points on the client's head and chest, while the client is focused on a specific emotional or physical problem. The theory is that tapping the energy meridians and voicing positive affirmation works to clear the emotional block that is restricting the electromagnetic energy that flows through the body.

**Bach flower remedies:** The Bach flower remedies are a type of "vibrational, or energy medicine" developed in the 1920s by Edward Bach, an English doctor and homeopath. Because Bach flower remedies do not contain any of the original substance used, only its "vibrational pattern," they are considered to be different from homeopathic remedies (which contain minute amounts of the original substance). The most common types of remedies for fear and phobia includes rock rose (to treat genuine, overwhelming terror), cherry plum (to treat panic with loss of self-control), aspen (to treat vague, spooky fear that is not directed at anything specific), red chestnut (to treat fear for another's safety), star of Bethlehem (to ease fear related to a past trauma), and larch (to treat related issues such as lack of confidence).

## HOMEOPATHY

Fears and phobias tend to fall into a chronic category, often going back to childhood, so homeopathic remedies should be administered by an experienced homeopathic practitioner, ideally in combination with additional psychological support such as behavioral therapy. The remedies listed below are included to give an overview of some of the possible homeopathic remedies that can be helpful.

**Arsenicum album:** If sufferers are perfectionists and crave surroundings that are as neat and orderly as possible, Arsenicum album may be helpful. This tendency can be so marked, that patients are driven from their sickbeds to tidy up their rooms, since the distress caused by looking at a mess is untolerable. Specific fears include a fear of death and illness, and a specific phobia about coming into contact with germs.

**Lycopodium:** If there is a fear of speaking in public or giving a presentation, Lycopodium may be used. Although sufferers are very anxious before the event, once it arrives and everything goes well their confidence tends to build. Symptoms include anxiety and fear that cause great distress in the digestive tract, leading to acidity in the stomach, bloating, gas, and anxiety-related diarrhea.

**Argentum nit:** This is a strong candidate for treating anyone who has a morbid fear of heights (especially crossing bridges), where there may be a paradoxical impulse to jump. It can also be very helpful in treating fear and anxiety that develops as an important event approaches, especially if it causes someone to talk compulsively. This remedy also soothes the digestive tract when diarrhea and flatulence is triggered by fear and anxiety.

**Phosphorus:** This remedy may be helpful in treating a fear of the dark. Sufferers are emotionally reactive and labile, and respond well to reassurance and attention. Feeling fearful and panicky also tends to trigger hot flashes.

## HERBALISM

Experiencing fears and phobias can be a very normal experience. However, they can be disruptive to daily life if they get out of control. Extreme fears and phobias should be evaluated by a doctor, as there are many helpful medications and services available.

**St. John's wort:** When feelings of fear are paired with anxiety and/or depression, St. John's wort can be helpful at relieving symptoms. Current clinical studies show St. John's wort relieves symptoms of mild to severe depression (with or without anxiety), obsessive compulsive disorder (OCD), and attention deficit-hyperactivity disorder (ADHD), all of which are conditions where feelings of fear and anxiety are prevalent. Begin taking 300 mg of the herb standardized to 0.3% hypericin three times daily. It may take four to six weeks before any improvements are noticed; however, most people notice changes relatively quickly. St. John's wort can cause symptoms of photodermatitis, sensitivity to light, and mania in people with bipolar disorder. It also increases the metabolism of some drugs, so check with a doctor for contraindications before taking it.

**Ginseng:** This herb has been used for centuries to increase vitality and reduce fatigue. It is indicated for adrenal "fatigue" due to stress and overwork, leading to emotional and physical exhaustion. Experiencing fear can elevate stress levels, and vice-versa. Take 100 mg of a ginseng capsule daily, or take 3 ml of tincture twice daily. You can also drink a decoction made by steeping 1 tbsp of dried, cut, or powdered root per cup of water for 10–15 minutes twice daily.

**Nervous system supportive formula:** Make an herbal combination (using dried herbs or tinctures) made up of 20% kava kava, 20% Siberian ginseng, 20% St. John's wort, 20% schisandra, 10% oats, and 10% catnip. Add a few drops of lavender and orange essential oils to flavor, relax, and uplift. These herbs will relieve symptoms of depression, fear, and anxiety, tonify and soothe the nerves, and nourish and lift the spirit. Drink a decoction made by boiling 1–2 tsp of dried herb per cup of water for 5–10 minutes, or take 2–3 ml of tincture twice daily. Check with a medical herbalist if you decide to incorporate kava as part of this formula; kava can have adverse liver effects an may not be appropriate for your case.

# HYPERACTIVITY AND ADHD

## DIAGNOSIS

All children go through periods of heightened activity from time to time, and this is generally nothing to worry about. However, children who are prone to hyperactivity, are easily distracted, and have poor concentration levels may have attention deficit hyperactivity disorder (ADHD, also known as attention deficit disorder, ADD). The name ADHD refers to the two different groups of symptoms associated with this illness: hyperactivity (behavioral problems) and attention deficit (learning problems). Most affected children have a mixture of both, but some may only have one type of symptom. If your child is not particularly hyperactive, for example, they may still be diagnosed as having ADHD, but it will be called "ADHD without hyperactivity."

ADHD can begin to manifest when children are very young. Affected children will be restless, constantly on the go, often clumsy, and always seeking attention. At school, teachers find them untidy, disorganized, and forgetful. They find it hard to sit still or concentrate on one task, so learning is often a challenge. It is hard to judge how many children have ADHD, because different experts classify the condition in different ways. The cause of the condition is unknown, and there may be a number of different factors at work. Genetics, stress, and diet may all contribute to problems.

## SYMPTOMS

- Hyperactivity
- Difficulty concentrating
- Forgetfulness
- Clumsiness
- Spontaneous behavior
- A need to be the center of attention

## TREATMENT GOAL

Only a child psychiatrist, an educational psychologist, or a pediatrician can diagnose ADHD. Treatment should involve behavior management, counseling or psychotherapy, special help at school, and possibly medication.

## CONVENTIONAL MEDICINE

**Behavioral therapy:** General strategies that help to manage hyperactivity include reinforcing good behavior, brief timeouts for unacceptable behavior, making eye contact during speech, and allowing a child expression of activity in a safe environment.

**Ritalin®:** The type of medications used to treat ADHD are psycho-stimulants. The first choice is methylphenidate or Ritalin®, which accounts for over 90% of medications used for hyperactivity in children. Ritalin® is addictive and has side effects such as appetite suppression, insomnia, and slowing growth.

**Straterra®:** Atomoxetine (Straterra®) is a non-addictive medication that is also available, and in general, it has less severe side effects.

**Lifestyle modifications:** Although the official opinion on diet is that it has no effect on hyperactivity, many doctors and sufferers do not agree. The Feingold diet, which eliminates additives and certain food groups, has been well researched and seems to be worthwhile. Some supplements may also help in diminishing hyperactivity. These include fish oil, at a dose of about 1–4 g daily, a B-complex vitamin, and magnesium. Taurine, tyrosine, and tryptophan may also be helpful in encouraging the body to relax.

## TRADITIONAL CHINESE MEDICINE

**Herbs:** Mix 12 g of Chai Hu (hare's ear root), 15 g of Bai Shao (white peony root), 18 g of Fuling (poria), 12 g of Suan Zhao Ren (sour Chinese jujube seed), 30 g of Zhen Zhu Mu (mother of pearl), 30 g of Dai Zhe Shi (hematite), 15 g of Di Huang (Chinese foxglove), 12 g of Shan Zhu Yu (Asiatic cornelian cherry fruit), 15 g of Shan Yao (Chinese yam), 12 g of Zi Xie (water plantain rhizome), 12 g of Dan Pi (cortex of tree peony root), and 12 g of Sang Shen Zi (mulberry root bark). Place the herbs in a ceramic pot and add 3 cups of water. Bring to a boil and simmer for 30 minutes. Strain and drink 1 cup twice a day.

**Acupuncture:** A well-trained acupuncturist will assess a patient's health to determine whether an underlying condition is contributing to symptoms. Generally, sessions once a week are recommended, beginning with a full course of treatment made up of 12 acupuncture sessions.

**Acupressure:** Press the Nei Guan point, which is located in the center of the wrist on the palm side about 2 inches below the crease. The San Yin Jiao point is in the center of the inside of the leg, about 3 inches above the anklebone. Press these points for about one minute.

**Diet:** Chinese dietary therapy recommends adding calming and cooling foods to the diet. Apples, barley, cucumbers, aubergines, mung beans, mandarin oranges, pears, spinach, strawberries, licorice, marjoram, and peppermint are a few suggestions. Eat foods that help you to sleep and have a calming effect, such as chamomile tea and rice porridge. Eat a balanced diet and have regular meals that include fresh vegetables to keep bowel movements regular.

## NATUROPATHY

**Diet:** Eating a natural, whole food diet is essential for a healthy nervous system. Include brewer's yeast, green leafy vegetables, and whole grains in your meals to obtain essential nutrients, especially B-complex vitamins. Some sufferers have iron deficiency, which can be replenished by taking 1 tbsp of blackstrap molasses a day. Eat unsweetened yogurt, organic chicken, and turkey for their tryptophan content, an important amino acid involved in making serotonin, which has a calming affect on the body. Avoid all processed sugars and junk foods. These will play havoc with your blood sugar levels, which can cause hyperactivity. Foods rich in essential fatty acids nourish the nervous system and have been shown to help with hyperactivity. Such foods include wild Pacific salmon, sardines, trout, ground flaxseeds, walnuts, and almonds. Avoid all preservatives and artificial colors, which are toxic to the nervous system and contribute to hyperactivity.

**Supplements:** Take 100 mg of B-complex vitamins a day to nourish the nervous system. Also take 100 mg of vitamin B6 a day, which is essential for the synthesis of serotonin, a hormone important for causing a calming effect. A good multivitamin/multimineral, taken as directed on the label, provides the basic nutrients for proper brain function (consult a practitioner about a good-quality product). Take 3,000 mg of fish oils a day to obtain essential fatty acids that nourish the brain and nervous system. A calcium/magnesium complex can help relax the nervous system. Take 500 mg of calcium and 250 mg of magnesium twice a day. Also take 300 mg of phosphatidylserine a day; it is found in high concentrations in brain cells and helps them function properly.

**Herbs:** Drink chamomile tea, made by pouring boiling water over 2–3 heaped tsp of flowers and steeping them for 10 minutes, to calm the nervous and digestive systems. Chamomile tinctures and pills should be taken according to the directions on the pack. Alcoholic tincture may be the most potent form for internal use. Kava kava has been used traditionally as a nervine, a substance that balances the nervous system. A typical dosage of kava when used for treatment of anxiety is 300 mg a day of a product standardized to contain 70% kavalactones. Lemon balm is taken orally for its calming effect, and the standard dosage of lemon balm is 1.5–4.5 g of dried herb daily; extracts and tinctures should be taken according to instructions on the label. Passionflower has calming properties. The proper dosage of passionflower is gained by drinking 1 cup of a tea three times a day, made by steeping 1 tsp of dried leaves in hot water for 10–15 minutes. You can also take 200 mg a day in pill form. Ginkgo brings blood and oxygen to the brain. The standard dosage of ginkgo is 40–80 mg three times daily of a 50:1 extract standardized to contain 24% ginkgo-flavone glycosides.

## HOMEOPATHY

Homeopathy can play a very positive role in treating hyperactivity and ADHD, but the best results will be obtained by consulting an experienced homeopathic practitioner for constitutional treatment. Some homeopaths specialize in treating children who are struggling with this condition, and so it is well worth enquiring if a homeopath in your area has this kind of experience. Even if this is not the case, a homeopath is generally able to treat conditions of this kind, but will want to gain as complete a picture as possible of your child's emotional, mental, and physical health before attempting to select the most appropriate homeopathic prescription. When treatment is effective, there should be an overall improvement in your child's heath, and mood and energy levels will become more stable.

## HERBALISM

See Anxiety (p. 828), Panic Attacks (p. 870), and Stress (p. 885) for additional herbal remedies.

**Relaxing tea formula one:** Combine equal parts of dried California poppy flowers and seeds, oat seeds, chamomile, lavender, and marshmallow root. Infuse 1 tsp of the combined herbs per cup of water for 5–10 minutes and drink. Add a little honey to sweeten if needed. This blend of herbs is suitable for children and can be used daily to treat hyperactivity. The formula is mildly sedating, nourishing, reduces spasms, soothes digestion, and calms the spirit, especially at times of stress.

**Relaxing tea formula two:** Combine equal parts of dried passionflower, catnip, lemon balm, and chamomile. Infuse 1 tsp of the combined herbs per cup of water for 5–10 minutes and drink. Add honey or sugar to sweeten if needed. This combination of herbs is suitable for children. It also calms the nerves, is mildly sedative to induce sleep and relaxation, relieves spasm and inflammation, and is especially good at easing gas and cramping in the digestive system.

# INSOMNIA

## DIAGNOSIS

Insomnia involves having problems falling asleep at night, waking up during the night, and erratic sleeping patterns. Insomnia can be a long- or short-term problem.

Transient or short-term insomnia lasts for a few days and can be triggered by a sudden change in your circumstances, such as moving into a new home, or anxiety about an upcoming stressful event. You may find it difficult to sleep because it is too hot or too cold, too noisy, or too light in your bedroom. An illness can also temporarily change your sleeping habits, and certain prescription drugs can disturb your sleep. Jet lag or shift-work can disrupt the body clock, which tells you when to sleep and when to get up. Sleep patterns can be severely affected by consuming too many stimulants, such as alcohol, caffeine, and nicotine.

Another type of insomnia is called "learned insomnia." After a few sleepless nights, people can become apprehensive about going to bed because they fear they will not be able to get to sleep. This anxiety usually does make it difficult to sleep, which begins the cycle over again. Other people are affected by "night terrors," which occur during deep sleep and may be caused by stress, or when normal sleep patterns have been broken. Nightmares can also make people feel stressed and anxious about the thought of going to sleep.

## SYMPTOMS

- Difficulty falling asleep
- Waking up in the middle of the night and not being able to drift back to sleep
- Tiredness
- Feeling stressed and anxious about the thought of going to sleep

## TREATMENT GOAL

Try to determine the cause of the insomnia, and eliminate contributory factors, such as stress or too many stimulants before bed. Treatment involves encouraging normal sleeping patterns and developing strategies to prevent insomnia from occurring.

## CONVENTIONAL MEDICINE

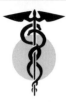

**Sleep hygiene techniques:** "Sleep hygiene" techniques involve looking at diet and medications, and identifying any factors that may be contributing to poor sleep, or an inability to sleep. It is also important to go to bed at a consistent time every night and avoid daytime naps.

**Stimulant medications:** Many stimulant medications, such as diet pills and drugs used to treat attention deficit hyperactivity disorder (ADHD), can cause insomnia. Children with ADHD are at particularly high risk of developing insomnia. Asthma medications, and all medications mixed with caffeine, can also cause insomnia. Some antidepressants, some blood pressure medications, and cold medicines can also lead to disturbed sleep.

**Pharmaceutical sleeping aides:** Medications can be used for a short period of time (a maximum of three weeks) to induce sleep. These will generally make you sluggish in the morning, and all are potentially addictive. Temazepam (Restoril®), zolpidem (Ambien®), and zaleplon (Sonata®) are the most common sleeping aides prescribed.

**Natural sleeping aides:** These can be successful in treating insomnia. Natural sleeping aides include melatonin, at a dose of 3 mg, and 5-hydroxytryptophan, at a dose of 150 mg at bedtime. Plants such as valerian, kava, chamomile, and passionflower can also help you to sleep.

## TRADITIONAL CHINESE MEDICINE

**Herbs:** The herbs listed below are available from Chinese pharmacies or online. To prepare a formula, place the herbs in a glass or ceramic pot and add 3 cups of water. Bring the mixture to a boil and simmer for 30 minutes. Strain the liquid and drink 1 cup twice a day.

• To treat insomnia associated with a deficient or weak constitution: Mix 12 g of Yuan Zhi (Chinese senega root), 12 g of Suan Zhao Ren (sour Chinese jujube seed), 15 g of Fu Shen (poria spirit), 15 g of Bai Zhu (white atractylodes rhizome), 15 g of Ye Jiao Teng (fleeceflower vine), and 6 g of Gan Cao (licorice).

• To treat insomnia associated with stress and anxiety: Mix 10 g of Chai Hu (hare's ear root), 12 g of Bai Shao (white peony), 12 g of Bai Zhu (white atractylodes rhizome), 15 g of Fuling (poria), 5 g of Bo He (field mint), 12 g of Dang Gui (Chinese angelica), 5 g of Gan Cao (licorice), and 12 g of Zi Su Ye (perilla leaf).

**Acupuncture:** A doctor of traditional Chinese medicine will first want to identify the cause of insomnia, which can be related to other serious illness. Treatment will then focus on the cause. You may have acupuncture once or twice a week and each session will last for 30 minutes. Progress will be monitored to determine how many sessions may be needed.

**Acupressure:** The Nei Guan point is in the center of the wrist on the palm side, about 2 inches above the crease. The Shan Yin Jiao point is on the inside of the leg, about 3 inches above the center of the anklebone. Apply moderate pressure to these points with the tip of your finger.

**Diet:** Eat foods that have a calming effect and may help you to sleep, such as chamomile tea, peppermint, rice porridge, pears, and mandarin oranges. Foods that nourish the blood, such as black sesame seeds, red beans, black beans, spinach, fish, and carrots, are also good. In addition, food that is cooling, such as watermelon, green vegetables, tofu, and Chinese jujube dates, is recommended. Avoid hot, spicy food.

## NATUROPATHY

**Diet:** Do not overeat at dinner and avoid having late meals. Also eliminate caffeine, including all caffeinated beverages such as colas and other carbonated drinks, as well as chocolate. If this is too difficult, limit your caffeinated beverages to the morning only. Helpful foods include turkey and tuna, which contain L-tryptophan to induce sleep.

**Supplements:** Take 1,200 mg of calcium at bedtime. Another supplement that can be helpful in promoting sleep is melatonin. Some researchers have found it to be as effective as tryptophan in promoting sleep, and it does not produce side effects. It is available in 2 mg capsules; take one a night for two weeks. Discontinue taking them if no results are produced.

**Herbs:** Try taking 2 capsules of valerian one hour before bedtime to help you sleep. You can also drink 1 cup of passionflower tea before bedtime.

**Lifestyle modifications:** Stop smoking, or at the very least do not smoke within a few hours of going to bed, as nicotine is a stimulant. It is important to avoid any form of stimulation before bedtime, including doing work, reading, or doing anything that is likely to cause anxiety. Do not take naps even if you are tired during the day. Instead develop regular sleep patterns by going to bed and getting up at virtually the same time every day. Get regular exercise, but avoid exercise in the evening close to bedtime. Finally, consult a doctor regarding any medications you may be taking, as some can cause insomnia.

## HOMEOPATHY

 The remedies suggested below may be helpful in managing mild to moderate complaints of insomnia. More established and severe sleep problems may also benefit from some of this advice, but if insomnia begins to disrupt your overall quality of life, consult an experienced homeopathic practitioner.

**Coffea:** If a poor sleep pattern develops after drinking too much coffee or other caffeinated drinks during the day, or too late at night, try Coffea. Irritating and infuriating symptoms include feeling physically exhausted, but mentally alert. Sleep, when achieved, is fitful and so light that you are woken up by the slightest sound.

**Aconite:** If sleep patterns have been affected by a recent traumatic incident, use Aconite. Triggers may include experiencing or witnessing an accident, or receiving bad news. Symptoms include severe restlessness, and frequently waking up feeling fearful, breathless, shaky, and panicky. Sleep is also likely to be disturbed by nightmares or very vivid dreams.

**Lachesis:** This remedy can be especially helpful in easing poor sleep patterns that are related to premenstrual syndrome, where symptoms build in severity from mid cycle until a period begins. The difficulty and distress of trying to sleep can produce a real aversion to going to bed, and sufferers tend to stay up late as a result. There is also an unpleasant jolting sensation throughout the body just as you begin to lose consciousness.

**Ignatia:** If a previously healthy sleep pattern has been upset by bereavement, try Ignatia. When this remedy is called for, symptoms include repeated yawning, sighing, and muscle twitching.

**Nux vomica:** Try this remedy for easing sleep problems that set in as a result of living in the fast lane. Symptoms include tension in muscles that refuse to relax at night, an alert mind that refuses to switch off, and a tendency to fall into a sound sleep just before the alarm goes off. Additional triggers include relying on too much caffeine to keep going during the day, and alcohol to unwind at night.

**TIP:** MAKE SURE YOUR BEDROOM IS CONDUCIVE TO SLEEP
Choose curtains or blinds that block out light adequately, ventilate the room so that it feels fresh but not too chilly or hot, and minimize noise as much as possible. Above all else, avoid the temptation to watch television when in bed.

## HERBALISM

 Once any underlying medical conditions that may cause insomnia have been ruled out, a variety of herbal remedies can be used to improve sleep quality. Herbal medicines that are used to treat insomnia work by generally relaxing and calming the person so that he or she can reach a state that is conducive to sleep. Ideally, begin "preparing" for sleep 30–45 minutes before bed by taking calming herbs while sitting and reading, taking a bath, or doing deep breathing exercises.

**Relaxing herbal formula:** Lavender is a gentle sedative that is aromatic and cooling. Lavender flowers have antispasmodic, carminative, nervine, and anti-inflammatory properties. Oat seeds nourish and calm the body and spirit. They contain a variety of minerals that can improve the function of the nervous system, especially in times of exhaustion. Valerian will soothe and ground one's energy with its sweet and earthy flavor, and is especially helpful if you are restless and irritated. Chamomile is excellent for individuals who are sensitive, restless, and irritable, making it a wonderful herb for fussy children. Chamomile's slightly sweet flowers will also soothe digestion and are mild sedatives. Catnip will also sedate and soothe. It is excellent for relieving restlessness and insomnia related to colds and flu, and is safe for use by children. Create a soothing tea or tincture by combining equal parts of each herb in dried or tincture form. Drink 2–3 cups of an infusion make from 1 tbsp of the combined herbs per cup of water before bed, or take 5–10 ml of a combined tincture 30 minutes before bedtime.

# NICOTINE WITHDRAWAL

## DIAGNOSIS

Quitting smoking can reduce your risk of serious life-threatening diseases and increase your life expectancy. Those who decide to give up smoking, however, face two challenges: breaking the habit of smoking and overcoming the addiction to nicotine. When you smoke, nicotine moves into the small blood vessels around your lungs, and from there it travels to your brain and the rest of your body. Nicotine contains various chemicals that have a stimulating effect on the body, releasing good feelings that can become addictive. When someone stops smoking, the body goes through nicotine withdrawal, in which case you experience severe nicotine cravings.

Nicotine withdrawal is usually the worst in the first 24–48 hours of quitting. Although the physical withdrawal from nicotine is a temporary condition, it can cause serious discomfort while it lasts. As well as craving cigarettes, you may experience irritability and anxiety, difficulty concentrating, increased appetite, restlessness, coughing, and dizziness. Most people experience some symptoms but rarely all. Symptoms gradually decline in intensity over time, and the worst tend to be over within a couple of weeks.

## SYMPTOMS

- Cravings for cigarettes
- Irritability and impatience
- Change to sleeping patterns, including insomnia
- Fatigue
- Poor concentration
- Hunger pangs
- Withdrawal cough
- Constipation

## TREATMENT GOAL

There is a range of products that can support those trying to quit smoking. Conventional and complementary therapies can also provide support, and provide advice on coping techniques to help you deal with symptoms and overcome cravings.

## CONVENTIONAL MEDICINE

Conventional treatment of nicotine withdrawal primarily involves nicotine replacement to gradually phase it out of the patient's system.

**Nicotine replacement:** Nicotine gum, patches, and lozenges are available to support those trying to give up smoking. They are available over the counter, and the specific instructions of each product should be followed. A nicotine inhaler is also available by prescription.

**Modifying behavior:** The above products encourage patients to taper their doses of nicotine, and this can be supported by replacing smoking behavior with a healthier option. For example, if cigarette breaks were taken as a means of stress reduction and getting away from a hectic environment, then leaving the environment, chewing on a piece of nicotine gum, and practicing deep breathing is a good replacement therapy. Eventually, as the nicotine gum dose is tapered, breaks can be taken for deep breathing only. Several instructional audio tapes are available commercially on breathing and meditation.

**Medication:** Buprion (Zyban™) is available to minimize the side effects of depression linked to nicotine withdrawal. Medication can also decrease cravings and may be used with nicotine patches while nicotine is being gradually phased out of the system. A newer medication, verenicline (Chantrix™), has recently been released. This decreases the pleasure response obtained from cigarettes by blocking nicotine receptors.

**Other therapies:** Hypnosis and acupuncture both have specific treatments for supporting those quitting smoking that are very effective in some people.

## TRADITIONAL CHINESE MEDICINE

**Herbs:** Mix 10 g of Chai Hu (hare's ear root), 12 g of Bai Shao (white peony), 12 g of Bai Zhu (white atractylodes rhizome), 15 g of Fuling (poria), 5 g of Bo He (field mint), 12 g of Dang Gui (Chinese angelica), 5 g of Gan Cao (licorice), and 12 g of Zi Su Zi (perilla hips). Place these herbs in a ceramic pot and add 3½ cups of water. Bring the mixture to a boil and simmer for 30 minutes. Strain and drink 1 cup twice a day for three to seven days.

**Acupuncture:** An experienced practitioner will recommend having 30-minute sessions once or twice a week. The duration of the treatment will depend on the individual. You may stop smoking immediately or you may stop gradually, but treatment may help you to control your nicotine cravings.

**Acupressure:** Pressing the Nei Guan and Tai Yang points may help to calm the spirit and reduce the craving. The Tai Yang point is situated at the temple in the depression between the lateral end of the eyebrow and the eyelid. The Nei Guan point is in the center of the wrist on the palm side, about 2 inches above the crease.

**Diet:** Detoxifying foods (which clean heat) are recommended to help with nicotine withdrawal. These foods include purslane, mung beans, wild chrysanthemum flowers, crab, and honeysuckle flowers. Fruits such as pears, cranberries, blueberries, and bananas are also helpful, as are red beans and bamboo shoots. Avoid foods that are rich and fatty, as they have dry and warm properties.

## NATUROPATHY

**Diet:** Blood sugar levels drop in many people when they first quit smoking, contributing to many side effects such as headaches, dizziness, and an inability to concentrate. Blood sugar can be controlled through your diet to help decrease many of these symptoms. Eat a protein product every two to three hours to keep your blood sugar levels from dropping, keep your metabolism strong, and prevent you from gaining weight. Smokers also tend to have multiple nutritional deficiencies, which can also be rectified by following a whole food diet that includes whole grains, lean meats, and fresh organic vegetables and fruits. Drink an 8 oz glass of freshly squeezed orange juice every two to three hours for the first four to five days after quitting smoking. This will keep blood sugar from dropping, will clear nicotine out of your body, and provide a good amount of vitamin C, which is commonly depleted in smokers. However, do not drink orange juice if you are using a nicotine patch or gum, because you want to keep nicotine in your body. Other foods that are high in vitamin C include citrus fruits and juices, broccoli, peppers, strawberries, collard greens, mangoes, onions, radishes, and avocados.

**Supplements:** A high-quality multivitamin/multimineral will provide your body with some of the nutrients depleted by smoking (consult a practitioner about a good-quality product). This, combined with a good diet, will help you minimize the fatigue that can often occur during nicotine withdrawal. Follow the instructions on the label. Antioxidants should be taken to help the body rid cells of free radicals, which can damage healthy tissue and eventually cause more harm. Vitamin C (taken at 2,000–4,000 mg a day in divided doses), alpha lipoic acid (100–200 mg a day), coenzyme Q10 (60–100 mg a day), and vitamin E (400 IU a day) are additional supplements that may be helpful. N-acetyl cysteine (NAC) also helps to detoxify the body and rejuvenate the lungs. Take 500–1,000 mg a day. Also take 10–20 mg a day of zinc, which is another nutrient that is heavily depleted in smokers, along with 4 g of fish oils a day.

**Herbs:** Valerian, skullcap, passionflower, and oat berries help calm the nervous system and decrease irritability. A tincture combining these herbs may help this purpose. Combine ½ tsp of valerian rhizome, ½ tsp of skullcap leaves, 1 tsp of fresh oat berries, and ½ tsp of passionflower in tincture form and take 1 dropper (60 drops) two to three times a day. Those with serious health conditions, or who are taking prescription drugs for mood or neurological disorders, should consult a qualified professional before taking valerian. Kava is a herb that is used widely to treat nervous anxiety, tension, agitation, and insomnia, all of which are common symptoms in those suffering from nicotine withdrawal. A typical dosage of kava when used for treatment of anxiety is 300 mg a day of a product standardized to contain 70% kavalactones. However, it is best to take this herb under the supervision of a physician, and you should not take pharmaceutical tranquilizers while taking kava. Chamomile calms the nervous and digestive systems. Make a tea by pouring boiling water over 2–3 heaped tsp of flowers and let them steep for 10 minutes. Chamomile tinctures and pills should be taken according to the directions on the label. An alcoholic tincture may be the most potent form for internal use. Lemon balm can also be taken orally for its calming effect. The standard dose is 1.5–4.5 g of dried herb daily; extracts and tinctures should be taken according to instructions on the label. Ginkgo, which brings blood and oxygen to the brain, can be taken in capsule form at a dose of 40–80 mg three times daily, or as a 50:1 extract standardized to contain 24% ginkgo-flavone glycosides. Dandelion root and milk thistle will help protect your liver from toxins and strengthen the liver to rid toxic chemicals due to smoking. A typical dosage of dandelion root is 2–8 g three times daily of dried root, 250 mg three to four times daily of a 5:1 extract, or 5–10 ml three times daily of a 1:5 tincture in 45% alcohol. The standard dosage of milk thistle is 200 mg two to three times a day of an extract standardized to contain 70% silymarin, or 1–2 ml of a tincture a day.

**Exercise:** This is perhaps the safest and most effective method of managing stress, avoiding weight gain, and easing nicotine withdrawal. Cardiovascular exercise combined with calming exercise such as walking several times per week can be very beneficial. Exercise reduces edginess and improves circulation. It also releases endorphins, the "feel good" hormones. So, when the urge to smoke strikes, go for a run, lift weights, or go for a walk.

**Stress-reduction techniques:** Mind-body breathing exercises, physical exercise, yoga, T'ai chi, self-hypnosis, massage, meditation, and biofeedback are just some of the stress reduction techniques used to treat anxiety due to nicotine withdrawal. Try different techniques and determine which routine you can stick with even when your schedule becomes hectic.

## HOMEOPATHY

Homeopathic treatment can help to significantly ease irritability and mood swings, which are symptoms of nicotine withdrawal. However, for the best results, treatment should be administered by an experienced practitioner, who will prescribe to get your whole system into a state of optimum balance and health. The remedies outlined below can help ease more acute episodes of distress and irritability that withdrawal from nicotine can trigger.

**Nux vomica:** This remedy has the potential to detox the body, helping to ease symptoms of nausea, disturbed sleep, and constipation. It can be particularly helpful to those who rely on stimulants (such as caffeine and recreational drugs) to keep going, and sedatives (such as alcohol and conventional drugs) to relax. Symptoms include irritability and an emotional short fuse, and sufferers tend to feel worse after waking, but improve as the day goes on.

**Tabacum:** Symptoms of trembling and dizziness that are associated with nicotine withdrawal may respond well to this remedy. Additional symptoms include sweating and nausea, and an unpleasant amount of saliva produced by the salivary glands. Patients feel indifferent and lethargic, and are unable to concentrate. A stubborn constipation may also contribute to an overall feeling of toxicity.

**Chamomilla:** If frustration and irritability trigger tantrums that feel out of control, use Chamomilla. You may get hot and bothered as a result of anger, and pace around the room feeling beside yourself with tension. One cheek often looks flushed and red.

**Ignatia:** If twitchiness and mood swings are associated with nicotine withdrawal, use Ignatia. When under stress, sufferers tend to sigh a lot and brood on negative thoughts. Headaches that set in as a result of withdrawal from tobacco may also respond well to this remedy. Symptoms include lots of yawning, and possibly vomiting in response to a sharp pain at the side of the head.

## HERBALISM

Herbs can support the whole body and mitigate some of the symptoms associated with quitting smoking. Herbs should be used in addition to conventional pharmaceuticals, behavioral modification, acupuncture, and psychological approaches.

**Sedative herbs:** The anxiety associated with nicotine withdrawal can be calmed by using any of the herbs recommended to treat anxiety (p. 828), panic attacks (p. 870), and insomnia (p. 859). Drinking a calming tea of hops, skullcap, passion flower, or chamomile when there is an intense urge to smoke can provide calming substances and a healthier substitute for cigarettes. You can also take valerian capsules before bed to help relieve insomnia associated with nicotine withdrawal, and its effects could linger enough to help ease anxiety during the day.

**Herbal tonics:** For many people, nicotine withdrawal can cause a variety of symptoms that affect many different body systems. In such situations, it is useful to use tonics or adaptogens, plants that are known for their ability to affect the whole body, probably because of their hormone-producing, antioxidant, or anti-inflammatory effects. Common tonics are Asian or Korean ginseng, American ginseng, eleuthero, rhodiola, and ashwaganda. The ginsengs are often very expensive and as such can be subject to adulteration by other, cheaper plants. For this reason, many experts recommend using standardized extracts of ginseng, or buying ginseng products only from reputable suppliers. A standardized extract of Asian ginseng, G115, has been studied extensively and is generally dosed at 100–200 mg a day. It can be purchased in most stores or pharmacies that sell herbal medicines. The nuances involved in choosing an adaptogen are best resolved by a medical herbalist. For example, for people who are going through nicotine withdrawal, Asian ginseng might be a good choice (see Post-Traumatic Stress Disorder for more information on Asian ginseng, p. 875). For others, a slightly more calming tonic such as American ginseng or rhodolia might be more suitable. As mentioned above, check with a medical herbalist to determine which herbs will be most useful for your specific condition.

# PANIC ATTACKS

## DIAGNOSIS

Panic attacks are feelings of intense fear and anxiety that come on without any warning, and often have no apparent trigger. They result from an exaggeration of the body's normal response to fear, stress, or excitement. When faced with a situation perceived as a threat, the body gears itself up for danger by producing adrenaline, known as the "fight or flight" hormone. When adrenaline floods into your body, muscles tense up, breathing becomes faster, the heart pumps harder, you sweat more, digestion slows, and salivary glands dry up, causing a dry mouth. Panic attacks can be very frightening experiences.

In some people, attacks are linked to fear about an illness, a major life change, or being in a crowd or a confined space. In others, panic attacks are associated with extreme excitement. They tend to come on suddenly, generally last between 5 and 10 minutes, and can occur several times a day. Sometimes, however, people will experience one panic attack and never have another one again.

## SYMPTOMS

- Feeling terrified, tense, and anxious
- Feeling detached, both from the body and surroundings
- Fear of dying or going mad
- Feeling out of control
- Feeling unable to breathe
- Rapid breathing
- Pounding heartbeat and pains in the chest
- Sweating
- Feeling faint, dizzy, or nauseous
- Tingling or numbness in the extremities
- Alternating sensations of being too hot or cold
- Weak bladder

## TREATMENT GOAL

Treatment involves identifying triggers of panic attacks and confronting the emotional issues behind them. Coping strategies can also be developed to prevent attacks from occurring, or to lessen their severity.

## CONVENTIONAL MEDICINE

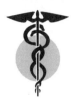

The first step is to make sure that an underlying illness is not contributing to panic attacks. Specifically, hyperthyroidism (see p. 567) can cause anxiety and panic. Drug abuse and heavy alcohol consumption can also lead to panic disorders, during active use or withdrawal. Some over-the-counter medications may also contribute to panic attacks. Consult a doctor to rule out these conditions.

**Cognitive behavioral therapy:** Most people benefit from cognitive behavioural therapy, which involves exposing the affected person to a feared situation, first in the imagination and then in reality, until he or she can tolerate the situation without symptoms. This should be conducted by a psychiatrist or counselor, and can be used in conjunction with medication. Psychodynamic psychotherapy is another treatment that can be offered by a psychiatrist or a counselor. It is based on the concept that mental processes outside of conscious awareness contribute to the panic attack and that dealing with these alleviates panic episodes.

**Medication:** Selective serotonin reuptake inhibitors (SSRIs) can be used to treat panic and depression. Escitalopram (Lexapro®) seems to be one of the best for helping with anxiety. Tricyclic antidepressants are also used, and benzodiazepines can be used as a secondary treatments. They are addictive but highly effective and sometimes necessary for treating severe panic.

**Complications:** Treatment programs should take into account co-existing diseases such as cardiac or respiratory illnesses. In these cases, a panic disorder may result in serious secondary damage during a full-blown attack. A strong therapeutic plan should be on hand to treat episodes of panic.

## TRADITIONAL CHINESE MEDICINE

**Herbs:** The raw herbs listed below are available from Chinese pharmacies or online. To prepare a formula, place the herbs in a ceramic or glass pot and add 3 cups of water. Bring the ingredients to a boil and simmer for 30 minutes. Strain the liquid and drink 1 cup twice a day.

• To treat Qi stagnation: This formula can regulate energy flow in the body to help patients who have panic attacks, are unable to think clearly, and have stiff facial expressions. Mix 12 g of Fa Ben Xia (pinellia rhizome), 10 g of Hou Po (magnolia bark), 15 g of Fuling (poria), 12 g of Zi Su Gen (perilla), 6 g of fresh ginger, and six pieces of Da Zhao (Chinese jujube).

• To nourish and tonify the heart, spleen, and kidney: This formula can help those who suffer from panic attacks associated with fatigue, insomnia, excessive sleeping, diminished memory, or loss of appetite. Mix 10 g of ginseng, 15 g of Bai Zhu (white atractylodes rhizome), 15 g of Fuling (poria), 12 g of Yuan Zhi (Chinese senega root), 12 g of Dang Gui (Chinese angelica root), 12 g of Long Yan Rou (longan), 15 g of Shu Di Huang (Chinese foxglove cooked in wine), 12 g of Mai Men Dong (ophiopogon tuber), and 5 g of Gan Cao (licorice).

**Acupuncture:** It is helpful to have a regular series of treatments before the onset of a panic attack. Acupuncture will help resolve the underlying causes of the condition.

**Acupressure:** Press the Nei Guan and Tai Yang points while having a panic attack to help calm down the spirit, and reduce the sensation of panic. The Tai Yang point is situated at the temple in the depression between the lateral end of the eyebrow and the eyelid. The Nei Guan point is in the center of the wrist on the palm side, about 2 inches above the crease.

**Diet:** Eat food that is nourishing to the spleen, kidney, and blood, such as beef, polished rice, sweet potatoes, potatoes, string beans, wheat, red beans, black beans, spinach, fish, carrots, radishes, and black sesame seeds. Foods that have a calming effect such as chamomile tea, peppermint, rice porridge, pears, and mandarin oranges are also recommended. Avoid hot, spicy food, such as chilli peppers and garlic.

## NATUROPATHY

**Breathing exercises:** Deep breathing relaxes the mind, calms the nervous system, and improves mental focus and energy. Deep breathing requires imitating the breathing patterns of a child—they breath from the belly not the chest. To deep breath properly, find a comfortable, quiet area. Stand with your knees slightly bent or sit straight with your buttocks touching the back of your seat. Breath in through your nose to a count of five, hold for two seconds, and exhale to a count of five. While breathing in, your stomach, rather than your chest, should expand outward. When breathing out, your stomach should flatten.

**Bach flower remedies:** The Bach flower remedies are a type of "vibrational, or energy medicine," developed in the 1920s by Edward Bach, an English doctor and homeopath. Because Bach flower remedies do not contain any of the original substance used, only its "vibrational pattern," they are considered to be different from homeopathic remedies (which contain minute amounts of the original substance). The most common types of remedies for panic attacks include cherry plum (to treat panic with loss of self-control), aspen (to treat vague, spooky fear that is not directed at anything specific), red chestnut (to treat fear for another's safety), star of Bethlehem (to ease fear related to a past trauma), and larch (to treat related issues such as lack of confidence).

**Relaxation movements:** T'ai chi is a form of stress reduction and exercise that involves specific body movements and deep breathing. Yoga can also help with relaxation and stress reduction. It primarily involves deep breathing, stretches, and meditation.

---

**TIP: DRINK A HERBAL TEA**

Mix ½ oz each of dried lavender, oats, linden flower, catnip, and lemon balm. Use 4 tsp of this mixture per quart of boiling water. Pour the water over the herbs and steep for about 10 minutes. Strain and drink while the tea is still warm. You can drink up to 6 cups of this drink per day after meals.

---

## HOMEOPATHY

The following remedies can help ease symptoms of panic, stress, and anxiety that develop in response to an obvious trigger, such as giving a presentation, a job interview, a first date, or exams. Established, severe, and recurrent panic attacks are best treated by an experienced homeopathic practitioner.

**Phosphorus:** If you experience "free-floating" panicky feelings that attach themselves to any focus of anxiety, use phosphorus. Feeling tense and panicky can lead to exhaustion, but may be relieved by sympathy and reassurance. Feelings of anxious panic are especially noticeable in the early evening.

**Aconite:** If feelings of panic sweep up quickly and dramatically, causing a great deal of restlessness, shaking, and trembling, try Aconite. This is a particularly appropriate remedy for feelings of distress and panic that are associated with witnessing or being involved in an upsetting or traumatic event. Symptoms are often at their most intense and distressing when you wake up.

**Argentum nit:** If panic develops in connection with anticipatory anxiety, and is associated with mental and emotional restlessness that causes you to talk incessantly, use Argentum nit. Symptoms include palpitations and trembling, and a craving for sweet things. The stomach is also likely to be very upset and be affected by diarrhea.

**Gelsemium:** This remedy is also a suitable choice to treat panic attacks associated with anticipatory nerves, especially if they cause you to become withdrawn, brooding, and quiet. Symptoms tend to build slowly and gradually, and become more intense as the stressful event gets closer, making you feel exhausted, drained, weak, and shaky.

**Lycopodium:** This is an appropriate remedy for those who are able to hide panicky, anxious feelings well and appear to be confident and in control under stress. However, there tends to be strong feelings of anxiety and tension in the stomach, causing acid to wash up into the throat when belching. Feelings of tension and pain also lead to alternating bouts of diarrhea and constipation, as well bloating and loud rumbling and gurgling sounds in the belly.

## HERBALISM

There are many herbs that can be useful for calming symptoms associated with panic attacks, including anxiety and an increased heart rate. In addition to the remedies below, any of the anti-anxiety, sedative, or relaxing herbs recommended in Anxiety (p. 828), Insomnia (p. 859), Fears and Phobias (p. 850), and Hyperactivity (p. 855) may be useful.

**Passionflower:** This herb is used to calm many types of nervous hyperactivity, including panic attacks. It is available in capsule form, as a tincture, or as raw herbs that can be infused to make a tea. The recommended dose of passionflower varies, depending on the person and the severity of symptoms, and it may take several weeks before overall anxiety levels have improved and the frequency of panic attacks have lessened. Capsules are generally dosed at ½–1 g, tinctures at ½–2 ml, and a tea can be made from 1–2 g; all forms should be taken three times daily. Some people feel too sedated when taking passionflower, or any of the other herbs in this section. Be cautious if you are also taking psychoactive medications such as antidepressant medications, as these can increase the effect of passionflower.

**Kava kava:** This herb is used to relieve insomnia, stress, and anxiety, and can be useful for panic attacks. Boil 1 tsp of root per cup and drink, or take 30 drops of 1:1 tincture, twice daily, but only under the guidance of a medical herbalist because of recent reports of liver toxicity in certain individuals.

# POST-TRAUMATIC STRESS DISORDER

## DIAGNOSIS

The term post-traumatic stress disorder (PTSD) is used to describe a range of psychological symptoms that may result from experiencing or witnessing a traumatic or life-threatening event, such as a natural disaster or military combat. Other incidents that can trigger this disorder include road accidents, muggings, and sexual or physical assaults. It can also occasionally follow a particularly difficult childbirth. Most survivors of trauma will go on to live normal lives once time has passed, but for others, just hearing news of shattering events can have a lasting impact. This highlights the fact that people who have not been directly involved in a trauma may still experience high levels of distress. Sufferers may relive events through flashbacks or nightmares, and have difficulty sleeping as a result. Those with PTSD feel estranged or detached from those around them.

## SYMPTOMS

- Feeling numb
- Emotional and physical reactions
- Changes in behavior
- Nightmares
- Intense distress when reminded of the trauma
- Easily startled
- Disturbed sleep patterns
- Feeling irritable and aggressive
- Poor concentration
- Feeling guilty, as though responsible for the event
- Avoiding memories
- Feeling detached
- Feeling there is no point in planning for the future

## TREATMENT GOAL

It can be very helpful for people to share their experiences with others who have been through similar problems. Treatment involves psychological therapy to come to terms with causes, and restore quality of life.

## CONVENTIONAL MEDICINE

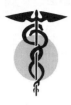

**Psychotherapy:** The primary treatment for PTSD is psychotherapy. Specific techniques include anxiety and stress management with relaxation techniques, cognitive behavioral and exposure therapy (which involves exposing the affected person to a feared situation, first in the imagination and then in reality, until he or she can tolerate the situation without symptoms), group therapy, education, and play therapy for children.

**EMDR:** A technique known as eye movement desensitization and reprocessing (EMDR) is relatively new and promising. In this technique, a person focuses on the therapist's finger movement while visualizing the traumatic event. The goal is to maintain a deep state of relaxation while working through a traumatic event.

**Lifestyle modifications:** Avoid drugs and alcohol, as many people with PTSD have concomitant substance abuse disorder. A healthy diet and good nutrition also support other behavioral and medication therapies.

**Medication:** Selective serotonin reuptake inhibitors (SSRI), specifically Paxil® and Zoloft®, are used to treat this condition. Effexor®, another SSRI, has also been used for PTSD. Serotonin has a calming effect on the body and reduces feelings of aggression and anxiety. Anti-anxiety medication such as BuSpar® and benzodiazepines have also been used to treat PTSD.

## TRADITIONAL CHINESE MEDICINE

**Herbs:** The following formula can reduce the stress to your liver, which, according to traditional Chinese medicine, is the organ that is most sensitive to traumatic stress. Mix 12 g of Chai Hu (hare's ear root), 15 g of Bai Shao (white peony), 12 g of Dang Gui (Chinese angelica root), 8 g of Bo He (field mint), 15 g of Bai Zhu (white atractylodes rhizome), 12 g of Yu Jin (turmeric tuber), 12 g of Xiang Fu (nut grass rhizome), 12 g of Long Yan Rou (longan), and 8 g of Gan Cao (licorice). To prepare the formula, place the herbs in a glass or ceramic pot and add 3 cups of water. Bring the mixture to a boil and simmer the ingredients for 30 minutes. Strain and drink 1 cup twice a day. These herbs are available from Chinese pharmacies or online.

**Acupuncture:** Regular treatments can be useful. Sessions once or twice a week are recommended, starting with one full course of 12 sessions. Further courses will be determined as progress is monitored.

**Acupressure:** Press the Shen Men, Hegu, Tai Yang, and Feng Chi points with moderate to heavy pressure for one minute and repeat. These points should be pressed when you feel an episode coming on. The Shen Men point is located on the inside of the wrist, just above the crease in the first depression at the base of the thumb. The Hegu point is located on the back of the hand in the depression between the thumb and first finger. The Tai Yang point is situated at the temple in the depression between the lateral end of the eyebrow and the eyelid. The Feng Chi point is at the back of the head at the base of the skull, about 2 inches from the center point.

**Diet:** Food that is calming and good for the liver, heart, and kidney is recommended, including chives, duck, plums, grapes, tangerines, egg yolk, celery, rice porridge, persimmon, adzuki beans, watermelon, black soybeans, lychees, and hawthorn fruit. Eat foods that have a calming effect and help you to sleep, such as chamomile tea, peppermint, pears, and mandarin oranges. Also eat plenty of fresh vegetables to keep the bowel movements regular. Foods that nourish the blood, such as black sesame seeds, red beans, black beans, spinach, fish, radishes, and carrots, will also help. In addition, foods that are cooling such as green vegetables, tofu, and Chinese jujube dates can be added to your diet. Hot and spicy foods should be avoided.

## NATUROPATHY

 There are no natural cures for PTSD, but there are some natural recommendations that may help ease some of the symptoms of the condition, such as general restlessness, insomnia, aggressiveness, and depression.

**Diet:** Keep your blood sugar levels balanced by eating small, frequent meals throughout the day. Make sure to eat only when you are calm, however, as eating while depressed or angry may worsen symptoms. Include whole grains such as oats, quinoa, or brown rice with every meal. These foods contain high levels of B vitamins and fiber, and increase your body's ability to make serotonin (neurotransmitters have a calming effect on the body and ease aggression and anxiety). The B-vitamins are calming to the nervous system and the fiber keeps your bowels movements regular. Calcium and magnesium also produce a calming effect. Sea vegetables, green leafy vegetables, nuts, and yogurt are good sources of these nutrients. Caffeine, refined sugars, and alcohol can make symptoms worse and should be avoided.

**Supplements:** 5-hydroxytryptophan (5-HTP) increases serotonin levels, which have a calming effect on the body. Take 50–100 mg two to three times daily, but do not take 5-HTP if you are on anti-depressant medications. Taking 500 mg of calcium and 250 mg of magnesium will also help calm the nervous system. Chromium can be taken at a dose of

200 mcg twice a day to help balance blood sugar. Those who suffer from PTSD often have symptoms that inhibit the production of digestive juices. Betaine hydrochloride supports stomach acid levels and helps with digestion. Take one to two capsules with each meal. Digestive enzymes also help your body to digest food more effectively, reducing irritation. The enzymes include lipases that digest fat, proteases that digest proteins, and amylases that digest starch. Take 2 capsules or tablets of a full spectrum enzyme product with each meal.

**Herbs:** Kava is an herb that is used widely in Europe to treat nervous anxiety, tension, agitation, and insomnia. Take 200–250 mg twice a day, but do not take pharmaceutical tranquilizers while taking kava. It is best to take this herb under the supervision of a doctor. Valerian is an herbal tranquilizer that is best known as a remedy for insomnia. It calms the nervous system, balances mood swings, and is not habit forming. Take 300 mg in capsule form or 0.5–1.0 ml of a tincture two to three times a day. People with serious health conditions, or who are taking prescription drugs for mood or neurological disorders, should consult a qualified professional before taking valerian. Passionflower relaxes the nerves and can be used during the day without causing drowsiness. Take 250 mg of a capsule or 0.5 ml of tincture three times a day. Lemon balm can be taken for its calming effect to help reduce anxiety levels. The standard oral dose is 1.5–4.5 g of dried herb daily. Extracts and tinctures should be taken according to instruction on the label.

**Manage stress:** Regular exercise, particularly cardiovascular activity combined with calming exercises, such as walking, can help you manage your stress levels. Massage therapy, shiatsu, and other forms of bodywork can also relax muscle tension, relieve stress, and improve sleep.

## HOMEOPATHY

Ideally, this condition requires a combination of professional homeopathic treatment and psychological support. However, the most appropriately selected of the following remedies can provide helpful temporary relief at an acute level while seeking medical help.

**Aconite:** This remedy can help to relieve feelings of terror or panic that are triggered by witnessing or being involved in a traumatic incident, or receiving very bad news. Symptoms such as trembling, breathlessness, and hyperventilation develop violently and rapidly, with feelings of anxiety and fear are so strong that sufferers are convinced they are about to die. Patients may also experience disturbed sleep, or go to sleep feeling fine, but wake up in the night feeling extremely anxious and fearful.

**Ignatia:** To temporarily relieve a strong emotional reaction to an upsetting or traumatic event, try Ignatia. Classic symptoms include heightened emotions, and patients alternate between laughing and crying. Sighing and sobbing are also prevalent, and there is an associated irritability and a desire to be alone to reflect on one's feelings. This remedy is particularly suitable for providing emotional support for those who are grieving and coping with the early stages of loss.

**Arnica:** If you are in denial about an emotional and/or physical shock, try Arnica. Patients assert that everything is all right and reject rather than accept help and support.

## HERBALISM

 Herbs can help with some of the symptoms of this disorder while more definitive treatments, such as special psychotherapeutic therapies, are pursued. For example, any of the herbal hypnotics (see Insomnia, p. 859) would be effective to help people suffering from PTSD that affects sleep.

**Tonics:** Herbal tonics, also called adaptogens, are often used to help strengthen the whole body and make it more resistant to the anxiety and overall stress of this disorder. Common tonics are Asian or Korean ginseng, American ginseng, eleuthero (also called Siberian ginseng), and ashwaganda. Most herbal tonics have a variety of effects on several different body systems. For example, they may act as an anti-inflammatory and antioxidant, and affect hormones such as cortisol secreted by the hypothalamus, pituitary, and adrenal glands. The ginsengs are often very expensive and as such can be subject to adulteration by other, cheaper plants. For this reason, many experts recommend using standardized extracts of ginseng, or buying ginseng products only from reputable suppliers. A standardized extract of Asian ginseng, G115, has been studied extensively in medical research and is generally dosed at 100–200 mg daily. It can be purchased in most stores or pharmacies that sell herbal medicines. A tincture of various herbal tonics is often dosed at 60–180 drops (1–3 droppers full) daily. Water-based infusions or decoctions of these tonics may be effective, though many of the important phytochemicals are not very soluble in water; standardized extracts and alcohol or glycerin tinctures are usually the most effective forms. When taking Asian ginseng, the conventional recommendation is to take the herbal tonic daily for three weeks, followed by one week of a ginseng "holiday," and repeated as necessary. Asian ginseng may cause a decrease in blood sugar, so people with diabetes who are taking oral hypoglycemic medication or insulin should be careful. Also, Asian ginseng may either raise or lower blood pressure, so people with blood pressure abnormalities should monitor their blood pressure closely when beginning ginseng therapy.

# SEASONAL AFFECTIVE DISORDER (SAD)

## DIAGNOSIS

Seasonal affective disorder (SAD) is a condition where sufferers experience seasonal changes of mood and behavior, such as depression. During the winter months, the change in the quality and quantity of light, specifically fewer daylight hours, has an effect on the outlook of some people. The exact causes of SAD are still unclear. Most research looks at the effect of light on the brain. When light hits the eye, particularly the retina, messages are passed to the hypothalamus gland, which releases serotonin and melatonin, which are neurotransmitters that control sleep patterns, appetite, libido, body temperature, mood, and energy levels. If we are not exposed to enough light, these functions slow down, leading to symptoms of fatigue, disturbed sleep, an inability to concentrate, and low libido. Around 20% of cases are fairly mild (known as the "winter blues," or sub-syndromal SAD), but 2–5% of cases are severe, and patients are unable to function without treatment.

## SYMPTOMS

- Lethargy or fatigue
- Sleep problems
- Depression and feeling sad and low
- Overeating, especially a craving for carbohydrates
- Irritability and tension
- Concentration problems
- Loss of libido
- Feeling under the weather
- Period problems

## TREATMENT GOAL

Treatment involves developing strategies to compensate for lack of sunlight during winter months to relieve symptoms. Light therapy is the most effective treatment, and helps about 80% of patients.

## CONVENTIONAL MEDICINE

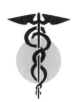

**Light therapy:** This type of treatment involves using a light box to expose patients to a full spectrum light at 2,500 lux (a measure of light intensity) or greater. Patients should receive treatment for two hours a day at 2,500 lux, or one hour a day at 10,000 lux. An alternative technique is known as dawn simulation, where a full spectrum lamp is used to create an artificial dawn for 60–90 minutes in the early morning.

**Antidepressants:** This type of medication is used in patients that are unresponsive to light therapy, or when light therapy is not acceptable to a patient. Selective serotonin reuptake inhibitors (SSRIs) are generally used. Serotonin has a calming effect on the body and reduces feelings of aggression and anxiety. No one SSRI seems to be more beneficial than another, but the atypical SSRI mirtazapine has the side effect of increasing appetite.

**Lifestyle modifications:** Eat a high-protein diet that excludes processed foods and is low sugar and caffeine. This can help to increase the effectiveness of other therapies. Winter holidays, or in extreme cases, relocation to a sunnier area may be advisable if possible. St. John's wort has been shown to be effective when taking 300 mg of a 30% hypercium extract; however, consult with a herbalist or doctor of integrative medicine before using this if you are taking other medication. Taking 2–4 g of fish oil a day also helps to combat depression. Stress management techniques, such as exercise or meditation, are also recommended as adjunct treatments.

## TRADITIONAL CHINESE MEDICINE

**Herbs:** The herbs listed below are available from Chinese pharmacies or online. To prepare a formula, place the herbs in a ceramic or glass pot and add 3 cups of water. Bring the ingredients to a boil and simmer for 30 minutes. Strain the liquid and drink 1 cup twice a day.
• To treat SAD associated with fatigue and body weakness: Mix 10 g of ginseng, 12 g of Bai Zhu (white atractylodes rhizome), 15 g of Shan Yao (Chinese yam), 12 g of Huang Qi (milk-vetch root), 15 g of Fuling (poria), and 3 g of Gan Cao (licorice).
• To treat SAD associated with kidney deficiency: Mix 12 g of Ji Shen (jilin root), 15 g of Di Huang (Chinese foxglove), 15 g of Dan Shen (salvia root), and 12 g of Shan Zhu Yu (Asiatic cornelian cherry fruit), 15 g of Shan Yao (Chinese yam), 15 g of Fuling (poria), 12 g of Sang Shen Zi (mulberry fruit-spike), and 12 g of Tu Si Zi (Chinese dodder seed).

**Acupuncture:** To treat SAD, a well-trained acupuncturist will assess the patient's general health to identify the internal condition that may be contributing to the problem. The practitioner will then treat the original or underlying condition. One course of treatment will consist of 12, 30-minute acupuncture sessions once or twice a week. The number of courses needed depends on a patient's individual progress.

**Acupressure:** Press the Hegu points with strong pressure and the Nei Guan point with moderate pressure for one to three minutes, and repeat. The Hegu point is located on the back of the hand between the thumb and first finger. The Nei Guan point is found in the center of the wrist on the palm side, about 2 inches above the crease.

**Diet:** Eat a well-balanced diet that includes fresh vegetables and fruit such as pears, cranberries, blueberries, bananas, mung beans, red beans, bamboo shoots, and purslane. Eat foods that nourish the blood such as black sesame seeds, radishes, spinach, fish, and carrots. Also, choose food that is cooling such as watermelon, green vegetables, tofu, and Chinese jujube dates. Avoid hot and spicy food, including chili peppers, garlic, and lamb.

## NATUROPATHY

Naturopathic treatment involves normalizing serotonin and melatonin levels to regulate mood and sleeping patterns.

**Supplements:** The body creates vitamin D when it is exposed to the sun, and consequently vitamin D levels in the body drop during the winter months. Taking 500–1,000 IU of vitamin D supplements daily may help to ease symptoms of SAD. Melatonin, a hormone produced in the pineal gland, plays a major role in regulating the daily biological clock, sleep patterns, and core body temperature at night. Taking low doses of melatonin (1–3 mg two to three hours before bedtime) has been shown to be effective in treating SAD. 5-hydroxytryptophan (5-HTP) is effective in increasing levels of serotonin in the body. Take 100–200 mg at night on an empty stomach or with a protein-free snack. Vitamin B6 is an important co-factor involved in the production of serotonin. Vitamin B6 deficiency should be considered when diagnosing SAD, particularly in the elderly, who may suffer from vitamin deficiencies. Take 250 mg daily early in the day. Do not take vitamin B6 within six hours of taking 5-HTP because it may interfere with the latter's conversion to serotonin. Eicosapentaenoic acid (EPA) and docosahexaenoic acid (DHA), which are omega-3 fatty acids, also play a role in the synthesis on serotonin, and there is encouraging data about their use in depressive disorders. Take 700 mg and 500 mg a day respectively.

**Herbs:** St. John's wort has been shown to be effective in treating severe depression and the depressive symptoms of SAD. Take 300–900 mg daily on an empty stomach. St. John's wort can increase sensitivity to sunlight, so minimize your exposure to the sun when taking it to avoid getting a sunburn.

**Essential oils:** Various essential oils can be used to reduce stress and promote relaxation. Use 5 drops of all or some of the oils below in a steam inhalation, add them to your bath water, or incorporate them into a massage oil, using almond or apricot oil as a base. Petitgrain oil can be uplifting, balancing, calming, and refreshing. Bergamot oil has a fresh, sweet, fruity scent. It is often described as being like sunshine in a bottle, and has an uplifting, cheerful effect. Do not apply it directly to the skin. Neroli oil has a light, sweet floral fragrance. It has a balancing tonic effect on the nervous system and can be relaxing and uplifting. It is great for treating anxiety, nervous tension, and depression. Jasmine's heady aroma is considered emotionally warming and is very useful for relieving sexual anxiety and fear.

## HOMEOPATHY

This problem appears to vary in its severity. It is estimated that 2% of the population may experience a severe form of depression, fatigue, and disturbed sleep, while an additional 20% may suffer from a less severe manifestation of the condition. Both situations can benefit from homeopathic attention and support. Since this is likely to be a recurring problem (although the severity of symptoms may vary from one year to another), it falls into a chronic category and is best treated by an experienced homeopathic practitioner. The remedies described below give an idea of some of the choices available, and are not intended to encourage self-prescribing.

**Sepia:** If symptoms of the blues are accompanied by mental, emotional, and physical exhaustion, non-existent libido, and a general sense of indifference to things that would normally stimulate and excite, Sepia may be used. Patients may feel more positive after aerobic exercise.

**Natrum mur:** If you are feeling withdrawn and depressed, and also crave carbohydrates and salt, Natrum mur may be helpful. Patients may weep when alone, since crying in front of anyone else feels humiliating. Displays of affection and sympathy are not well received as sufferers tend to keep a stiff upper lip.

## HERBALISM

 See Depression (p. 839) for more details about St. John's wort and other herbs that may be helpful in treating SAD.

**St. John's wort:** St. John's wort can be useful for treating seasonal affective disorder. It seems to be most effective for mild-to-moderate depression rather than more severe cases. St. John's wort can be taken in many forms. It is possible to purchase tinctures, standardized extracts, tablets, or the dried herb (the above-ground parts) in order to make a tea. Many products will be standardized to one of the compounds, hypericin, that was originally thought to account for much of its antidepressant activity. Most clinical trials have used an extract standardized to 0.3% hypericin dosed at 300 mg three times daily. Should you decide to use a tablet, choose one that is standardized to 0.9 mg of hypericin and take a 1.5 g tablet three times a day. For optimal effect in treating SAD, begin the daily use of St. John's wort two months before your symptoms usually start. This may be in late September or October as the amount of daylight starts to wane.

# STRESS

## DIAGNOSIS

Stress generally describes feelings of frustration, anger, or anxiety. It tends to be an inevitable component of modern living, and affects everyone from time to time. Common triggers include work, study and exams, relationship problems, financial worries, and feeling unable to cope. When we find ourselves in a stressful situation, the nervous system goes on red alert. The brain sends signals to the adrenal glands to release more adrenalin into the system. This has multiple effects on the body, causing muscles to become tense, and the heartbeat and breathing rate to speed up. This rush of adrenalin also causes energy to flow away from the digestive system, which often leads to the nagging aches and upset stomachs characteristic of stress. Stress is a normal part of everyday life, but learning how to control stress is important. Try to find ways of dealing with stress to neutralize the dangerous effects it can have on your health.

## SYMPTOMS

- Irritability
- No sense of humor and many negative thoughts
- Difficulty concentrating and memory loss
- Feeling defensive and constantly worrying
- Tightness in neck and shoulders
- Insomnia and sleep problems
- Sweating
- Breathlessness
- Loss of appetite and/or binge eating
- Stomach problems
- Constipation and/or diarrhea
- Headaches
- Cramps and spasms
- Loss of libido

## TREATMENT GOAL

Treatment involves examining your lifestyle and pinpointing any particularly stressful area. Conventional and complementary therapies can help you to develop a strategy for dealing with stress to prevent long-term problems, such as depression and other serious medical disorders.

## CONVENTIONAL MEDICINE

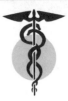

Treatment of stress involves learning techniques to modify your response to stressful situations and making lifestyle changes to reduce day-to-day stress. Stress affects the cardiac, immune, gastrointestinal, and hormonal systems greatly and, if any compromise in these areas exists, then evaluation by a healthcare professional is warranted.

**Meditation:** Formal stress reduction instruction has been initiated in several major hospitals. The most well known is Jon Kabat Zin's mindfulness based stress reduction program. This relaxation technique utilizes mindfulness meditation, which involves expanding one's consciousness to identify subtle emotions. Other forms of meditation are available, which help the mind to divert attention from problematic emotional responses and decrease mental chatter. Simple techniques such as relaxation breathing and repeating a focus word or mantra are forms of meditation that help to modify the stress response, not just while performing the meditation, but also during everyday activities. Meditation for 20 minutes a day is optimal.

**Other therapies:** Progressive muscle relaxation involves the systematic contraction and relaxation of major muscle groups, and can also be helpful for relaxation and stress reduction. Biofeedback involves the machine-based detection of tension responses, and can help a person learn to sense the physical signs of stress and modify them. Hypnosis uses verbal suggestions to relax the mind and body. A newer technique, known as Heart Math, uses heartbeat responses to emotions as a guide to reduce stress. Psychological counseling and behavior modification also have a role in the treatment of chronic stress.

**Lifestyle modifications:** Chronic stress depletes B-complex vitamins and magnesium in the body, so it is advised that you replace these through supplements during periods of stress. A practitioner who can measure adrenal hormones may also be helpful in evaluating the adrenal depletion that can occur with unremitting chronic stress. Adequate sleep and regular meals with little sugar or processed foods are mandatory during periods of stress to avoid physical side-effects. Regular exercise is one of the primary techniques to combat stress.

## TRADITIONAL CHINESE MEDICINE

**Herbs:** Mix 12 g of Chai Hu (hare's ear root), 15 g of Bai Shao (white peony), 12 g of Yu Jin (turmeric tuber), 6 g of Bo He (field mint), 12 g of Gou Ji Zi (wolfberry), 15 g of Fuling (poria), 15 g of Bai Zhu (white atractylodes rhizome), and 5 g of Gan Cao (licorice). Place the herbs in a ceramic pot and add 3 cups of water. Bring the mixture to a boil and simmer for 30 minutes. Strain the liquid and drink 1 cup twice a day. The herbs are available from Chinese pharmacies or online.

**Acupuncture:** Acupuncture is a relaxation process so is very helpful in dealing with stress. Regular treatments once a week can be useful to relieve symptoms and restore balance in the body. You may need long-term treatment depending on the severity of the condition.

**Acupressure:** To release stress, try pressing the Tai Yang points. With your eyes closed, put your thumbs on the depression at the temples. The Nei Guan point, located in the center of the wrist on the palm side, about 2 inches below the crease, can also be helpful. Each point can be pressed with moderate pressure for one to two minutes, released, and then pressed again. Repeat three to five times.

**Diet:** Eat foods that have a calming effect and help you to sleep, such as chamomile tea, peppermint, rice porridge, pears, and mandarin oranges. Eat plenty of fresh vegetables to keep bowel movements regular, and cut down on your caffeine intake. Fruits such as cranberries, blueberries, and bananas are recommended, along with mung beans, red beans, bamboo shoots, and purslane. Avoid food that is rich and fatty.

## NATUROPATHY

**Diet:** Balance your blood sugar levels by eating small meals frequently throughout the day. Unbalanced blood levels can lead to a stressed stomach or aggravate an existing condition. Include whole grains such as oats, quinoa, or brown rice with every meal. These foods contain high levels of B-vitamins and fiber, and increase your body's ability to make serotonin, which has a calming effect on the body and eases anxiety. B-vitamins are also calming to the nervous system and the fiber keeps your bowels moving. Increase your B-vitamin intake by consuming brewer's yeast, brown rice, and leafy green vegetables. Calcium and magnesium also have a calming effect on the body. Sea vegetables, green leafy vegetables, nuts, and yogurt can provide you with a good amount of these nutrients. Caffeine and refined sugars in alcohol can make symptoms worse, so avoid them. They will cause blood sugar imbalances and increase stressed stomach symptoms.

**Supplements:** 5-hydroxytryptophan (5-HTP) increases serotonin levels, to produce a calming effect in the body. Take 50–100 mg two to three times daily, but do not take 5-HTP if you are on antidepressant medications. Take 500 mg of calcium and 250 mg of magnesium a day to help calm the nervous system, and 200 mcg of chromium twice a day to help balance blood sugar. Digestive enzymes, such as lipases that digest fat, proteases that digest proteins, and amylases that digest starch, help you digest food more effectively to reduce irritation. Take two capsules or tablets of a full spectrum enzyme product with each meal. Betaine hydrochloride supports stomach acid levels and helps with digestion. Take one to two capsules with each meal. Probiotics also help digestion and prevent overgrowth of candida and other harmful microbes. Take a product containing four billion active organisms daily of Lactobacillus acidophilus and bifidus.

## HOMEOPATHY

 Stress is a complex condition. With this in mind, the advice included below is given with a view to helping ease mild stress-related symptoms that have developed recently. Severe, established problems that are related to excessive stress levels should be treated by an experienced homeopathic practitioner.

**Arnica:** If aching, tense muscles make it really difficult to get comfortable and drift off into a sound, refreshing sleep, try Arnica. It can also be especially helpful for those who have decided to combat high stress levels by going to the gym and have overdone it, making every muscle achy and sore.

**Arsenicum album:** Perfectionists and high achievers who push themselves to meet impossibly high, self-set standards can often benefit from this remedy. Symptoms include extreme restlessness at night and in the early hours of the morning, which interferes with sound sleep. When highly stressed, sufferers may become anxious about health issues, and show signs of becoming obsessive or compulsive. The digestive system is also affected by nausea and queasiness at the thought or smell of food, and diarrhea may develop when feeling uptight and tense.

**Nux vomica:** This is a classic remedy for treating stress, especially in those who have relied on poor lifestyle choices to keep the pace. Symptoms that respond well to this remedy include problems switching off mentally when trying to sleep (even though the body is tense and exhausted), tension headaches, and feeling genuinely hungover when waking up.

**TIP: USE AVENA SATIVA**
If a particularly stressful period at work and/or at home has left you feeling exhausted and strung out, take a diluted Avena sativa tincture to restore the nervous system. Consult a homeopath regarding the recommended dosage, which should be diluted in a small glass of water and taken daily for up to a month.

**Lycopodium:** If tension and stress particularly affects the stomach and gut, resulting in acidity, heartburn, and bloating, and causing you to alternate between constipation (due to tension) and diarrhea (due to anxiety), try Lycopodium. Sufferers lack confidence when highly stressed, and become domineering and sarcastic in an attempt to hide their vulnerability.

## HERBALISM

 Herbs are best used in combination with lifestyle changes to address the fundamental causes of stress in your life. Herbal medicines can serve as sedatives and calmatives to ease the symptoms of stress, help to improve sleep, and decrease anxiety. See Anxiety (p. 828) for additional recommendations.

**Herbal sedatives and calmatives:** Chamomile is a gentle and safe herb that acts as a mild sedative. One of the active constituents in the flowers, apigenin, calms nerves and relieves anxiety. Drinking an infusion made from 1 tsp of flowers per cup of water several times a day can be very helpful. Allow the flowers to steep for 10 minutes while covered to prevent the loss of important volatile oils. Alternatively, take 60–120 drops (1–2 droppers full) of an alcohol-based or glycerin tincture two to three times daily for its calming effects.

**Lemon balm and lavender:** Lemon balm and lavender are two other mild sedatives. The entire herb and leaves of lemon balm can be infused with hot water. Use 2 tsp of plant material per cup of water and drink several times a day. Use an aromatherapy distiller to spread the calming scent of lavender essential oil throughout the air. With every breath, your tension will evaporate and stress levels will ease. Lavender lotions and oils can be purchased and massaged into the temples to achieve relaxation. Be careful not to get the oil or lotion in your eyes; if you do, wash it out with water immediately.

**Tonics:** Herbal tonics, also called adaptogens, are often used to help strengthen the whole body and make it more resistant to the negative effects of stress. Common tonics are Asian or Korean ginseng, American ginseng, eleuthero, and ashwaganda. See Post-Traumatic Stress Disorder for information on their use (p. 875).

# TICS AND TWITCHES

## DIAGNOSIS

A tic is a rapid and repeated contraction of a group of muscles, which results in movement (a motor tic) or the production of a sound (a vocal tic). Motor tics usually involve the muscles of the face (especially around the eye), head, and neck, producing movements such as blinking, facial twitching, and shrugging of the shoulders. They can, however, affect other parts of the body. Common vocal tics include grunting and clearing the throat.

Tics and twitches usually develop during childhood and tend to affect boys more often that girls. As many as one in four children will develop a "transient" or "simple" tic, which subsides with age, at some point during their school years. Although most children do grow out of tics, they occasionally continue into adulthood. The cause of them is unknown, but it is thought that there is a genetic predisposition to the condition. Tics have also been linked with psychological conditions such as obsessive compulsive disorder (OCD). An extreme form manifests as Tourette's syndrome, which is characterized by multiple, dramatic tics, both motor and vocal.

## SYMPTOMS

- Repeated, uncontrollable movement of a muscle in the body, particularly the face
- Commonly manifests as repeated blinking or facial twitches
- Making sounds, such as grunting, repeatedly and uncontrollably

## TREATMENT GOAL

Most tics are mild, do not require much treatment, and usually fade with age. Conventional and complementary therapies involve identifying the cause of the movement and ruling out any complications. Psychological support and counseling may also help those with severe tics deal with the distress that can accompany this condition.

## CONVENTIONAL MEDICINE

Conventional treatment of tics primarily involves educating patients about the condition, prescribing medication if necessary, and providing psychological support.

**Medications:** Patients with mild symptoms often do not need medication to treat the condition, as it often subsides. If medications are required they usually fall into the category of sedatives and neuroleptics (antipsychotics). Haloperidol (Haldol®) is effective, but it is reserved for severe cases as it has many side effects, some of which are long-term and do not resolve when the medication is stopped. It does, however, reduce tics and obsessive behavior in 80–90% of cases. Fluphenazine is a similar medication, which can be given intramuscularly every two to three weeks. It is an antihypertensive and a milder drug, and is usually used to treat tics that accompany Tourette's syndrome or attention deficit hyperactivity disorder (ADHD). Risperidone can sometimes be used along with selective serotonin reuptake inhibitor (SSRI) drugs to reduce tics. It is a milder neuroleptic, which has side effects such as sedation. Clonazepam is a benzodiazepine (in the Valium® family) that can be used to control tics, but is addictive. Methylphenidate (Ritalin®) is another medication that can be used to control tics, and is also used to treat ADHD. It can, however, make tics worse if given in excessive doses.

**Non-drug therapies:** Psychotherapy can help to control tics, and it is important to manage any behavioral or psychological complications associated with a tic disorder. Strategies to support pharmaceutical treatment include stress reduction therapies, such as meditation. Excluding processed foods and high sugar foods from the diet is also beneficial, as are certain supplements such as magnesium aspartate, taurine, and 5-hydroxytryptophan.

## TRADITIONAL CHINESE MEDICINE

**Herbs:** Consult a Chinese medicine doctor for a herbal formula for tics and twitches. In the meantime you can try taking Chuan Xiong Cha Tiao Wan and Liu Wei Di Huang Wan herbal pills, available from Chinese pharmacies or online.

**Acupuncture:** A practitioner will perform an evaluation and make a diagnosis to determine the cause of the condition from a Chinese medicine perspective. You may be advised to have a full course of acupuncture consisting of 12 sessions to treat the underlying cause.

**Acupressure:** Press the Feng Chi, Xue Hai, and Tai Chong points. The Feng Chi points are at the back of the head at the base of the skull, about 2 inches on either side of the center point. The Xue Hai point is on the inside of the leg in the depression just above the knee. The Tai Chong point is on the sole of the foot in the depression between the first and second toe, at the base of the large toe. Press these points with the tip of the fingers for one minute. Press the Xue Hai and Tai Chong points while in a sitting position.

**Diet:** Eat foods that have a calming effect, such as chamomile tea, peppermint, rice porridge, pears, and mandarin oranges. Eat a balanced diet that includes fresh vegetables to help keep bowel movements regular.

## NATUROPATHY

**Diet:** Tics and twitches are often caused by mineral imbalances. Eat plenty of foods that contain potassium and magnesium. These minerals are needed to conduct the nerve impulses that control muscle movements. Leafy green vegetables such as spinach, parsley, and lettuce, as well as broccoli, peas, lima beans, tomatoes, and potatoes (especially potato skins) all have significant levels of potassium, as do oranges and other citrus fruits, bananas, apples, avocados, raisins, and apricots (particularly dried). Whole grains, wheat germ, seeds, and nuts are also high in potassium and magnesium. Fish such as flounder, salmon, sardines, and cod are rich in potassium, and many meats contain even more potassium than sodium, although they often have sodium added as salt. The B-vitamins are essential for the health of the nervous system, and adding nutritional yeast, whole grains, and dark green vegetables daily to your diet will provide sufficient B-complex vitamins. Niacin (vitamin B3) is especially important for the nervous system and has been effective in alleviating tics. Good sources of niacin include brown rice, peanuts, lean meats, poultry, fish, and milk. Avoid caffeine and simple sugars, which cause nervous system abnormalities.

**Supplements:** Take a multivitamin, following dosage instructions on the label, to provide your body with the nutrients necessary for a healthy nervous system (consult a practitioner about a good quality product). Essential fatty acids are also important for the development and proper nourishment of the entire nervous system. Take 500 mg of docosahexaenoic acid (DHA) from a fish oil with 100 mg of gamma-linolenic acid (GLA), which is found in evening primrose oil and blackcurrant or borage oil.

**Herbs:** Drink a tea or take a tincture of chamomile, hops, lady's slipper, passion flower, skullcap, wood betony, St. John's wort, or valerian. These herbs have a sedative effect on the nervous system. To make a tea, add 1 cup of boiling water to 1 tsp of herbs and drink, or take 20 drops of herbal tincture diluted in liquid daily. You can also take vitamin C to help the immune system and reduce stress damage to nerves.

## HOMEOPATHY

 If there is no underlying condition causing tics or twitches, and if they are not a side effect or reaction to a conventional medicine, they are most likely due to tension and stress. If symptoms have become chronic, consult an experienced homeopathic practitioner as well as a conventional physician. However, short-term or mild symptoms that develop as a result of an obvious stress trigger may be relieved by choosing the most appropriate of the homeopathic remedies below.

> **TIP:** REDUCE YOUR CAFFEINE INTAKE
> Drink no more than two small cups of coffee a day. Also watch out for "hidden" sources of caffeine, such as cola drinks.

**Nux vomica:** If nervous tics and twitches have developed in response to working and/or playing too hard, and you have been consuming too much caffeine and alcohol, and smoking cigarettes to keep up, try Nux vomica. When this remedy is indicated, sleep patterns and the digestive system are negatively affected by this lifestyle, and the degree of muscular tension present is likely to lead to tension headaches and tooth grinding from clenching the jaw at night.

**Ignatia:** If trembling and twitching is linked to feeling overwhelmingly emotional and tense, and you move quickly from bouts of sobbing to hysterical laughter when under pressure, try Ignatia. Tightness and tension of the muscles leads to constant sighing, and possibly bouts of hiccuping.

**Belladonna:** This is a remedy worth considering if muscular twitching is especially prevalent at night when trying to sleep. Symptoms include a tendency to jerk awake just as you are about to drift off to sleep, and teeth grinding.

> **TIP:** BEGIN RELAXATION THERAPY
> Take up a form of relaxation that appeals to your temperament. Potential choices include meditation, progressive muscular relaxation, autogenic training, bio-feedback, yoga, or T'ai chi.

## HERBALISM

Herbal remedies can address the spasms occurring in the muscles, as well as hyperactivity in the nerves. Also refer to Muscle Cramps (p. 663) and Anxiety (p. 828) for more information on herbs that are also useful for treating tics and twitches.

**Muscle relaxant herbs:** Cramp bark is excellent at relieving cramping, twitchy muscles. Khella is used to relieve muscle spasms. Chamomile is a wonderful herb for the relief of nervous tension and irritability, which are almost always involved in tics and twitches. Chamomile gently sedates while inhibiting inflammation and spasm in the muscles. Combine equal parts of tinctures of all these herbs and take 2–3 ml every three hours to help with tics and twitches. Use this herbal formula in addition to following an active health program of muscle stretching, moderate exercise, and good nutrition.

**Jamaican dogwood:** This herb is indicated for muscle pain and spasm combined with nervous irritability and nerve pain, making it an excellent choice to treat tics and twitches. It also demonstrates analgesic and sedative properties, relieving pain while it soothes the nerves. This herb is potentially toxic and should only be used in low doses and under the guidance of a medical herbalist. Take only 5 drops of tincture twice a day.

**Sedative herbs:** Kava root is used to relieve stress, anxiety, and spasms, and can help in cases of tics and twitching. Drink a decoction made by boiling 1 tsp of root per cup of water, or take 30 drops of 1:1 tincture twice daily. This herb should only be used under the guidance of a medical herbalist because of recent reports about liver toxicity in certain individuals.

# FIRST
# AID

# BEE AND WASP STINGS

## DIAGNOSIS

Bee and wasp stings often cause one or more red bumps that are usually itchy and sometimes painful. There is often a small hole in the middle of the sting, perhaps with the end of the stinger sticking out. Stingers are effective weapons because they deliver a venom that causes pain when injected into the skin. The pain is usually sharp to begin with and then subsides to a dull ache. The affected area may be very sensitive to the touch, even up to a few days after the sting has occurred. The body responds to stings by trying to flush the venom from the system. This often results in redness, swelling, and inflammation. The area around the sting is also likely to be very itchy.

Although they are distressing, bee and wasp stings are only serious if an allergy to insect venom exists. Bee and wasp stings are more likely to cause an allergic reaction than other kinds of insect stings. Reactions can be mild or severe, or even potentially life-threatening. Stings can also become infected if they are scratched. If a rash or swelling develops, consult a doctor.

**DANGER**: An allergic reaction can sometimes cause swelling inside the mouth. Seek immediate emergency assistance if there is any dizziness, nausea, pain in the chest, choking or wheezing, or difficulty breathing following a bee or wasp sting.

## SYMPTOMS

- Sharp needling pain, that turns into a throbbing ache
- Red, itchy skin
- Localized tenderness
- Localized swelling
- Occasionally, swelling inside the mouth, which leads to breathing difficulties

## TREATMENT GOAL

To ensure that a life-threatening allergy is not present, and resolve any symptoms of pain, itchiness, and discomfort.

## CONVENTIONAL MEDICINE

Conventional treatment involves reducing pain, and treating any allergic reactions or side effects caused by the venom.

**Remove the stinger:** If the stinger is still in the skin, gently remove it. Do not crush the stinger as doing this will release more venom from the stinger's venom sac.

**Topical treatments:** Apply an ice pack to the sting, but do not compress the affected area. A topical coolant and analgesic such as lidocaine spray may be used, and aloe vera gel can be applied to the sting to relieve the pain.

**Antihistamines:** If the area is severely swollen and itchy, diphenhydramine (Benadryl®) should be given orally. Adults should take 50 mg and children can take 1 mg per 2 lb of body weight.

**Antibiotics:** If the sting becomes infected, it may lead to cellulitis, which is the inflammation of the connective tissue underneath the skin. This is treated with antibiotics, which work against staphylococcus bacteria.

**Treating an allergic reaction:** If someone stung shows any signs of breathing difficulties or shock, they should seek emergency medical help. Patients may be given respiratory support with oxygen or a breathing mask as needed. They may be given salbuterol to treat wheezing, and an intravenous steroid such as methylprednisolone. Antihistamines, which are commonly used to treat allergy symptoms, and epinephrine, a hormone that can combat the chemicals released by the body in an allergic reaction, may also be given intravenously. Some or all of these measures may be needed depending on the severity of the reaction. Moderate allergic reactions are also treated with epinephrine, which can be given with an "epi pen" (available by prescription).

## TRADITIONAL CHINESE MEDICINE

**Herbs:** The herbs needed to make the formulas below are available from Chinese pharmacies or online.
• Jin Yin Hua tea: Mix 5 g of Jin Yin Hua (honeysuckle flower), and 3 g of Bo He (field mint) in a teapot. Add boiling water and let the herbs steep for a few minutes. Drink this tea throughout the day.

• Herbal bath: Mix 15 g of Jin Yin Hua (honeysuckle flower), and 15 g of Jing Jie (schizonepeta stem and bud). Boil these two ingredients in 5 cups of water for five minutes. Strain the liquid and add to your bathwater. Soak in this herbal bath once a day until the pain subsides.

**Acupuncture:** Treatment aims to clear the inflammation and relieve discomfort by stimulating certain meridian points. Acupuncture can also regulate a patient's circulation, and help maintain skin health.

**Acupressure:** Press the Tai Yang point at the temple in the depression between the lateral end of the eyebrow and eyelid. Also press the Hegu point, located on the back of the hand between the thumb and first finger. The Feng Chi points, found at the back of the head at the base of the skull, about 2 inches on either side of the center point, are also helpful. Press each point gently for about one minute.

**Diet:** Eat food that is gentle and strengthens the immune system, such as green vegetables, aubergines, radishes, mung beans, bitter melon, purslane, and pear. Green tea is also beneficial since it has a gentle cleansing effect. Avoid seafood, and fatty and spicy foods. Eat fresh vegetables and fruits such as cranberries, blueberries, bananas, red beans, and bamboo shoots.

## NATUROPATHY

**Diet:** Eat two to three servings of brightly colored foods, such as carrots, berries, green vegetables, or squash, a day to soothe skin irritation and inflammation. Cod, salmon, mackerel, avocados, and wheat germ are rich in omega-3 fatty acids, which help reduce inflammation. Avoid sugars, refined carbohydrates, junk food, and carbonated beverages, all of which will worsen inflammation and skin irritation.

**Supplements:** Take 1,000 mg vitamin C three times a day to help boost the immune system and reducing inflammation. Take 1,000 mg of bioflavonoids twice a day to reduce swelling and alleviate pain. Also take 500 mg of quercitin three times a day to alleviate inflammation of the skin.

**External herbal applications:** Lavender can relieve pain and itchiness and also repels insects. Rub fresh lavender leaves, tincture, or essential oil into the affected area. You can also try applying calendula ointment or cream, available widely from health stores, to the affected area twice a day to heal skin wounds and soothe irritation. Aloe vera gel also has soothing and healing properties. Break off an aloe leaf and apply the gel to the affected area, or purchase aloe vera gel from a health food or natural health store. To prevent stings from occurring, try a natural insect-repellent spray that contains one or all of the following: sweet basil, holy basil, sage, and/or thyme. This type of spray can be found in some health food stores.

> **TIP:** AVOID ATTRACTING BEES
> Avoid using fragrances, including hair spray, scented soaps, lotions, and oils, and keep soft drinks and sweet foods covered. Do not wear brightly colored clothing, particularly floral patterns. If a bee does land on you, blow on it gently to encourage it to move on without startling it.

## HOMEOPATHY

Homeopathic intervention can be of great help in treating bee or wasp stings, if an underlying allergy does not exist. If an allergic reaction does occur, immediately seek emergency conventional treatment to prevent the situation from escalating.

**Apis:** This remedy can be used to treat bee or wasp stings that show the classic symptoms of localized inflammation and swelling. The affected area is likely to be raised and look puffy, feel worse for contact with warmth in any form, and feel soothed by exposure to cool applications.

**Ledum:** If the affected area feels cold and slightly numb, but is also made more comfortable by applying cool compresses or cool bathing, try Ledum. When this remedy is indicated, the stung area is red and swollen, and a prickling sensation is felt.

**Urtica urens:** If stings trigger strong burning sensations around the edge of the affected area, use Urtica urens. There is also localized itchiness and a stitch-like discomfort that is aggravated by contact with cool air and cool bathing. This remedy can also be effective in easing lingering and itchy sensations that refuse to clear up as a result of a bee sting.

> **TIP:** USE URTICA URENS TINCTURE
> Stings that trigger short-term itchiness or a stinging sensation can be locally soothed by applying a cotton wool pad soaked in a diluted solution of Urtica urens tincture to the affected area. Apply this as often as feels soothing until the inflammation and discomfort has subsided. This treatment can be combined with taking Urtica urens.

**Borage:** The leaves of borage can be made into a poultice and applied to the site of a bee sting to calm the reaction and stop the pain, redness, and swelling. Borage is the source of omega-6 oils, which may explain why a poultice is soothing for the skin. To make a poultice you will need about 1 oz of fresh, whole leaves, or 1 oz of dried leaves (available in stores that sell herbal medicines). Place the leaves in a pot and add a few cups of hot water until the leaves are just covered. Let the leaves stand for 5–10 minutes and, once the mixture has cooled to the point that it will not burn your skin, remove the whole fresh leaves, squeeze out some of the excess liquid, and place them on the sting. Dried leaves will have to be strained before you can place a mass of wet plant material on the site of pain and inflammation. Leave the poultice in place for 10–15 minutes; it can be covered with Saran™ or similar plastic and then an elastic bandage to keep it in place if you need to move around. Unpurified, unprocessed borage should not be ingested as it contains pyrrolizidine alkaloids, which can cause liver toxicity.

**Arnica:** This is an excellent herb to use on the skin to treat bee and wasp stings. Prepare a poultice or compress of arnica flowers that are either growing wild or that you have purchased from a local herbal medicine store. Place 2–3 g of the flowers in about 150 ml of hot water and allow them to steep for 5–10 minutes. To make a poultice, allow the plant material to cool enough so that it will not burn your skin and place it on top of the affected area. To make a compress, strain the flowers, soak a clean piece of gauze or cloth in the liquid, and apply the cloth to the sting. Do not ingest arnica unless it has been made into a homeopathic form. Occasionally, dermatitis will develop with arnica, or, for that matter, any plant that is applied topically. Discontinue use if this occurs.

# BLACK EYE

## DIAGNOSIS

A black eye is caused by the rupturing of small blood vessels around the eye, which causes blood to leak into surrounding tissues and collect under the surface of the skin. This manifests as an area of red, purple, and black bruising. Bruising around the eye tends to be darker than on other parts of the body because the skin around the eye is thin. Most frequently, black eyes are caused by being hit or punched in the eye. Depending on where the blow lands, one or both eyes may be affected. A blow to the nose can also cause the tissue around the eyes to swell, as a nasal injury causes fluids to collect in the loose tissues of the eyelids. Surgical procedures to the face, such as a facelift or nose surgery, can also trigger black eyes. The majority of injuries are minor, and most black eyes will heal on their own in a few days. They can also appear after a head injury, and may be due to bleeding from a fracture at the base of the skull. Although blurred vision or difficulty opening the eyes because of swelling may occur, more serious visual problems due to black eyes are rare. If you have any double vision or see flashing lights, seek emergency medical attention.

## SYMPTOMS

- Swelling and bruising around the eye
- The skin around the eye may be broken
- The affected area becomes blue, black, or purple

## TREATMENT GOAL

To ease the pain and reduce swelling, apply a cold compress to the area as soon as possible. A pack of frozen peas wrapped in a tea towel is ideal.

## CONVENTIONAL MEDICINE

**Rest and ice:** If a black eye does not have any complications that require emergency care, the first step is to treat it with rest and ice. Apply ice to the injury as soon as possible after it occurs to constrict the blood vessels and decrease bruising, swelling, and any puffiness. Ice should be applied for 20 minutes every two hours for the first 24 hours following the injury. Do not apply ice directly to the skin, but instead wrap it in a cloth and hold it against the eye as a compress. Rest, especially from sporting activities, is also needed to avoid further injury.

**Do not use aspirin:** If you need to use medication for pain reduction, avoid using substances that cause bleeding such as aspirin.

**When should I see a doctor?** If the injury that has caused the black eye is severe, and there is possible damage to the surrounding bones, seek immediate professional help as fractures to the face and eye area can be very serious. Any change in vision also needs further evaluation.

## TRADITIONAL CHINESE MEDICINE

**Herbs:** Mix 15 g of Bai Zhu (white atractylodes rhizome), 18 g of Fuling (poria), 15 g of Mu Gua (Chinese quince fruit), 15 g of Shan Yao (Chinese yam), 12 g of Ji Shen (jilin root), and 12 g of Dan Zhu Ye (lophatherum stem and leaves). To make a decoction, place the herbs in a ceramic pot and add 3 cups of water. Bring the ingredients to a boil and simmer for 30 minutes. Strain the liquid and drink 1 cup three times a day. The herbs needed for this formula are available from Chinese pharmacies or online.

**Acupuncture:** Treatment can help by enhancing spleen and kidney energy. Consult an experienced practitioner to determine your treatment options and develop a treatment plan.

**Acupressure:** Wash your hands, close your eyes, and press the Cuan Zhu, Si Bai, Tai Yang, and Tong Zi Liao points while in a sitting position. Place your index finger gently on the Cuan Zhu point, found on the inside end of the eyebrow, apply moderate pressure for one minute, and then press the temple for one minute with your thumb. The Si Bai point is located directly under the pupil in the depression below the eye socket bone. The Tai Yang point is found at the temple in the depression between the lateral end of the eyebrow and eyelid. The Tong Zi Liao point is located about ½ inch from the outside corner of the eye. Press these points with gentle to moderate pressure.

**Diet:** Eat foods that promote circulation such as mustard greens, water spinach, towel gourd (found in Chinese groceries), mung beans, and honey. Foods that are good for the spleen and kidney are ham, potato, string beans, and sweet potato. Drinking green tea also helps.

## NATUROPATHY

**Diet:** Eating foods such as green, leafy vegetables, apples, and citrus fruits, which are rich in vitamin C, will help blood capillaries heal quickly. It is best to eat these foods raw, as vitamin C, as well as the enzymes these foods provide, are destroyed by heat. Other brightly colored foods such as peppers, berries, and carrots contain bioflavonoids, which help to heal all kinds of bruises. Flaxseed oil will help reabsorb the blood from bruises, reducing inflammation. Eat a salad of fresh, raw vegetables dressed with lemon juice and 2 tbsp of flaxseed oil daily. Salmon, walnuts, and other seeds have a similar effect. Exclude sugars, refined carbohydrates, hydrogenated oils, and trans-fatty acids found in fried foods and junk foods from your diet as they interfere with the healing process and promote inflammation.

**Supplement:** Take 1,000 mg of vitamin C three times a day to heal blood vessels and connective tissue found throughout the body. Bioflavonoids work synergistically and similarly to vitamin C, and should be taken at a dose of 500–1,000 mg three times a day. Take 50 mg of grapeseed extract twice a day to promote tissue healing, and 3,000 mg of fish oils a day to heal and decrease inflammation. Vitamin K is involved in the blood clotting process. Take 1 mg twice a day for two weeks to treat an acute bruise, and then 500 mg daily until the bruise has healed.

**Herbs:** Take 500 mg of bromelain three times a day for its natural anti-inflammatory effects. Apply compresses of fennel, chamomile, calendula blossoms, and peppermint to soothe and heal the injury.

**TIP:** USE A CLAY PACK

To reduce the swelling, apply cool, medicinal clay packs or quark packs, renewing them every half-hour. Add a few drops of horsetail tincture to the clay for an even better effect. To draw out toxins and speed up healing, alternate the clay pack with a cabbage leaf poultice.

## HOMEOPATHY

The following homeopathic first aid measures can play a positive role in gently, but efficiently, speeding up recovery from a black eye. It is, however, important that the injury is first assessed by a doctor or optometrist. If the black eye is severe, there is a risk that further complications may develop, such as damage to the eyeball, or a concussion.

**Arnica:** This remedy is generally the first choice to treat a black eye. It can promptly heal bruised tissue by promoting the swift re-absorption of blood. It also assists the body in coming to terms with the psychological shock that is involved in any accident or trauma.

**Ledum:** If Arnica helps relieve the trauma of a black eye in the first 24 hours, but then fails to help any further, Ledum may help to resolve the condition, provided, of course, that the symptoms fit. It is appropriate if there is a numb, cool sensation around the bruised area, which is temporarily soothed by the application of a cool or cold compress. Symptoms also include stabbing, tearing sensations in the bruised tissues, and a severe amount of swelling and tenderness in the area.

**Symphytum:** This is a specific remedy that is indicated for minor trauma that involves the eyeball (once, of course, a doctor has checked out the situation). Classic injuries of this kind include a blow to the eye from a tennis ball. In this sort of situation, this is the remedy to consider if Arnica has initially helped with swelling around the site of injury, but pain stubbornly persists.

> **TIP:** APPLY A SOOTHING CREAM
> If the skin around the eye socket is not abraded or cut in any way, gently apply arnica cream to the bruise to reduce inflammation, pain, and tenderness. Lacerated areas are better treated with a combination of calendula and hypericum cream, which promotes the production of healthy new tissue. Arnica cream can set off inflammation when applied topically to broken skin.

## HERBALISM

Applying ice and anti-inflammatory herbs, such as chamomile and comfrey, to an eye immediately after a trauma has occurred can prevent or lessen swelling and bruising. Once a black eye has appeared, herbal medicines may be helpful, but more than anything, the body will have to slowly remove the accumulated blood. Any herb or other substance has the potential to irritate the eye, so care should be taken to keep the eye closed when applying compresses. Also keep ointments and salves away from the eye. If irritation does occur, flush the eye with cool water and discontinue using the herb.

**General advice:** Apply a bag of ice wrapped in a soft cloth to the black eye for 15–20 minutes. Remove the ice and rest for 30–45 minutes and then reapply the ice. Repeat this process for the first 24–48 hours following the injury.

**Chamomile:** This herb possesses calming properties and anti-inflammatory effects, making it a good choice for a variety of medical conditions. To treat a black eye make a compress by steeping approximately 2–5 g of dried chamomile flowers in 200 ml of boiling water for 10 minutes. Strain the mixture and allow it to cool in the refrigerator. Soak a washcloth in the mixture, squeeze out the excess liquid, and wrap the cloth around a small handful of ice in a plastic bag. Place the compress over the injured area for 15–20 minutes several times a day. If you begin to notice redness or irritation around the application site, discontinue using chamomile. Do not use chamomile if you are allergic to plants in the daisy family.

**Comfrey:** This is a good choice for treating bruises when applied topically on unbroken skin. Purchase and use an ointment that contains 5–20% comfrey root extract. When used topically there has been little evidence of adverse reactions; however comfrey root should not be taken internally because it has been shown to cause serious liver disease.

# BLISTERS

## DIAGNOSIS

A blister is a raised area of skin that becomes filled with a clear, sterile fluid. Blisters affect everyone at one time or another, and are usually caused by friction when something rubs against the skin. For example, they commonly occur on the feet when breaking in new shoes. Blisters generally heal naturally and do not require treatment, especially if they are unbroken. The fluid contained inside a blister forms a protective barrier to stop infection, and as new skin grows beneath the blister, this fluid is slowly absorbed by the body, and the skin on top dries and peels off. Any kind of burn, including sunburns, can also cause blisters. Certain medical complaints may also cause blisters to appear on different parts of the body. These include eczema (p. 73), shingles (p. 956), chickenpox (p. 919), and impetigo (p. 99), where the blisters fill with pus rather than the usual clear fluid. In such cases the underlying condition needs to be treated to resolve the blisters. If a blister becomes red, hot, filled with pus, or painful, seek medical advice as it may have become infected. Avoid touching or scratching blisters, and keep them clean to prevent infection.

## SYMPTOMS

- A fluid-filled bump on the skin, particularly the feet
- The surrounding area may be red and sore
- Occasionally, the area is hot and very painful

## TREATMENT GOAL

To protect the blister to avoid it breaking and becoming infected. Treatment also involves clearing any infections that may have occurred. Preventive measures can also be taken to avoid blisters from forming.

## CONVENTIONAL MEDICINE

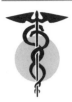

Non-infectious blisters are usually caused by burns, bites, or friction on the skin. Sometimes, however, they can be a symptom of a viral, bacterial, or skin infection. In each case, the cause of the blister should be defined and if an underlying illness is identified, it needs to be treated in order for the blister to resolve.

**To treat a non-infectious blister:** These types of blisters form when the body tries to protect itself from an external irritant. They should generally be left alone, as they will heal slowly by themselves. The area should always be kept clean, but it does not have to be bandanged.

**To treat an infectious blister:** If redness and swelling occur in the skin area surrounding the blister, it is a sign of infection. Medical care should be sought and an appropriate treatment administered to resolved the underlying condition. For example, a blister caused by herpes can be treated with an antiviral drug such as acyclovir (see Herpes, p. 739), but this is ofen unnecessary. If a blister has resulted from impetigo (see p. 99) or an infection of the skin, it should be treated with antibiotics.

## TRADITIONAL CHINESE MEDICINE

**Herbs:** The herbs listed below are available from Chinese pharmacies or online.
• Jin Yin Hua tea: Mix 5 g of Jin Yin Hua (honeysuckle flower), and 3 g of Bo He (field mint) in a teapot. Add boiling water and let the herbs steep for a few minutes. Drink this tea throughout the day for five to seven days.
• Herbal bath: Mix 15 g of Jin Yin Hua (honeysuckle flower), and 15 g of Jing Jie (schizonepeta stem and bud). Boil these two ingredients in 5 cups of water for five minutes. Strain the liquid and add to your bathwater. Soak in this herbal bath once a day until the blister subsides.

**Acupressure:** Press the Tai Yang, Hegu, and Feng Chi points gently for about one minute once a day. The Tai Yang point is located at the temple in the depression between the lateral end of the eyebrow and eyelid. The Hegu point is located on the back of the hand between the thumb and first finger. The Feng Chi points are at the back of the head at the base of the skull, about 2 inches on either side of the center point.

**Diet:** Generally, light, fresh food is recommended, such as turnips, celery, spinach, aubergine, purslane, wax gourd, bitter melon, and mung beans. Avoid eating ginger, chilies, mustard greens, and mutton as they are pungent and irritating, and increase heat in the body and may make blisters worse.

## NATUROPATHY

**Prevention:** It is important to minimize friction to prevent blisters from forming. For example, make sure your shoes are the right size and shape and that they fit properly. There should be a ½ inch space between your longest toe and the end of your shoe. Be sure that you have enough room to wiggle your toes inside the shoe, and that your heel does not slip when you walk. Inspect the inside of your shoes for seams or worn areas that might produce extra friction. Wear socks made from synthetic blends that include a soft, wicking fabric such as Coolmax® products. Do not wear cotton socks as they absorb moisture and are usually rough in texture. Ensure that socks do not have bulky stitching at the toes or heels. Apply petroleum jelly or talcum powder to your feet to keep them dry and further reduce friction.

**Treatment:** The following steps can minimize the chance of infection in a blister. Small blisters can usually be treated without puncturing them. If you can leave the blister intact, only follow steps 1, 3, 7, 8, 9, and 10 of the treatment. Diabetics should always seek medical attention for blisters and should not follow these steps. Wash your hands with disinfectant soap and water (1); put on latex gloves (2); clean the blister and surrounding area using a disinfectant soap or solution (3); sterilize the tip of a needle by soaking it for at least three minutes in a disinfectant solution, or heating it until it glows red and then cools (4); make a small puncture at the base of the blister, leaving the roof of the blister attached so that it can continue to protect the skin (5); use a gloved finger to gently push the fluid out (6); apply antibiotic ointment to a piece of gauze and cover the wound (avoid drying products such as alcohol, 7); cut a hole the size of the blister in a piece of moleskin (8); cover the blister with the moleskin so that the blister rests in the middle of the hole and the adhesive sticks to the skin around the blister (9); and replace the bandage daily and check for signs of infection such as heat, pain, swelling, or pus on or around the blister (10).

## HOMEOPATHY

The following remedies can help to speed up recovery from a mild to moderate blister that has developed in response to a very minor burn or scald, friction, or an infection such as chickenpox. Also see the homeopathic recommendations for cold sores (p. 37).

**Urtica urens:** To treat mild blistering associated with a stinging inflammation around the affected area, use Urtica urens. The area is aggravated by cool bathing and touch. This remedy can be taken orally in tablet form, and a diluted herbal tincture can be used topically to bathe the blisters.

**Cantharis:** If mild to moderate blistering develops very rapidly, is associated with severe smarting and burning pain, and is extremely sensitivity to touch, try Cantharis. Unlike symptoms that call for Urtica urens, those that respond well to Cantharis are temporarily soothed by bathing in cool water.

## HERBALISM

Most small blisters do not need to be ruptured; the body will quickly heal of its own accord. When treating larger blisters, or blisters that have broken, the most important thing is to keep the area clean and dry. There are a few herbs that may also be helpful.

**Tea tree oil:** This can be used topically as an antifungal and antibacterial agent. Apply a thin layer of tea tree ointment (containing 5–10% tea tree oil) to the affected area as needed. Make sure you cover the area with a clean bandage after application. The antiseptic properties of the tea tree oil will help keep the area free of infection, while the other ingredients in the ointment will soothe the skin and keep the bandage from sticking. Dermatitis is the only significant side effect associated with the prolonged and repeated topical use of tea tree oil.

**Aloe vera:** The clear gel-like substance that oozes from freshly cut leaves of aloe has been used for many years to treat a wide array of skin conditions. To treat a blister, apply the gel from a fresh cut aloe leaf directly to the affected area. If fresh leaves are not available, there are a variety of gels and lotions containing aloe vera that can be purchased at a local health food store or pharmacy.

**Calendula:** Also known as marigold, holly gold, and Mary bud, calendula can be applied topically to a blister as an ointment three to four times daily. Use an ointment with a 2–5% concentration of calendula if possible. Calendula has very few contraindications and causes few adverse reactions when used topically. There is a small potential for an allergic reaction on the skin; should this occur, discontinue using calendula immediately.

**Slippery elm:** The bark of elm produces a slippery, mucus-like substance with medicinal properties. Mix 1 tsp of the powdered root with about ¼ cup of boiling water to make a paste. Allow the paste to cool and spread it directly on the affected area. Leave the paste on for 5–10 minutes, and repeat two to three times a day. Adverse reactions to slippery elm when applied topically are rare, but if the blister worsens, or you notice new symptoms, discontinue use and consult a medical herbalist.

# BRUISES

## DIAGNOSIS

A bruise occurs when small blood vessels under the surface of the skin are broken and blood leaks out and causes discoloration and tenderness in the surrounding tissue. They often appear after an injury to the skin, such as a direct hit or blow to the skin or from banging into an object. A bruise is usually a deep purple color at first and then starts to fade after a few days, taking on yellowish-green and brown tinges as the healing process starts.

Some people are naturally more likely to bruise than others, for example, because they are thinner and do not have as much flesh on their bodies. However, if you suddenly develop lots of bruises, or start to bruise for no apparent reason, consult a doctor. Unusual bruising is sometimes a symptom of an underlying blood disorder. Bruises do not just happen under the surface of the skin; they can also occur deeper in the tissues or organs. Although bleeding in these places is not visible, symptoms of swelling and pain may emerge. If you are worried that you may have internal bruising from an injury or accident, consult your physician.

## SYMPTOMS

- Purple, black, or red marks following an injury or fall
- The marks will begin to fade to a yellow or green color
- Pain, tenderness, and swelling in the affected area
- The area may feel hot to the touch

## TREATMENT GOAL

The extent of the injury should be assessed to ensure that more serious complications, such as a fracture, have not been sustained. Conventional and complementary therapies involve relieving the pain and tenderness in the area, and encouraging the bruise to fade and heal as quickly as possible.

## CONVENTIONAL MEDICINE

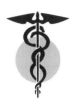

**Rest, ice, and elevation:** Apply an ice pack to the injury as soon possible. Wrap the ice in a cloth so that it does not damage the skin, and hold it against the affected area for 20 minutes every hour for the first 24 hours following the injury. Also rest the affected body part to prevent further injury and keep it as elevated as possible to encourage the body to reabsorb the blood.

**To treat frequent or unexplained bruising:** In some cases, a simple solution such as including more vitamin C in your diet helps (generally, about 500 mg a day is needed as a supplement). Taking regular aspirin or NSAIDs and certain herbs such as ginkgo, ginger, ginseng, garlic, and feverfew may predispose some people to easy bruising as can very high doses of certain supplements (for example, more than 3 g a day of Vtiamin C, or more than 6 g a day of fish oil). In other cases, a coagulation or clotting disorder may be present and should be evaluated. Such disorders are often genetic and most (but not all) are mild. They are diagnosed by blood tests.

## TRADITIONAL CHINESE MEDICINE

**Herbs:** According to traditional Chinese medicine, bruises are caused by blood stagnation, and herbs that are proven to remove blood stagnation are generally used to treat this condition. Mix 12 g of Sang Shen Zi (mulberry fruit-spike), 12 g of Chi Shao (red peony root), 12 g of Haui Niu Xi (achyranthes root), 12 g of Dan Shen (salvia root), and 15 g of Ji Xue Teng (millettia root). To make a decoction, place the herbs in a ceramic pot and add 3 cups of water. Bring the ingredients to a boil and simmer for 30 minutes. Strain the liquid and drink 1 cup two to three times a day. Consult a TCM practitioner for advice before using these herbs, and do not use this formula if you have heart disease or a blood disorder. The herbs listed are available from Chinese pharmacies or online.

**Acupuncture:** In some case, acupuncture can be a beneficial treatment method for this condition as it promotes circulation. If the bruising is chronic and long-term, regular sessions are usually recommended. Consult an experienced practitioner to determine whether acupuncture is appropriate for your individual condition.

**Acupressure:** Press the Hegu points, located on the back of the hands between the thumbs and first fingers, with firm pressure. Press the Nei Guan points, found on center of the palm side of each wrist, about 2 inches above the crease, with moderate pressure for one to three minutes and repeat. Pressure may reduce or take the edge off the pain.

## NATUROPATHY

**Diet:** Foods such as green, leafy vegetables, apples, and citrus fruits are rich in vitamin C and will help blood capillaries heal quickly. It is best to eat these foods raw, as vitamin C, as well as the enzymes these foods provide, are destroyed by heat. Other brightly colored foods such as peppers, berries, and carrots contain bioflavonoids, which help to heal all kinds of bruises. Flaxseed oil will help reabsorb the blood from bruises, reducing inflammation. Eat a salad of fresh, raw vegetables dressed with lemon juice and 2 tbsp of flaxseed oil daily. Salmon, walnuts, and other seeds have a similar effect. Avoid sugars, refined carbohydrates, hydrogenated oils, and trans-fatty acids found in fried foods and junk foods as they interfere with the healing process and promote inflammation.

**Supplement:** Take 1,000 mg of vitamin C three times a day to heal blood vessels and connective tissue found throughout the body. Bioflavonoids work synergistically and similarly to vitamin C, and should be taken at a dose of 500–1,000 mg three times a day. Take 50 mg of grapeseed extract twice a day to promote tissue healing, and 3,000 mg of fish oils a day to heal and decrease inflammation. Vitamin K is involved in the blood clotting process. Take 1 mg twice a day for two weeks to treat an acute bruise, and then 500 mg daily until the bruise has healed.

**Herbs:** Take 500 mg of bromelain three times a day for its natural anti-inflammatory effects. Apply arnica oil topically to the affected area, but not to broken skin, for its anti-inflammatory benefits. Apply compresses of fennel, chamomile, calendula blossoms, and peppermint to soothe and heal the injury.

## HOMEOPATHY

The following remedies can help to ease the pain and tenderness of a mild to moderate amount of bruising. Self-prescribing is appropriate only if a bruise has been sustained from a minor accident or injury. More serious traumas, or a tendency to develop spontaneous bruises, are best treated by an experienced homeopathic practitioner plus a conventional medical opinion. Also refer to the remedies recommended in Black Eye (p. 901).

**Ruta:** This remedy is particularly appropriate for treating the pain and discomfort that result from bruising the periosteum (the sheath-like membrane that covers the bones). This kind of injury is most likely to occur on an area of the body where the skin in very thin, such as the shins.

**Arnica:** If bruising has occurred as a result of a minor accident or fall, use Arnica. It is effective in reducing the swelling of bruised tissue, and also helps the system to come to terms with the psychological shock that accompanies even the most minor of falls.

**Bellis perennis:** If deep bruising has been sustained, for example, as a result of a heavy fall or a blow, try taking Bellis perennis. It can also be used in situations where deep bruising has occurred as a consequence of surgery or childbirth, and where Arnica has helped initially, but failed to resolve the bruising.

## HERBALISM

 If you bruise easily and often without any apparent cause, you may have a serious medical condition and should consult your doctor. For a typical injury that may lead to a bruise, applying ice is the best treatment. Although there are very few herbs that help with bruising per se, there are several that have anti-inflammatory properties and can have a soothing effect when incorporated into a cold compress. A preventive strategy often works best, so apply ice and the herbs as described immediately after any blunt trauma. Once a bruise has appeared, the body will have to slowly remove the accumulated blood.

**Chamomile:** This herb possesses calming properties and anti-inflammatory effects, making it a good choice for a variety of medical conditions. To treat a bruise, make a compress by steeping approximately 2–5 g of dried chamomile flowers in 200 ml of boiling water for 10 minutes. Strain the mixture and allow it to cool in the refrigerator. Soak a washcloth in the mixture, squeeze out the excess liquid, and wrap the cloth around a small handful of ice in a plastic bag. Place the compress over the injured area for 15–20 minutes several times a day. If you begin to notice redness or irritation around the application site, discontinue using chamomile. Do not use chamomile if you are allergic to plants in the daisy family.

**Comfrey:** This is a good choice for treating bruises when applied topically on unbroken skin. Purchase and use an ointment that contains 5–20% comfrey root extract. When used topically there has been little evidence of adverse reactions; however, comfrey root should not be taken internally because it has been shown to cause serious liver disease.

# BURNS

## DIAGNOSIS

Burns can be caused by the sun, fire, hot surfaces, chemicals, radiation, and/or electricity. When the skin becomes burned, nerve endings are damaged, which causes intense feelings of pain. Burns can also affect the body's electrolyte balance, temperature, joint function, and dexterity. As well as damaging the skin, serious burns can affect muscles, bones, nerves, and blood vessels.

Burns are classified according to their degree of severity. First degree burns, which are the most common type of burn, involve damage to the top layer of skin, the epidermis, and present as reddening and soreness but no blistering. They are painful, but not serious. Second degree burns damage two layers of skin, the epidermis and dermis underneath, and are very red, raw, and blistered. They are considered minor if they involve less than 15% of the body's surface in adults, and less than 10% in children. Third degree burns, also referred to as full thickness burns, are extremely serious, and involve damage to all the layers of skin and sometimes blood vessels and nerves as well. These kinds of burns cause the skin to look charred and blackened. Third degree burns should be treated by emergency medical services.

## SYMPTOMS

### FIRST DEGREE BURNS
- Painful burning sensation on the skin
- Skin is hot and sensitive to touch
- Skin is red and raw

### SECOND DEGREE BURNS
- Skin is red, raw, and blistered
- Skin appears moist
- Clothing may be stuck to the skin

### THIRD DEGREE BURNS
- Skin is blackened
- Difficulty breathing
- Result in severe scarring

## TREATMENT GOAL

Treatment involves relieving the pain and soreness caused by the burn and promoting healing with as little scarring as possible. If the burn appears to be anything more than superficial, seek medical help immediately.

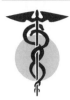

## CONVENTIONAL MEDICINE

First degree burns usually heal within a week or two, and anything more severe should be evaluated by a doctor. Patients that have serious burns should be taken to the hospital where specialized treatment can be administered to resuscitate, block pain, prevent infection, and deliver oxygen when necessary.

**Cool the skin:** The skin should be cooled to reduce its temperature and thereby stop any further burning of the skin. Run cool water over the area for 20 minutes. Do not put an ice cube directly on the burn, as this may cause further skin damage.

**Topical treatment:** Bacitracin ointment, a topical antibiotic, is commonly used to treat superficial wounds. Burns are usually covered with petrolatum gauze. Some doctors use collagenase, an enzyme that promotes the production of collagen, to treat second degree, partial thickness, burns second or third degree burns, which take months to heal.

**Debridement and skin grafting:** A doctor will remove dead tissue to prevent an infection from occurring. Skin grafting may also be necessary to help cover the wound.

**Treating chemical and electrical burns:** Chemical burns may be treated differently from case to case depending on the substance that has caused the burn. Consult a doctor for advice. Electrical burns are of particular concern because they can sometimes involve electrocution, affecting cardiac and other essential body functions. After removing the source of the electricity, make sure that the breathing and heart rate of the patient are not compromised. If this is the case, begin cardio-pulmonary resuscitation (CPR) and call for an ambulance.

## TRADITIONAL CHINESE MEDICINE

**Herbs:** Mix 5 g of Jin Yin Hua (honeysuckle flower), and 3 g of Bo He (field mint) in a teapot. Add boiling water and let the herbs steep for a few minutes. Sip the tea throughout the day for five to seven days. You can also use apply Chinese medicine oil, such as Wan Hua oil, to the area. These herbs and oils are available at Chinese pharmacies or online.

**Diet:** Generally, light, fresh food that dispels dampness and heat is recommended. These foods include mung beans, watermelon, lotus root, purslane, wax gourds, red beans, bananas, and grapefruit. Avoid foods that promote heat and dampness such as pepper, dried garlic, cloves, dried ginger, green peppers, leeks, liver, mustard greens, mutton, and green onions, as these may make the burn worse.

**TIP:** APPLY GINGER
Crush fresh ginger, squeeze out the juice, and apply it to the burn with a cottonwool ball to reduce pain and help reduce swelling and blistering.

## NATUROPATHY

**Diet:** Drink plenty of fluids and electrolyte drinks to avoid dehydration. Brightly colored foods, such as berries, citrus fruits, papaya, carrots, and squash contain high amounts of bioflavonoids, which strengthen the immune system and assist in healing. Most of these foods also contain high levels of vitamin C, which contributes to tissue healing. Essential fatty acids found in fresh salmon, cod, walnuts, and flaxseeds are equally important for tissue repair.

**Supplements:** Vitamin E helps tissue to heal and is an excellent antioxidant. Take 400 IU of mixed tocopherol vitamin E a day, or apply a vitamin E oil or cream to the affected area. These substances can be purchased in most health food stores. Take 1,000 mg of vitamin C, to promote skin healing. L-glutamine is helpful in preventing infections from burns and also assists in tissue healing. Take 500 mg three times a day. Zinc is essential for skin healing and increasing immune function. Take 30 mg of zinc a day. Zinc can deplete the body's stores of copper, so 3 mg of copper should be taken with this supplement.

**Essential oils:** Lavender oil is one of the only essential oils that can be applied directly to the skin without dilution. Lavender oil will take the sting out of the burn, and heal it quickly. Its calming aromatherapy properties will also help to ease the emotional upset of a painful burn. Apply 3–5 drops of oil to the affected area and spread it with a gauze pad.

**TIP:** USE HONEY TO EASE PAIN
Uncooked, raw, natural honey (found in health food stores) eases the pain of a mild burn. Its antimicrobial and hydrating properties work to keep the area free of infection and well-moisturized. Gently apply a thick coat of honey to the burn and cover it with gauze to keep the honey from getting on to clothing. Apply honey twice a day until the area is no longer sensitive.

## HOMEOPATHY

 The following remedies can be helpful in stimulating a prompt recovery from a minor domestic burn that covers a surface area of less than 1 inch in diameter. A burn that is more severe than this falls outside the remit of home prescribing and requires professional medical attention. Also refer to Sunburn (p. 965) for additional remedies that may relieve minor burns.

**Arnica:** This is a useful all-purpose homeopathic remedy for calming the shock of even a minor accident. Patients tend to deny needing any help, and just want to get on with things with a minimum of fuss. This, of course, is a common symptom of minor shock, which can be associated with burns.

**Cantharis:** If there is a severe burning sensation around the affected area and blisters form rapidly, use Cantharis. Because of the high degree of inflammation and smarting, being touched causes great distress, while bathing the burn in cool water provides temporary relief.

**Urtica urens:** To treat minor burns that sting and are accompanied by slight signs of blistering, use Urtica urens. Unlike minor burns that respond well to Cantharis, those that respond well to this remedy feel more sensitive and uncomfortable when bathed in cool water.

## HERBALISM

**Aloe vera:** Most people will tell you that nothing soothes a burn better than cooling aloe vera. The clear gel-like substance that oozes from freshly cut leaves of aloe has been used for many years to treat a wide array of skin conditions. To treat a burn, apply the gel from a fresh cut aloe leaf directly to the affected area. If fresh leaves are not available, there are a variety of gels and lotions containing aloe vera that can be purchased at a local health food store. Some aloe vera gels contain alcohol as a base to contribute to its cooling effect. Be aware that alcohol will sting on any open skin, so avoid any alcohol-based gels if a burn is accompanied by a break in the skin.

**Calendula:** Also known as marigold, holly gold, and Mary bud, calendula can be applied topically to a burn in the form of an ointment three to four times daily. Use an ointment with a 2–5% concentration of calendula if possible, which should be readily available at your local health food store. Calendula has very few contraindications and causes few adverse reactions when used topically. There is a small potential for an allergic reaction on the skin; should this occur, discontinue using calendula immediately.

**Slippery elm:** The bark of elm produces a slippery, mucus-like substance with medicinal properties. Mix 1 tsp of the powdered root with about ¼ cup of boiling water to make a paste. Allow the paste to cool and spread it directly on the burn. Leave the paste on for 5–10 minutes, and repeat two to three times a day. Adverse reactions to slippery elm when applied topically are rare, but if the burned area worsens, or you notice new symptoms, discontinue use and consult a medical herbalist.

# CHICKENPOX

## DIAGNOSIS

Chickenpox is a highly infectious viral disease. It can affect people of all ages but it usually develops in children under the age of 10. It manifests as a rash of small red spots that appear on the scalp and face, or sometimes the torso, which then spread to the rest of the body. There can also be spots in the mouth and ears. The spots develop into blisters that are intensely itchy, and may scar if scratched. Yellow scabs form after a couple of days, which eventually drop off. The amount of spots that develop varies from patient to patient; some have just a few while others are covered from head to toe.

Chickenpox is spread either by droplets of saliva or by contact with the fluid that oozes from the blisters. It can only be caught by coming into direct contact with someone who has it. It takes between 10 and 21 days for the illness to incubate, and the patient is most infectious before the rash even appears and until the blisters have all scabbed over. Chickenpox generally lasts about a week. Once you have had the disease you are generally immune for life.

**DANGER:** If the patient still feels unwell once the scabs have healed, complains of headaches, or feels drowsy, call a doctor immediately. Rarely chickenpox can lead to encephalitis (inflammation of the brain).

## SYMPTOMS

- Feeling under the weather or cranky
- Headache, sore throat, and general malaise
- Raised temperature and mild fever
- Loss of appetite
- Swollen lymph glands
- Rash of small red spots on the scalp and face, which spreads to the rest of the body

## TREATMENT GOAL

Therapies involve making the patient feel as comfortable as possible, relieving frustrating symptoms of itchiness, and preventing scratching and scarring.

## CONVENTIONAL MEDICINE

Chickenpox is becoming more rare as the varicella vaccine is now recommended for children, which prevents the virus from developing. When chickenpox does occur, treatment is generally to relieve symptoms until the virus has run its course. One important exception is that any newborn whose mother develops chickenpox up to five days before delivery to two days after delivery should receive an anti-chickenpox immunoglobulin.

**Reduce fever:** Acetaminophen (Tylenol®) can be administered to bring down a fever. Aspirin should not be used by those under 16 as it has been linked to the development of Reye's syndrome, a lethal disease that affects the liver and other body organs.

**Relieve itchiness:** An antihistamine (Benadryl® or Periactin®) or hydroxyzine can be used to relieve itchiness. Taking soothing baths to which baking soda or Aveeno® have been added is also helpful. Topical calamine, chamomile, or calendula lotion is also soothing.

**Antivirals:** The antiviral acyclovir may be used to lesson symptoms in adolescents and adults. It is also recommended for all immuno-compromised people (those whose immune systems are not working well), and for those who have been on steroids, who have serious lung infections, or who suffer from chronic skin disorders. Valacilovir (Valtrex®) or famiciclovir (Famvir®) are also used for this purpose.

**Antibiotics:** If a secondary skin infection occurs, antibiotics are prescribed. Usually antibiotics that target the bacteria streptococcus are appropriate.

## TRADITIONAL CHINESE MEDICINE

**Herbs:** Mix 5 g of Jin Yin Hua (honeysuckle flower), and 3 g of Bo He (field mint) in a teapot. Add boiling water and let the herbs steep for a few minutes. Sip the tea throughout the day for 10–30 days. These herbs and oils are available at Chinese pharmacies or online.

**Acupuncture:** Consult a doctor of traditional Chinese medicine for advice as to whether or not to use acupuncture in treating chickenpox, since it is highly contagious. Acupuncture may be able to help clear the heat and rash from the skin by stimulating certain meridian points. Treatment can also regulate circulation to help maintain skin health.

**Acupressure:** Press the Tai Yang, Hegu, and Feng Chi points with gentle pressure for about one minute every day. The Tai Yang point is located at the temple in the depression between the lateral end of the eyebrow and eyelid. The Hegu point is located on the back of the hand between the thumb and first finger. The Feng Chi points are at the back of the head at the base of the skull, about 2 inches on either side of the center point.

**Diet:** Eat light, fresh food such as turnips, celery, spinach, aubergines, purslane, wax gourds, and mung beans. Gentle foods, such as organic green vegetables, radishes, bitter melon, and pears, can strengthen the immune system. Green tea is also beneficial since it has a gentle cleansing effect. Avoid ginger, chilies, mustard greens, and mutton, as they are pungent and irritating and increase heat in the body, which may make the condition worse. Also avoid seafood, and fatty and spicy food.

## NATUROPATHY

The following therapeutic suggestions apply to both adults and children unless otherwise specified.

**Diet:** Drink raw fruit and vegetable juices. These cool the system and hydrate the skin. Lemon juice is considered to be especially beneficial. Drink lots of water (about two 8 oz glasses of water every hour throughout the day) to prevent dehydration. Avoid all dairy products until the skin lesions have resolved, as dairy is a major allergen and may worsen symptoms. A soup prepared from carrots and coriander has been found to be beneficial in the treatment of chickenpox. Use about 100 g of carrots and 60 g of fresh coriander cut into small pieces and boiled. Eat this soup once a day.

**Supplements:** The dosages provided in this section are for adults only. The supplements are also available from health food stores for children and the instructions on the label should be followed. Take 400 IU of vitamin E a day to promote healing and provide the body with powerful antioxidants. Applying vitamin E oil to the skin is also beneficial in treating chickenpox as it makes the marks left by the virus fade more quickly. Take 25,000 IU of vitamin A twice a day to boost the immune system and also help with skin healing. Pregnant women should not take more than 10,000 IU of vitamin A a day. Vitamin C, which can be taken at 1,000 mg three times a day, also helps to stimulate the immune system and it is important for tissue healing. Bioflavonoids work similarly and synergistically with vitamin C. Take 500–1,000 mg two to three times a day. Also take 15,000 IU of beta-carotene a day to heal tissue and stimulate the immune system.

**TIP:** ADD NEEM LEAVES TO YOUR BATH
Soak 2 cups of neem leaves in a tub of warm water for 30 minutes. Add cool water and some ginger and soak in the tub for 30 minutes to relieve itchiness.

**Herbs:** Apply sandalwood oil to the rash until the scabs start to fall off to help reduce scarring. You can also sip on a tea made from mildly sedative herbs, such as chamomile, marigold, and lemon balm, several times a day. This can help to relieve the distress caused by itchiness.

---

**TIP:** USE BAKING SODA

Baking soda is a popular remedy to control the itchiness caused by chickenpox. Add some baking soda to a glass of water and sponge the affected area with the liquid. The soda will dry on the skin to keep the patient from scratching the lesions.

---

## HOMEOPATHY

The following remedies described below can be helpful in easing the marked itchiness associated with chickenpox and in shortening the duration of an acute episode.

**Aconite:** This remedy can be useful during the first, feverish stage of chickenpox. Restlessness and fear may develop quickly and severely at night, and a fever may be accompanied by thirst and dry skin. It is an appropriate remedy to use before the chickenpox rash has actually appeared. Once a rash develops, you will need to change the remedy used.

**Belladonna:** This remedy can also be used to ease a fever associated with the early stage of chickenpox that develops rapidly and severely. Symptoms include a high fever with bright red skin that radiates heat and irritability. Once a rash develops, another remedy is likely to be needed.

**Ant tart:** If a rash is very slow to emerge, and if chickenpox is associated with a persistent cough, use Ant tart. When the rash does develop, spots tend to be large, have a bluish-tinge, and leave a red mark behind as they heal. There is also a thick, unpleasant coating on the tongue. Becoming overheated or bathing makes symptoms more distressing, while contact with cool air and coughing up phlegm from the chest brings a sense of relief.

**Rhus tox:** To treat spots that are maddeningly itchy at night in bed, causing distress and restlessness, use Rhus tox. Spots may be moist and blistery at first, and then become crusty. Resting and undressing make the rash more irritating, while rubbing and changing position provide temporary relief.

Avoid bathing your child during the feverish stage of this illness, since hot baths make a rash more irritated and itchy. Instead, sponge your child down in a comfortably warm room, making sure they do not get chilled in the process. Once the spots have become crusty and dry, be careful not to knock them off when towel drying.

**Pulsatilla:** This remedy is appropriate for treating the later stage of chickenpox, especially where the spots are slow to appear, and/or linger longer than is expected. Symptoms include feeling chilly but disliking hot, stuffy conditions, and having a dry mouth and white-coated tongue but not feeling thirsty. Children who are normally cheerful and content when well may become weepy and clingy when suffering from chickenpox.

**TIP:** USE CALENDULA TINCTURE
The extreme itchiness and irritation caused by chickenpox can be eased by applying a diluted tincture of Calendula to a saturated cottonwool pad and placing it on the affected areas. Dilute one part of tincture to 10 parts of boiled, cooled water. For a prolonged soothing effect, apply Calendula cream following the tincture.

## HERBALISM

Chickenpox is a manifestation of the herpes virus and many of the herbs recommended for viral infections (such as flu p. 550, mumps p. 952, and measles p. 947) may help to decrease the severity and duration of chickenpox by boosting the immune system. The common complaint with chickenpox is, of course, itchiness. Herbal therapies can be very beneficial in relieving this symptoms. Also refer to Pruritus (p. 129) for additional herbs that help to relieve itchiness.

**Oatmeal:** This herb is the first choice of therapy for treating a variety of skin conditions, including itchiness due to chickenpox. Oatmeal is inexpensive, widely available and can be used without worry, as there are virtually no known side effects. To treat chickenpox, which commonly affects large areas of the body, an oatmeal bath is most effective. Run a warm bath and add approximately 1 cup of finely ground oatmeal (grind oatmeal in a food processor or coffee grinder—it is also available commercially in this form as Aveeno®). Soak in the tub to allow the oatmeal to lightly coat the skin and relieve the itchiness and irritation associated with chickenpox. This method is particularly effective because chickenpox lesions can be extensive and sometimes hard to reach, so topical treatments can be difficult to administer.

**Burdock root:** This herb has a soothing effect on the skin. Try adding a handful of ground burdock root to an oatmeal bath to increase the effect of oatmeal.

**Elderberry:** The fruit of this plant can be used to treat chickenpox. Specific formulations of elderberry juice can be bought at your local health food store—raw elderberry juice can be quite toxic and is not recommended. Although cooking the berry destroys most of these toxins, it is still not considered safe. The recommended preparation of elderberry juice is the specific, store-bought formulation, which eliminates the problem with toxicity. Take the formulated juice orally at the onset of symptoms for three to five days. Diarrhea and vomiting have been reported with use of elderberry juice, although this side effect is greatly decreased with specific formulations.

**Astragalus:** This herb is well known for its immune-stimulating effects. Astragalus root can be used as a tea, or taken in capsule form at 500 mg three times a day. It should not be taken if you are on blood-thinning drugs, immunosuppressive drugs, or have an autoimmune disorder, such as lupus or rheumatoid arthritis.

# CUTS

## DIAGNOSIS

Cuts can either be minor injuries, involving minimal bleeding, or more severe, incurring significant blood loss. Either way, it is important to control the bleeding and prevent infection. Many people accidentally cut themselves on household items, or while operating machinery. Children are also prone to cuts when playing or participating in sports. Lacerations are caused by blunt objects that tear or crush the skin, particularly around bony areas of the body such as fingers or knees. These types of injuries also tend to result in swelling and leave jagged edges, so problems with healing may occur. Incised wounds are caused by objects with sharp edges, such as knives or scissors, which slice into the skin. These types of cuts tend to be deeper, damaging underlying tissue. Sharp-edged objects can also pierce the skin, resulting in a stab or puncture wound. Minor cuts, where the skin does not gape open, should be washed carefully (under cold running water, if possible) and gently patted dry. You can also sponge the wound clean.

**DANGER:** If the bleeding does not stop after 10 minutes or the wound is gaping and may need stitches, go to the emergency room of your nearest hospital.

## SYMPTOMS

- Bleeding from an open wound
- Stinging or throbbing pain
- There may be swelling around the area

## TREATMENT GOAL

To stop the bleeding as soon as possible, to encourage the cut to heal, and to prevent the wound from becoming infected.

## CONVENTIONAL MEDICINE

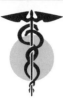

Blood loss following a cut can be minimal to severe, depending on the area where the injury has occurred and the vessels cut. A cut artery constitutes a medical emergency, since a pumping artery can release the entire blood supply in a short period of time.

**Apply pressure:** Remove any clothing around the cut and immediately apply direct pressure to the area from which blood is flowing. This should be done using a cloth folded under the hands. If possible, apply a sterile dressing and bandage it in place by wrapping it with tape or gauze so that some amount of pressure is continually applied to the wound. If the bleeding continues, the injured area should be raised to above the level of the heart. Continue to place dressings over the bandage as they become saturated, rather than removing one and replacing it. Of course, if a heavy amount of bleeding occurs, you should call an ambulance.

**Keep the area clean:** Wounds should be kept clean and dry. Waterproof bandages are helpful, and an antiseptic such as Neosporin® or Bacitracin® can also be applied.

**Tetanus shot:** If the wound has occurred in an area that is dirty, get a tetanus booster if it has been more than 10 years since your last one. This will prevent tetanus, a serious disease of the central nervous system caused by the infection of a wound by soil-dwelling bacteria, from developing.

**Diet and supplements:** The rate at which a wound heals is influenced by a patient's nutritional status, especially his or her zinc levels. It may be helpful to take 40 mg of zinc daily, and assure that the diet is high in protein and fresh fruit and vegetables. Large amounts of processed foods and sugar should be avoided.

**Antibiotics:** If redness and heat spread around the immediate area of the cut or if the cut becomes purulent, it should be assessed to determine whether it is infected. If this is the case, antibiotic therapy is required.

## TRADITIONAL CHINESE MEDICINE

**Herbs:** Chinese herbs are not used to treat cuts.

**Acupuncture:** This method of treatment is not used to treat ordinary cuts. For the treatment of severe cuts, acupuncture may help with the healing process. Consult a doctor of Chinese medicine for advice.

**Acupressure:** This method of treatment is not used to treat cuts.

**Diet:** There is no specific dietary advice other than maintaining a healthy and well-balanced diet that includes plenty of fresh fruit and vegetables, and grains. Also drink plenty of water every day.

## NATUROPATHY

**Diet:** Foods such as green, leafy vegetables, apples, and citrus fruits are rich in vitamin C and will help blood capillaries heal quickly. It is best to eat these foods raw, as vitamin C provides enzymes that are destroyed by heat. Other brightly colored foods, such as peppers, berries, and carrots, contain bioflavonoids, which help to heal all kinds of cuts. Avoid sugars, refined carbohydrates, hydrogenated oils, and trans-fatty acids found in fried foods and junk foods, as they interfere with the healing process and promote inflammation.

**Supplements:** Vitamins A, C, and E, as well as zinc are traditionally used to treat minor wounds and cuts. They can be taken orally or applied topically. Take 15,000 IU of vitamin A a day, 1,000 mg of vitamin C three times a day, 400 IU of vitamin E a day, and/or 15–30 mg of zinc a day. Creams that contain these ingredients are available from natural food stores.

**Herbs:** Gotu kola is thought to have general wound-healing properties, as well working to prevent or treat heavy scars. The recommended dose is 20–60 mg three times a day of an extract standardized to contain 40% asiaticoside, to be taken for two to three weeks. The aloe vera plant has long been used to treat skin conditions. Remove an outer leaf from a plant, slice it lengthways, and then apply the clear, thick gel inside the leaf to the skin two to three times daily. You can also purchase aloe vera gel from good health food stores. Calendula is also helpful for treating minor wounds and rashes, and contains antimicrobial properties. Apply a calendula salve, found in health food stores, to the injured area two to three times daily.

## HOMEOPATHY

The following remedies can encourage a minor wound to heal promptly and efficiently. Treating minor injuries of this kind is also a good way of familiarizing yourself with acute homeopathic prescribing.

**Arnica:** This should be the first remedy you reach for after a minor accident or trauma, and is especially well indicated in situations where cuts and bruises have occurred together. Although it can be taken appropriately as an internal remedy, never apply arnica cream to an open wound; use calendula cream instead.

**Hypericum:** This remedy can be used after arnica if a cut has occurred on an area of the body that is especially rich in nerve supply, such as the fingers or toes. Symptoms include intermittent pains that shoot through the injured area, which tends to be hypersensitive and very tender.

**Staphysagria:** This remedy is specifically used to heal incised wounds. An episiotomy (cutting tissue to enlarge the vagina) as a result of childbirth is an excellent example of the kind of wound that calls for Staphysagria. It is appropriate for wounds that involve sharp stinging pains, and that are sensitive to touch. It can also be used to ease residual pain once stitched areas have healed.

## HERBALISM

 **Tea tree oil:** This is perhaps the best and most effective herbal therapy for treating cuts owing to the oil's antibacterial and antifungal properties. Apply a thin layer of tea tree ointment or salve that contains 5–10% tea tree oil to the cut for the first day or two. Tea tree can be strong, especially on open skin, and after one or two days the body is generally able to fight off any lingering bacteria on it own. Dermatitis is the only significant side effect associated with the prolonged and repeated topical use of tea tree oil.

**Calendula:** This herb is valued for its anti-inflammatory and wound-healing properties, which are due to the flavonoids, carotenes, carotenoid pigments, and volatile oils contained in the plant. Steep the flowers in hot water, let them cool slightly, and then soak a clean cloth or piece of gauze in the liquid and apply it to the affected area as a compress. A poultice can also be made, which involves applying warm or hot (but not hot enough to burn the skin) masses of plant material to the affected area.

**Comfrey:** This herb contains the constituent allantoin, the same active compound secreted by maggots to dissolve wound secretions and promote healing. To use comfrey, prepare a decoction of the freshly peeled root and leaves and apply it as a compress. Add 2 oz of fresh, peeled root to 4 cups of water and boil for five to seven minutes. Add 2–4 oz of fresh leaves and let them steep for 5–10 minutes. When the decoction has cooled to a warm temperature, strain the decoction and soak a clean cloth or piece of gauze in the liquid. Hold the cloth against the cut for 10–15 minutes. The compress can also be covered in gauze and wrapped with a bandage to hold it in place.

# HANGOVER

## DIAGNOSIS

Alcohol is a toxic substance, and drinking it to excess has a detrimental effect on the body. A hangover is a condition that develops after a period of heavy drinking, and the symptoms, which include headaches, fatigue, and nausea, are largely due to the by-products that alcohol leaves in your system. It can take the body up to 24 hours to break down the toxins and recover. The most serious consequence of heavy drinking is dehydration. The liver, which needs water to get rid of the toxins found in alcohol, uses the body's reserves to deal with the extra strain. This means that water is taken from other organs, including the brain, which accounts for the throbbing headaches associated with a hangover. Waking up with a thick head and a raging thirst is your body's way of telling you that it lacks sufficient fluids to perform normally. Alcohol causes your blood sugar levels to drop, which can contribute to the general feeling of malaise. Alcohol also acts as an irritant to the lining of the stomach, which is why drinking can cause nausea or even ulcers if you drink heavily on a regular basis.

## SYMPTOMS

- Dehydration
- Fatigue
- Headache
- Sensitivity to light and sound
- Trembling
- Red eyes
- Muscle aches
- Vomiting
- Disturbed sleep
- Extreme thirst
- Dizziness
- Depression, anxiety, and irritability

## TREATMENT GOAL

The primary goal is to rehydrate the body, which will ease many of the symptoms. Regular heavy drinking can sometimes indicate psychological problems, and treatment should involve dealing with issues that prompt you to drink if this is the case.

## CONVENTIONAL MEDICINE

**Prevention:** Factors such as the type of alcohol drunk, genetics, nutritional status, and hydration seem to affect the intensity of a hangover. Drinking to the extent of feeling drunk, however, usually means a hangover is likely to occur. There are several steps you can take to prevent this, or lessen alcohol's side effects. Avoid drinking on an empty stomach or when overly tired, and avoid intense physical activity while drinking. Taking vitamin B6 prior to drinking also seems to lessen the effects of a hangover. Brown or red alcohol seems to incur worse hangovers than white/clear alcohol, as many dark, fermented alcohols have toxic by-products including methanol, aldehydes, and heavy metals. Drink plenty of water when drinking alcohol, and afterwards, to decrease the intensity of the hangover by hydrating the body.

**Diet:** If you are experiencing a hangover, avoid eating  grapefruits (and drinking their juices) as they have properties that decrease the liver's ability to clear the by-products of alcohol. Fatty meals should also be avoided. Avoid saunas as they can dehydrate you further and cause you to become overheated. Exercise is encouraged as long as you stay adequately hydrated.

**Herbs:** Some herbal products may help clear the hangover by enhancing the liver's ability to remove toxins. Liver detoxifiers sold in herb shops (Liv 52 is one example) may help if taken on a regular basis. Glutathione and milk thistle may also be helpful.

**Medications:** A drug called tolfenamic acid may help to relieve the symptoms of a hangover, and is safer to use than acetaminophen and ibuprofen. These pain relievers can usually be taken safely, however, unless extremely large amounts of alcohol have been consumed.

## TRADITIONAL CHINESE MEDICINE

**Herbs:** Mix 5 g of Ye Ju Hua (wild chrysanthemum flower) and 3 g of Shen Gan Cao (raw licorice) in a teapot. Add boiling water and let the herbs steep for a few minutes. Drink the tea three to four times a day. The herbs are available from Chinese pharmacies or online.

**Acupuncture:** Treatment can be useful for a hangover. Consult a practitioner who will recommend a certain number of sessions and advise on the frequency of treatments.

**Acupressure:** Use the tip of your thumb to press the Hegu, Tai Yang, and Feng Chi points with strong pressure for one to two minutes. The Hegu point is located on the back of the hand in the depression between the thumb and the first finger. The Tai Yang point is found at the temple in the depression between the lateral end of the eyebrow and the eyelid. The Feng Chi points are at the back of the head at the base of the skull, about 2 inches on either side of the center point.

**Diet:** Eating fresh strawberries can help to relieve a hangover. In general, pears, cranberries, blueberries, and bananas are recommended, along with mung beans, red beans, bamboo shoots, and purslane. Avoid foods that are rich and fatty as these increase heat in the body, worsening symptoms.

## NATUROPATHY

**Diet:** Always eat a big meal before drinking alcohol. Foods that are high in protein and fat will slow the absorption rate of alcohol into your bloodstream. Alcohol flushes fluids out of the body, leading to dehydration and magnifying other hangover symptoms such as headaches and tiredness. Drink water before, during, and after a night of drinking to counter alcohol's diuretic effects. Drinking Gatorade® is another effective method of replacing lost electrolytes and hydrating the body. Avoid drinking coffee as it is a diuretic and may lead to further dehydration. Bananas are an excellent source of potassium, a mineral that is lost when drinking alcohol. Magnesium, which helps control blood sugar levels, is reduced by alcohol. Bananas can help replace magnesium as well as vitamin C, which will make you feel better. Eat one banana before drinking alcohol and another afterwards. Also eat a slice of bread or some crackers spread with honey, or any other food that is high in fructose, after a heavy drinking session. The fructose (a natural sugar) helps the body burn off alcohol faster. Other good sources of fructose are apples, cherries, and grapes. You can also try eating an umeboshi plum—these have long been reputed to cure hangovers. They are available at Asian markets and health food stores.

**Supplements:** B-complex vitamins may be helpful in restoring energy after a night of heavy drinking. Take a high potency B-100 before drinking, before bedtime, and again the next day if you are hungover. Vitamin C helps relieve hangover symptoms and boosts the immune system. Take 1,000 mg before drinking, and 1,000 mg after. N-acetyl-cysteine (NAC) helps your liver detoxify by making glutathione. Take 1,500 mg before drinking and 1,500 mg when you wake up the next day.

**Herbs:** Ginger can help settle an upset stomach and ease feelings of nausea. In fact, some studies have shown that ginger may be up to three times more effective for treating nausea than common over-the-counter medications. Take 1–4 g daily in pill form or drink ginger tea until the hungover feeling dissipates. Do not take more than 1 g of ginger a day if you are pregnant.

## HOMEOPATHY

This condition well illustrates the value of homeopathic prescribing in treating an acute ailment that has been triggered by an obvious cause. Appropriate holistic measures can shorten the duration and severity of a hangover, and support the self-healing and self-balancing mechanisms of the body. If hangovers are becoming a regular feature of life, attention needs to be paid to lifestyle issues that may benefit from professional advice and support.

**Coffea:** Symptoms that respond well to this remedy include nervy exhaustion and a severe, crushing headache. Hangover symptoms are made more severe by drinking a strong cup of coffee, while warmth and rest feel helpful and restorative.

### TIP: REST, SLEEP, AND RE-HYDRATE

These should be the priorities if you are suffering from a hangover. Replacing fluid is a necessity due to the dehydrating effect of alcohol, but do not force yourself to eat if you feel queasy. If you do feel hungry, opt for light items that are easy to digest, such as soups, salads, fruit smoothies, and natural, bio-yogurt. Avoid fatty foods that will put extra strain on the liver, which will already be under considerable stress.

**Nux vomica:** This is a classic cure if symptoms have developed as a result of overindulging in alcohol, food, and cigarettes. Sufferers are irritable and have an emotional short fuse due to lack of sleep, constipation, and a queasy headache that lodges at the back of the head. Vomiting may also be a symptom, but it tends to be unproductive and does not bring relief.

**Bryonia:** If a hangover is a result of low-grade or severe dehydration, use Bryonia. Headaches are likely to be severe and are generally located in the front of the head. The scalp may also feel very sensitive and painful. When this remedy is appropriate, symptoms intensify with the slightest movement. Rest and keeping still for as long as possible brings relief, as do long drinks of water.

### TIP: ADD GRAPEFRUIT ESSENTIAL OIL TO A BATH

Grapefruit has a reputation for encouraging the body to detoxify. If you are hungover, add a few drops of grapefruit essential oil to warm bathwater, or invest in a good-quality commercially produced bath or shower gel that includes this essential oil.

## HERBALISM

Dehydration is perhaps the salient cause of a hangover. Although there is no specific herbal therapy that has been proven to cure a hangover, there are many theories regarding which herbs are most effective. Fresh, clean water is perhaps the most important aid. A hangover is often associated with nausea and headaches, and these symptoms may be alleviated with the herbal therapies recommended below.

**Turmeric:** This herb contains compounds called curcuminoids that may be effective in easing a headache associated with a hangover. Try drinking a few drops of turmeric tincture diluted in a glass of water. You can also steep a small amount of fresh turmeric rhizome (1–3 g) in boiling water for 10–20 minutes. Allow to cool and drink two to three times a day.

**Mints:** Peppermint and spearmint are common herbs used to treat nausea and other gastrointestinal disturbances. Many of the medicinal properties from plants in the mint family come from a class of compounds called essential, or volatile, oils, such as menthol, carvone, and limonene. Steep a handful (1–3 g) of mint leaves in a pot of boiling water, allow the liquid to cool, and drink two to three times a day while you have symptoms. It should be noted that the volatile oils disappear quickly when heated, so your mint tea may be more effective if you cover it while the herbs are steeping. It is also possible to buy a small bottle of the essential oil of peppermint. One drop of the essential oil taken under the tongue may be enough calm your digestive tract and stop the nausea. Do not take any essential oil internally for long periods of time or in high doses because it can have adverse effects on the liver.

**Milk thistle:** This herb has a long history of use for liver disorders. Some people take capsules of milk thistle prior to an expected heavy night of drinking, or afterwards to prevent the untoward effects of alcohol. Milk thistle seems to work best when taken as an extract standardized to 70% silymarin, at a total dose of 200–420 mg per day.

# HEATSTROKE

## DIAGNOSIS

Heatstroke occurs when the body cannot disperse excess heat in the normal way and becomes overheated within a relatively short period of time. It is a serious condition and some cases can be life threatening, incurring loss of consciousness and requiring urgent medical attention. An abnormally high body temperature can be caused by a variety of factors. It can result from prolonged exposure to a climate with high temperatures, humidity, and strong sunlight. Too much physical exertion, or overdoing it during a sports activity, particularly in hot, humid climates, can also result in heatstroke. Sunburn, a lack of fluids or salt in the system, and excessive alcohol consumption in hot surroundings can also trigger this condition.

Certain groups of people are particularly at risk of developing heatstroke, including the elderly and infirm, babies and small children, people who are overweight, and pregnant women. Anyone with cardiovascular or lung diseases and people taking certain types of medication, such as beta-blockers, are also more at risk.

**DANGER**: If your body temperature rises to over 104°F, a medical emergency exists. Once body temperatures rise above 107°F, cell damage to the brain, liver, kidneys, and skeletal muscle often occurs, as well as bleeding disorders.

## SYMPTOMS

- Headache
- Feeling unwell, tired, and dizzy
- Nausea
- Aches and pains
- Face becomes flushed and dry
- Diminished urination
- Feeling faint
- Feeling confused

## TREATMENT GOAL

It is important to first rule out any life-threatening symptoms, such as an abnormally high temperature, or un-consciousness. Treatment then involves cooling the patient down as much as possible, and restoring the balance of fluids and salts in the body.

## CONVENTIONAL MEDICINE

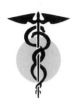

**To treat heat exhaustion:** Heat exhaustion occurs when a person is overheated, but does not have a fever and remains mentally alert and conscious. Place the patient in a cool, shaded area, and feed them ½ liter of fluid an hour to re-hydrate them. If possible, add ½ tsp of salt to each liter of water to prevent any complications developing as a result of low sodium in the body.

**To treat heatstroke:** Heatstroke occurs when a person is overheated and has a fever, and his mental status and possibly his vital signs are compromised. The patient should be transported to a hospital where intravenous resuscitation and support is available. Remove the patient's clothes and place him in a cool, well-ventilated room. His body temperature should be monitored carefully, with the goal being to lower it to 102°F or less over a 30–60 minute period. Spray the patient with cool mist, and if possible place fans around the body. The use of ice packs is controversial as they may constrict the blood vessels and cause shivering, thus driving the temperature back up. Sometimes treatment for low blood pressure and seizures is required, as these conditions may accompany severe heat stroke. Acidosis, a life-threatening condition that results from a lack of insulin in the system, is another complication, which needs to be addressed in the hospital. Most people recover from heatstroke completely in 48 hours.

## TRADITIONAL CHINESE MEDICINE

**Herbs:** The herbs listed below are available from Chinese pharmacies or online.
• Jin Yin Hua tea: Mix 5 g of Jin Yin Hua (honeysuckle flower), and 3 g of Bo He (field mint) in a teapot. Add boiling water and let the herbs steep for a few minutes. Drink this tea throughout the day for 10–30 days.
• Herbal decoction: Mix 12 g of Tai Zi Shen (pseudostellaria), 15 g of Mai Men Dong (ophiopogon tuber), 5 g of Shen Gan Cao (raw licorice), and 5 g of Bo He (field mint) in a glass or ceramic pot. Add 3 cups of water, bring the ingredients to a boil, and simmer for 30 minutes. Drink 1 cup twice a day.

**Acupuncture:** Treatment can be helpful and can be combined with herbal remedies. A session to treat heatstroke will last for 30 minutes and the sooner you receive acupuncture the more effective it will be.

**Acupressure:** Use the tip of your finger to apply moderate pressure to the Ru Zhong, Qu Chi, and Hegu points for one to two minutes. With the elbow flexed, the Qu Chi point is on the outside of the elbow at the lateral end of the crease. The Hegu point is located on the back of the hand in the depression between the thumb and the first finger. The Ru Zhong point is in the center of the nipple.

**Diet:** Watermelon and pears help rehydrate those suffering from heatstroke. Drinking plenty of water is also recommended. In general, eat light, fresh food such as turnip, celery, spinach, aubergines, purslane, wax gourds, mung beans, bitter melon, tofu, radishes, and celery. Green tea is also helpful since it has a gentle cleansing effect. Avoid food that has heat and warming properties, such as hot chili peppers, ginger, mustard greens, beef, and lamb, as well as fried food, and fatty and greasy food.

## NATUROPATHY

The best naturopathic treatment for heatstroke is prevention by keeping the body cool.

**Diet:** Eat a plain, light diet that primarily consists of fruit and vegetables. Celery, cucumber, watermelon, and oranges are particularly useful due to their high water content. Use salt freely to keep electrolytes in check. Electrolytes are various ions, such as sodium, potassium, or chloride, required by cells to regulate the electric charge and flow of water molecules across the cell membrane. Hydrate the body well before becoming thirsty. Drinking lots of fluids before, during, and after exertion in the heat is vital. Continue drinking plenty of liquids such as water or sports drinks every 15 minutes. In general, avoid caffeine, hot drinks, and alcohol while in the heat or while exercising, as they keep you hot and contribute to dehydration.

**Prevention:** When in the sun or while exercising, wear light, loose clothing, such as cotton, so that sweat can evaporate. Better still, get clothing that is best suited to exercise in hot weather such as Coolmax® products, which wick away moisture from the body to keep temperatures low. Also wear a hat that provides shade and allows ventilation. If you feel yourself begin to become hot and tired, stop activity and try to cool off. Move to a cool place indoors or in the shade.

## HOMEOPATHY

It must be stressed that heatstroke is a potentially serious condition if it occurs in a severe form, and complementary therapies are only appropriate for very mild cases. If there are any signs that heatstroke is progressing to a serious problem, seek conventional medical assistance and treatment.

**Belladonna:** If symptoms develop rapidly after being overexposed to the sun, take Belladonna. Symptoms include a throbbing headache that is eased by loosening the hair and letting the head bend backwards, and pulsating pains that radiate down from the head. The skin will also look bright red and feel extremely dry and hot to the touch.

**Glonoin:** This remedy can also relieve mild symptoms of heatstroke that involve a nasty headache, but in cases where pain and discomfort is intensified rather than eased by bending the head back. Symptoms develop rapidly, and are relieved by contact with cool air, but made worse if an ice pack is applied to the head. Pains are also likely to move in an upward direction, are made more intense by jarring movement, and eased by undressing.

**Carbo veg:** This remedy can treat symptoms of faintness that develop as a result of mild dehydration caused by heatstroke. Patients have an "air hunger," or a need to be fanned with cool air to feel comfortable. Being in stuffy surroundings makes symptoms more distressing, while sipping cool drinks and resting with the feet elevated in a cool room provides a sense of relief.

**TIP: STAY OUT OF THE SUN**
Avoid exposure to the sun when its effects are at their strongest. This is generally between 11 a.m. and 3 p.m.

## HERBALISM

Heatstroke is a very serious condition, marked by an extremely high body temperature, a cessation of sweating, and eventual collapse and coma. This occurs if there is exposure to high temperatures for an extended period of time and should be distinguished from heat exhaustion, which is a condition characterized by weakness, nausea, dizziness, and profuse sweating that results from physical exertion in a hot environment. Immediate referral to an emergency room is necessary if there is any suspicion of heat stroke; do not waste any time with home remedies that may delay medical treatment. You can begin to give fluids and cool the person during transit to the hospital.

**Peppermint and chamomile:** If you are suffering from heat exhaustion, where you are overheated but remain mentally alert, keep hydrated and take every measure to cool the body down. If you are experiencing any nausea or gastrointestinal distress, add peppermint or chamomile to a hydrating solution or water to help ease symptoms. The pleasant flavor of peppermint may also make it easier to drink adequate quantities of water.

# INSECT BITES

## DIAGNOSIS

Insect bites are particularly common during the summer months. Insects that bite include mosquitoes, gnats, midges, horseflies, ants, spiders, fleas, and lice. The most obvious sign of a bite is a red bump on the skin, or several bumps that show up as a rash (fleas, for example, often bite several times). Bites tend to be itchy and are sometimes painful. The skin around a bite can also become red and swollen. It is wise to avoid scratching bites as much as possible as this can cause them to become infected. Bites are generally not dangerous, provided there is no allergic reaction. Biting insects, however, can spread diseases such as malaria, yellow fever, Lyme disease, and typhus. If the bite appears to worsen rather than improve over time, consult a doctor.

**DANGER**: Bites can sometimes cause an allergic reaction. Call for an ambulance if you notice symptoms of dizziness, nausea, pains in the chest, choking or wheezing, and/or difficulty breathing. A life-threatening situation can develop if the victim goes into shock.

## SYMPTOMS

- A raised, red bump on the skin, or several bumps clustered together
- A small hole may be visible in the center of the bump
- The area is itchy and swollen, and may be painful

## TREATMENT GOAL

Treatment involves easing symptoms of itchiness, pain, and swelling, and preventing an infection from developing. There are several strategies available to prevent bites from occurring.

## CONVENTIONAL MEDICINE

Conventional treatment involves alleviating pain, treating or preventing an allergic reaction, and dealing with any side effects of a bite.

**Remove the insect:** If it is still present, the stinger or in some cases the insect should gently be removed without crushing or squeezing the area of the bite. Use a straight-edged object (such as a credit card) to scrape away the stinger. To treat tick bites, it is essential to remove the tick without compressing the body parts. Apply gentle traction until the tick comes out. If a red rash appears around the tick bite within one to three weeks and begins to spread, consult a doctor, as it could be a sign of Lyme disease.

**Topical treatments:** Apply an ice pack wrapped in a cloth to the bite. Calamine lotion, hydrocortisone cream (0.5%), or a baking soda paste (made from baking soda and water) can be applied after the ice and thereafter three times a day as needed.

**Antihistamines:** Diphenhydramine (Benadryl®), which is commonly used to treat symptoms of allergic reactions, may be needed if severe itching is present.

**Treating an allergic reaction:** Observe the victim for any signs of breathing difficulty, excessive swelling, dizziness, or shock. If any of these symptoms are present, go to a hospital immediately. Moderate allergic reactions are also treated with epinephrine, which can be injected with an "epi pen." A doctor will evaluate the patient's airways, breathing, and circulation and treat any complications.

## TRADITIONAL CHINESE MEDICINE

**Herbs:** Combine 15 g of Jin Yin Hua (honeysuckle flower) and 15 g of Jing Jie (schizonepeta stem and bud). Boil the ingredients in 5 cups of water for five minutes, strain the liquid, and add it to a container that is large enough to bathe the affected area. Soak the bite in this herbal bath once a day for as long as required. These herbs are available from Chinese pharmacies or online.

**Acupuncture:** Stimulating certain meridian points on the body can regulate a patient's circulation and help maintain skin health. Consult an experienced practitioner to form a treatment plan.

**Acupressure:** Press the Tai Yang, Hegu, and Feng Chi points gently for about one minute twice a day. The Tai Yang point is at the temple in the depression between the lateral end of the eyebrow and the eyelid. The Hegu point is located on the back of the hand between the thumb and first finger. The Feng Chi points are at the back of the head at the base of the skull, about 2 inches on either side of the center point.

**Diet:** Eat a balanced diet that includes fresh vegetables and reduce your coffee intake, since caffeine dehydrates the skin. Fruit such as pears, cranberries, blueberries, and bananas are recommended. Mung beans, red beans, bamboo shoots, and purslane are also good. Avoid food that is rich and fatty, as it has drying and warming properties that can make symptoms worse.

## NATUROPATHY

**Supplements:** Take 3–5 g of omega-3 essential fatty acids a day as they have anti-inflammatory properties that may help protect against the extreme reaction of anaphylaxis and other allergic responses to insect bites. Quercetin, when taken before being bitten, can lessen the severity of an allergic response. If you have a history of an allergy to bees, wasps, or other insects, consider taking 250 mg of quercetin supplements three times a day. Vitamin C, which can be taken at 500–1,000 mg three times a day, is essential for healing and a strong immune system to avoid infection. Bioflavonoids work synergistically with vitamin C and have anti-inflammatory properties. Take 250–500 mg two to three times a day.

### TIP: USE AN APPLE CIDER VINEGAR SOLUTION
To relieve the discomfort of insect bites, make up a solution of water and apple cider vinegar in a 1:1 ratio and apply it to the bite for a few minutes. Rinse with warm water.

**Topical herbs:** There are a variety of herbs that can be used topically to prevent insect bites from occurring, or encourage existing bites to heal. Arnica can be used as a topical herb to treat inflammation from insect bites. Place 3 drops on the bite and massage it into the affected area. Lemon balm, which is another traditional treatment for relief of insect bites or stings, can be applied in the same way. You can also apply aloe vera gel to the affected area for two weeks, or until it is healed, to relieve inflammation. Calendula cream is used as a natural insect repellent, and also soothes skin irritations. Comfrey cream promotes tissue healing, and tea tree oil can be used as an antiseptic to prevent infection. Citronella is a lemon-scented plant that has long been used as an insect repellent. It is also the active ingredient in several commercial insect repellents that you can apply to either your skin or clothing. Pure citronella oil can be irritating to the skin and should never be ingested. If you want to use the oil, dilute it by adding several drops to a vegetable oil base. You can then rub the diluted oil directly on your skin. Citrus essential oil has aromatic qualities that repel insects. Dilute it by adding several drops of essential oil to a vegetable oil base, and experiment by using different combinations of essential oils together to customize your own insect repellent. Lemongrass is a cousin of citronella and has many of the same insect-repelling compounds. If you have access to the fresh herb, simply crush some and rub it directly on your skin. Plantain is also excellent for bug bites and can also be rubbed directly on the skin.

## TIP: APPLY A POULTICE
Mash up a clove of garlic and place the poultice on the affected area. This will prevent an infection from developing. You can also use a wet tea bag as a poultice. The tannic acid in tea helps to reduce the swelling associated with insect bites. Black tea is the most effective.

## HOMEOPATHY

The following remedies can be helpful in stimulating the recovery from an insect bite in those who do not have a history of allergic reactions.

**Ledum:** Use this remedy to treat stings that cause the affected area to feel cool to the touch. Discomfort is considerably relieved by contact with cool air, applying cool compresses, and cool bathing. The skin that has been stung is also likely to look red and slightly swollen.

**Apis:** This remedy can be used to treat bites that show symptoms of localized inflammation and swelling. The affected area is likely to be raised and look puffy, feel worse for contact with warmth in any form, and feel soothed by exposure to cool applications.

**Urtica urens:** If bites trigger strong burning sensations around the edge of the affected area, use Urtica urens. There is also localized itchiness and a stitch-like discomfort that is aggravated by contact with cool air and cool bathing. This remedy can also be effective in easing lingering and itchy sensations that refuse to clear up.

## TIP: USE LAVENDER ESSENTIAL OIL
Diluted lavender essential oil can be immensely soothing and healing when applied to skin affected by an insect bite. Dilute a few drops in a vegetable oil base before applying it directly to the skin.

**Staphysagria:** If insect bites cause severe irritation, itchiness, and localized stinging sensations that trigger strong feelings of irritation and anger, use Staphysagria. The least touch to the affected area is uncomfortable, while warmth and scratching give temporary relief. This remedy can also play a useful role as a prophylactic when used by those who know that they tend to attract midge bites.

---

**TIP:** USE INSECT REPELLENT

Take preventive steps by using an insect repellent on the skin. There are many formulas available that are made from natural ingredients.

---

## HERBALISM

Additional remedies to those described below are listed in Bee and Wasp Stings (p. 896).

**Stinging nettle:** Although it seems counterintuitive to put stinging nettles on an insect sting, this plant may be beneficial. The suggested dosage is to drink a tea made from 1–2 g of the leaf two to three times daily. Many health food stores now sell stinging nettles in standardized extracts as freeze-dried capsules. You may find this a more convenient mode of delivery; simply follow the dosage instructions on the back of the bottle. In addition, the underside of the fresh cut leaf of the nettle plant can be applied to the affected area. While this is a good option, obtaining the fresh cut leaf may be difficult. Stinging nettles may cause upset stomach and nausea, and there is the potential for an allergic reaction.

**Chamomile:** This herb can help calm the inflammation and irritation associated with insect bites. Make a poultice from a handful of fresh chamomile flowers and apply it directly to the affected area. Do not use chamomile if you are allergic to plants in the daisy family.

**Thyme:** This herb may help to relieve the sting of insect bites when used topically. Apply 1 drop of the essential oil directly to the insect bite. It can also be incorporated with other oils, such as apricot kernel oil, that help nourish and moisturize the skin. Thyme oil has been associated with a few toxic reactions when taken internally, so only use the oil topically to treat insect bites.

# JELLYFISH STINGS

## DIAGNOSIS

Jellyfish can be a hazard when swimming in warm waters. Stings usually occur when someone swimming or wading in the ocean accidentally comes into contact with a jellyfish. The stingers on these animals are located at the ends of tentacles and contain poisons that can be toxic to humans. In most cases, however, the poisons only cause injury to the part of the skin that comes into contact with the jellyfish tentacles. A sting causes an intense pain in the affected area. There will be a distinct red mark on the skin, which may appear as a raised rash, indicating the site of the sting. This will be followed by a burning sensation and localized swelling in the area. The marks can last from days to weeks, and severe stings can cause the affected skin to peel off as it heals. Very rarely, symptoms can be serious, resulting in breathing difficulties and unconsciousness. Stings around the eyes can also be serious, leading to abrasions that can harm the eyesight.

**DANGER**: Seek emergency medical help if a victim is experiencing severe swelling or difficulty breathing or swallowing. Any stings on the eyes, face, mouth, or genitals should also be assessed by a doctor.

## SYMPTOMS

- Intense pain at the site of the sting
- A red mark on the skin
- Burning sensation
- Localized swelling

## TREATMENT GOAL

Treatment involves ruling out a serious allergic reaction, and relieving local symptoms of pain and discomfort.

## CONVENTIONAL MEDICINE

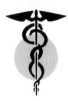

**Rinse the area:** Move away from the jellyfish and immediately rinse the area of the sting with salt water. Do not use fresh water as it may activate the stinging substance even further, causing more toxins to be released. Also apply white vinegar to inactivate any remaining toxin so that further injury does not occur.

**Remove any tentacles:** The stung area should be examined to determine whether any tentacles are embedded in the skin. These should be removed with gloved hands or tweezers if available. The area should also be immobilized as much as possible.

**Medications:** A non-steroidal anti-inflammatory drug (NSAID) such as ibuprofen may be used for pain relief. Topical 5% hydrocortisone cream can be applied to the area, and diphenhydramine (Benadryl®), which is an antihistamine commonly used to treat allergies, may also be taken to relieve itchiness.

**To treat an allergic reaction:** Generally, only the box jellyfish of Australia releases a serious poison that requires victims to take an antidote at a hospital. However, anyone who appears very ill, has an altered mental state, is vomiting, or is experiencing severe swelling should be taken to a hospital. Allergic reactions and shock are potential problems that need to be treated immediately. Once at the hospital, the area is rinsed with a normal saline solution, acetic acid (vinegar) is applied, and any stingers are removed. Medications such as epinephrine and steroids may be given at the hospital, and antihistamines and steroid creams may be prescribed when the patient is discharged.

## TRADITIONAL CHINESE MEDICINE

**Herbs:** Combine 15 g of Jin Yin Hua (honeysuckle flower) and 15 g of Jing Jie (schizonepeta stem and bud). Boil the ingredients in 5 cups of water for five minutes, strain the liquid, and add it to a container that is large enough to bathe the affected area. Soak the bite in this herbal bath once a day for as long as required. The herbs are available from Chinese pharmacies or online.

**Acupuncture:** Sessions can relieve the immediate pain of jellyfish stings. Stimulating certain meridian points can regulate a patient's circulation and help maintain skin health.

**Acupressure:** Press the Tai Yang, Hegu, and Feng Chi points gently for about one minute twice a day. The Tai Yang point is at the temple in the depression between the lateral end of the eyebrow and the eyelid. The Hegu point is located on the back of the hand between the thumb and first finger. The Feng Chi points are at the back of the head at the base of the skull, about 2 inches on either side of the center point.

**Diet:** Eat food that is gentle and strengthens the immune system, such as green vegetables, aubergines, radishes, mung beans, bitter melon, purslane, and pears. Foods that dispel dampness and heat are also recommended, such as watermelon peel, lotus root, wax gourds, red beans, bananas, and grapefruit. Avoid food that promotes heat and dampness, such as pepper, dried garlic, cloves, dried ginger, green peppers, leeks, liver, and green onions. Also, avoid seafood, and fatty and spicy foods.

## NATUROPATHY

**Jellyfish sting treatment:** Rinse the affected area with seawater, as fresh water will increase the pain. Do not rub the wound or apply ice to it. For classic jellyfish stings, apply topical vinegar or isopropyl alcohol. Remove any tentacles embedded in the skin with tweezers. Shaving cream or a paste of baking soda or mud can also be applied to the wound. Shave the area with a razor or knife and reapply vinegar or alcohol. The shaving cream or paste prevents nematocysts (stinging cells) that have not been activated from discharging toxins during removal with the razor. Immobilize the extremity that has been stung because movement may cause the venom to spread. If a jellyfish stings you in the eye, irrigate the eye with 1 gallon of fresh water. If you are stung in the mouth, rinse the mouth with vinegar diluted to one-quarter of its strength. However, do not use vinegar if oral swelling or difficulty swallowing occurs.

## HOMEOPATHY

The following remedies can be helpful in stimulating recovery from a jellyfish sting.

**Staphysagria:** If stings cause severe irritation, itchiness, and localized stinging sensations that trigger strong feelings of irritation and anger, use Staphysagria. The least touch to the affected area is uncomfortable, while warmth gives temporary relief.

**Ledum:** Use this remedy to treat stings that cause the affected area to feel cool to the touch. Discomfort is considerably relieved by contact with cool air, applying cool compresses, and cool bathing. The skin that has been stung is also likely to look red and slightly swollen.

**Apis:** This remedy can be used to treat stings that show symptoms of localized inflammation and swelling. The affected area is likely to be raised and look puffy, feel worse for contact with warmth in any form, and feel soothed by exposure to cool applications.

**Urtica urens:** If a sting triggers strong burning sensations around the edge of the affected area, use Urtica urens. There is also localized itchiness and a stitch-like discomfort that is aggravated by contact with cool air and cool bathing. This remedy can also be effective in easing lingering and itchy sensations that refuse to clear up.

## HERBALISM

Herbal therapy can be used to treat symptoms of pain, irritation, and infection. Tea tree oil and aloe vera can be applied to treat post-sting symptoms. Also, see Bee and Wasp Stings (p. 896) for additional herbal treatments that could be helpful for jellyfish stings.

**Tea tree oil:** Apply a thin layer of tea tree ointment or salve that contains 5–10% tea tree oil to the sting for the first day or two. Tea tree can be strong, especially on open skin, and after one or two days the body is generally able to fight off any lingering bacteria on its own. Dermatitis is the only significant side effect associated with the prolonged and repeated topical use of tea tree oil.

**Aloe vera:** The clear gel-like substance that oozes from the fresh-cut leaves of aloe has been used for years to treat a wide array of skin conditions such as burns, bites, stings, and generally dry, scaly skin. To treat a sting, simply take the gel from a fresh-cut leaf and apply it directly to the affected area. If fresh leaves are not available, there are a variety of gels and lotions containing aloe vera that can be purchased at your local health food store, pharmacy, or stores that specialize in herbal medicines. Some aloe vera gels contain alcohol as a base to contribute to its cooling effect. Be aware that alcohol will sting on any open skin, so avoid any alcohol-based gels if your sting is accompanied by breaks in the skin.

# MEASLES

## DIAGNOSIS

Measles (rubeola) is one of the most contagious viral diseases, although the number of cases has largely decreased with widespread vaccination. The first signs of the disease are a hacking cough, runny nose, high fever, and watery red eyes. Small red spots with blue-white centers may also form inside the mouth. A rash then spreads to the rest of the body, taking on a reddish-brown and blotchy appearance. The rash usually first develops on the forehead and then travels down over the face, neck, and body to the feet.

Measles is spread by airborne droplets of saliva, and the incubation period of the disease is usually one to two weeks. Patients are infectious from four days before the onset of a rash until five days after the rash appears. Recovery usually takes about one week. Anyone who has not already had measles can be infected, but once a person has had the disease he or she is immune for life. Occasionally, complications with pneumonia can develop from the measles, and in some cases the disease can be fatal.

**DANGER**: There are two forms of measles, rubeola and German measles (rubella). Rubella is less severe but can cause developmental malformations in a fetus. If you are pregnant and come into contact with someone infected with measles, contact your doctor immediately for advice and reassurance.

## SYMPTOMS

- A fever and temperature of 102°F
- A cold and sore throat
- A hacking cough
- Red eyes and increased sensitivity to light
- A rash of clear red spots around the ears, which spreads to the body

## TREATMENT GOAL

As measles is caused by a virus, symptoms typically resolve on their own without treatment. Conventional and complementary therapies can help to make patients more comfortable, relieving symptoms until the virus has run its course.

## CONVENTIONAL MEDICINE

Measles is generally a benign self-limiting, acute illness. Treatment involves reducing the fever and pain, and relieving itchiness.

**Medication:** Acetaminophen (Tylenol®) can be taken to relieve pain and lower fever. Aspirin should not be used by those under 16 years old because it has been linked to the development of Reye's syndrome, a lethal disease that affects all organs of the body. If joint pain is a problem, non-steroidal anti-inflammatory drugs (NSAIDs) such as Motrin® can be used. To prevent children from scratching, trim their fingernails or consider dressing very young children with mittens. Skin rashes can be soothed using starch baths and calamine lotion. Diphenhydramine (Benadryl®) can also be given to treat itchiness.

**If you are exposed to the virus while pregnant:** Measles is clinically significant because it is the only known virus that can cause developmental malformations in a fetus. Almost all fetuses that are infected during the first 16 weeks of pregnancy are affected. Unfortunately, it continues to circulate and newborns infected with rubella remain a problem. Pregnant women who are exposed to measles, particularly in the first trimester, are at risk. In this case, immunoglobulin, an antibody that identifies and neutralizes viruses, can be given, but although this shortens the duration of the disease in the mother, it does not seem to prevent defects in newborns. An infant born with measles is contagious for up to a year.

## TRADITIONAL CHINESE MEDICINE

**Herbs:** Make a herbal bath using 15 g of Jin Yin Hua (honeysuckle flower) and 15 g of Jing Jie (schizonepeta stem and bud). Mix the ingredients, add 5 cups of water, and boil for five minutes. Strain the liquid and add it to your bathwater. Soak your body once a day, for as long as required. The herbs are available from Chinese pharmacies or online.

**Acupuncture:** Measles is a highly contagious condition, so acupuncture is not always appropriate, as the patient will have to be exposed to the public to receive treatment. However, stimulating certain meridian points can help by regulating circulation and helping to maintain skin health.

**Acupressure:** Press the Tai Yang, Hegu, and Feng Chi points gently for about one minute twice a day. The Tai Yang point is at the temple in the depression between the lateral end of the eyebrow and eyelid. The Hegu point is located on the back of the hand between the thumb and first finger. The Feng Chi points are at the back of the head at the base of the skull, about 2 inches on either side of the center point.

**Diet:** Drink plenty of water every day and choose foods that nourish the body's Yin and replenish Qi, such as coriander, spinach, and water chestnut. Eat food that is gentle and strengthens the immune system, such as organic green vegetables, aubergines, purslane, and pears. Drinking green tea is also helpful since it has a gentle, cleansing effect. Avoid food that has heat and warming properties, such as hot chili peppers, beef, lamb, and deep-fried and fatty, greasy food. Also avoid raw and/or cold food.

## NATUROPATHY

**Diet:** A child suffering from measles should sip on water all day. Teas and juices are also helpful as they keep the throat moist, lower fever, and keep the child hydrated. Soups and fruit juice made into ice pops can also be soothing. Feed these to your child throughout the day instead of solid food. Eliminate fats while the child is sick with measles, as they are extremely difficult to digest when suffering from this condition.

**Supplements:** Vitamin C supports the immune system and helps fight infection. Give a child 200 mg three times a day. Children can also take 10 mg of zinc a day to help boost the immune system and promote healing. Vitamin A aids in healing the mucous membrane inside the throat and mouth. Give your child 5,000 IU of vitamin A a day.

**Herbs:** Herbs can help to alleviate many of the distressing symptoms associated with measles, including fever, itchiness, eye sensitivity, and coughing. A fever can be relieved with the help of teas made from catnip, yarrow, and linden. Mix 20 drops of a tincture of each herb in hot water and give it to your child to drink. Relieve itchy skin by using antipruritic herbs, such as chickweed. To make an infusion, steep 2–4 oz of dry herbs in 6–8 cups of hot water for 15 minutes. Strain the liquid, add it to bath water, and soak the body for 20 minutes. Distilled witch hazel can also be dabbed on to itchy skin to immediately, although temporarily, soothe the skin. Eye strain due to photosensitivity is a common symptom of measles, so most patients prefer to be in a darkened room. An eyebright wash or a chamomile compress will ease such discomfort, but not replace the need for reduced light. To make an eyebright wash, dilute 10–20 drops of a tincture in 2 oz of lukewarm water and pour it by the side of the eye while standing over a sink twice a day. A chamomile compress can be made by boiling 1–2 tsp of the dried herb in 500 ml of water for 10 minutes. Let the liquid cool and moisten a piece of cotton or wool gauze with the solution. Wring it out and place it over the affected eye. Make sure the patient gets plenty of rest and that the lights in his or her room are dimmed.

## HOMEOPATHY

Any of the following remedies can play a positive role in speeding up recovery from, and easing the distress of, a mild episode of measles.

**Aconite:** This remedy is appropriate if symptoms such as feverishness develop sudden and dramatically, triggering restlessness and anxiety. The eyes are likely to be very sensitive, and a harsh croupy cough and runny nose may also be present. This remedy is most appropriate at the initial stage of infection (usually within the first 24–48 hours). Once this stage has passed and the symptoms have moved on, it will be necessary to change the choice of homeopathic remedy accordingly.

**Belladonna:** This is an alternative remedy that may be indicated in the early, feverish stage of illness. Symptoms include a rapidly developing high fever that results in bright red, hot, dry skin. During the feverish stage the pulse may be rapid, and there may be a throbbing headache. This remedy is most helpful in the stage before the rash has fully developed.

**Bryonia:** If the feverish phase is very slow to develop, and the skin has a deeply flushed appearance, use Bryonia. Symptoms include a persistent, dry, tickly cough and a frontal headache that is made more intense by the slightest movement.

**Pulsatilla:** This remedy is often helpful in treating the later, more established stage of this illness, once a rash has fully developed. There may be symptoms of catarrh and a dry mouth and coated tongue due to nasal congestion at night. Any mucus present is characteristically thick, bland, and greenish-yellow in color. When ill a normally placid child tends to become weepy and clingy.

---

**TIP:** DO NOT FORCE A PATIENT TO EAT

Avoid forcing food on your child if he or she is in the feverish stage of measles and does not have an appetite. It is far more important that he keeps his fluid intake up and stays hydrated. This will help sustain a patient's temperature to reasonable boundaries, while eating at this stage can raise the temperature.

---

## HERBALISM

Measles was once a common childhood illness, but due to the widespread use of childhood vaccines there has been a sharp drop in the number of cases. Measles are caused by a viral infection, and many herbs may be used to help augment the immune system.

**Blessed thistle:** This herb is used to help fight infections and may even possess anti-cancer properties, although research into both claims is still lacking. Blessed thistle is best taken as a tea. Steep 1–3 g of the flowering tops of this plant in 1 cup of water and drink two to three times daily while symptoms persist. A tincture of blessed thistle may also be used. Add several drops of tincture to juice or water and drink two to three times a day. You can often find blessed thistle in local health food stores in a combination call Essiac tea, which includes burdock root, Indian rhubarb, sheep sorrel, slippery elm bark, watercress, red clover, and kelp. This may also be helpful in treating measles.

**Astragalus:** Also known as milk vetch, astragalus has long been used in traditional Chinese medicine for its immune-stimulating effects. Astragalus root can be used as a tea, or taken in capsule form. If you choose to take the capsule, take 500 mg three times daily. Astragalus should not be taken if you are on blood-thinning drugs, immunosuppressive drugs, or have an autoimmune disorder, such as lupus or rheumatoid arthritis.

**Elderberry:** This herb may be effective in treating measles. Specific formulations of elderberry juice can be bought at local health food stores. It is recommended that this be taken orally at the onset of symptoms for three to five days. Raw elderberry juice can be quite toxic and is not recommended. Although cooking the berry destroys most of these toxins, it is still not considered safe. The recommended preparation of elderberry juice is the specific, store-bought formulations, which eliminate this problem with toxicity. Diarrhea and vomiting have been reported with use of elderberry juice, although this side effect is greatly decreased by taking specific formulations.

**Garlic:** This herb is purported to have antiviral properties, and generally boosts the immune system. Take garlic capsules, which can be found at local health food stores, or eat a couple of fresh cloves a day. The probable effective dosage for a child is based on what has been determined for adults, so use 500 mg of a capsule twice a day if the child can take capsules, or one-half to one full clove garlic hidden in food per day.

# MUMPS

## DIAGNOSIS

Mumps is one of the most common childhood illnesses, but many children are now vaccinated against the disease. Mumps is a viral infection that causes the salivary glands in the cheeks and neck (the parotid glands) to swell and become sore. The virus is contagious for about one week before symptoms of the disease emerge, which can make it difficult to track down the source of infection. It is spread through airborne droplets that are breathed in, and the virus is then passed into the bloodstream and circulated around the body. The first signs of the virus are a high fever, headache, and loss of appetite. The glands then become increasingly swollen over a period of one to three days. The pain is made worse by talking, swallowing, chewing, or drinking. Either both the left and right glands become swollen, or the virus may only affect one side.

Although the swollen glands and high temperature caused by mumps are unpleasant, the most serious complications involve the possible infection of other organs. In the case of adult men with mumps, the disease infects the testicles, causing swelling, pain, soreness, and a high temperature. A less rare complication of mumps is meningitis, which may appear 3–10 days after the onset of mumps.

## SYMPTOMS

- Feeling under the weather
- Raised temperature
- Swollen glands and neck
- Swollen face
- Earache
- Inability to chew and/or swallow
- Nausea
- Swollen joints

## TREATMENT GOAL

There is no cure for mumps. Treatment involves bed rest and relieving symptoms to make the patient as comfortable as possible until the virus has run its course.

## CONVENTIONAL MEDICINE

The primary treatment for mumps is through vaccination, and over 90% of adults have been vaccinated against the virus. If you suspect that you have the mumps, consult a doctor—it is now a rare disease so another condition may be causing symptoms. Usually, mumps is a benign virus that can be allowed to run its natural course (this usually takes two weeks). Resting and drinking lots of fluids are an important part of treatment, as with any viral illness.

**Acetaminophen:** The first choice of drug in the treatment of mumps is acetaminophen, which can lower a fever and relieve pain.

**To treat testicular swelling:** In teenagers or adults suffering from mumps, particularly males, severe joint pain and swelling, as well as testicular pain and swelling, may occur. Prednisolone is sometimes prescribed to treat this complication. If significant pain and swelling of the testicles is present, a testicular bridge (available from drug stores) can be used to support the scrotum. A drug known as interferon alpha 2b has been used to prevent infertility in men who experience severe swelling of the testicles.

## TRADITIONAL CHINESE MEDICINE

**Herbs:** Mix 8 g of Jin Yin Hua (honeysuckle flower), 6 g of Jing Jie (schizonepeta stem and bud), and 12 g of Ban Lan Gen (isatis root). Boil these herbs in 2 cups of water for five minutes. Strain the liquid and drink. The herbs are available from Chinese pharmacies or online.

**Acupuncture:** Mumps is a highly contagious condition, so acupuncture is not always appropriate as the patient will have to be exposed to the public to receive treatment. However, acupuncture is usually effective. A practitioner may recommend 30-minute sessions once to three times a week.

**Acupressure:** In a sitting position, use your thumb to press the Hegu, Qu Chi, and San Yin Jiao points with strong pressure for about one minute two or three times a day. The Hegu point is located on the back of the hand between the thumb and first finger. With the elbow flexed, the Qu Chi point is located in the depression on the outside of the bend at the lateral end of the crease. The San Yin Jiao point is located on the inside of the leg, about 3 inches above the anklebone.

**Diet:** Drink plenty of fresh water every day and eat light, fresh food such as turnips, celery, spinach, aubergines, purslane, wax gourds, and mung beans. Avoid food that has heat and warming properties, such as hot chili peppers, beef, lamb, mustard greens, and ginger. Also, avoid deep-fried food, and eat less fatty and greasy foods, since they create more heat. Bitter melon, watermelon, adzuki beans, tofu, and radishes are also good choices.

## NATUROPATHY

**Diet:** Feed your child soft foods, since children with mumps have a hard time chewing. Soups and fruit juice ice pops can be soothing, and can be fed to a child throughout the day instead of solid food. Eliminate fats while the child is sick as they are extremely difficult to digest with this condition.

**Supplements:** Vitamin C supports the immune system and helps fight infection. Give a child 200 mg three times a day. Children can also take 10 mg of zinc a day to help boost the immune system and promote healing. Quercetin has anti-inflammatory and antiviral properties. Give a child 500 mg a day.

**Herbs:** Arnica tincture can help to relieve headaches when it is rubbed on the temples or forehead. However, be sure to keep tincture away from eyes and any areas of broken skin. Chamomile tea can be beneficial if your child is feeling restless, as it encourages the body to relax. Give 1 cup of tea twice a day.

### TIP: APPLY A COMPRESS TO SWOLLEN GLANDS
Apply a warm or cold compress to ease the discomfort of swollen glands. Children should also be kept isolated until the swelling has subsided.

## HOMEOPATHY

Any of the following homeopathic remedies can help minimize the distress of an acute episode of mumps.

**Jaborandi:** This remedy is appropriate if swollen and tender glands make it difficult for a patient to move his or her jaw. As a result, talking, eating, and drinking tend to cause great distress. The patient is also likely to look flushed and feverish and

have a strong thirst.

**Phytolacca:** This remedy can be helpful if stiffness and tension in the glands makes swallowing very difficult, a situation that is made worse by a persistent feeling of dryness in the throat. The latter becomes especially noticeable when talking or eating.

**Mercurius:** Take this remedy to shift lingering symptoms once the feverish stage has subsided. Symptoms include an increased amount of saliva in the mouth that causes drooling at night, and a nasty, metallic taste in the mouth. Sweatiness, restlessness, and distress tend to be especially prevalent during the night.

## HERBALISM

The number of mumps cases has dramatically decreased due to the effective use of childhood vaccines. In addition to the remedy below, see Measles (p. 947) for herbal therapies that may also be effective for mumps due to their antiviral properties.

**Poke root:** This herb can be helpful in patients with mumps dues to its ability to cleanse the lymph nodes. Poke root contains triterpenoids and saponins, which are responsible for many of its therapeutic effects. To use poke root, boil ½ tsp of the root in 1 liter of water for 10–15 minutes and drink 1 cup of the liquid two to three times a day. You can also take ½–1 ml of tincture mixed with juice or water two to three times a day. Poke root is a very strong herb and care should be taken not to use it too much; it would be best to consult a medical herbalist prior to beginning therapy with poke root. Common side effects include diarrhea, nausea, and vomiting, and more serious side effects have also been noted.

# SHINGLES

## DIAGNOSIS

Shingles (also known as herpes zoster) is triggered by the same virus that causes chickenpox. It is an infection of the nerves that manifests as a painful, blistering rash that often appears in a band around the chest and the back. After the chickenpox virus has been contracted and run its course, it travels along the nerve paths to the roots of the nerves, where it becomes inactive and lies dormant. In most people, it remains inactive. When the virus is reactivated, however, often many years after the initial chickenpox infection, it travels via the nerve paths to the skin, causing an outbreak of shingles. It is not known what factors trigger a reactivation of the virus. Shingles is contagious and may itself cause chickenpox in those who have not had the disease before. Shingles generally affects the elderly, and those with an immune deficiency. Occasionally, it can also cause complications. The rash can become infected, vision can be affected if there is a rash near the eyes, and the senses can also be affected, though it is usually attributed to some decrease in immunity.

## SYMPTOMS

- Sharp pains under the surface of the skin
- A rash of red sores located along nerve pathways
- Itchy blisters, which eventually burst and scab over
- Fever and enlarged lymph nodes

## TREATMENT GOAL

Treatment involves rest and keeping the rash uncovered so that fresh air can circulate to it. Measures can also be taken to relieve symptoms of pain and itchiness, and prevent scarring from occurring.

## CONVENTIONAL MEDICINE

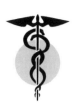

**Antivirals:** The primary treatment for shingles is one of the oral antivirals that are effective against the herpes virus. These include acyclovir (Zovirax®), valacyclovir (Valtrex®), and famicyclovir (Famtrex®). If they are taken within the first 72 hours of the onset of the rash, they can shorten the duration of the disease and the symptoms of pain and swelling. A topical antiviral agent known as Vidarabine is used if shingles have affected the eyes.

**Cold compress:** Apply a wet compress of cold tap water to the affected area for 20 minutes four to eight times a day to encourage the rash to resolve.

**Pain relief:** Tylenol®, Motrin®, or in severe cases, codeine may be needed to relieve pain. A lidocaine skin patch may also be given for pain relief.

**Preventive measures:** If you are infected, avoid young children, pregnant women, and anyone with a compromised immune system to avoid passing the virus to them. Stress reduction is also recommended as it helps prevent outbreaks. More rest may be required during an outbreak of shingles as well. The FDA has approved a vaccine called Zostavax® to help prevent shingles. It is given to adults over 60 and has been shown to cut the incidence of shingles by 64%.

**To treat post-herpetic neuralgia:** If pain and nerve symptoms exist after the rash is gone, it is treated with lidocaine and a medication known as Neurontin®. A natural topical ointment, such as Zostrix®, that contains capsaicin, a substance derived from peppers, may be helpful in relieving itchiness. It is also important to keep the affected area clean.

## TRADITIONAL CHINESE MEDICINE

**Herbs:** The herbs and creams listed below are available from Chinese pharmacies or online.
• External herbal creams: Jin Huang Gao and Si Huang Gao are both external herbs that are available in cream form. Apply either cream, since they have similar effects, once or twice a day.
• External herbal wash: Mix 30 g of Zi Hua Di Ding (Yedeon's violet), 18 g of Pu Gong Ying (dandelion), 30 g of Huang Bai (phellodendron), 30 g of Bai Jiang Cao (patrinia), and 30 g of Jin Yin Hua (honeysuckle flower). Place the herbs in a ceramic pot and add 6 cups of water. Boil the mixture for 5 minutes, and then simmer for 10 minutes. Strain

the decoction, add 6 more cups of water, and boil the herbs a second time. Use the decoction to wash the affected skin once or twice a day.

**Acupuncture:** Treatment is appropriate for both the acute and chronic stages of shingles. For acute conditions, the treatment will focus on resolving the virus and reducing the pain. The practitioner will use needling techniques that release toxins, in order to stop itchiness and prevent the condition from becoming chronic. At a chronic stage, treatment will regulate immunity, or rebuild your internal balance by tonifying some of your deficient organs or reorganizing the disordered energy. In a chronic treatment plan, patients can undergo acupuncture sessions for a few months or even years, depending on the severity of the condition.

**Acupressure:** Acupressure is not recommended for this condition.

**Diet:** Foods to be avoided include ginger, chilies, mustard greens, and mutton, as they are pungent and irritating and increase heat in the body, which may make the condition worse. Generally light, fresh food is recommended. Examples include turnips, celery, spinach, aubergines, purslane, wax gourds, and mung beans.

> **TIP:** DRINK DAIKON RADISH JUICE
> Wash and cut some daikon radishes into small chunks and juice them in a blender. Drinking the juice may help heal the shingles.

## NATUROPATHY

**Diet:** Include foods in your diet that are high in B-vitamins, including wheat germ, brewer's yeast, eggs, and whole grains, as they are healing to the nervous system. Brightly colored fruit and vegetables such as squash, carrots, berries, and oranges have high amounts of bioflavonoids and vitamins A and C, which will help resolve inflammation and blisters of the skin, and boost the body's immune system. Avoid meats, fried foods, sugar, chocolate, and carbonated beverages, as they suppress the immune system and interfere with the healing process. Drinking green vegetable juice every day will flood your body with essential nutrients to alkalinize the body and boost immunity.

**Supplements:** Take 1,000 mg of vitamin C four times a day for increased immune support and to reduce stress damage to nerves. Zinc also helps support the immune system and can be taken at 30 mg a day. Take 200 mg a day of selenium to help resolve the viral infection, and 3,000 mg of L-lysine a day as it can help heal and perhaps suppress herpes virus infections. B-vitamins are essential for nerve health and can be taken at 100 mg three times a day. Vitamin B12 injections, administered by a qualified practitioner, are essential to help the body recover more quickly and reduce pain associated with shingles. Proteolytic enzymes are thought to benefit cases of shingles caused by the herpes zoster virus by decreasing the body's inflammatory response and regulating the immune response to the virus. Take two to three capsules on an empty stomach twice a day.

**TIP:** TAKE AN OATMEAL BATH

Colloidal oatmeal is a type of finely ground oatmeal. You can make your own by grinding oatmeal in a food processor. Add several cups of colloidal oatmeal to your bath water to relieve itchiness. Oatmeal can be slippery when wet, so use caution when getting into and out of the bathtub.

**Herbs:** Take 500 mg of olive leaf extract four times a day for its potent antiviral benefits. Lomatium root is used for immune support and also has antiviral effects; take 500 mg four times a day. You can also take 300 mg of St. John's wort in capsule form, or 4 ml as a tincture, three times a day for its antiviral properties.

**TIP:** DO NOT SCRATCH

Although it is hard to resist scratching, refrain as much as possible. When you scratch, you increase the risk that the blisters will become infected from dirt under the fingernails. It is also important to keep blistered areas clean. Use soap and water to help prevent any bacterial infections from developing.

## HOMEOPATHY

Any of the following homeopathic options can be helpful in easing the pain and distress of a bout of shingles.

**Rhus tox:** This remedy can be helpful for relieving intense pains that are especially distressing in bed at night, causing severe restlessness. Pains may be limited to the left side of the body, or move from the left to right side. The affected areas of skin itch and burn, and pain and discomfort is especially troublesome following contact with cold drafts of air.

**Mezereum:** If painful, itchy sensations constantly change position when scratched, try Mezereum. When this remedy is well indicated, lesions take on a thick, crusty texture and may discharge a sticky liquid. Irritation and general discomfort are made generally more intense by contact with warm water.

**Ranunculus bulbosus:** If burning, shooting, stitching pains are severe enough to bring tears to the eyes, use Ranunculus bulbosus. Symptoms include neuralgic pains that linger long after the bluish-tinged eruptions have superficially cleared. Movement (especially moving the arms) aggravates pain and discomfort, and can be eased by sitting in a position that allows the body to bend forward.

**TIP:** USE HYPERICUM

A soothing infusion of diluted Hypericum tincture can be applied to a cool compress in order to ease pain. Follow this with an application of Hypericum cream for added benefit.

## HERBALISM

 **Chili pepper:** Recent research has propelled the chili pepper and its primary active ingredient, capsaicin, into the spotlight. Capsaicin has been shown to be useful for many types of aches and pains, including those associated with shingles. Creams and ointments can be found in health food stores. Look for one containing 0.025–0.075% capsaicin and apply it to the affected area three to four times daily. A mild tingling sensation is normal with the application of capsaicin products; it may last for a day or two before the pain begins to disappear. An intense burning or itching sensation is not normal so discontinue use if these adverse reactions are present. Also be sure to wash your hands after applying any capsaicin-containing product to the skin.

# SHOCK

## DIAGNOSIS

Shock is a life-threatening condition that occurs when the heart is not able to pump enough blood to carry the necessary oxygen and nutrients to different parts of the body. It requires emergency medical treatment. Shock can be linked to any condition that reduces blood flow and is classified according to the cause. Cardiogenic shock is associated with heart problems; hypovolemic shock is caused by an inadequate volume of blood in the body; anaphylactic shock is triggered by an allergic reaction; septic shock is associated with an infection; and neurogenic shock is caused by damage to the nervous system. Symptoms of shock typically include anxiety or agitation; confusion; cool, clammy skin; chest pain; shallow breathing; and unconsciousness. Shock is also associated with very low blood pressure.

**DANGER**: Shock is life-threatening and requires immediate emergency assistance. First aid for shock includes laying the person down, raising the legs to help blood return to the heart, stopping any bleeding, ensuring warmth, and performing cardiopulmonary resuscitation (CPR) if needed. Emergency medical staff will administer oxygen and intravenous fluids to help raise blood pressure.

## SYMPTOMS

- Breathing becomes either very slow or very fast
- Frequent unconsciousness
- Pale skin
- Clammy skin and sweating
- Dizziness, confusion, or disorientation
- Shaking and trembling

## TREATMENT GOAL

Severe shock requires immediate emergency treatment. Call emergency services, check the victim's breathing, and loosen any tight-fitting clothes. Keep the patient as warm and comfortable as possible, and stay close until help arrives.

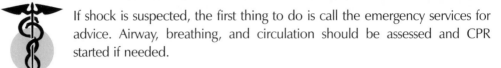

## CONVENTIONAL MEDICINE

If shock is suspected, the first thing to do is call the emergency services for advice. Airway, breathing, and circulation should be assessed and CPR started if needed.

**Position the victim:** Place the victim in a reclining position with the feet raised higher than the head. Do not do this, however, if it causes pain, if the person is unconscious, or if they have an injury to the head. If the patient is vomiting or bleeding from the mouth, he or she should be placed on his or her side instead of the back, and kept still.

**Make the patient comfortable:** Tight clothing should be loosened, but keep the victim warm using a blanket. Do not give the patient fluids or food.

**Emergency treatments:** The victim should be transported to a hospital where intravenous fluids will be given, along with an assessment to determine the cause of shock. The victim's blood pressure, cardiac, and respiratory levels are taken and assistance is given as needed to keep the victim's vital signs normal.

## TRADITIONAL CHINESE MEDICINE

If you are experiencing shock, you should go to the emergency room of the nearest hospital immediately.

**Herbs:** Several Chinese herbal medicines, such as 6 g of ginseng, 12 g of Mai Men Dong (ophiopogon tuber), and 8 g of Qin Pi, can help with recovery from this condition. However, these herbs should only be used after the initial condition has been stabilized.

**Acupuncture:** Consult a doctor of traditional Chinese medicine regarding a treatment plan and prognosis. If acupuncture is deemed appropriate, treatment will generally be administered once or twice a week for several months to help you recover from shock.

**Acupressure:** Press the Ren Zhong acupressure point, found in the center of the depression between the base of the nose and upper lip. Press this point with the tip of the finger or thumb with strong pressure for one minute and repeat two to three times a day.

**Diet:** If you are recovering from shock, eat light foods that are well cooked and easily digested. Avoid food that has heat and warming properties, such as hot chili peppers, ginger, mustard greens, beef, and lamb, as well as fried food, and fatty and greasy food.

## NATUROPATHY

Shock is considered a medical emergency and an ambulance should be called immediately. The following naturopathic treatments may help a patient to recover after the victim has received the proper emergency care.

**Prevention:** To help prevent shock, those with heart disease and other conditions that may predispose them to shock should be treated appropriately. If you have allergies, avoid allergens that may trigger anaphylactic shock, and carry an epi pen to administer epinephrine if an allergic reaction occurs.

**Supplements:** Oxidative stress (damage to cells caused by the body's normal use of oxygen) may play a role in shock. Several studies have suggested that treatment with antioxidants that help rid the body of free radicals (harmful by-products of the oxidative process) may protect against some types of shock. Other nutrients may also be protective. L-Carnitine may be helpful in treating cardiogenic, septic, and hypovolemic shock. Take 500 mg three times a day. Take 100 mg twice a day of coenzyme Q10 (CoQ10), an antioxidant that may be beneficial in treating hypovolemic and septic shock and may improve blood flow. Nicotinamide (a form of vitamin B3) taken at 2–4 g a day may help protect against bacterial endotoxin, which causes septic shock. Glutamine added to parenteral nutrition (nutrients given through the veins when someone cannot take oral nutrition) may protect the intestines and prevent complications from septic shock. If a dose can be tolerated, take 20–30 mg in divided doses. Consult a naturopathic physician about parenteral administration.

## HOMEOPATHY

Shock constitutes a medical emergency and demands immediate medical treatment. Examples of this kind of medical condition include anaphylactic shock that has set in as a result of a severe allergic reaction, or symptoms of shock that have developed as a consequence of significant blood loss. This type of condition clearly goes beyond the remit of first aid prescribing. However, once the emergency situation has been dealt with, homeopathic treatment may still be of value in helping the patient to come to terms with the trauma. Prescribing of this kind is best delivered by an experienced homeopathic practitioner. The following are some possible homeopathic remedies that may be considered as treatment.

**Arnica:** This is the primary remedy to consider after a trauma of any kind occurs to help the body come to terms with systemic shock.

**Aconite:** This remedy can be appropriate in treating residual panic and anxiety that have been triggered by the experience of being very seriously ill. Common symptoms include flashbacks of the traumatic episode accompanied by shaking, trembling, and palpitations, and a general feeling of terror. When this remedy is helpful symptoms arise quickly and suddenly.

**Ignatia:** If trauma has triggered a very emotionally labile state, consider using Ignatia. Signature symptoms include sudden mood changes with bouts of tears following laughter. When this remedy is helpful, there is a tendency to sigh repeatedly and generally feel highly emotionally charged.

## HERBALISM

Shock is a medical emergency, and herbal therapy is not indicated for this condition. However, herbal remedies may be helpful in assisting the body to recover from shock. Appropriate treatments will depend on the type of shock experienced, for example, septic or hypovolemic. Consult a medical herbalist, as this is a complicated and severe situation. The herbs below may be recommended as they are supportive and act as anti-oxidants for the circulatory system.

**Bilberry:** This herb has no side effects and is packed with antioxidants. A suggested dose is 50–120 g of berries two to three times a day. If it is difficult to find fresh or dried berries look for the extract and take 80–160 mg diluted in juice or water.

**Hawthorn:** Take a tea, tincture, or standardized extract of hawthorn to support the circulatory system. These can be purchased in health food stores and taken as directed on a daily basis.

# SUNBURN

## DIAGNOSIS

The painful inflammation, redness, and blistering of the skin caused by over-exposure to the sun is known as sunburn. Almost everyone has been sunburned, or will become sunburned, at one time or another. In severe cases, blood vessels as well as skin cells can become damaged. Repeated sunburns increase the risk of developing skin cancer, and can also cause signs of premature aging such as wrinkles. Burns result from the ultraviolet (UV) radiation produced by the sun, and can happen within 30 minutes of exposure. UVA and UVB are different wavelengths in the light spectrum. UVB is more damaging to the skin and is linked to skin cancer, while both UVA and UVB are responsible for premature aging and sunburn. Tanning beds also produce UVA and UVB rays and improper tanning bed use can cause sunburn.

The sun is at its strongest between 11 a.m. and 3 p.m., and should be avoided as much as possible during these hours. Remember that it is possible to get burnt on overcast days too, as clouds do not block out UV rays. The sun is also stronger in regions close to the equator, and places at high altitudes. Many light-skinned and fair-haired people burn more easily and are at greater risk of getting sunburned. Always use a sunscreen with a high protection factor when you are outside for extensive periods, and be sensible when it comes to how long you expose your skin to the sun.

## SYMPTOMS

- Areas of bright red skin
- Skin may radiate heat and feel hot to the touch
- Burning skin that is painful to touch
- Blistering and peeling skin
- In severe cases, faintness, nausea, and vomiting

## TREATMENT GOAL

The best treatment is prevention by protecting your skin from the sun and UV exposure. If a sunburn does occur, conventional and complementary therapies involve relieving the pain and discomfort of inflamed skin, and preventing blistering and peeling as much as possible.

## CONVENTIONAL MEDICINE

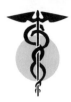

**Prevention:** Sunburn is best avoided. Apply a waterproof sunscreen with SPF30 and UVA blockage to your skin at least 20 minutes before going out in the sun. A plant called *Plypodium leucotomos*, found in a product called Heliocare®, has been used for many years to prevent sunburn and associated skin damage. Heliocare® can be taken orally and used in conjunction with sunscreen.

**Pain relief:** Once a sunburn has occurred, treatment involves relieving pain and inflammation, and caring for the skin. Aspirin or non-steroidal anti-inflammatory drugs (NSAIDs) can be used to manage the pain, and cool topical soaks can also provide relief when applied during the first 24 hours. Lotions that aid skin repair and soothe the burn include Sarna® (which contains menthol and camphor), pramoxine lotion, and Aveeno® anti-itch, which is a combination of pramoxine, calamine, and camphor. If a lotion is refrigerated before being applied it is more soothing.

**To treat blisters:** If blisters develop, medical treatment should be sought to evaluate the extent of the burn. Blisters should not be popped, as they are a method the body uses to protect itself (see Blisters, p. 906).

## TRADITIONAL CHINESE MEDICINE

**Herbs:** The following herbal remedies are available from Chinese pharmacies or online.
• Ru Yi Gao: This external herbal medicine is a paste that can be applied gently to the skin twice a day to relieve sunburn.
• Jin Yin Hua tea: Combine 5 g of Jin Yin Hua (honeysuckle flower) with 3 g of Bo He (field mint) in a teapot. Add boiling water and let the herbs steep for a few minutes. This tea can be sipped throughout the day for 10–30 days to assist the healing process. It can also help to prevent infection from occurring. Jin Yin Hua tea can be used in combination with Ru Yi Gao.

**TIP:** DRESS APPROPRIATELY
Wear light, loose clothing, such as cotton, so sweat can evaporate. Better yet, get clothing suited to exercise in hot weather, which wicks away moisture from the body to keep temperatures low.

**Diet:** Drink plenty of water and eat fresh fruit and vegetables, such as bitter melon, watermelon, mung beans, tofu, radishes, and celery. Avoid food that has heat and warming properties, such as hot chili peppers, beef, and lamb. Also avoid deep-fried food, and eat less fatty and greasy foods, as they also create more heat in the body.

## NATUROPATHY

**Diet:** Eat a plain, light diet that primarily consists of vegetables and fruits. Celery, cucumber, watermelon, and oranges are particularly beneficial because their high water content will keep you hydrated. Drinking lots of fluids before, during, and after exposure to heat is vital. Sip on water or sports energy drinks every 15 minutes, as hydration will speed up the healing process and keep the body cool while you are in the sun. Do not drink alcohol, hot drinks, or beverages with caffeine while in the sun; they increase the rate of dehydration.

**Supplements:** Vitamin A nourishes the skin and destroys free radicals, which can harm cells in the body. Take 50,000 IU thoughout the day, but do not take more than 10,000 IU a day if you are pregnant. Vitamin E aids in tissue repair and helps heal scar tissue. Take 400 IU a day. Also take 4,000 mg of vitamin C throughout the day to help with tissue repair of the skin.

**Herbs:** Calendula cream has been used for many years to soothe sunburns. Apply a small amount of a cream containing calendula two to three times a day. Using oatmeal can also heal and cool the skin. Use a soap made from oatmeal, available from most health food stores, or wrap oatmeal in one or two cheese cloths, tie them with string, and add them to your bath water.

**TIP:** USE SUNSCREEN
Use sunscreen to prevent sunburn. Natural brands are available in most health food stores.

## HOMEOPATHY

Any of the following homeopathic remedies can be helpful in supporting the body in recovering from a case of mild to moderate sunburn. A severe sunburn may require conventional medical therapy, but you can also seek advice from a homeopathic practitioner.

**Belladonna:** If symptoms of sunburn, including bright red, throbbing, hot skin, develop rapidly, use Belladonna. Additional symptoms include a pounding headache, and feeling irritable and short-tempered. Being exposed to chilled air, and an inability to perspire make discomfort worse, while resting while slightly propped up under light covers feels soothing.

**Carbo veg:** If sunburn is combined with a feeling of exhaustion that nears the point of collapse, consider using Carbo veg. The body tends to feel cold, while the head feels hot. There may also be low-grade dehydration, which tends to make symptoms worse, while contact with cool air or being fanned feels soothing.

**Glonoin:** When this remedy is helpful the affected areas of skin look and feel flushed and itchy, and symptoms set in rapidly after over-exposure to the sun. Classic symptoms include a throbbing headache that is temporarily soothed by contact with cool, fresh air, and made more uncomfortable by using an ice pack.

> **TIP:** USE URTICA URENS CREAM
> Applying Urtica urens cream to the affected area can do a great deal to ease the heat, discomfort, and general inflammation of a mild bout of sunburn.

## HERBALISM

**Aloe vera:** Most people will tell you that nothing soothes a burn better than cool aloe vera gel. The clear gel-like substance that oozes from the fresh-cut leaves of aloe has been used for years to treat a wide array of skin conditions such as burns, bites, stings, and generally dry, scaly skin. To treat burns, simply take the gel from a fresh-cut leaf and apply it directly to the affected area. If fresh leaves are not available, there are a variety of gels and lotions containing aloe vera that can be purchased at your local health food store, pharmacy, or stores that specialize in herbal medicines. Some aloe vera gels contain alcohol as a base to contribute to its cooling effect. Be aware that alcohol will sting on any open skin, so avoid any alcohol-based gels if your burn is accompanied by breaks in the skin.

# SUNSTROKE

## DIAGNOSIS

Sunstroke is a very serious condition and in some cases can even be life-threatening. It often occurs when someone is in a hot climate that has higher temperatures that those they are used to. It can be exacerbated by dehydration, and exertion, for example, by engaging in a sporting activity. The first signs are often dizziness, fatigue, a headache, rapid pulse, rapid breathing, and muscle cramps. The condition becomes serious if the skin is flushed and the person is no longer sweating, has a high body temperature, is confused, or loses consciousness. If the body is unable to reduce its own temperature by sweating, it can rise to as high as 107°F in some cases. When the body temperature rises even a couple of degrees it can have a significant effect on the way the metabolism works, and an extreme rise can cause many of the body's vital systems, including the heart, lungs, kidney, and brain, to fail.

## SYMPTOMS

- Throbbing headache
- Feeling dizzy and sick
- Thinking you are going to pass out
- Feeling very ill and unwell
- Feeling incredibly hot
- Flushed face and red skin
- Falling unconscious
- Sense of fatigue and the need to lie down
- The next day you may feel like you have a bad hangover with a headache and nausea

## TREATMENT GOAL

Treatment involves relieving symptoms by cooling the patient down and restoring fluids to the body.

## CONVENTIONAL MEDICINE

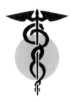

**To treat heat exhaustion:** Heat exhaustion occurs when a person is overheated, but does not have a fever and remains mentally alert and conscious. Place the patient in a cool, shaded area, and feed her ½ liter of fluid an hour to re-hydrate her. If possible, add ½ tsp of salt to each liter of water to prevent any complications developing as a result of low sodium in the body.

**To treat sunstroke:** Sunstroke occurs when a person is overheated and has a fever, and their mental status and possibly their vital signs are compromised. The patient should be transported to a hospital where intravenous resuscitation and support is available. Remove the patient's clothes and place them in a cool, well-ventilated room. Their body temperature should be monitored carefully, with the goal being to lower it to 102°F or less over a 30–60 minute period. Spray the patient with cool mist, and if possible place fans around the body. The use of ice packs is controversial as they may constrict the blood vessels and cause shivering, thus driving the temperature back up. Sometimes treatment for low blood pressure and seizures is required, as these conditions may accompany severe heat stroke. Acidosis, a life-threatening condition that results from a lack of insulin in the system, is another complication, which needs to be addressed in the hospital. Most people recover from sunstroke completely in 48 hours.

## TRADITIONAL CHINESE MEDICINE

**Herbs:** Mix 5 g of Jin Yin Hua (honeysuckle flower), and 3 g of Bo He (field mint) in a teapot. Add boiling water and let the herbs steep for a few minutes. Drink throughout the day when in a hot climate as a preventive measure.

**Acupuncture:** Treatment may be needed every day for a few days to help recovery from sunstroke. Needles will be left in for 20–30 minutes during each session. Consult an experienced practitioner for advice on a treatment plan.

**Acupressure:** Press the Feng Chi and Hegu points with the tip of your finger or thumb for one minute, and repeat twice a day. The Hegu point is located on the back of the hand between the thumb and first finger. The Feng Chi points are at the back of the head at the base of the skull, about 2 inches on either side of the center point.

**Diet:** Drink plenty of water every day and eat fresh fruit and vegetables, including bitter melon, watermelon, mung beans, tofu, radishes, and celery. Avoid food that has heat and warming properties, such as hot chili peppers, beef, and lamb. Also avoid deep-fried food, and eat less fatty and greasy foods since they also create more heat in the body, which can make symptoms worse.

## NATUROPATHY

The best naturopathic treatment for sunstroke is prevention. There are various methods of keeping cool in the heat, but if you do start to feel overheated by the sun, move to a cool place indoors or into the shade and loosen your clothing.

**Diet:** Eat a plain, light diet that primarily consists of fruit and vegetables. Celery, cucumber, watermelon, and oranges are particularly useful due to their high water content. Add salt to your food freely to keep electrolytes in check, unless you suffer from kidney disease or hypertension. Electrolytes are any of various ions, such as sodium, potassium or chloride, required by cells to regulate the electric charge and flow of water molecules across the cell membrane. Drink plenty of water and make sure that your body stays hydrated. Drinking lots of fluids in the heat is vital. Replacing any water, salt, and potassium lost by the body due to sun exposure will help prevent sunstroke from occurring. Eliminate caffeine, hot drinks, and alcohol from your diet, as they keep you hot and contribute to dehydration.

**Prevention:** Wear light, loose clothing, such as cotton, so that sweat can evaporate. Better yet, get clothing that is best suited to hot weather, which wicks away moisture from the body to keep temperatures low. Also wear a hat that provides shade and allows ventilation.

**TIP:** USE SUNSCREEN
Use sunscreen to prevent sunburn, which can hinder the skin's ability to cool itself.

## HOMEOPATHY

Severe sunstroke requires prompt medical attention as potentially serious problems can arise. Even the mildest cases will need to be monitored closely to make sure that patients are not at risk of developing more serious complications. This becomes an even greater priority in cases that affect the very young or the elderly. However, the following homeopathic remedies can be used alongside any conventional medical support that may be needed to encourage recovery.

**Belladonna:** Consider using this remedy to treat sunstroke symptoms that develop swiftly and dramatically. Symptoms include bright red, hot, dry skin, and throbbing pains. Headaches are also common, and pulsating pains radiating from the head down the body. Sufferers become irritable and crotchety when feeling unwell.

**Veratrum album:** If symptoms of sunstroke include localized burning sensations, as well as an associated feeling of being icy cold, use Veratrum album. Nausea is likely to accompany a headache, and patients generally feel faint and chilled.

## HERBALISM

 Sunstroke is a medical emergency and must be treated by a medical professional in an emergency setting. Do not delay medical treatment by instituting home remedies, although you should try to cool down the patient and administer liquids.

**General advice:** Once the very first signs of sunstroke appear, go indoors as fast as possible and begin self-help measures. Replacing fluids must be a priority. Also loosen any restrictive clothing around the neck and waist in order to help the body cool down and become more comfortable.

# WHIPLASH

## DIAGNOSIS

Whiplash is an injury to your neck that results when your head is thrown backwards, putting the muscles, ligaments, and sometimes the vertebrae in the neck under stress and temporarily throwing them out of alignment. It usually follows a forceful impact from behind, and most commonly results from a car accident. It generally manifests as headaches and stiffness in the neck and back of the head, and symptoms usually appear within a couple of days following the accident. This may be because the inflammation around a bruised muscle can take a while to build up. It can take two to three weeks for an injury involving the muscles to heal, and even longer if ligaments have been torn. If you have whiplash, avoid sporting activities and/or carrying heavy bags to allow your body to recover properly.

**DANGER**: Consult a doctor if you experience memory loss or periods of unconsciousness following an injury to the head or neck. Other serious symptoms include severe pains in the back of the head, tingling in the shoulders or arms, or a sensation of heaviness in the arms.

## SYMPTOMS

- Pain and stiffness, which can last for several days
- Pain is sometimes intense and sometimes mild
- Pain spreads down from the head to the neck, shoulders, chest, and arms
- Swollen and tender neck

## TREATMENT GOAL

Mild cases of whiplash should improve in a couple of days. Treatment involves restoring the normal range of motion to the neck to prevent further complications, as well as relieving pain and discomfort.

## CONVENTIONAL MEDICINE

Immediate medical treatment of whiplash is to exclude serious injury to the nerves, spinal cord, and backbone. A reduction of long-term disability and resolution of symptoms are thereafter sought.

**Compresses:** Generally, applying an ice pack to the injury for 20 minutes each hour for the first 24 hours is helpful. Following that, moist, heated compresses can be used several times daily as needed for pain relief. Try applying castor oil to a washcloth, warming it in the microwave, and placing it directly over the neck. Although there is no research to support it, this technique can sometimes be very helpful.

**Pain relief:** A high dose of methyl prednisone is given for immediate pain relief. A first dose should be given intravenously, and then oral doses can be taken for the following 24 hours. It is recommended that the drug be administered within eight hours of the injury. Non-steroidal anti-inflammatory drugs (NSAIDs), such as ibuprofen and naproxen, can then be used to relieve pain as needed. Muscle relaxants are also effective at relieving pain, and cyclobenzaprine, methocarbamol, and carisoprodol are most commonly prescribed. These drugs interact with antidepressants and may be contraindicated in thyroid disease, so it is advisable to pay close attention to the side-effect profile before taking them. All of these drugs also cause sedation. Magnesium, which naturally relaxes muscles and has fewer side effects, can be taken as an alternative. It should be taken as glycinate or aspartate salt.

**Physical therapy:** Physical therapy or chiropractic manipulation of the neck is helpful for many people suffering from whiplash. Returning to normal activity is encouraged, generally while taking NSAIDs to reduce inflammation and encourage healing.

**Neck support:** A soft cervical collar can provide an injured neck with good support. However, patients are encouraged to restore the neck's range of motion, and collars should not be used for more than two weeks.

## TRADITIONAL CHINESE MEDICINE

**Herbs:** Consult a doctor of Chinese medicine for advice on whether herbal medicine is appropriate, and to determine the best formula for your individual condition.

**Acupuncture:** The discomfort associated with whiplash can be eased through acupuncture. Treatment can also help the healing process. An experienced practitioner will begin with a course of 12 acupuncture sessions once or twice a week.

**Acupressure:** If you have whiplash, always consult a doctor before you attempt any self-massage or acupressure.

**Diet:** As general practice, eat a well-balanced diet that includes plenty of fruits, vegetables, and grains. Drink plenty of water as part of your daily routine. Have fresh food, but avoid shrimp, beef, lamb, and chili peppers, since they increase heat in the body.

## NATUROPATHY

**Diet:** Add raw wheat germ to your cereal every morning. Wheat germ is the best dietary source of vitamin E, which plays an important role in rebuilding muscle tissue. Wheat germ also contains magnesium to help relax tense neck muscles. Eating rolled-oats muesli with organic raisins, organic grated apple, and raw sunflower seeds can also be helpful. Oats provide silica for tissue building and B-vitamins to relax muscles and nerves of the neck. Eating nuts will provide added nutritional support for recovery from whiplash. Pecans are an excellent source of vitamin E, and cashews and almonds are rich in magnesium. All nuts provide protein and essential fatty acids. Eat plenty of green, organic vegetables for their high nutrient content, which includes vitamin E and magnesium. The most common and tastiest are spinach, leeks, kale, and broccoli.

**Supplements:** Take 400 IU a day of vitamin E to support the healing of the nervous system. Magnesium relaxes the muscles around the neck. Take 500 mg twice a day. Take 2,000–4,000 mg of vitamin C a day to promote collagen synthesis, which helps with tissue healing. Chondroitin sulfate, which can be taken at 400 mg three times a day, treats and heals damaged joints. Glucosamine sulfate works synergistically with chondroitin sulfate. Take 500 mg three times a day.

**Herbs:** Take 300 mg of boswellia three times a day to decrease inflammation and alleviate pain. Butterbur, which can be taken at 75 mg twice a day, has anti-inflammatory and anti-spasmodic effects. Ginger has been traditionally used for its anti-inflammatory effects and can help alleviate pain. Take 4 mg in two divided doses. Horsetail contains silica, which is excellent to help rebuild tissue. Take 3 cups of horsetail tea or 15 drops of tincture diluted in water three times daily for a couple of weeks. A compress of fresh comfrey leaf pulp reduces pain and speeds healing. It encourages cell regrowth in connective tissue and bones, and absorbs the pooled blood from bruises. To make a compress, soak a clean cotton or wool cloth in an infusion of comfrey, wring it out, and apply it to the affected area. You can also try adding 5 drops each of arnica, comfrey, and thyme essential oils to a hot bath to stimulate blood flow to the area. This speeds healing and repairs damaged tissue.

---

**TIP:** TRY PROLOTHERAPY

This type of therapy may help injured tissue and reduce pain. Prolotherapy treatment involves injections of chemical irritant solutions into the area around injured ligaments. These solutions cause tissue to grow, increasing the strength and thickness of ligaments. This tightens up the joint and relieves the burden on associated muscles, stopping muscle spasms and reducing pain. Consult a practitioner with training in prolotherapy about receiving injections.

---

## HOMEOPATHY

Homeopathic remedies can help to speed up the healing process of whiplash, but ideally they should be used alongside conventional medical treatment. When appropriately selected, a homeopathic remedy can help relieve pain, stiffness, and discomfort.

**Arnica:** This remedy can help the body deal with the psychological and physical effects of an accident of this kind. In addition, it can ease initial localized pain and stiffness.

**Hypericum:** This remedy can follow Arnica if the latter has helped initially but does not provide sustained relief. Hypericum can help to heal damaged nerve tissue, and also has the potential to reduce inflammation and pain. Symptoms include shooting, lightning-like pains that travel down the arm.

**Rhus tox:** If pain and stiffness is noticeably eased by limbering up or by contact with warmth, try Rhus tox. Symptoms tend to be worse when resting, and when exposed to cold and damp. Rhus tox can also follow Arnica if that fails to provide sustained relief. Pain and stiffness become aggravated when in bed at night, leading to restlessness and emotional despondency.

## HERBALISM

There are many herbs that can help relieve the muscle pain and spasm of whiplash. If the symptoms have not lessened within two weeks, there may be a more extensive injury involving the spinal joints and inter-vertebral discs. Below is a short list of herbs that are helpful in treating muscle stiffness, soreness, pain, and inflammation associated with whiplash. For more options, see Back Pain (p. 604) and Neck Pain (p. 672).

**Blue cohosh:** This herb is a good choice for decreasing spasm and guarding the injured muscles associated with whiplash. The medicinal properties are due to the alkaloids and glycosides the herb contains. Use blue cohosh when muscle pain has an aching, heavy quality. Take it as a tea by steeping 1 g of dried herb in 1 cup of water. Drink two to three times a day. This herb can also be taken in tincture form: mix 3 ml in 8 oz of juice or water and drink two to three times a day. Blue cohosh should not be used if you have angina.

**Cramp bark:** A more appropriate name for this herb would be "anti-cramp bark" due to its ability to relieve pain and spasm. Use it to treat muscle pain that is worse in the evening and from resting on the affected part.

**Jamaican dogwood:** This herb demonstrates analgesic and sedative properties, relieving pain while it soothes the nerves. Jamaican dogwood is potentially toxic and should only be used in low doses and under the supervision of a herbalist. Take 5 drops of tincture twice a day.

# GLOSSARY

**acupoint**

Anatomical points on the body that are used in acupressure and acupuncture. There are several hundred points on the body, which are distributed along the meridians (channels through which Qi, the body's vitalizing energy, flow). The points used to treat a condition may or may not be close to the part of the body where symptoms are experienced.

**acupressure**

Involves using fingers, hands, elbows, and feet to apply firm pressure to acupoints on the surface of the body. Acupressure stimulates the flow of energy (Qi) in the body's meridian system to bring relief.

**acupuncture**

The practice of inserting needles into various acupoints to stimulate the body's healing responses and help restore its natural balance.

**acute condition**

A condition that has a limited life span and a clear initial, middle, and final phase of illness. Examples of acute conditions include colds, flu, and hangovers.

**antibiotic**

A drug that kills or slows the growth of bacteria. Antibiotics are part of a larger group of drugs called antimicrobials, which also includes antiviral, antifungal, and antiparasitic drugs. These drugs are used to treat infections.

**bacteria**

Microscopic single-celled organisms that can exist either as independent organisms or as parasites. Many pathogens are bacteria.

**biofeedback**

A form of alternative medicine that involves raising a patient's awareness of bodily processes, such as blood pressure, heart rate, and muscle tension, so that the patient is able to gain physical control over physical processes that were previously thought to be automatic.

**bioflavonoid**

A type of phytochemical that acts as a potent antioxidant, helping the body rid itself of toxins and fight infection. The best food sources of bioflavonoids are citrus fruits, berries, broccoli, cherries, grapes, papaya, plums, tomatoes, tea, and red wine.

**chronic condition**

A condition that involves symptoms that flare up repeatedly. Examples include asthma, eczema, and migraines.

**compress**

A pad of soft fabric soaked in a herbal infusion or decoction and applied to a painful area. Compresses can be hot (which are generally used to relieve cramps and other muscle problems) or cold (which are used if the skin feels hot to the touch and for headaches). Compresses should be continually refreshed to keep the affected area warm or cool as required.

## conventional medicine

A type of health therapy that uses detailed scientific knowledge and academic research to diagnose and treat disease. The emphasis is on fighting and destroying disease through the use of drugs and surgery.

## decoction

A herbal remedy made by boiling, simmering, and then straining powdered or crushed root, bark, or seeds. Decocting is a vigorous method of extracting the active constituents from the tougher parts of a herb.

## diagnosis

The process of identifying a medical condition or disease by its signs and symptoms, and through the results of tests and/or examinations.

## enzyme

Proteins that accelerate chemical reactions in the body to convert one type of molecule into another. For example, lactase is the enzyme that converts lactose into glucose and galactose.

## essential fatty acids (EFAs)

Beneficial fats found in oily fish, such as salmon, sardines, tuna, and mackerel, and nuts and seeds. EFAs include omega-3s (such as eicosapentanoic acid, EPA, and docosahexenoic acid, DHA) and omega-6s. They are essential for a healthy nervous system and brain function.

## essential oil

A concentrated solution containing volatile aromatic compounds extracted from plants.

## herb

Plant of which the leaves or stems are used for medicine, or for their scent or flavor. Herbal medicine includes extracts from a part of a plant, such as the leaves, roots, and berries, which can be used in a variety of forms.

## herbal tonic

A liquid herbal remedy that restores and increases body tone.

## herbalism

A health therapy that uses plant remedies to treat disease. Herbalism centers on the belief that plants have a vital energy that is beneficial to the body and can help to boost self-healing abilities.

## holistic medicine

A system of health care that looks at the whole person, including physical, nutritional, environmental, emotional, social, spiritual, and lifestyle factors, when treating ailments.

## homeopathy

A health therapy in which a highly dilute amount of a substance is administered to boost the body's healing process. Homeopathy works on the principle that "like cures like," and practitioners prescribe substances with characteristics that are common to the symptoms of the specific illness.

## hormones

Chemicals that are produced by organ systems in the body. Hormones are released directly into the bloodstream to carry a signal from one part of the body to another.

**hydrotherapy**
A health therapy that involves using water to ease pain and treat a disease.

**immune system**
The body's mechanism for defending itself against illness. Cells, organs, and tissues are arranged in an elaborate communication network to detect and respond to an invading pathogen, and to prevent bacteria and viruses from entering the body.

**infection**
A condition in which the body is invaded by a pathogen (a bacterium, fungus, or virus), which multiplies and interferes with the normal functioning of the bodily systems.

**junk food**
A term used for any food that is perceived to be unhealthy or have poor nutritional value. Examples include, but are not limited to, foods that are high in sugar such as candy and carbonated drinks, and salty foods such as potato chips and French fries.

**mind–body therapy**
A health therapy that relies on innate, instinctual resources rather than medication to bring about healing. It combines "talk" therapy with body movements, such as touch and postural alignment, to increase body awareness and positive energy.

**moxibustion**
A technique used in traditional Chinese medicine in which a stick or cone of burning moxa is used to warm acu-

puncture points, but removed before it burns the skin. Moxibustion stimulates and strengthens the body's energy (Qi) and encourages it to flow smoothly.

**multivitamin/multimineral**
A supplement that contains more than one vitamin and/or mineral. They are available in many forms, and a health practitioner can recommend a reliable brand.

**naturopathy**
A health therapy that encourages healing on all levels. It aims to strengthen the body's immune system and make it more resilient to disease through diet and lifestyle choices.

**ointment**
A viscous, semisolid preparation that is used topically on the skin. An ointment is oil-based whereas a cream is water-based.

**pathogen**
A biological element that causes disease or illness. Pathogens disrupt the normal physiological workings of the body's systems.

**phytochemical**
Biologically active compound found in food that plays a vital role in keeping the body healthy.

**poultice**
A hot paste made by mixing herbs with boiled water. Poultices are applied directly to the skin and are mainly used to draw out pus and reduce inflammation.

**probiotics**
Supplements that contain beneficial bacteria. Probiotics help keep bad bacteria in

the gut under control and at a level that allows for healthy digestion.

## Qi

The body's motivating energy, according to traditional Chinese medicine. Good health is dependent on Qi moving in a smooth and balanced way through a series of meridians (channels) beneath the skin. The flow of Qi can be disturbed by a number of factors, including anxiety, stress, poor nutrition, hereditary factors, infections, and trauma.

## side effect

An adverse reaction. Unwanted, negative consequences can be associated with both pharmaceutical and herbal medicines.

## sitz bath

A bath in which only the hips and buttocks are immersed in water to stimulate circulation and benefit the abdominal organs. Herbal infusions are often added to the water to provide additional benefits.

## standardized extract

A solution made by extracting and purifying the active compound of a plant.

## supplement

Pills, capsules, or powders that can be taken to enhance health. They include nutrients such as vitamins, minerals, essential fatty acids, amino acids, and protein that may be missing or not consumed in sufficient quantity in the diet.

## symptom

The physical manifestation of disease. For example, a cold manifests through symptoms of sneezing and/or a runny nose.

## tincture

A solution of a medicinal substance steeped in alcohol. Tinctures can be made from fresh or dried plants, although fresh plants are preferred as they contain a higher concentration of the active ingredients.

## traditional Chinese medicine

A health therapy that includes herbalism, acupuncture, acupressure, dietary therapy, and exercises in breathing and movement, such as T'ai chi.

## virus

A microscopic particle that can infect the cells and multiply to cause diseases such as chickenpox, measles, and mumps.

## vitamins

Nutrients required for essential metabolic reactions in the body. Most vitamins are obtained through food sources. In humans, there are 13 vitamins: vitamin A, C, D, E, and K, and eight B vitamins.

## whole foods

Any food that is natural, unprocessed, and unrefined. Examples include fruits and vegetables and unpolished grains.

## Yin and Yang

A concept of Chinese philosophy that describes two primal opposing but complimentary forces found in all things in the universe. Yin is the darker element, and Yang is the brighter element.

## CONVENTIONAL MEDICINE

American Medical Association (AMA)
515 North State Street
Chicago, IL
60610
Tel: 1 (800) 621-8335
Website: www.ama-assn.org
Unites physicians to work on the most important professional and public health issues.

American Public Health
Association (APHA)
800 I Street, NW
Washington, DC
20001
Tel: 1 (202) 777-2742
Email: comments@apha.org
Website: www.apha.org
A professional association dedicated to improving the public's health through education and advocacy.

American Health Care Association (AHCA)
1201 L Street NW
Washington, DC
20005
Tel: 1 (202) 842-4444
Website: www.ahca.org
A non-profit federation of affiliated state health organizations.

## TRADITIONAL CHINESE MEDICINE

American Association of Oriental
Medicine (AAOM)
PO Box 162340
Sacramento, CA
95816
Tel: 1 (916) 443-4770
Website: www.aaom.org
Represents and advocates on behalf of practitioners in order to ensure that the wellbeing of the public is protected, and to ensure that providers are given their rightful place in the health care system.

American Chinese Medicine
Association (ACMA)
Email: info@americanchinesemedicine
association.org
Website: www.americanchinesemedicine
association.org
Dedicated to introducing safe and effective Chinese medicine to patients and the public in the United States and around the world.

## NATUROPATHY

American Association of Naturopathic
Physicians (AANP)
4435 Wisconsin Avenue NW
Suite 403
Washington, DC
20016
Tel: 1 (866) 538-2267
Email: member.services@
naturopathic.org
Website: www.naturopathic.org
Strives to expand access to naturopathic medicine nationwide.

American Naturopathic Medical
Association (ANMA)
PO Box 96273
Las Vegas, NV
89193

Tel: 1 (702) 897-7053
Website: www.anma.com
A non-profit organization dedicated to
exploring new frontiers of mind, body,
medicine, and health.

## HOMEOPATHY
American Association of Homeopathic
Pharmacists (AAHP)
5112 Wilshire Drive
Santa Rosa, CA
95404
Tel: 1 (800) 478-0421
Email: info@homeopathicpharmacy.org
Website: www.homeopathicpharmacy.org
Aims to create a better understanding
and appreciation of homeopathic
medicines by both professionals
and consumers.

National Center for Homeopathy
801 North Fairfax Street
Suite 306
Alexandria, VA
22314
Tel: 1 (703) 548-7790
Email: info@homeopathic.org
Website: www.homeopathic.org
Provides general education to the public
about homeopathy, and specific
education to homeopaths, to make
homeopathy available throughout the
United States.

North American Society of
Homeopaths (NASH)
PO Box 450039
Sunrise, FL
33345-0039
Tel: 1 (206) 720-7000
Email: nashinfo@homeopathy.org
Website: www.homeopathy.org

Works to enhance the role of the
homeopathic profession as an integral
part of health care delivery.

## HERBALISM
American Herbalists Guild
141 Nob Hill Road
Cheshire, CT
06410
Tel: 1 (203) 272-6731
Email: ahgoffice@earthlink.net
Website: www.american
herbalistsguild.com
Promotes cooperation between herbal
practitioners and other health care
providers, integrating herbalism into
community health care.

American Herbal Products
Association (AHPA)
8484 Georgia Avenue
Suite 370
Silver Spring, MD
20910
Tel: 1 (301) 588-1171
Email: ahpa@ahpa.org
Website: www.ahpa.org
Promotes the responsible commerce of
herbal products to ensure that consumers
have informed access to goods.

## GENERAL
American Chiropractic Association (ACA)
1701 Clarendon Boulevard
Arlington, VA
22209
Tel: 1 (703) 276-8800
E-mail: memberinfo@acatoday.org
Website: www.amerchiro.org
Preserves, protects, improves, and
promotes the chiropractic profession and
services for the benefit of patients.

American Health Planning
Association (AHPA)
7245 Arlington Boulevard
Suite 300
Falls Church, VA
22042
Tel: 1 (703) 573-3103
Email: info@ahpanet.org
Website: www.ahpanet.org
A non-profit organization committed to
health policies and service systems that
promote quality, assure equal access, and
advocate reasonable costs.

American Holistic Health
Association (AHHA)
PO Box 17400
Anaheim, CA
92817-7400
Tel: 1 (714) 779-6152
Email: mail@ahha.org
Website: http://ahha.org/
Dedicated to promoting the holistic
principles of honoring the whole person
(mind, body, and spirit) and encouraging
people to participate in their own health.

American Holistic Medical
Association (AHMA)
PO Box 2016
Edmonds, WA
98080
Tel: 1 (425) 967-0737
Website: www.holisticmedicine.org
Supports practitioners in their professional
development as healers and educates
physicians about holistic medicine.

American Hospital Association (AHA)
One North Franklin
Chicago, IL
60606-3421

Tel: 1 (312) 422-3000
Website: www.aha.org
Leads, represents and serves hospitals,
health systems, and other related
organizations that are accountable to the
community and committed to health
improvement.

American Alternative Medical
Association (AAMA)
2200 Market Street
Suite 329
Galveston, TX
77550-1530
Tel: 1 (409) 621-2600
Email: office@joinaama.com
Website: www.joinaama.com
Promotes an enhanced professional
image and prestige among doctors of
traditional and non-traditional therapies
and methodologies.

American Mental Health Counselors
Association (AMHCA)
801 North Fairfax Street
Suite 304
Alexandria, VA
22314
Tel: 1 (703) 548-6002
Website: www.amhca.org
Enhances the profession of mental health
counseling through licensing, advocacy,
education, and professional development.

American School Health
Association (ASHA)
7263 State Route 43
PO Box 708
Kent, OH
44240
Tel: 1 (330) 678-1601
Email: asha@ashaweb.org

Website: www.ashaweb.org
Unites the many professionals working in schools who are committed to safeguarding the health of children.

American Social Health Association (ASHA)
PO Box 13827
Research Triangle Park, NC
27709
Tel: 1 (919) 361-8400
Website: www.ashastd.org
Dedicated to improving the health of individuals, families, and communities, with a focus on preventing sexually transmitted diseases and their harmful consequences.

Craniosacral Therapy Association of North America (CSTA/NA)
852 Don Diego Avenue
Santa Fe, NM
87505
Tel: 1 (505) 820-1335
Email: info@craniosacraltherapy.org
Website: www.craniosacraltherapy.org
Preserves the integrity of craniosacral therapy and maintains standards for practitioners, teachers, and students of biodynamic craniosacral therapy.

Complementary Alternative Medicine Association (CAMA)
Email: cama@camaweb.org
Website: www.camaweb.org
A provider of quality education and accurate information about complementary/alternative medicine.

International Association of Mind-Body Professionals (IAMBP)
31441 Santa Margarita Parkway

Suite A140
Rancho Santa Margarita, CA
92688
Tel: 1 (949) 589-9166
Website: www.mindbodypro.com
Dedicated to bridging the gap between traditional and non-traditional health and wellness through better understanding of Western and Eastern philosophies and the mind-body connection.

Pan American Health Organization
Pan American Sanitary Bureau
Regional Office of the World Health Organization
525 Twenty-third Street, N.W.
Washington, DC
20037
Tel: 1 (202) 974-3000
Website: www.paho.org
Works to improve health and living standards of the countries of the Americas.

US Food and Drug Administration (FDA)
5600 Fishers Lane
Rockville, MD
20857-0001
Tel: 1 (888) 463-6332
Website: www.fda.gov
Responsible for protecting the public health by assuring the safety, efficacy, and security of human and veterinary drugs, biological products, medical devices, the food supply, cosmetics, and products that emit radiation.

World Health Organization (WHO)
Website: www.who.int
The United Nations' specialized agency for health dedicated to the attainment by all peoples of the highest possible level of health.

# INDEX

BT
11/07

615.5
D

1000 cures for 200
ailments.

| DATE | | | |
|---|---|---|---|
| | | | |
| | | | |
| | | | |
| | | | |
| | | | |
| | | | |
| | | | |
| | | | |
| | | | |
| | | | |
| | | | |
| | | | |